ELSEVIER'S

Medical Laboratory Science
Examination Review

ELSEVIER'S

Medical Laboratory Science

Examination Review

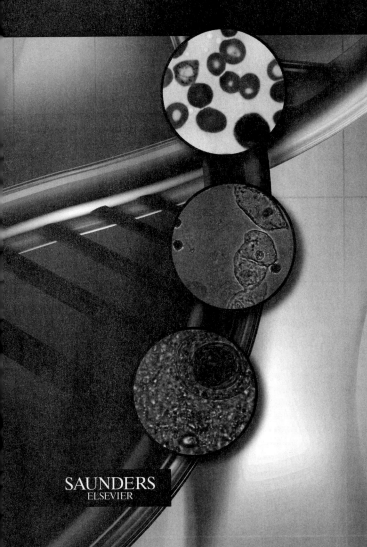

Linda J. Graeter
Associate Professor
Medical Laboratory Science Program
University of Cincinnati
Cincinnati, Ohio

Elizabeth G. Hertenstein
Assistant Professor
Medical Laboratory Science Program
University of Cincinnati
Cincinnati, Ohio

Charity E. Accurso
Assistant Professor
Medical Laboratory Science Program
University of Cincinnati
Cincinnati, Ohio

Gideon H. Labiner
Associate Professor
Medical Laboratory Science Program
University of Cincinnati
Cincinnati, Ohio

SAUNDERS
ELSEVIER

ELSEVIER
SAUNDERS

3251 Riverport Lane
St. Louis, Missouri 63043

Elsevier's Medical Laboratory Science Examination

ISBN: 978-1-4557-0889-5

Notices

Knowledge and best practice in this field are constantly changing. As new research and experience broaden our understanding, changes in research methods, professional practices, or medical treatment may become necessary.

Practitioners and researchers must always rely on their own experience and knowledge in evaluating and using any information, methods, compounds, or experiments described herein. In using such information or methods they should be mindful of their own safety and the safety of others, including parties for whom they have a professional responsibility.

With respect to any drug or pharmaceutical products identified, readers are advised to check the most current information provided (i) on procedures featured or (ii) by the manufacturer of each product to be administered, to verify the recommended dose or formula, the method and duration of administration, and contraindications. It is the responsibility of practitioners, relying on their own experience and knowledge of their patients, to make diagnoses, to determine dosages and the best treatment for each individual patient, and to take all appropriate safety precautions.

To the fullest extent of the law, neither the Publisher nor the authors, contributors, or editors, assume any liability for any injury and/or damage to persons or property as a matter of products liability, negligence or otherwise, or from any use or operation of any methods, products, instructions, or ideas contained in the material herein.

Library of Congress Cataloging-in-Publication Data
Elsevier's medical laboratory science examination review / [edited by] Linda J. Graeter, Elizabeth G. Hertenstein, Charity E. Accurso, Gideon H. Labiner. – First edition.
    p.; cm.
Medical laboratory science examination review
Includes bibliographical references and index.
ISBN 978-1-4557-0889-5 (pbk.: alk. paper)
I. Graeter, Linda J., editor. II. Hertenstein, Elizabeth G., editor. III. Accurso, Charity E., editor. IV. Labiner, Gideon H., editor. V. Title: Medical laboratory science examination review.
[DNLM: 1. Clinical Laboratory Techniques–Examination Questions. QY 18.2]
RB37
616.07′56–dc23

2014016504

Executive Content Strategist: Kellie White
Content Development Manager: Billie Sharp
Content Development Specialist: Betsy McCormac
Publishing Services Manager: Catherine Jackson
Senior Project Manager: Rachel E. McMullen
Design Direction: Maggie Reid

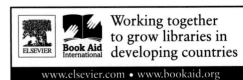

Printed in the United States of America

Last digit is the print number: 9 8 7 6 5 4 3

Brenda C. Barnes, PhD, MT(ASCP)SBB[CM]
Director, Medical Laboratory Science Program,
Associate Professor
Allen College
Waterloo, Iowa

Janelle M. Chiasera, PhD, MT(ASCP)
Chair, The Department of Clinical and Diagnostic Sciences,
Professor
The University of Alabama, Birmingham
Birmingham, Alabama

Sandy Cook, MS, MT(ASCP)
Assistant Professor
Clinical Laboratory Services
Ferris State University
Big Rapids, Michigan

Melanie J. Giusti, BS, MLS(ASCP)[CM]
Program Manager
Medical Laboratory Science Program
College of Allied Health Sciences
University of Cincinnati
Cincinnati, Ohio

Mark W. Ireton, MA, BS, MLS(ASCP)[CM]
Blood Bank Technologist II
Hoxworth Blood Center
University of Cincinnati
Cincinnati, Ohio

Paul R. Labbe, MS, MCLT
Vice President Information Resources
CompuNet Clinical Laboratories
Dayton, Ohio

Joel E. Mortensen, PhD, HCLD, FAAM
Department of Pathology and Laboratory Medicine
Cincinnati Children's Hospital Medical Center
Cincinnati, Ohio

Susan King Strasinger, DA, MLS(ASCP)
Faculty Associate
The University of West Florida
Pensacola, Florida

ACKNOWLEDGMENTS

We are grateful to all contributing authors and reviewers who dedicated time and effort during the development of this book. A special word of recognition and appreciation for their dedication to Medical Laboratory education is offered to Melanie Giusti, MLS(ASCP)^{CM}; Lara Kolar, MT(ASCP); John Landis, MS, MT(ASCP); Jennifer Macht, BS MT(ASCP), CHT (ABHI); Ryan McGough, MS, MT(ASCP); Erin Rumpke, MS, MT(ASCP); and Beth Warning, MS, MLS (ASCP)^{CM}.

Last but not least, our sincere thanks are extended to our Elsevier colleagues: Ellen Wurm-Cutter, Content Manager; Amy Whittier, Content Development Specialist; and all others at Elsevier who were involved in this project. Their assistance, thoughtful advice, and continued support were invaluable as we navigated through the various steps in completing the book.

The *Medical Laboratory Science Review* is intended to serve as a review tool for candidates who are preparing to sit for certification or licensure examinations in Medical Laboratory Science. However, the integral nature of this review book provides a review for individuals seeking to strengthen knowledge in the topics related to the clinical laboratory. Therefore this text can provide a multi-purpose review. The text is ideal for those preparing for Medical Laboratory Science (MLS) or categorical Technologist/Scientist (Blood Banking, Chemistry, Hematology, Microbiology, and Molecular Biology) certification examinations sponsored by the American Society of Clinical Pathology (ASCP) Board of Certification or for the American Medical Technologists (AMT)-supported certification examination. Additionally, this text will be helpful for those preparing for the Medical Laboratory Technology (MLT) certification examination, although the scope of some of the advanced topics are outside the required competencies for the MLT level. The outline format enhances learning and comprehension for each professional career entry track. Others who would benefit from using this review text to support their studies are those seeking advanced degrees, ASCP Specialist certification, Physician Assistant students, and Pathology Residents. Additional uses include serving as a reference book for students and educators, providing continuing education review and to refresh knowledge.

The book's preface is followed by review materials encompassing all major areas of the laboratory, divided into 11 chapters. Each chapter includes a comprehensive bulleted summary of didactic information. The chapter summary outlines provide a thorough but efficient review of key content information. Each chapter is followed by 30 to 100 multiple-choice questions. The questions include representation of the three question types (I, II, III) to enhance recall, interpretation, and problem-solving skills. Each question includes an explanation of the correct answer. The book's final section is a comprehensive practice examination designed using the ASCP Board of Certification guidelines.

The chapters and examination questions were written by Medical Laboratory educators and clinical experts, all of whom are recognized for expertise in their respective area of practice. All chapters and multiple-choice questions underwent a peer-review process as the content was developed.

The companion website—Evolve to accompany *Medical Laboratory Science Review*—was developed to enhance each candidate's preparation process by providing additional review materials. Students often benefit from a variety of study approaches when preparing for certification or licensure examinations. The Evolve website was created with that in mind and includes printable study worksheets and additional review materials. Students are able to generate individualized study files from these materials. The website also includes 1000 additional multiple-choice questions that are different from those in the book. From these materials, students can create additional practice examinations focusing on the content area of their choice.

EXAMINATION PREPARATION

Preparation for certification and licensure examinations is sometimes a daunting and intimidating process. We encourage students to recognize the time and effort placed in successfully completing their respective educational programs and the knowledge gained while doing so. Preparing for the examination then becomes a structured plan that provides for a review of the knowledge gained.

Shortly before program completion, thoroughly review the ASCP Board of Certification website. Be sure to review the requirements that must be met to sit for the examination, along with the recommended dates to submit the application. We encourage students to sit for the examination within 6 months of program completion. Students who wait longer tend to have a more difficult time reviewing and preparing for the examination. On the website, you will also find content outlines and a distribution of the content areas that will aid in your planning. Details are included about the cost, length, and structure of the examination. Review the examination preparation guide.

- Complete a practice examination or set of review questions. Record your answers on a separate piece of paper so that you can continue to practice with the same questions.
  - After reviewing missed questions, make a list of the specific content areas that were missed (e.g., anemias, streptococci, liver enzymes) and then design a study schedule using a calendar that allows more time to review the more challenging areas.
  - Plan 1 to 2 weeks for a thorough review of each content area.
- Create mini study guides for your more challenging or weaker areas. The study guides should include the following:
  - Graphical representations of a disease or process
  - Concise charts or tables
  - A brief paragraph explaining the topic or question or a short outline

Preparing the guides is an active learning exercise that will help in reviewing the specific content and in maintaining focus on weaker topics. It is human nature to gravitate toward favorite topics, but it is also necessary to focus on the areas that are more challenging. Compile the study guides in a binder organized by content area. The guides will be great tools to review the week before the actual examination

When studying the review questions or old examinations:

- Provide a rationale as to why you can rule out incorrect answers and rule in correct ones.
- Pay attention to small details that will help rule out a wrong answer.
- Writing your rationales out in sentence form is another great review tool.
- Create your own question rationales.

Practice, practice, practice! It is always helpful to address questions you previously reviewed. Use the questions in this text and those from the online companion site.

The day of the examination . . . breathe deeply! If you are not sure of the location of the testing center, take a test drive to the center a week before the examination. Have a scheduled plan for the day. Be well rested and be sure to eat a good meal before arriving at the testing center. If you have prepared, your efforts will be evident in your success!

NOTE: *Although it is this book's intent to properly prepare readers for their certification examination, use of this book alone does not guarantee passage of certification or licensure examinations.*

Color insert follows p. 20

Microbiology

Joel E. Mortensen and Linda J. Graeter

STAINED SMEARS

- Gram stain
  - Gram stain history
    - Developed by Hans Christian Gram in 1884
    - Became the major bacterial staining method
  - Most bacteria are stained by this method
    - Exceptions include *Legionella, Mycoplasma, Chlamydia,* and others
  - Gram stain procedure
    - Crystal violet
    - Gram's iodine
    - Decolorizer
    - Acetone and alcohol either alone or together
    - Safranin
  - Gram stain mechanism
    - Differences in the microbial cell wall are visualized
      - Cell walls of gram-negative cells have higher lipid content than gram-positive cells
    - Crystal violet penetrates both types
    - Iodine is added, forming the crystal violet–iodine (CV-I) complex (mordant)
    - Decolorizer dissolves the lipid layer from the gram-negative cells allowing the CV-I complex to wash out
    - Counterstain is applied to dye the decolorized gram-negative cells
  - Clinical utility
    - A true STAT test in microbiology
    - Judge adequacy of a specimen
    - Recognition specific morphologies
    - Indicate need for additional tests
    - Expand clinical diagnostic picture
  - Limitations
    - Only partial bacterial identification
    - Some organisms do not stain
    - "No organisms seen" does not rule out infection
    - Normal flora can mask pathogens
    - Human error
    - Organisms do not stain as expected
  - Diagnostic considerations
    - Cell identification
      - Epithelial cells
      - Polymorphonuclear (PMN) cells
      - Bacteria
  - Proper staining technique
    - Underdecolorization
    - Overdecolorization
  - Special considerations: Sputum specimens
    - >25 epithelial cells/lpf = saliva
    - Few epithelial cells, many PMN cells:—Specimen more likely to yield a pathogen
    - Examine properly stained area
    - Recognize normal oral flora
    - Report or reject
    - Sputum only, may not apply to aspirates or children
  - Special considerations: Urine
    - Urine specimens
      - 1 cell per oil immersion field = approximately 1×10^5 CFU/mL
      - Not commonly performed
  - Quantitation
    - No organisms seen
    - Few per slide = Rare
    - 0 to 2 per field = Few
    - 2 to 10 per field = Moderate
    - More than 10 per field = Many

GROWING BACTERIA IN THE LABORATORY—MEDIA

- Types of media
  - Bacteriology
    - Routine
    - Fastidious
    - Anaerobes
    - *Mycoplasma, Ureaplasma*
  - Mycobacteriology
  - Mycology
  - Virology
    - Viruses
    - *Chlamydia*
- Constituents of media
  - Agar
    - Gelatinous seaweed extract
    - 1% to 2% agar in plates
  - Nutrients
    - Hydrolyzed proteins

- Animal
- Plant
  - Carbohydrates, sugars
- Enrichments
  - Yeast extracts, blood
- Buffers
  - Stable pH for growth
- pH indicators
  - Neutral red: Red to colorless
  - Phenol red: Yellow to red
  - Thymol blue: Yellow to green/blue
  - Others
- Inhibitors
  - Dyes
    - Crystal violet, eosin, and methylene blue
  - Bile salts
    - Sodium deoxycholate
  - Sodium chloride
  - Sodium citrate
  - Antibiotics
- Selective
  - Contains inhibitory agents to all organisms except one being sought
  - Selects for certain organisms to the disadvantage of others
  - Example
    - Colistin nalidixic acid agar (CNA)
    - MacConkey agar
- Differential
  - Allows organism to be morphologically distinguished from other organisms with different characteristics
  - Examples
    - Sheep blood agar (SBA)
    - MacConkey agar
- Key media for routine aerobic cultures
  - Supportive
    - Blood agar
    - Chocolate agar
  - Selective/differential for gram-negative bacilli
    - MacConkey agar
    - Xylose lysine desoxycholate (XLD) or Hektoen (HE) for stool
  - Selective/differential for gram-positive organisms
    - CNA
    - Phenylethyl alcohol agar (PEA)
  - Examples
    - Blood agar
      - Casein peptones: Group of proteins from milk
      - Soybean peptones
      - 5% sheep blood
      - Approximately 1% agar-agar
      - Used for general growth of gram-positive and gram-negative aerobes
      - The most common supportive media because most organisms grow on it, but it is also differential because of hemolytic pattern

- Chocolate agar
  - Casein peptones
  - Meat peptones
  - Corn starch
  - Hemoglobin (V factor)
  - IsoVitaleX Enrichment (X factor)
    - Used for specimens from which fastidious organisms may be isolated
    - *Haemophilus* spp., *Neisseria* spp., *Brucella* or *Capnocytophaga* spp.
- MacConkey agar
  - Peptone base with lactose, crystal violet, and bile salts
    - Lactose to provide fermentable sugar (Lactose positive vs negative)
    - Crystal violet—inhibit gram-positive bacteria
    - Bile salts—inhibit gram-positive bacteria
  - Neutral red pH indicator
  - Selective for gram-negative organisms
  - Differential for lactose fermentation
    - Lactose positive
      - *Escherichia coli*: Dry, flat, dark pigment
      - *Klebsiella/Enterobacter*: Mucoid
      - *Citrobacter*: Late fermenter
      - *Serratia*: Late, red pigment (some)
    - Lactose negative
      - *Proteus*: Swarming
      - *Morganella, Providencia, Edwardsiella, Hafnia*
      - *Pseudomonas*
      - *Salmonella*
      - *Shigella*
  - Used for various patient and environmental samples
- XLD
  - Yeast extract
  - Sodium deoxycholate
    - Inhibits gram-positive organisms
  - Phenol red: pH indicator
  - Lactose and sucrose in excess, xylose in lower amounts
    - Lactose and sucrose to provide fermentable sugar
  - Lysine: Lysine decarboxylase
    - *Salmonella* decarboxylate the lysine shift the pH indicator to red
  - Sodium thiosulfate, ferric ammonium citrate
    - H_2S production
  - Yellow: Ferments the excess carbohydrates (or xylose only), causes large pH drop, yellow (*E. coli*)
  - Colorless or red: No fermentation, no H_2S (*Shigella* and *Providencia*)
  - Red with black center
    - Ferments xylose, produces low pH, then decarboxylates lysine, produces high pH
    - H_2S production (*Salmonella*)

- HE
  - Meat peptones and yeast extract
  - Bile salts
    - Inhibit gram-positive organisms
  - Lactose, sucrose, salacin
    - Lactose and sucrose to provide fermentable sugar
  - Indicators: Bromophenol blue and acid fuchsin
    - pH indicators
  - Ferric ammonium citrate for H_2S production
  - Differential for *Salmonella* and *Shigella*
  - Yellow-orange colonies: Lactose fermenter (*E. coli*)
  - Colorless/green colonies with unchanged medium: Non–lactose fermenter (*Shigella, Providencia*)
  - Black colonies: H_2S production (*Salmonella*)
- CNA
  - Casein peptones
  - Digest of animal tissue
  - Yeast and beef extract
  - Corn starch
  - 5% sheep blood
  - CNA: inhibits most gram-negative organisms
  - Used for samples with mixed flora
- PEA
  - Casein peptones
  - Soybean peptones
  - 5% sheep blood
  - Phenylethyl alcohol to inhibit gram-negative organisms
  - Some laboratories use CNA rather than PEA because of gram-negative breakthrough
- Key media for routine anaerobic
  - Basic: Blood agar
    - Agar base supplemented with 5% sheep blood, hemin, and vitamin
    - Agar base usually trypticase soy or brain heart infusion
    - Good nonselective medium for initial isolation of anaerobes
  - Selective for anaerobes: Supplemented PEA
    - Vitamin K and hemin are added to PEA agar
    - Suppresses growth of facultative gram-negative bacilli
    - All anaerobes grow well on this medium
  - Selective for gram-negative bacilli: Kanamycin-vancomycin–laked blood agar (K-V agar)
    - Aminoglycoside helps separate aerobes and anaerobes in mixed cultures
    - Limit the swarming of *Proteus* spp.
    - Kanamycin and vancomycin permit growth of only gram-negative anaerobes
    - Laked blood stimulates the growth of some anaerobes
- Back-up broth
  - Broth medium serves as a check for agar plates
  - Useful when the primary shows no growth
  - Chopped meat–glucose and thioglycolate broth are most common
  - Use should be limited to fluids and tissue
    - Not swabs

Growth Requirements—Other Important Components

- Atmosphere requirements
  - 3% to 5% CO_2
  - Room air
  - Increased CO_2 and N, decreased O_2
    - Microaerophilic: 5% O_2, 10% CO_2, 85% N
    - Anaerobic: 85% N_2, 10% H_2, 5% CO_2
- Temperature requirements
  - 35° C Room temperature (25° C to 30° C)
  - 42° C
  - 4° C
- pH and moisture requirements
  - pH
    - Most are 6.5 to 7.5
    - Buffers maintain pH of media
  - Moisture
    - 70% humidity is optimal for good growth
    - Prevents drying of media

STRUCTURE AND METABOLISM

- Bacteria are prokaryotes: Single-cell organisms lacking membrane-bound nuclei
- Eukaryotes are organisms with a defined nucleus
  - Mammalian and plant cells are eukaryotic
- Reproduction of prokaryotic cells is by binary fission
  - Simple division of one cell into two cells
  - DNA replication and formation of a separating membrane and cell wall
  - Can be approximately 20 minutes

Bacteria

- Cells must acquire nutrients, produce energy, and synthesize macromolecules
- It is important to study these areas so that bacteria can be isolated and identified in the laboratory
- Bacterial growth requirements
  - Nutrients acquired by active transport across the cell membrane from the environment
  - Requirements for all bacteria
    - A carbon source (for cellular constituents)
    - A nitrogen source (for proteins)
    - Energy source: Adenosine triphosphate (ATP) (to perform cellular tasks)
    - Trace elements
      - Iron
      - Calcium
      - Zinc

- Copper
- Manganese
- Cobalt
- Phosphorus
- Sulfur
- Potassium
- Magnesium
- Oxygen growth requirements
  - Obligate aerobe: Live and grow in air, cannot grow anaerobically
  - Facultative anaerobe: Can grow aerobically and anaerobically
  - Aerotolerant anaerobe: Grows better anaerobically, but can tolerate low levels of air
  - Obligate anaerobe: Grows only anaerobically, poisoned by air
  - Microaerophilic: Increased CO_2 or other enriched environment
- Bacterial metabolism
  - Production of ATP
    - Drives other metabolic processes
  - Substrates → glucose → metabolic pathway → energy
  - Fermentation versus respiration
    - Fermentation
      - Glucose is converted into pyruvate
      - Embdem-Meyerhof pathway or glycolysis
      - Fermentation is metabolism in the absence of O_2
      - Anaerobic
      - Net gain: 2ATP, $NADH_2$
      - Pyruvate can then enter several other cycles
      - End-products vary depending on cycle entered
    - Aerobic respiration
      - Glucose usage under aerobic conditions
      - Pyruvate enters Krebs cycle (tricarboxylic acid [TCA] cycle)
      - Nicotinamide adenine dinucleotide (NADH) and flavin adenine dinucleotide (FADH) enter the electron transport chain
      - Net gain: 38 ATP (including ATP from fermentation)
      - End-products: CO_2 and H_2O
    - Application to the clinical laboratory
      - Systems to detect fermentation or respiration
        - Acid detection (pH indicators)
        - Gas detection
        - Alcohol detection
  - Different carbon sources
  - Not all bacteria undergo respiration
    - Some lack the enzymes needed
    - Some cannot survive in O_2
  - Potential biochemical tests for organism identification
    - Tests based on presence or absence of these specific enzymes
- Cellular structure
  - Bacteria are prokaryotic
  - Bacteria are small (0.2-2 μm diameter, 1-6 μm length)

- Most bacteria are placed into two groups (determined by differences in the cell wall)
  - Gram-positive
  - Gram-negative
- Chromosome
  - Single, long, supercoiled, circular DNA molecule
  - Prokaryotic cell contains no nucleus
  - Attached to the cell membrane
  - Bacterial chromosomes contain genetic information to code for between 850 to 6500 products
    - Enzymes, proteins, and RNA molecules
    - Human chromosome contains approximately 30,000 genes
- Plasmids
  - Small, circular double-stranded DNA
  - Not part of the chromosome
  - May contain several to several hundred genes
  - One plasmid, multiple copies of same plasmid, or more than one type
  - Antibiotic resistance genes common
  - Can be exchanged between a donor and a recipient in conjugation
- Ribosomes
  - Sites of protein synthesis
  - A 70S prokaryotic ribosome comprises a 30S subunit and a 50S subunit
  - Estimated approximately 15,000 ribosomes in the cytoplasm of an *E. coli* cell
- Cell membrane
  - Bacterial membrane similar in structure and function to eukaryotic cell membrane
  - Membrane consists of proteins and phospholipids
  - Bilayer, with charged or polar groups facing outward and the noncharged portions in between
  - Selectively permeable
  - Many enzymes are attached to membrane
    - Metabolic reactions take place at membrane
- Bacterial cell wall
  - Cell wall defines the shape of bacterial cells
  - Main constituent is complex polymer—peptidoglycan
    - Many sugar molecules (polysaccharide) linked by small peptide (short protein) chains
    - Peptidoglycan is found only in bacteria
  - Thickness of the cell wall and its exact composition vary with the species of bacteria
  - Gram-positive cell walls have thick layer of peptidoglycan
  - Gram-negative walls have much thinner layer of peptidoglycan and an outer membrane
  - Within the cell wall of gram-negative bacteria is lipopolysaccharide (LPS)
    - Part of LPS protrudes from the cell surface—O antigen
- Cellular morphology and arrangement
  - Glycocalyx
  - Some bacteria have layer of material located outside cell wall

- Glycocalyx is a slimy, gelatinous material produced near the cell membrane and secreted outside of the cell wall
- Two types of glycocalyx
  - Slime layer: Not highly organized, not firmly attached
    - *Pseudomonas* and *Staphylococcus*
  - Capsule: Highly organized and firmly attached to the cell wall
    - Usually polysaccharides, may be combined with lipids and proteins
    - Protects from engulfment by white blood cells (WBCs)
  - Both may protect the bacterium from antibiotics
- Flagella
  - Enable bacteria to move in liquid environment
    - Water, intestinal tract, blood, or urine
  - Consist of three or more protein appendages twisted together
  - Number and arrangement of flagella are characteristic of species
  - Single flagellum at one end to multiple flagella covering the entire cell surface
- Pili
  - Pili or fimbriae are short, hairlike structures
    - Usually on external surface of gram-negative organisms
  - Much thinner than flagella, rigid structure, not associated with motility
  - Originate in cytoplasm and extend through the plasma membrane, cell wall, and capsule
  - Two types—sex pilus and attachment pilus
    - Adherence pili anchor to surfaces
      - Tissues in animal's body
      - Usually quite numerous
    - Sex pilus transfers genetic material
      - Cell possessing a sex pilus is donor cell
      - Attach to another cell (usually of the same species)
      - Genetic material, usually a plasmid, transferred through the hollow sex pilus
- Spores
  - Some bacteria form thick-walled structures
    - *Bacillus* and *Clostridium*
    - Means of survival when moisture or nutrients low
  - Formed during sporulation
    - Copy of the chromosome
    - Some cytoplasm enclosed in thick protein coats
  - Resistant to heat, cold, drying, most chemicals, boiling
  - Survive for many years in soil or dust
- Virulence factors
  - Bacteria that cause disease are termed pathogenic because of various factors
  - Examples
    - Exotoxins
    - Endotoxin

- Capsules
- Pili
- Other extracellular proteins
- Bacterial taxonomy: Shared morphologic, physiologic, and genetic traits
  - Species
    - Basic taxonomic group
    - Composed of related individuals with shared characteristics that resemble one another
    - Complete definition difficult
  - Genus (genera)
  - Family
  - Order
  - Class division
  - Kingdom
  - Bacterial names are binomial
    - Genus and species
    - Treated as Latin and written in italic
    - Genus can be abbreviated in written material after first used
      - *Staphylococcus aureus*
      - *S. aureus*
  - Name changes are designated with ( )
    - *Stenotrophomas (Xanthomonas) maltophilia*

FAMILY STAPHYLOCOCCACEAE

- General characteristics
  - Gram-positive cocci in clusters or tetrads
  - Catalase positive
  - Aerobic to facultative anaerobic
  - Nonmotile
- *Staphylococcus*: Greek *staphyle* means "bunch of grapes" and *coccos* means "granule"
- Genus *Staphylococcus*: General characteristics
  - All ferment glucose
  - Differentiated by coagulase test
  - Coagulase-positive are considered *S. aureus*
  - Coagulase-negative species
    - *Staphylococcus epidermidis*
    - *Staphylococcus saprophyticus*
  - Approximately 30 other species

Staphylococcus aureus

- Most clinically important
- Causes numerous infections
- Important hospital pathogen
- Antibiotic resistance has become a major issue (again)
- Epidemiology
  - Humans are natural reservoir for *S. aureus*
  - Asymptomatic colonization is far more common than infection
  - Colonization of nasopharynx and perineum skin occurs shortly after birth and recurs
  - Transmission occurs by direct contact with a colonized carrier
    - Carriage rates from 25% to 50%

- ○ Higher in injection drug users; patients with diabetes, dermatologic conditions, or long-term indwelling intravascular catheters; and health care workers
- Young children have higher rates
- Colonization may be transient or persistent
- Clinical disease
  - Causes suppurative (pus-forming) infections and toxin diseases
  - Infections can be superficial or invasive
    - ○ Superficial skin lesions: Boils, sties, furuncles, impetigo
    - ○ Invasive: Pneumonia, mastitis, arthritis, meningitis, osteomyelitis, and endocarditis
  - Toxin diseases: Food poisoning, scalded skin syndrome, toxic shock disease
    - ○ Scalded skin syndrome
      - ▪ Extensive exfoliative dermatitis (skin sloughing)
      - ▪ In adults, occurs in chronic renal failure and immunocompromised individuals
      - ▪ Mortality in adults can be as high as 50%
      - ▪ Localized = Bullous impetigo (large pustule)
      - ▪ Generalized = Profuse peeling of the epidermal layer of skin
    - ○ Toxic shock syndrome
      - ▪ Toxic shock syndrome toxin-1 (TSST-1) associated
      - ▪ Superantigen
      - ▪ Characteristic rash
      - ▪ Multisystem disease: High fever, hypotension, and shock
      - ▪ Identified in both sexes
      - ▪ Higher prevalence with tampon use
      - ▪ Most patients recover: 2% to 5% mortality
- Oxacillin-resistant *S. aureus*
  - Oxacillin-resistant *S. aureus* (ORSA) and methicillin-resistant *S. aureus* (MRSA) are resistant to antibiotics
    - ○ Methicillin, oxacillin, nafcillin, penicillin, and amoxicillin
    - ○ Frequently other agents
- Hospital acquired versus community acquired
  - Historically, among persons in hospitals and health care facilities who have weakened immune systems
  - Infections acquired by persons who have not been recently hospitalized are known as community-acquired (CA-ORSA) infections
  - Infections in the community are usually skin infections and occur in otherwise healthy people
  - May be more pathogenic than hospital-acquired (HA-ORSA) infection
- Pathogenesis and virulence factors
  - Carriage of the organism
  - Disseminated via hand to body sites and breaks in the skin
  - Eczema or minor dermatitis

- Abscess
- Fibrin wall around a core of organisms and leukocytes
- Pathogenesis
- Ability to elaborate proteolytic enzymes may facilitate the process
- Nondisseminated: Local disease (e.g., boils)
- Dissemination results in pneumonia, bone and joint infection
- Toxin disease: Either toxin alone or in combination with invasion
- Toxins
  - Enterotoxins
    - ○ Heat-stable exotoxins that cause diarrhea and vomiting
    - ○ Enterotoxins A and D are resistant to gastric and digestive acids
    - ○ Toxins are preformed in foods
    - ○ Symptoms (i.e., nausea, vomiting, abdominal pain, and cramping) appear 2 to 8 hours after ingestion and resolve within 8 hours
  - Enterotoxin F (TSST-1)
  - Epidermolytic toxin
    - ○ Sloughing of the skin
    - ○ Widespread systemic immune responses
  - Exfoliative toxin
    - ○ Similar to TSST-1 but a different site in skin
    - ○ Cytolytic toxins: Extracellular factors that affect red blood cells (RBCs) and WBCs
  - Hemolysins
    - ○ Alpha α-Hemolysin: Destroys RBCs, platelets, tissue
    - ○ Beta β-Hemolysin: Destroys RBCs
    - ○ Gamma δ-Hemolysin: Causes injury, less lethal
  - Leukocidin
    - ○ Panton-Valentine leukocidin: Exotoxin lethal to PMNs
    - ○ May suppress phagocytosis
  - Enzymes
  - Coagulase: Causes coagulation of surroundings
  - Hyaluronidase: Hydrolyzes hyaluronic acid in connective tissue
  - Lipase: Aids colonization by acting on sebaceous glands
  - Fatty acid–modifying enzyme: Breaks down antistaphylococcal lipids made by the host
  - Protein A
    - ○ In *S. aureus* cell wall
    - ○ Binds Fc portion of immunoglobulin (avoid phagocytosis)

Coagulase-Negative Staphylococci

- Clinically important
  - *Staphylococcus epidermidis*
  - *Staphylococcus saprophyticus*

- Normal flora of skin and mucous membranes
  - Approximately 30 other species

Staphylococcus epidermidis
- Infections
  - Predominantly hospital acquired
  - Predisposing factors
    - Catheterization, prosthetic heart valves, immunosuppressive therapy
  - Bacteremia
  - Endocarditis
  - Most common cause of hospital-acquired urinary tract infection (UTI)

Staphylococcus saprophyticus
- Normal flora of the mucous membranes of the urogenital tract
- Causes UTI
- Young, sexually active women
- Considered significant in urine cultures even if it is found in small numbers

Laboratory Diagnosis

- Media
  - Mannitol salt
  - CNA
  - PEA
  - CHROMagar—media containing patented chromogenic substrates that can be formulated to provide specific colors to develop in colonies of a particular genus or species
  - CHROMagar MRSA
- *S. aureus*
  - Colonies are medium to large, ivory to yellow, and beta-hemolyic
  - Catalase positive and coagulase positive
  - Mannitol salt positive
- *S. epidermidis*
  - Colonies are small to medium, nonhemolytic, white
  - Coagulase negative
  - Biochemicals required to identify
  - Often not speciated
- *S. saprophyticus*
  - Colonies are large, with approximately 50% producing a yellow pigment
  - Coagulase negative
  - Novobiocin resistant

FAMILY STREPTOCOCCACEAE

- Genus *Streptococcus*
  - Gram-positive cocci in chains or pairs
  - Catalase negative
  - Small, grayish colonies on sheep blood agar
  - Categorized by Lancefield groups
    - Alpha (α): conversion of hemoglobin to methemoglobin resulting in a green zone in the blood agar around a colony
    - Beta (β): Lysis of the sheep RBCs in the blood agar plates
    - Gamma (γ): Nonhemolytic
  - Classification
    - 85 species at present
    - Hemolytic pattern on 5% sheep blood agar
    - Serologic group (Lancefield) of the β-hemolytic group: A, B, C, D, F, G . . . T
    - Taxonomic/genetic related now used
  - β-Hemolytic streptococci
    - *Streptococcus pyogenes*: Group A
    - *Streptococcus agalactiae*: Group B
    - *Streptococcus* group C, F, G
  - Others
    - Many found predominately in animals

Streptococcus Species

Streptococcus pyogenes
- Group A *Streptococcus*
- Not the exact same as *S. pyogenes*, approximately 5% *Streptococcus anginosus*
- Spread from person to person
- Carriers do exist
- Clinical disease
  - Causes relatively common, significant diseases
  - Pharyngitis: "Strep throat"
  - Skin infections
  - Otitis
  - Sinusitis
  - Sepsis
  - Scarlet fever
  - Some less common diseases
    - Pneumonia
    - Meningitis
    - Fasciitis: Flesh-eating bacteria
  - Complications
    - Rheumatic heart disease
    - Glomerulonephritis
  - Rheumatic fever
    - Complication of pharyngitis
    - Can cause chronic, progressive damage to heart
    - Pathogenesis poorly understood
  - Acute glomerulonephritis
    - Complication of pharyngitis or cutaneous
    - Circulating immune complexes deposit in glomeruli
    - Inflammatory response causes damage
- Pathogenesis and virulence factors
  - Enters through the respiratory tract or skin contact
  - Either local disease or spread
    - Local disease alone or with *S. aureus*
    - Systemic spread leads to disease and complications
  - M protein and lipoteichoic acid for attachment
  - Hyaluronic acid capsule: Inhibits phagocytosis
  - Extracellular products

- Pyrogenic (erythrogenic) toxin, which causes the rash of scarlet fever
- Streptokinase
- Streptodornase (DNase B)
- Streptolysins
- Laboratory diagnosis
  - GPC in chains
  - Small, transparent, smooth, β-hemolytic colonies
  - Bacitracin susceptible
  - L-pyrrolidonyl arylamidase (PYR) positive
  - Latex or other grouping tests are usually used in clinical laboratories
- Susceptibility testing and treatment
  - *All* isolates are penicillin susceptible
  - Susceptibility testing not appropriate in almost all settings
    - Exceptions are penicillin-allergic patients
    - Manual method usually used

Streptococcus agalactiae
- Group B *Streptococcus*
- Normal flora in female genital tract and gastrointestinal (GI) tract
- Clinical significance
  - Neonatal sepsis and meningitis
  - UTI
  - Pneumonia in elderly
- Pathogenesis and virulence factors
  - In early-onset neonatal disease, organism is transmitted vertically from the mother
  - In late-onset (from 7 days to 3 months age) meningitis is acquired horizontally, in some instances as a nosocomial infection
  - Virulence
    - Capsule
    - Hemolysin
    - Hyaluronidase
    - Proteases
- Laboratory diagnosis
  - Grayish-white, slightly mucoid colonies
  - Small zone of β-hemolysis: Larger colony than group A
  - Hippurate and CAMP test positive
  - Latex or other grouping tests are usually used in clinical laboratories
- Susceptibility testing and treatment
  - All isolates are penicillin susceptible
  - Other agents are not always active
    - Susceptibility testing not appropriate in almost all settings
    - Exceptions are penicillin-allergic patients

Group D *Streptococcus*
- Normal flora
  - GI tract
  - Urogenital tract
- Group D antigen, although not always β-hemolytic
  - *Streptococcus gallolyticus*
  - *Streptococcus equinus*
- Clinical significance: Bacteremia and endocarditis

- Group D laboratory diagnosis
  - Small, white colonies with hemolysis on blood agar
  - *Enterococcus* and group D bile esculin positive
  - *Enterococcus* grows in higher NaCl concentration and is PYR positive
- α-Hemolytic streptococci
  - *Streptococcus pneumoniae*
  - Viridans group streptococci
  - Sometimes enterococcal species
  - Nutritionally variant streptococci

Streptococcus pneumoniae
- No Lancefield grouping
- Infects humans exclusively, no reservoir is found in nature
- Carrier rate of *S. pneumoniae* in the normal human nasopharynx is 20% to 40%
- Clinical disease
  - Pneumococcal pneumonia is most common in elderly, debilitated, or immunosuppressed
    - Often after viral infection damages the respiratory ciliated epithelium
    - Incidence peaks in the winter
    - Community-acquired pneumonia
  - Otitis media
  - Meningitis (most common cause in adults)
  - Septicemia
- Laboratory diagnosis
  - GPC in pairs, lancet
  - Colonies are round and usually wet, glistening, mucoid
  - α-Hemolysis
  - Optochin susceptible
  - Bile soluble
- Susceptibility and treatment
  - Susceptibility testing appropriate for isolates from normally sterile body sites
  - Most automated methods do not work well
  - Penicillin resistance an issue

Other α-Hemolytic Streptococci
- Viridans streptococci
- Normal flora
  - Upper respiratory tract
  - Urogenital tract
  - Clinical significance: Subacute bacterial endocarditis
- Identification
  - α-Hemolytic
  - Optochin resistance
  - Examples: *Streptococcus mutans, Streptococcus salivarius, Streptococcus anginosus* group, *Streptococcus gallolyticus* (bovis)
- Susceptibility testing and treatment
  - Some penicillin resistance has been reported
  - Susceptibility testing not usually appropriate because the isolates are rarely clinically significant
  - If the cause of true disease, susceptibility testing may be appropriate

FAMILY ENTEROCOCCACEAE

Enterococcus Species

- 38 species
- Most common isolates from humans
  - *Enterococcus faecalis*
  - *Enterococcus faecium*
  - *Enterococcus avium*
  - *Enterococcus casseliflavus*
  - *Enterococcus gallinarum*
- General characteristics
  - Gram-positive cocci typically in pairs and short chains
  - Facultative anaerobe
  - Catalase negative
- Epidemiology
  - Normal flora of the GI and urogenital tract of humans and animals
  - One of the top three nosocomial pathogens
- Clinical significance
  - UTI
  - Wounds
  - Abdominal and pelvic infections
  - Nosocomial infections
  - Endocarditis and bacteremia
- Virulence factors
  - Fimbriae: Attachment to epithelial cells
  - Adhesins: Attachment to intestinal tract
  - Bacteriocins: Inhibits growth of other intestinal bacteria
  - Gelatinase: Hydrolizes collagen and hemoglobin
- Laboratory diagnosis
  - Small, white colonies
  - α-Hemolytic or nonhemolytic, may be β-hemolytic
  - Both *Enterococcus* and group D are bile esculin positive
  - *Enterococcus* grows in higher NaCl concentration and PYR positive
- Susceptibility testing and treatment
  - Inherently resistant to cephalosporins
  - Less susceptible than streptococci to penicillin and ampicillin
  - Vancomycin (vancomycin-resistant enterococcus [VRE])
  - Resistant to trimethoprim and sulfamethoxazole
  - Most isolates should be tested but limited reporting
  - Treatment often limited to vancomycin, aminoglycosides, and maybe fluoroquinolones
  - Some newer agents may be useful: Linezolid, daptomycin

MISCELLANEOUS GRAM-POSITIVE COCCI

- *Abiotrophia*
- *Aerococcus*
- *Granulicatella*
- *Leuconostoc*
- *Micrococcus*
- *Pediococcus*
- General characteristics
- Uncommonly isolated
- Vitamin B_6/pyridoxyl is required for lab growth of *Abiotrophia* and *Granulicatella*
  - May be mistaken for *Staphylococcus* or *Streptococcus* spp.
  - Limited pathogenic potential but possible in the young, the old or the immunocompromised
  - May be difficult to identify, rule out *Staphylococcus* or *Streptococcus* may be all that is possible

AEROBIC GRAM-POSITIVE BACILLI

- Aerobic gram-positive bacilli represent a taxonomically and genetically diverse group of organisms
- As human pathogens, notable diseases include listeriosis, anthrax, erysipelas, and diphtheria, although incidence in North America is very low
- General characteristics
  - Similarities
    - Capable of growth in the presence of O_2
    - Retention of crystal violet after alcohol decolorization step of Gram stain thus appearing purple in color (gram-positive)
    - Rod shaped
    - Generally grow easily after 24 hours on nonselective agars such as SBA
  - General characteristics
  - Phenotypic diversity includes
    - Cell size
    - Approximately 0.2 to 1.5 μm wide, 0.5 to 10 μm long
    - Production of spores
    - Microscopic appearance may vary
    - Regular "rod" shape
      - Rounded, square, or slightly pointed ends
    - Coryneform with club-shaped cells arranged such that they resemble the letters V and L
    - Filamentous: Cells form long chains
    - Filamentous with rudimentary or true branching
- Initial grouping of aerobic gram-positive bacilli
  - Spore forming
    - *Bacillus* spp.
  - Non–spore forming
    - *Listeria, Erysipelothrix, Corynebacterium,* and others

Bacillus Species

- General characteristics
  - More than 50 species, all are found in soil
  - All *Bacillus* sp. form endospores
  - All are catalase positive
- Spore formation

- Endospores are unique to *Bacillus* spp. among aerobes
- Transition from vegetative cells to spores under harsh and desiccated environments preserves cell viability for long periods
- Not always evident in Gram smears, but visualization of spores confirms *Bacillus* genus
- Special stains are used to better visualize spores
- Spores can be "weaponized" for use as infectious aerosols in biological attack
  - Highly infectious

Bacillus cereus
- Most common disease is food poisoning
- Less common opportunistic infection
- Epidemiology
  - Common agent in food poisoning
  - Two forms of food poisoning
    - Diarrheal: Meat, 24 hours, self-limiting
    - Emetic: Fried rice, 10 hours, self-limiting
    - Above symptoms caused by two distinct toxins
  - Opportunistic disease
    - Serious ocular infection
    - Wound infection
- Pathogenesis and virulence
  - Food poisoning is toxin mediated
- Laboratory diagnosis
  - Colonies are large, spreading, beta-hemolytic
  - Catalase positive

Bacillus anthracis
- Most virulent and significant human disease
- Epidemiology
  - Zoonotic disease in herbivores (e.g., sheep, goats, cattle) follows ingestion of spores in soil
  - Human infection typically acquired through contact with anthrax-infected animals or animal products (no person-to-person spread)
  - Less typical is infection through intentional exposure (bioterrorism)
  - Clinical presentation: Anthrax
    - Cutaneous: Direct contact with infected material
    - Inhalation: Aspiration of spore aerosol (wool sorters disease)
    - Gastrointestinal: Eating of contaminated meat
- Anthrax: Cutaneous
  - Form most commonly encountered in naturally occurring cases
  - Incubation period: 1 to 12 days
    - Begins as a papule, progresses to a vesicular stage, then to a depressed black necrotic ulcer (eschar)
    - Edema, redness, or necrosis without ulceration may occur
  - Case-fatality
    - Without antibiotic treatment: 20%
    - With antibiotic treatment: 1%
- Anthrax: Inhalation
  - Begins as a "viral-like" illness, characterized by myalgia, fatigue, fever, with or without respiratory symptoms, followed by hypoxia

- Rhinorrhea (runny nose) rare
- Incubation period: 1 to 7 days (possibly ranging up to 42 days)
- Case fatality
  - Without antibiotic treatment: 97%
  - With antibiotic treatment: 75%
- Anthrax: GI
  - Abdominal distress, usually accompanied by bloody vomiting or diarrhea, followed by fever and signs of septicemia
  - GI illness sometimes seen as oropharyngeal ulcerations with cervical adenopathy and fever
  - Develops after ingestion of contaminated, poorly cooked meat
  - Incubation period: 1 to 7 days
  - Case-fatality: 25% to 60% (role of early antibiotic treatment is undefined)
- Anthrax: Complications
  - 5% develop meningitis
  - Coma and death occur 1 to 6 days after exposure
  - Recovery confers immunity
  - Vaccines available to high-risk groups
  - Antibiotics used after exposure
    - Ciprofloxacin, tetracycline (60-day treatment)
- Pathogenesis and virulence factors
  - Cutaneous infection remains localized
  - Inhalation and GI cases often proceed to bacterial sepsis with high morbidity and mortality
- Laboratory diagnosis
  - Colonies are medium to large irregular, gray. Medusa head projections, non-hemolytic
  - Catalase positive
  - If suspected, stop working with the isolate and contact State Health Laboratory

Listeria Species

- General characteristics
  - Appear on Gram stain as gram-positive short rods or coccobacilli
  - Grow aerobically
  - No spores
  - Not acid fast
  - Able to grow at 4° C, unlike many other bacteria
- Taxonomy and history
  - Six species; type species is *Listeria monocytogenes*, the most important to human disease
  - Found widespread in nature; habitat is soil and decaying vegetation, but carried by numerous humans and animals
- Epidemiology
  - Easy access to food processing and represents major threat to food chain
  - Most virulent of the *Listeria* and common human pathogen is *L. monocytogenes*
  - Disease: Listeriosis
    - Predominantly a food-borne illness (ingestion)

- Cutaneous: Occupational exposure
  - Meat processors and veterinarians
- High mortality rate
- Clinical disease
  - Affects high-risk populations
    - Elderly, immunocompromised hosts
    - Pregnant women and their babies
  - Complications of pregnancy
    - Placentitis and/or amnionitis
    - Infection passed to fetus (congenital)
      - Premature birth, abortion, or stillborn birth
      - Neonatal meningitis
  - Meningitis
  - Sepsis

Listeria monocytogenes
- Laboratory diagnosis
  - Gram smear of normally sterile body fluids with characteristic morphology
  - Culture recovery from appropriate specimens
    - Blood, cerebrospinal fluid (CSF), amniotic fluid, placenta, genital tract, stool, respiratory secretion
  - Recognition of aerobic gram-positive bacilli
    - β-Hemolytic (clear zone)
    - Biochemical profile
    - Motility characteristics: umbrella pattern
    - Growth at 4° C

Erysipelothrix
- Non–spore forming gram-positive rod
- Related to *Listeria* spp.
- *E. rhusiopathiae* is the species of clinical interest
  - Agent of swine erysipelas, widespread disease in pigs
  - Cause of erysipeloid, a cutaneous infection in humans occasionally acquired by contact with infected animals
- General characteristics
  - Small gram-positive bacilli (0.2-0.5 μm wide × 0.8-2.5 μm long)
  - Occur singly, in short chains or filaments
  - Aerobic or facultative anaerobic O_2 requirements
  - Nonmotile
  - Catalase negative
  - Wide temperature range growth on complex nutrient media such as SBA
- Epidemiology and clinical disease
  - Widespread in nature
  - Colonizes variety of animals, fish, and birds, but particularly pigs
  - Resists cold and alkaline environment
  - In animals causes erysipelas, ranging from cutaneous to systemic disease
  - In humans, erysipeloid is a cutaneous infection consisting of localized cellulitis after acquisition through skin abrasion, injury, or bite
    - Occupational hazard among animal handlers, farming personnel, veterinarians

- Lesions painful, with edema, inflammation, and possible local arthritis
- Systemic disease possible in immunocompromised individuals
- Laboratory diagnosis
  - Specimen of choice
    - Skin biopsy
  - Gram stain of suspect lesion
    - Pleomorphic gram-positive *Bacillus*
  - Cultivation
    - SBA with 5% to 10% CO_2
      - H_2S positive on Triple Sugar Iron Agar (TSI) slant

Corynebacterium Species

- A diverse group of gram-positive bacilli commonly referred to as coryneforms
- Differentiated by chemotaxonomic means such as analysis of cell wall components
- Exhibits a clublike morphology that reflects its name (*coryne* means "club" in Greek)
- General characteristics
  - Small gram-positive bacilli
  - May resemble Chinese letters
  - Characteristic colonial morphology: dry

Corynebacterium diphtheriae
- Epidemiology
  - Significant human pathogen is *C. diphtheriae*, which manifests as a respiratory disease or less commonly as a cutaneous infection
  - Acquired by person-to-person contact and spread through close contact with carriers who harbor organisms
  - Although a global pathogen, is rare in the United States because of childhood vaccination programs
- Clinical disease
  - Normally encountered as a respiratory ailment
  - Common symptoms include sore throat with low-grade fever
  - Adherent membrane of the tonsils, pharynx, or nose is a hallmark of disease
  - Swelling of neck is usually present in severe disease
  - Cutaneous diphtheria can occur and manifests as infected skin lesions but without a characteristic appearance
  - Complications
    - Myocarditis
    - Kidney and liver inflammation
    - Peripheral neuropathy
    - Airway obstruction
    - Death (occurs in 5% to 10% of respiratory cases)
- Pathogenesis and virulence factors
  - Invasion
    - Bacteria colonize and proliferate in local tissues of the throat, creating pseudomembrane
  - Toxigenesis

- Bacteria produce an exotoxin that causes the death of eukaryotic cells and tissues by inhibition of cell protein synthesis
  - Causes heart and nerve damage and is responsible for the lethal symptoms of the disease
  - Vaccination consists of a toxoid, which maintains the antigenicity of the toxin without the toxicity and prompts production of toxin-neutralizing antibody
  - Vaccination programs solely are responsible for the control of diphtheria in a population
- Laboratory diagnosis
  - Specimens
    - Throat and nasopharyngeal
    - Material under pseudomembrane useful
  - Media
    - General media: 5% SBA
    - Selective medium: Cystine-tellurite medium (CTBA), which selects against normal throat flora
      - *C. diphtheria* colonies are black to gray
    - Differential medium: Tinsdale, which allows recognition of suspected *C. diphtheriae*
      - *C. diphtheria* colonies are black with brown halos
  - Gram stain of sample
    - Gram-positive "Chinese letters" appearance
  - Biochemicals
    - Urease negative
    - Nitrate positive
    - Catalase positive
  - Toxin testing (tests for toxin phage)
    - In vivo: Culture and antitoxin in rabbit
    - In vitro: Immunodiffusion

Corynebacteria Other Than *Corynebacterium diphtheriae*

- Corynebacteria are widespread as normal flora on the skin and mucosal membranes of humans and animals
- Such infections range from local cutaneous to deep-seated systemic infections
- *Corynebacterium jeikeium*
  - Important in nosocomial or immunocompromised
  - Line-related infections
  - Antimicrobial resistance

Other Corynebacteria

- Because of the common presence of *Corynebacterium* on human surfaces, significance should be attached to their recovery only in the following cases
  - Isolated from otherwise sterile body sites
  - If clearly predominant in mixed flora culture results grown from well-collected sample
  - If recovered in high count ($>10^4$ cfu/mL) from urine as single organism
  - Significance is enhanced in the following cases
    - Multiple specimens positive for same organism
    - Coryneform bacteria seen on direct Gram stain with strong leukocytic reaction

FAMILY MYCOBACTERIACEAE

- General characteristics
  - Slim, rod-shaped organisms that are 1 to 10 μm long
  - Nonmotile and non–spore forming, obligate aerobes
  - Slow growing (3 to 40 days in culture)
  - Contain mycolic acids, complex, long-chain fatty acids
  - Possess a cell envelope with a high lipid content
  - Although mycobacteria are discussed in the section on gram-positive bacilli, it is important to note that with the exception of species classified as "rapid growers," mycobacteria do not stain with Gram reagents
  - All mycobacteria will stain acid fast with Ziehl-Neelsen or auromine O stains and are commonly referred to as an acid-fast bacillus (AFB)
- Acid-fast staining (Ziehl-Neelsen)
  - Step 1 exposes the smear to carbol fuchsin, a red dye
  - Step 2 involves decolorization with hydrochloric acid
  - Step 3 counterstains with methylene blue
  - An acid-fast organism resists decolorization and remains red, whereas non–acid fast organisms stain blue
- Cell wall structure
  - Mycolic acids are components of a variety of lipids found only in mycobacteria, *Nocardia,* and corynebacteria
  - The chain length of these mycolic acids is longest in *Mycobacterium*, intermediate in *Nocardia,* and shortest in *Corynebacterium* spp.
  - This explains why mycobacteria are generally acid fast, nocardia less acid fast, and corynebacteria are non–acid fast
  - Conversely, *Mycobacteria* will not stain with the Gram procedure and *Nocardia* and *Corynebacterium* will stain as gram-positive
- Epidemiology and clinical disease
  - The pulmonary disease tuberculosis, caused by *Mycobacterium tuberculosis* complex, is an enormous global problem
    - Estimated 1.7 billion people, one third of the world's population, are infected
  - 8.4 million new cases per year and 2 to 3 million deaths
  - Infection risk proportional to intensity of exposure
  - Infection does not usually lead to disease
  - *M. tuberculosis* is exclusively a human pathogen
  - *Mycobacterium bovis* is a closely related animal pathogen that causes a disease in people that is indistinguishable from tuberculosis (TB). It is acquired from the ingestion of infected meat or milk

Mycobacterium Species (Box 1-1)

Mycobacterium tuberculosis

- Natural history of *M. tuberculosis* infection
  - *M. tuberculosis* is acquired through the inhalation of droplet nuclei
  - The primary spread of the organism is via aerosol droplets from coughing
  - Bacteria not initially killed multiply in the phagosome of a macrophage, destroying the macrophage
  - Released organisms are ingested by other macrophages
  - Cytokines and chemokines produced attract other phagocytic cells, including monocytes, other alveolar macrophages, and neutrophils
  - These cells eventually form a nodular structure termed the tubercle or granuloma
  - The immunologic response to this infection is cellular (rather than humoral), and a delayed type hypersensitivity reaction develops against tuberculin protein that manifests a positive skin test reaction
  - Dissemination of the organism to the lymph nodes and bloodstream occurs with deposition in liver, spleen, kidney, bone, brain, meninges, and other parts of the lung with further granuloma formation. This is termed disseminated or miliary TB and on radiography shows multiple "millet seed"–like lesions
- Natural history of TB
  - Reactivation of TB results when persisting bacteria in a host suddenly proliferate, because the granuloma formation does not eradicate the organisms
  - 15% to 20% of primary disease reactivates at a later point, leading to caseous granuloma and cavity formation, during which the disease is highly contagious
  - Greatest risk for reactivation
    - Within 5 years of primary infection
    - Those at the extremes of age
    - Pregnant women, immunosuppressed patients
    - Malnourished population, alcoholics, and patients with diabetes
- Most common presentation of TB is as a chronic pulmonary disease
  - Chronic cough
  - Chest pain
  - Shortness of breath
  - Low-grade fever
  - Fatigue
  - Night sweats
  - Loss of appetite
  - Weight loss
  - Sputum production
- Immunity to TB
  - Infection is contained in 80% to 85% of people who recover without ever having symptoms of disease
  - Cell-mediated immunity develops 2 to 6 weeks after active infection (result of T cell, not B cell, proliferation)
  - At that point, delayed-type hypersensitivity response is demonstrable through a skin test; the antigen reagent is termed purified protein derivative, so the test is known as the PPD test
  - Patients who cannot raise a sufficient delayed-type hypersensitivity response will develop miliary (disseminated) TB
- Epidemiology and clinical disease
  - Increased risk for clinical disease after primary infection is found in young children, Native Americans, Native Africans, patients infected with the human immune deficiency virus (HIV), intravenous drug abusers
    - Infants and the very young have a high mortality rate from primary infections
  - Highest risk for incidence and reactivation
    - Former for current prison inmates
    - The homeless, the elderly
    - Foreign-born persons from TB-endemic areas
- Prophylaxis
  - Bacillus Calmette Guérin (BCG) vaccine is 70% effective in preventing infection in a specific population
  - BCG is not used in countries with a low incidence of TB because the ability to detect infection with *M. tuberculosis* with the PPD is lost
  - After a positive tuberculin test, isoniazid (INH) and other drugs are taken for 6 to 9 months or rifampin for 4 to 9 months to prevent disease
- Drug-resistant strains
  - Increased resistance to INH and other antituberculosis drugs noted in recent years; in *M. tuberculosis* resistance is due to mutation, not plasmid transfer
  - Multiple drug–resistant strains pose severe problems and are seen in populations with HIV infection
  - Most nontuberculous *Mycobacterium* spp. are generally more resistant to drugs than *M. tuberculosis*
- Laboratory diagnosis
  - Dual motivation in laboratory detection of *M. tuberculosis*
    - Diagnose and treat patient
    - Infection control
      - Stop contagion
      - Protect others

Nontuberculous *Mycobacteria*
Atypical Mycobacteria and Mycobacteria Other Than Tuberculosis (MOTT)

- Environmentally acquired, not transmitted person to person by respiratory means
- Generally infects those with weakened immune systems because of age, disease, or other factors

BOX 1-1   Isolation and Identification of *Mycobacterium*

- Mycobacterium characteristics
- Slim rod-shaped organisms that are 1-10 μm long.
- Nonmotile and nonspore forming, obligate aerobes
- Slow growing (3 to 40 days in culture)
- All Mycobacteria will stain "Acid-fast" with Ziehl-Neelson or auromine/rhodamine stains and are commonly referred to as Acid Fast Bacilli or AFB
- With the exception of the rapidly growing AFB, mycobacteria will not stain with the Gram's procedure
- Lab safety is a major concern due to the potential of infectious aerosols
  - Containment is crucial
    - Biosafety level 2 hoods
    - Gowns, gloves, and masks
    - Sealed centrifuge cups
    - Negative pressure room and BSL 3 containment desirable
- Mycobacterium Sample Preparation
- Common samples:
  - NF likely to be present in sputum, bronchial wash or lavage, skin lesions, urine, stool
  - Normally sterile body sites do not contain normal flora—pleural fluid, blood, spinal fluid, deep tissue biopsies
- The complex lipid AFB cell wall allows procedures that decontaminate normal bacterial flora but allow AFB to remain viable
- Decontamination
  - Bacterial flora eliminated or reduced
- Mycobacteria release from mucus
  - Concentration aids in detection of low numbers
  - AFB are largely protected from decontamination
  - Use of mildest procedure that controls decontamination rate advocated
  - Expect contamination rate of 3%-5%
  - No contamination means procedure is too harsh
  - AFB smear and culture follows decontamination

Specimen Processing for AFB
- Culture Media—Slanted media in tubes preferred for safety reasons.
- **Egg based (whole or yolks)—Lowenstein-Jensen (LJ)**
  - Preferred basic nonselective media
  - Gruft modification—Penicillin/Nalidixic acid—inhibitory to contaminants
  - Malachite green—inhibitory to routine bacteria
- **Agar based, conventional petri dish**
  - Middlebrook 7H10, 7H11 most popular
  - Salts, vitamins, cofactors, tween/glycerol
  - "Thin" plates for early detection of colonies—10-12 days, microscopically
  - Less commonly used than LJ slants for reasons of containment
- **Liquid media**
  - 7H9 media most common
  - Reduces turnaround time to average of 10 days
  - Used in BACTEC system (^{14}C labeled palmitic acid-detection of free $^{14}CO_2$), and other continuous monitoring automated systems
  - 0.5 mL PANTA (polymixin B, amphotericin B, nalidixic acid, trimeth/sulfa, azlocillin)—added to processed specimens to prevent specimens

- AFB liquid detection systems
- Specimen Processing
- AFB Staining Techniques
- Carbol fuchsin based
  - Heat fix suspension to slides
    - 15 min @ 80° C or 2 hr @ 65° C
  - Ziehl-Nielson "requires HEAT step during staining" (tedious)
  - Kinyoun "COLD" modification of ZN preferred method
  - Read on oil immersion (1000 ×)
- Auramine Rhodamine fluorescent stain
  - Organisms appear yellowish green against a black background
  - Can scan slide at low power (250 ×) and confirm at 400 ×
  - More sensitive for detection and faster scan of slide than ZN
  - Requires microscope with fluorescent optics
- Incubation
  - Most species require 35° C-37° C, 5%-10% CO_2
  - Dark, high humidity, loose caps
  - Optimally at least 2 media
- Examine weekly for growth
  - Hold cultures for 6-8 weeks
  - Lower incubation temperature if infection cutaneous due to possible mycobacteria other than TB (MOTT)
- Identification of Mycobacteria
- Growth Rate—time for visible colonies to appear:
  - Rapid ≤ 7 days
  - Slow > 7 days
- AFB Colony morphology
- *M. tuberculosis*
  - The color is typically buff, regardless of light
  - Texture of the colony is rough
- *M. avium complex*
  - Color is tan to buff regardless of light
  - Texture of the colony is smooth
- *M. kansasii*
  - Color is yellow or reddish yellow
  - Texture of the colony is smooth
  - AFB Colony morphology
- Pigment Production among MOTT
  - **Scotochromogens**: grow with a deep yellow pigment regardless of light
  - *M. scofulaceum, M. gordonae*
  - **Photochromogens**: develop yellow pigment only after exposure to light
  - *M. kanasii, M. marinum*
  - **Nonchromogens**: no pigment beyond tan to buff colonies regardless of light
  - *M. avium-intracellulare*
  - Note: *M. tb* complex produces buff colonies
- Pigment production among MOTT
  - Key Biochemical Tests
  - Niacin test
    - *M. tuberculosis* accumulates considerable niacin in media. + Test early sign that isolate may be tuberculosis
    - Niacin extracted and tested with strip for color development

BOX 1-1	Isolation and Identification of *Mycobacterium*—cont'd

- Semi Quantitative Catalase
  - *M. kansasii* positive
  - *M. scrofulaceum* positive
  - *M. tb* and *avium* negative
  - Hydrogen peroxide added
  - Positive test = bubbles rising above 45 mm from baseline
- Arylsulfatase
  - Rapid growers are only mycobacterium positive in 3 day test
  - Helps to differentiate from similar looking *Nocardia* species
- Nitrate reduction
  - *M. tb* and *M. kansasii* are positive, *M. avium* is negative
  - Red color on strip or reagent test is positive

- Additional identification methods for mycobacteria
- GLC or HPLC
- Analysis of long-chain fatty acids
- Most health departments and CDC prefer method
- Genetic probes
  - DNA probes specific for hybridization for rRNA sequences—use chemiluminometer
  - Only single colony of organism needed
  - Rapid and specific detection of organism
  - Available for *M. tuberculosis, avium, intacellulare, kansasii* and *gordonae*

Species	Niacin	Semi Quant Catalase	Nitrate reduct.	Aryl sulfatase	Tween hydrol
M. tuberculosis	+	-	+	-	-
M. kansasii	-	+	+	-	+
M. scrofulaceum	-	+	-	-	-
M. avium complex	-	-	-		-
M. gordonae	-	+	-	V	+
M. fortuitum	-	+	+	+	V

- Can cause TB-like, cutaneous, or leprosy-like diseases
- Are not susceptible to certain common antituberculosis antibiotics
- *M. avium* complex (MAC) is the most commonly associated HIV-related systemic bacterial infection and manifests as a pulmonary pathogen, much like TB
- *M. avium* infection not associated with acquired immunodeficiency syndrome is quite rare
- Treatment of *M. avium* involves a long-term regimen of multiple drug combinations, because this organism does not always respond to the drug regimens used to treat *M. tuberculosis*
- *Mycobacterium kansasii:* Pulmonary disease in compromised hosts (individuals infected with HIV)
- *Mycobacterium marinum:* Cutaneous disease from contact with contaminated water
- *Mycobacterium scrofulaceum:* Cervical adenitis in children (contaminated raw milk, soil, daily products)
- *Mycobacterium fortuitum, Mycobacterium chelonae, Mycobacterium abscessus:* Primarily skin and soft tissue disease in various hosts
- *Mycobacterium leprae:* Agent of leprosy

Other Nontuberculous Mycobacteria
- *Mycobacterium gordonae*
  - *Mycobacterium* spp. commonly found in tap water
  - Generally nonpathogenic
  - Can confuse the reading of AFB smears if care not taken in sample preparation

General Collection Guidelines and Diagnosis

- Sterile body site areas can be set up directly onto culture media
  - CSF, pleural fluid, deep tissue biopsies
- Nonsterile sites require special processing: Decontamination and digestion
  - Sputum, bronchial washings, bronchoalveolar lavage, skin biopsy
  - Likely to be overgrown with routine bacteria
  - AFB resists decontamination and digestion because of cell wall lipid content, whereas routine bacteria are destroyed
- AFB: Safety precautions
  - Avoid direct contact with organism
  - Aerosols present greatest hazard
  - Class 2 biosafety hood
    - Maintenance: Airflow checks
    - High-efficiency particulate absorption (HEPA) filters: Sterile air current
  - Sealed centrifuge buckets
  - Gown, gloves, masks, foot covers
  - Keep doors closed when specimens are open—slight negative air pressure created by hood
- Laboratory diagnosis of TB
  - AFB visible by Ziehl-Neelsen or fluorochrome smears of sputum or appropriate sample
  - Recovery by culture (the gold standard) either on conventional AFB media or that which uses radiometric detection (BACTEC)

- Prolonged incubation time required (up to 8 weeks)
- Biochemical characterization
- Nucleic acid assays (NAA)
  - Represent rapid diagnosis of TB
  - Sensitivity of the NAA is approximately 95% in patients with a positive AFB smear, but only 50% in smear negative cases (U.S. Food and Drug Administration data)
- Nontuberculous mycobacteria (atypicals, MOTT)
  - Classified into Runyon groups based on
    - Presence or absence of pigmentation
    - Pigment production: Light dependent or not
    - Growth rate: Slow or fast
  - Chromatography techniques allow species-level identification of mycobacteria based on their cellular fatty acid and/or mycolic acid profiles (reference laboratories)
  - Specific DNA molecular probes are available for species identification
  - BCG used outside the United States as an attenuated vaccine
- Nontuberculous mycobacteria (MOTT)
  - All other species not in the *M. tuberculosis* complex
  - Present everywhere, generally environmental
  - Usually not transmitted person to person
  - Pathogenicity varies and often depends on host immune status (opportunistic infection)
  - Runyon: Four groups based on growth rate, pigment production, and reaction of pigment to light
- *M. avium* complex (MAC)
  - Complex includes *M. avium* and *Mycoplasma intracellulare*
  - Most commonly isolated AFB among the MOTT
  - Ubiquitous in nature
  - Acquired by inhalation or ingestion
  - Patients with HIV are particularly at risk
  - Nonphotochromogens: No pigment
  - Smooth, cream-colored colonies
  - Greater drug resistance than *M. tuberculosis*
- Rapid growers
  - *M. fortuitum-chelonae* complex
  - Grow in 7 days or less on solid media
  - Can grow in routine media and stain as gram-positive cells with diphtheroid-like morphology
  - Acquired from environmental sources or nosocomially during surgery from contaminated objects or fluids
  - Enter by inoculation into the skin
  - Can also cause chronic pulmonary infections
- *M. leprae*
  - Cause of leprosy, which is also termed Hansen's disease
  - Chronic disease of the skin, mucous membranes, tissue
  - Rare in the United States, but cases exist in Texas and Louisiana
- Spread person to person through inhalation or contact with infected skin
  - Silent phase: Multiplication of bacilli
  - Intermediate phase: Peripheral nerves, sensory impairment
- Organism can be grown in the footpads of mice and nine-banded armadillos, not on artificial media
    - Diagnosis usually made by clinical findings and observation of AFB on direct smear of lesions

FAMILY ENTEROBACTERIACEAE
(BOXES 1-2 AND 1-3)

- Largest, most heterogeneous group of clinically important bacteria
- General characteristics
  - Most are normal flora of the GI tract
  - Gram-negative bacilli
  - Facultative anaerobes
  - Colony morphology is similar for most
    - Large, gray, spreading colonies
    - Only *Klebsiella* and *Enterobacter* are mucoid
  - All Enterobacteriaceae
    - Ferment glucose
    - Reduce nitrates to nitrites (rare exceptions)
    - Oxidase negative
    - Most are motile by peritrichous flagella
- Serologic classification
  - Cell-associated antigens
    - O: Somatic antigens (heat stable)
      - Polysaccharide of the LPS
      - Associated with endotoxin release
    - K: Capsular antigens (heat labile)
      - Capsular polysaccharide
      - Strains with K are more pathogenic
    - H: Flagellar antigens (heat labile)
      - Flagellar protein antigens
      - Responsible for motility
- Clinical disease
  - Based on the clinical infections produced
    - Opportunistic
      - Normal flora
      - Cause infections outside of natural habitat
    - Primary intestinal
      - *Salmonella*
      - *Shigella*
      - *Plesiomonas*
      - *Yersinia enterocolitica*
  - Opportunistic genera
    - *Citrobacter*
    - *Edwardsiella*
    - *Enterobacter*
    - *Escherichia*
    - *Hafnia*
    - *Klebsiella*
    - *Morganella*

BOX 1-2 | Tests Used in the Identification of Enteric Gram-Negative Bacilli

Routine Enterobacteriaceae

Memebers of the family Enterobacteriaceae are usually divided into lactose fermenters (+) and non-lactose fermenters (-)

Lactose +

E. coli—dark

Klebsiella—mucoid

Enterobacter—mucoid

Citrobacter—late

Serratia—late, red pigment

Lactose –

Proteus—swarming

Morganella

Providencia

Edwardsiella

Hafnia

Important Biochemical Tests

o-Nitrophenyl-p-D-galactopyranoside (ONPG)

Some lactose fermenters lack permease and so are "slow" or "late"

Non-lactose fermenters lack both

ONPG tests for β-galactosidase

The substrate is complexed to galactose

Cleavage causes a color change

Positve: E. coli

Negative: Salmonella enteritica

Decarboxylase tests

Detects decarboxylation of specific amino acids

Alkaline end products result

Ornithine decarboxylase (ODC)

Ornithine → Putrescine

Lysine decarboxylase (LDC)

Lysine → Cadaverine

Arginine dihydrolase (ADH)

Arginine → Citrulline

Decarboxylase tests

Medium starts purple

Fermentation shifts medium acid—indictor to yellow

Decarboxylation shifts the pH alkaline—indicator to **purple**

Mineral oil "traps" alkaline end products

Control tube lacks amino acid—yellow

Simmons Citrate

Ability of organism to use sodium citrate for metabolism and growth

Indicator—bromophenol blue

Only streak slant

Light inoculum

Blue—positive (rise in pH)

Green—negative (no change)

Positive: Klebsiella pneumoniae and Proteus mirabilis

Negative: Escherichia coli and Shigella dysenteriae

Urease Production

Ability of bacteria to hydrolyze urea to ammonia and CO_2

Ammonia release causes pH change

Positive—bright pink

Urease—method

Streak slant

Incubate 37° C

Light orange to red positive

Yellow/no change—negative

Positive: Proteus spp.

Negative: E. coli

Indole

Ability to metabolize tryptophan by testing for indole

Indole + aldehyde yields a red color

Indole—spot test

Saturate filter paper with reagent

Rub portion of colony onto paper

Rapid development of color is positive test

Positive: E. coli

Negative: E. cloacae

Methyl Red and Voges-Proskauer (MR/VP)

Glucose metabolism and metabolic products

Lactose is degraded into glucose and galactose

Glucose used through Embden–Meyerhof–Parnas (EMP pathway) to produce pyruvic acid

Pyruvic acid use produces many mixed acids

Enterics take two separate pathways

Mixed acid pathway and butylene glycol pathway

Two tests for end-products of these pathways

Methyl Red test and Voges-Proskauer

Escherichia coli is MR + and VP−

Enterobacter aerogenes and Klebsiella pneumoniae are MR− and VP+

Pseudomonas aeruginosa is MR− and VP−

Gelatinase

Used to determine the production of proteolytic enzyme that digests gelatin

Positive: Proteus vulgaris

Negative: Enterobacter aerogenes

Carbohydrate fermentation

Various media used to determine the ability of bacteria to ferment specific carbohydrates

The fermentation pattern can then be used as part of an identification scheme

Motility Test

Single stab of the organism into the gelatin tube

Incubate at 37° C for up to 7 days

Movement away from initial stab line is positive motility

Positive: E. coli

Negative: K. pneumoniae

Identification of Enterobacteriaceae

Identification is a process or flow

1. Growth on media

2. Gram stain

3. Lactose fermentation

4. Oxidase

5. Basic biochemical tests

Identification of Enterobacteriaceae

API 20E

The API-20E test kit is designed for the identification of enteric bacteria

Plastic strip holding twenty mini-test tubes is inoculated with saline suspension of a pure culture

Rehydrates the dessicated medium in each tube

Incubated 18-24 hours at 37° C

Continued

BOX 1-2	Tests Used in the Identification of Enteric Gram-Negative Bacilli—cont'd

The reactions are converted to a seven-digit code
The code is fed into the manufacturer's database
Identification usually as genus and species
Identification of gastrointestinal pathogens
   Screen stool cultures
   Normal flora in lower bowel $=10^7$/mL
   Anaerobes, diptheroids, enterococcus, streptococcus, enterics, yeasts
   Anaerobes/aerobes at 1000/1
   Determine which colonies deserve further attention
Initial Screening Steps
   Detect suspicious colonies amongst numerous normal flora organisms
   Lactose fermenter vs. non-lactose fermenter
   Growth on selective media
   H_2S producing colonies
   Non-sorbitol fermenters—E. coli O157
   Beta hemolytic enteric organisms
   Oxidase positive—suspected non-Enterobacteriaceae
Suspected Enterobacteriaceae
   Conventional identification
   Automated identification
   Screening tubes
   TSI and LIA
Triple Sugar Iron (TSI) or KIA
   Screening ID of enteric pathogens
   Identical except TSI sucrose, KIA does not
   Detects ability to produce gas and acid from fermentation and H_2S
   Both are used as slants:
   Slant—aerobic
   Butt—anaerobic
   0.1% glucose, 1% sucrose, 1% lactose, phenol red, ferrous sulfate
   Detects fermentation:
   If glucose is the only one fermented, the small amount of acid that is produced on the slant will be oxidized to a neutral product
   Slant remains alkaline (red)
   Butt—acid is not oxidized and turns yellow
   If lactose and sucrose are also fermented, there is so much acid that both the slant and butt become yellow
   TSI—5 Reactions

No fermentation
   Alkaline slant/Alkaline butt (K/K) or (K/NC)
   Non-enterics—able to degrade peptones
Only glucose fermentation
   Alkaline slant/Acid butt (K/A)—red/yellow
   Too much acid in butt to revert to alkaline
Lactose (sucrose) fermentation
   Acid slant/Acid butt (A/A)—all yellow
H_2S production—Black
Gas production—bubbles or split media
Lysine Iron Agar (LIA)
   Lysine, glucose, ferric ammonium citrate, sodium thiosulfate
   Primarily used to detect lysine use
   Good tool when used with TSI to screen stools for pathogens
Suspected non-Enterobacteriaceae
Vibrio
Aeromonas
Campylobacter
Tests for other enteric pathogens
Growth on specialized medium
Oxidase and catalase
Gram stain
Suspected Campylobacter
   Growth on specialized media at 42° C
   Atmosphere 5% O_2, 10% CO_2, 85% N_2
   Oxidase and catalase positive
   Curved gram-negative bacilli
   Sea gull shape
   Stains very lightly
   Hippurate hydrolysis positive
Suspected Vibrio and Aeromonas
   Beta hemolytic on Blood agar
   Comma-shaped gram-negative bacilli
   Non-lactose fermenter on MacConkey agar
   Thiosulfate citrate bile sucrose agar (TCBS)
   Yellow green colonies
   Oxidase and catalase positive
   API or commercial systems usually identify

From Tille PM: Bailey & Scott's diagnostic microbiology, ed 13, St Louis, 2014, Mosby.

- - - Proteus
  - Providencia
  - Serratia
- Clinical disease
  - Most cause opportunistic and nosocomial infections
    - UTI
    - Pneumonia
    - Wound infections
    - Catheter colonization
  - Isolated from almost all body sites
- Laboratory diagnosis
  - Oxidase negative
  - Colony morphology and Gram stain
  - Culture: Use supportive and selective media to recover pathogens
    - MacConkey agar
    - XLD
    - Hektoen

- Biochemical tests: Many
- Lactose fermentation and utilization of carbohydrates are key biochemical tests
  - All ferment glucose, so lactose is used for initial differentiation
- Rarely, laboratories use traditional tube tests
- More often use spot tests or limited workup on some specimen types
- Commercially available in kits
  - API test strips
  - Most large laboratories use automated identification systems
    - Vitek (bioMerieux)
    - MicroScan (Dade)
    - Phoenix (BD Bioscience)
- Enteric pathogens
  - Food-borne
    - Salmonella

BOX 1-3 | Biochemical Differentiation of Representative Enterobacteriacae

	Escherichia coli	Ewingella americana	H. alvei	Plesiomonas shigelloides *oxidase +	Shigella sonnei	Other Shigella	S. enteritidis	S. typhi	Edwardsiella tarda	C. freundii	C. braakii	C. koseri (formerly diversus)	K. pneumoniae	K. oxytoxa	E. cloacae	E. aerogenes	Cronobacter sakazakii	Pantoea agglomerans (was Enterobacter)	S. marcescens	S. odorifera biotype 2	P. vulgaris	P. mirabilis	Morganella morganii	P. rettgeri	P. stuartii	Yersinia enterocolitica
Indole	+	−	−	+	−	V	−	−	+	−	−(v)	+	−	+	−	−	−	−(v)	−	V	+	−	+	+	+	V
Methyl red	+	+	−(v)	V	+	+	+	+	+	+	+	+	V	−(v)	−	−	−	V	V	+(v)	+	+	+	+	+	+
Voges Proskauer	−	+	+(v)	−	−	−	−	−	−	−	−	−	+	+	+	+	+	+(v)	+	+	−	V	−	−	−	−
Simmons' citrate	−	+	+	−	−	−	+	−	−	+	+(v)	+	+	+	+	+	+	V	+	+	−(v)	+(v)	−	+	+	−
Hydrogen Sulfide (TSI)	−	−	−	−	−	−	+(v)	+w	+	+	+(v)	−	−	−	−	−	−	−	−	−	+	+	−	−	−	−
Urea	−	−	−	−	−	−	−	−	−	−(v)	−(v)	+(v)	+	+	+(v)	−	−	−(v)	−(v)	−	+	+	+	+	−(v)	+
Motility	V	+(v)	+	+	−	−	+	+	+	+	+	+	−	−	+	+	+	+	+	+	+	+	V	+	+(v)	−
Lysine decarboxylase	+(v)	−	+	+	−	−	+	+	+	−	−	−	+	+	−	+	−	−	+	+	−	−	−	−	−	−
Arginine dihydrolase	−(v)	−	−	+	−	V	+(v)	−	−	+(v)	+	+	−	−	+	−	+	−	−	−	−	−	−	−	−	−
Ornithine decarboxylase	+(v)	−	+	+	+	−	+	−	+	−	+	+	−	−	+	+	+	−	+	−	−	+	+	−	−	+
Phenylalinine deaminase	−	−	−	−	−	−	−	−	−	−	−	−	−	−	−	−	−	+(v)	−(v)	−	+	+	+	+	+	−
Gas from D–glucose	+	−	+	−	−	−	+	−	+	+	+	+	+	+	+	+	+	−(v)	−	−	+	+	+	−	−	−
Lactose	+	+(v)	−	V	−	−	−	−	−	+(v)	+	V	+	+	+	+	+	−(v)	−	+	−	−	−	−	−	−
Sucrose	V	−	−	−	−	−	−	−	−	+(v)	−	−(v)	+	+	+	+	+	+(v)	+	+	+	−	−	−	V	−
D–Mannitol	+	+	+	−	+	+	+	+	−	+	+	+	+	+	+	+	+	+	+	+	−	−	−	+	−(v)	+
Adonitol	−	−	−	−	−	−	−	−	−	−	−	+	+	+	−(v)	+	−	−	−(v)	+(v)	−	−	−	+	−	−
Inositol	−	−	−	+	−	−	−	−	−	−	−	−	+	+	−(v)	+	−	−(v)	V	+	−	−	−	+	+	−
D–Sorbitol	+(v)	−	−	−	−	V	+	+	−	+	+	+	+	+	+	+	−	−(v)	+	+	−	−	−	−	−	+
L–Arabinose	+	−	+	−	+	V	+	−	−	+	+	+	+	+	+	+	+	+	−	+	−	−	−	−	−	+
Raffinose	V	−	−	−	−	V	−	−	−	−(v)	−	−	+	+	+	+	+	−(v)	−	+	−	−	−	−	−	−
L–Rhamnose	−	−(v)	+	−	+(v)	−(v)	+	−	−	+	+	+	+	+	+	+	+	+	−	+	−	−	−	+(v)	−	−
KCN, growth in	−	−	+	−	−	−	−	−	−	+	+	−	+	+	+	+	+	−(v)	+	−	+	+	+	+	+	−
Gelatin (22°C)	−	−	−	−	−	−	−	−	−	−	−	−	−	−	−	−	−	−	−(v)	+	+	+	+	−	−	−
DNase	−	−	−	−	−	−	−	−	−	−	−	−	−	−	−	−	−	−	+	−	−	−	−	−	−	−

From Tille PM: Bailey & Scott's diagnostic microbiology, ed 13, St Louis, 2014, Mosby.

- o E. coli
- o Campylobacter
- o Yersinia
- Human to human
  - o Shigella
  - o Salmonella typhi
  - o Helicobacter pylori
- Water-borne
  - o Vibrio
  - o Aeromonas
  - o Plesiomonas
- Enterobacteriaceae pathogens
  - Salmonella
  - Shigella
  - E. coli
  - Yersinia
  - Plesiomonas
- Serotyping
  - Antigens: Heat stable
    - o A, B, C, etc.
    - o 98% of human isolates are A through G
  - H antigens: Heat sensitive
    - o 1, 2, 3, etc.
  - Vi (K) antigens: Virulence antigens
    - o Heat sensitive
    - o May mask O antigens
    - o Boil to remove Vi, retype

- Epidemiology
  - Naturally occur in poultry products and reptiles
  - Food-borne infections account for 1.3 billion cases of acute diarrhea with 3 million deaths worldwide
  - Ingestion of contaminated food, water, or milk
  - 40,000 cases annually in the United States
  - Centers for Disease Control and Prevention (CDC) and reports: In recent years a notable increase in cases related to a multidrug-resistant *Salmonella typhimurium*
    - o Case-fatality and hospitalization rates for this strain are twice that of other *Salmonella* spp.
- Clinical disease: Gastroenteritis
  - Most common type of illness
  - Diarrhea, low fever, nausea
  - Symptoms last 1 to 3 days
  - Positive stool cultures
  - No systemic involvement
- Clinical disease: Bacteremia/septicemia
  - Nontyphoidal bacteremia
  - *Salmonella choleraesuis*
  - High spiking fever
  - Positive blood cultures
  - Few GI symptoms
  - Particularly invasive
- Clinical disease: Enteric fever
  - *S. typhi*: Typhoid fever

- ○ Most serious
- ○ Fever and GI involvement
- ○ Positive blood cultures during first week
- ○ Positive stool cultures during second week
  - • Carrier state
    - ○ Carry bacteria asymptomatically after infection
    - ○ Can shed organism unknowingly
    - ○ Typhoid Mary
- • Pathogenesis
  - • Ingested in food
  - • Survive passage through the gastric acid
  - • Invade the mucosa of the small and large intestine
    - ○ Produce toxins
  - • Invasion of epithelial cells stimulates release of cytokines, which induce an inflammatory reaction
  - • Inflammatory response causes diarrhea
    - ○ May lead to ulceration and destruction of the mucosa
  - • May disseminate from intestines to systemic disease
- • Laboratory diagnosis
  - • Lactose negative
  - • H_2S positive: Black colonies
  - • Triple Sugar Iron Agar (TSI): Alkaline/acid, H_2S, gas
    - ○ Butt is acid as a result of glucose fermentation
  - • Methyl red, citrate, lysine decarboxylase, ornithine decarboxylase, arginine dihydrolase positive
  - • Must confirm with serotyping
  - • Reportable organism

Shigella Species

- • Serotyping (O antigen)
  - • A: *Shigella dysenteriae* (12 serotypes)
  - • B: *Shigella flexneri* (6 serotypes)
  - • C: *Shigella boydii* (23 serotypes)
  - • D: *Shigella sonnei* (1 serotype)
  - • Groups A to C are physiologically similar; *S. sonnei* can be differentiated biochemically
- • Epidemiology
  - • Human to human (fecal-oral route)
    - ○ Very communicable
    - ○ Food—inoculated by humans
  - • *S. sonnei*: Most common in the United States
  - • *S. dysenteriae*: Least recovered in the United States
    - ○ Most severe
    - ○ Third World countries
- • Clinical disease
  - • Acute infection with onset of symptoms within 24 to 48 hours of ingestion
  - • Average duration of symptoms in untreated adults is 7 days
    - ○ Organism may be cultivated from stools for 30 days or longer
  - • Two basic clinical presentations
    - ○ Watery diarrhea associated with vomiting and mild-to-moderate dehydration

- ○ Dysentery characterized by a small volume of bloody, mucoid stools, and abdominal pain
- • Pathogenesis
  - • Resist gastric acidity
  - • Requires very few organisms to infect
    - ○ 10 to 200 organisms
    - ○ Organism resistant to acid
  - • Cytotoxin (Shiga toxin) causes inflammation and ulcerative lesions
    - ○ Destroys epithelial cell
    - ○ Bloody, mucus-laden stools
- • Laboratory diagnosis
  - • Lactose negative
  - • TSI: Alkaline/acid, no gas, no H_2S
  - • Urease negative
  - • Confirm with serotyping
  - • Report to health department

Escherichia coli

- • May cause several types of diarrheal illnesses
- • Enterohemorrhagic *E. coli* is most important
  - • *E. coli* O157:H7
  - • Hemorrhagic colitis: Pediatric
  - • Can lead to hemolytic uremic syndrome: Build-up of toxin in kidneys
  - • Bloody diarrhea with no PMNs
  - • Fever absent
  - • Water-borne or food-borne: Often transmitted via ground beef
- • Laboratory diagnosis
  - • All *E. coli*
    - ○ Ferment glucose, lactose, and xylose
    - ○ Indole and Methyl Red positive
    - ○ No H_2S or urease
    - ○ Citrate negative
    - ○ Motile or nonmotile strains
  - • *E. coli* O157:H7
    - ○ MacConkey with sorbitol (SMAC)
      - ▪ Does not ferment sorbitol (i.e., clear colonies)
    - ○ Typical *E. coli* reactions
      - ▪ Indole
      - ▪ Confirm identification with routine system
    - ○ Confirm with serotyping: O or H
    - ○ Reportable organism

Yersinia Species

- • Clinically significant species
  - ○ *Yersinia pestis*: Plague
  - ○ *Yersinia enterocolitica*
  - • Epidemiology: *Y. enterocolitica*
    - ○ Food-borne and water-borne illness
    - ○ Blood transfusions
- • *Y. enterocolitica*
  - • Clinical disease

- Gastroenteritis: May resemble appendicitis
- Seasonal and ethnic, chitterlings (small intestines of pig or other animals)
- Laboratory diagnosis
  - Grows better at 25° to 30° C
  - Small, lactose-negative colonies on MacConkey agar
  - Cefsulodin-irgasan-novobiocin (CIN) agar may be used: produce pink colonies with red center
  - TSI: Acid/acid, no gas
  - Routine identification system

Plesiomonas shigelloides

- Epidemiology
  - Water-borne gastroenteritis: Freshwater
  - Mostly in tropics
  - Clinical disease
    - Usually mild watery diarrhea
    - Human trial unsuccessful in setting up disease
- Laboratory diagnosis
  - Routine culture conditions
  - Gram-negative bacilli
  - Growth on blood agar: No hemolysis
  - Non–lactose fermenter on MacConkey agar
  - Positive oxidase and indole most important initial screening tests
    - Routine identification system

MISCELLANEOUS ENTERIC PATHOGENS

- *Campylobacter*
- *Vibrio*
- *Aeromonas*
- *Helicobacter pylori*

Family Campylobacteraceae

- *Campylobacter*
  - At least 18 species and subspecies in *Campylobacter*
- *Arcobacter*
  - Four species in *Arcobacter*

Campylobacter Species

- Curved or S-shaped
- 0.5 to 5.0 μm long × 0.5 to 1.0 μm wide
- Gram-negative, non–spore forming rods
- Motile
  - Single, polar flagellum
- Generally microaerophilic

Arcobacter Species

- Curved or S shaped
- 0.2 to 0.9 μm wide, 1 to 3 μm long
- Gram-negative, non–spore forming bacilli
- Motile
  - Single, polar flagellum
  - Grow at 15° to 30° C

- Variable from 35° to 42° C
- Generally aerobic

Campylobacter jejuni

- Epidemiology
  - *C. jejuni* most common
  - Food-borne gastroenteritis
    - Poultry and raw milk
    - Water
  - One of most common causes of human bacterial gastroenteritis in numerous parts of the United States
- Clinical disease
  - Diarrhea, cramps, abdominal pain, fever within 2 to 5 days of exposure
  - Bloody stool with high WBC count
  - Lasts for 7 to 10 days
  - Can be fatal
- Pathogenesis and virulence
  - Susceptibility of host and strain virulence key
  - Ingestion of contaminated food or water
  - Penetrate the GI tract mucous lining
    - Motility and shape
  - Adhere to the gut enterocytes and release toxins
    - Enterotoxin and cytotoxins
- Laboratory diagnosis
  - Special atmosphere and temperature
    - 42° C
    - 5% O_2, 10% CO_2, 85% N_2
  - Campy blood agar
    - *Brucella* agar base with antibiotics
    - Other selective media: Cefoperazone Vancomycin Amphotericin (CVA), Skirrow Medium
  - Curved gram-negative bacilli
    - Sea gull shape
  - Stains very lightly
  - Nonhemolytic, flat, gray, mucoid
  - Oxidase and catalase positive
  - Darting motility on wet preparation
  - Hippurate hydrolysis positive
  - Usually identified as *Campylobacter* spp.

FAMILY VIBRIONACEAE

- 10 genera, including *Vibrio*

Vibrio

- 76 species currently recognized
  - *Photobacterium damselae* previously classified as *Vibrio* and shares ecology
- Oxidase-positive, facultative anaerobic, non–spore forming, gram-negative bacilli
- Comma-shaped cells
- Typically found in saltwater
- All members of genus are motile by single, polar flagellum

Vibrio cholerae

- Epidemiology
  - Water-borne illness
  - Found in plankton of fresh, brackish, and salt water
  - Attached primarily to copepods in the zooplankton
  - Coastal outbreaks usually follow zooplankton blooms
- Pathogenesis and virulence
  - Colonizes the GI tract
  - Attaches to villi by pili
  - Secretes a two-part toxin, cholera toxin
  - Toxin causes increased cyclic adenosine monophosphate (cAMP) synthesis
  - Massive fluid efflux: Diarrhea
- Clinical disease
  - Cholera
    - Massive fluid loss: Death within 24 hours
    - "Rice water stools": WBCs and blood absent
  - Treatment
    - Replace fluids, antibiotics
- Laboratory diagnosis
  - Comma-shaped gram-negative bacilli
  - Non–lactose fermenter on MacConkey agar
  - Thiosulfate citrate bile sucrose agar (TCBS)
    - Yellow-green colonies
  - Oxidase and catalase positive
  - String test positive

Halophilic Vibrio Organisms

- Require 1% to 2% NaCl for growth
- Cause gastroenteritis, wound infections, septicemia
- *Vibrio parahaemolyticus:* Gastroenteritis from seafood
- *Vibrio vulnificus:* Septicemia from raw shellfish (lactose fermenter)
- *Vibrio alginolyticus:* Wound and ear infections

FAMILY AEROMONADACEAE

- Diseases mainly in fish and amphibians
  - Frogs
    - Red leg
    - Fatal internal hemorrhaging
  - Fish
    - Develop ulcers, tail rot, fin rot, and hemorrhagic septicemia

Aeromonas hydrophila

- Epidemiology and clinical disease
  - Organism ubiquitous in fresh and brackish water
  - Water-borne illnesses
    - Gastroenteritis
    - Wound infections
  - Exposure to water, fish hook injuries
    - Bacteremia
      - Most often in young or old

- Pathogenesis and virulence factors
  - Produces aerolysin
    - Cytotoxic enterotoxin
    - Causes tissue damage in fish and amphibians
  - Unclear pathogenesis in humans
- Laboratory diagnosis
  - Routine culture conditions
    - Grows on MacConkey and blood agar
    - Usually β-hemolytic
  - Gram-negative bacilli (straight)
  - Lactose fermenter
  - Positive oxidase and indole good screening tests
  - API or routine identification system

FAMILY HELICOBACTERACEAE

- *Helicobacter, Sulfuricurvum, Sulfurimonas, Sulfurovum, Thiovulum, Wolinella*

Helicobacter

- 29 species of *Helicobacter* recognized
  - Exact mode of transmission is unknown
  - Higher rate in undeveloped countries
- Clinical disease
  - One of the most transmitted human infections
    - Gastroenteritis
    - Peptic ulcers
    - Associated with gastric cancer
- Pathogenesis and virulence factors
  - Burrows into gastric mucosa
  - Urease
    - Converts urea to ammonia and bicarbonate
    - Ammonia neutralizes stomach acid
    - Ammonia is toxic to the epithelial cells
  - Protease, catalase, and phospholipases
  - Damage to epithelial cells
    - Elicits powerful immune response (ulcer)
    - Tissue biopsy is an important specimen in some settings
- Laboratory diagnosis
  - Curved gram-negative bacilli
  - Growth on blood agar in 3 to 5 days
  - 35° C with high humidity
  - Microaerophilic: 5% O_2, 10% CO_2, 85% N_2
  - Positive: Oxidase, catalase, urease
  - Not usually grown
    - Urease test on biopsy
    - Direct stain
    - Stool antigen test

FAMILY NEISSERIACEAE

- More than 20 genera
- General characteristics
  - Aerobic gram-negative diplococci

- Oxidase and catalase positive
  - *Neisseria elongate:* Catalase negative, rod shaped
- Human reservoir
  - Respiratory and urogenital tract
  - Sexual transmission *(Neisseria gonorrhoeae)*
- *N. gonorrhoeae* and *Neisseria meningitidis* are the primary pathogens

Pathogenic *Neisseria* Species

Neisseria gonorrhoeae
- Epidemiology
  - Sexually transmitted by carrier
  - Causes gonorrhea
- Clinical disease
  - Males: Acute urethritis with dysuria and urethral discharge
    - Not commonly asymptomatic
  - Females: Colonizes endocervix causing
    - Vaginal discharge
    - Dysuria
    - Abdominal pain
    - Untreated may lead to pelvic inflammatory disease (PID)
  - Other sites of infection include
    - Eyes
    - Throat
    - Rectum
  - Can disseminate if untreated
    - Less than 1% of infections
    - Purulent arthritis and septicemia
- Laboratory diagnosis: Culture
  - Rapid transport critical for recovery
    - Direct plating to selective media at the bedside
    - Use of transport systems for *Neisseria gonorrhoeae*
  - Selective media to inhibit other bacteria and yeast
    - Modified Thayer-Martin (MTM) or other selective medium
    - Chocolate agar: Allows growth of other saprophytes
  - Incubation:
    - 3% to 7% CO_2 incubator at 35° to 37° C
    - Humidity is important
- Laboratory diagnosis: Identification
  - Gram-negative diplococci (some may appear as tetrads)
  - Small gray, translucent, raised colonies
  - Grows on chocolate, but usually not on blood agar
  - Catalase and oxidase positive
    - Cysteine trypticase agar (CTA) sugar oxidation: glucose positive

Neisseria meningitidis
- Epidemiology
  - Human reservoir
    - Upper respiratory tract of 3% to 30% of asymptomatic individuals
  - Respiratory transmission
  - Mainly affects adolescents in overcrowded environments
    - College dormitories and the military
  - Vaccine an important control measure
- Clinical disease
  - First or second leading cause of community-acquired meningitis in the United States
  - Also causes sepsis, conjunctivitis, disseminated organ infections, pneumonia without meningitis
  - Many strains of *N. meningitidis;* clinically the most important are A, B, C, Y, and W135
- Laboratory diagnosis: Specimen collection and processing
  - CSF
    - An amount greater than 1 mL of CSF is hand carried to the laboratory
    - Specimen should not be refrigerated
    - CSF specimen may be centrifuged
    - Gram stain is prepared from the sediment
    - Sediment is inoculated to chocolate and blood agar
  - Blood
    - Conventional blood culture systems
  - Skin scraping
    - Petechiae may yield viable or stainable organisms
    - Cut open lesion and collect fluid on swab
- Laboratory diagnosis: Identification
  - Gram-negative diplococci found intracellularly and extracellularly
  - Grow well on sheep blood and chocolate agar
  - Grow on Thayer Martin selective agar
  - Catalase and oxidase positive
  - Cysteine trypticase agar (CTA) sugar oxidation: glucose and maltose positive

Other (Nonpathogenic) *Neisseria* Species

- *Neisseria lactamica*
- *Neisseria flavescens*
- *Neisseria sicca*
- Clinical significance
  - Normal flora of human upper respiratory tract
  - Cause occasional infections
  - Occasionally isolated from blood, genital tract, and CSF
  - Identification not appropriate unless isolated from systemic site or pure culture

FAMILY ALCALIGENACEAE
- General characteristics
  - Small (0.2-0.7 μm) coccobacilli
  - Fastidious, obligate aerobes that require nicotinic acid
  - *Bordetella pertussis* and *Bordetella parapertussis* are nonmotile, *Bordetella bronchiseptica* is motile

- Human respiratory tract is the only source of *B. pertussis* and *B. parapertussis*
- Others infect birds and other mammals

Bordetella pertussis

- Epidemiology
  - Worldwide 60 million cases with 500,000 deaths
  - Endemic in most populations
    - Cycle often—3 to 4 years
  - Majority of cases in the United States occur in August to November
  - No evidence of long-term carriage
    - Immunity from vaccine or infection is not lifelong
    - Protection wanes after 3 to 5 years
    - Immunity is undetectable by 12 years
  - Subclinical infections in adults may be common
  - Adults usually the index cases in infants
  - Vaccine for adolescents recently approved
- Clinical disease
  - Typical upper respiratory tract infection for 1 week
  - Paroxysmal cough (out, out, out, whoop)
    - Not always present
  - Long recovery
- Laboratory diagnosis
  - Direct fluorescent antibody (DFA) on nasal specimen
  - Culture of nasal specimen
  - Polymerase chain reaction
  - Serologic tests
    - Not generally available
    - Not helpful during acute phase
    - Difficult to interpret

FAMILY PASTEURELLACEAE

Pasteurella multocida

- Reported in 1878 in fowl cholera–infected birds
- 1880: Louis Pasteur
- Most common species of *Pasteurella* isolated from humans
- Grows on blood and chocolate
  - No growth on MacConkey agar
- Oxidase and catalase positive
- Indole positive
- Epidemiology
  - Oral cavity of cats and dogs
  - Causative agents of several economically significant veterinary diseases
    - Cattle, buffaloes, sheep, goats, poultry, turkeys, rabbits, horses, and camels
    - Serious infectious diseases such as fowl cholera, bovine hemorrhagic septicemia, and porcine atrophic rhinitis

- Clinical disease
  - Most human infections are wound infections/cellulitis after cat bites
    - Pain, swelling, and serosanguinous drainage at the wound site
  - Septic arthritis and osteomyelitis may occur after deep puncture wounds
  - Serious infections may occur in compromised hosts
  - Respiratory tract infections
  - Bacteremia, endocarditis
  - Central nervous system (CNS) infection
  - Eye infections after cat and dog scratches
- Laboratory diagnosis
  - Clinical history important
  - Specimens
    - Pus, wound swab, tissue, sputum, blood
  - Growth requirements
    - Growth on blood and chocolate agar
    - No growth on MacConkey agar
    - Incubate for 24 hours in CO_2, at 35° C
  - Small, short, gram-negative bacilli
  - Colonies
    - Gray-green, convex, nonhemolytic, odor
  - Biochemicals
    - Oxidase and catalase positive
    - Indole positive
    - Urease negative
    - Commercial systems usually appropriate for *P. multocida*

Other *Pasteurella* Species

- *Pasteurella canis*
- *Pasteurella dagmatis*
  - Found in mouths of canines
- *Pasteurella caballi*
- Infections associated with dog bites
  - Upper respiratory tract of horses
  - Horse bite wounds

Haemophilus Species

- Genus includes
  - *Haemophilus influenzae*
  - *Haemophilus aegyptius*
  - *Haemophilus haemolyticus*
  - *Haemophilus parainfluenzae*
  - *Haemophilus ducreyi*
- New genus *Aggregatibacter*
  - *Haemophilus segnis*, *Haemophilus aphrophilus*, and *Actinobacillus actinomycetemcomitans*
- Most members are nonpathogenic or opportunistic pathogens
- Three major pathogenic species
  - *H. influenzae*

- *H. aegyptius*
- *H. ducreyi*
- *Haemophilus:* Derived from Greek for "blood lover"
- Require growth factors present in blood
  - X Factor: Hemin, hematin
  - V Factor: Nicotinamide adenine dinucleotide (NADH) NADH
  - XV Factor strip test
- Both are found in chocolate agar
- Gram-negative pleomorphic coccobacilli or bacilli
- Nonmotile
- Aerobic or facultative anaerobic
- Oxidase and catalase positive
- Obligate parasite of mucous membranes of humans and mammals

Haemophilus influenzae

- Often found as part of normal upper respiratory tract flora in humans
- Spread by droplets and close contact
- Clinical disease
  - Especially in children
    - Meningitis
    - Septicemia
    - Epiglottitis
    - Pneumonia
    - Otitis
  - Vaccine: Single biggest impact on pediatrics in last 20 years
- Pathogenesis and virulence
  - Polysaccharide capsule
    - Seven serogroups: a to f and e′
    - Capsule type b (Hib) is the most clinically significant and virulent
    - Immunoglobulin A (IgA) proteases
  - Outer membrane proteins
  - Adherence factors
- Laboratory diagnosis
  - Grows on chocolate agar
    - Requires factors X and V
  - Requires 3% to 5% CO_2
  - Satellites around *S. aureus* on SBA
  - Small translucent colonies
  - Gram-negative coccobacilli

Haemophilus aegyptius

- Conjunctivitis: "Pink eye"
- Brazilian purpuric fever
  - Recurrent conjunctivitis
  - High fever
  - Vomiting
  - Septicemia
  - Shock
  - Mortality as high as 70%
- Laboratory diagnosis
  - Requires factors X and V
  - Grows on chocolate in 3% to 5% CO_2
  - Biochemical differentiation required

Haemophilus ducreyi

- Not normal flora: Sexually transmitted disease (STD)
- Genital tract pathogen
- Genital chancres, ulcers
- Epidemiology
  - Chancroid is rare in the United States
    - Localized endemic outbreaks occur in isolated STD and prostitution populations
  - Annual global incidence approximately 6 million per year
  - Chancroid more common in areas of low socioeconomic status such as Africa, Asia, and the Caribbean
  - More common in areas where the prevalence of HIV is high
- Laboratory diagnosis
  - 3% to 5% CO_2
  - High humidity
  - Must be plated immediately
  - Blood agar with X factor
    - Does not need V factor
    - Chocolate agar
    - Fastidious, will not satellite on blood agar
  - 2 to 10 days needed for growth
  - Gram-negative coccobacillus: "School of fish" pattern
  - Gray, yellow, or tan colonies
    - Nonmucoid
  - Catalase negative, oxidase positive
  - Nucleic amplification is definitive test

Miscellaneous *Haemophilus* Species

- Examples: *H. parainfluenzae, H. haemolyticus*
- Normal flora in humans that occasionally cause upper and lower respiratory tract infections
- May lead to systemic infections resulting from invasion of blood and tissue

Related Organisms

Aggregatibacter aphrophilus

- Includes both species formally known as factor V–independent (*H. aphrophilus*) and factor V–dependent (*H. paraphrophilus*) strains

Aggregatibacter segnis

- Formerly *H. segnis*

Eikenella corrodens

- General characteristics
  - All oxidase-positive, fastidious gram-negative bacilli
  - Part of mouth flora in 40% to 70% of humans
- Clinical disease
  - Frequently in infections from human bites
  - May be mixed infections
- Laboratory diagnosis

- Gram-negative coccobacilli
- Requires increased CO_2 for growth (3%-10%)
- Oxidase positive
- Catalase, urease, indole negative
- Usually pit the agar during growth

Kingella **Species**

- General characteristics
  - Four species in genus
  - Epidemiology
    - Flora of the pharynx in young children
    - Transmitted from child to child
- Clinical disease
  - Osteomyelitis
  - Bacteremia
  - Endocarditis
  - Joint infections
- Laboratory diagnosis
  - Fastidious short gram-negative coccobacillus
  - Joint fluid into blood culture bottles
  - Identification with Remel Rapid NH

FAMILY LEGIONELLACEAE

Legionella pneumophila

- *L. pneumophila* is the primary pathogen
  - 14 serotypes
  - 01 most common
- General characteristics
  - Non–acid-fast, nonsporulating, and noncapsulated bacilli
  - Aerobic fastidious gram-negative bacilli; difficult to stain
  - Nonfermentative
  - Oxidase and catalase positive
  - Produces β-lactamase
- Epidemiology
  - Ubiquitous, natural sources
    - Lakes, ponds, rivers
  - Human-made sources
    - Cooling towers, air-conditioning units, hot tubs/spas, plumbing fixtures
  - Illness acquired from breathing in organism; no human-to-human transfer
- Clinical disease
  - Described in 1976
  - Epidemic of American Legion members
  - Two diseases
    - Legionnaire's disease
      - Pneumonia: Fever, chills, cough, myalgia, headache, chest pain, sputum
      - Can have a high mortality rate (30%) if not treated
      - Symptoms depend on person—asymptomatic to life-threatening
    - Pontiac fever
      - Milder form of disease, more like influenza, no pneumonia, 0% mortality

- Can cause epidemics and isolated cases
- Occurs sporadically (community-acquired) or as an epidemic
- Predisposing factors—both forms
  - Immunocompromised
  - Increased age
  - Heavy smoking
  - Exposure to high concentration of organisms
    - Showers
    - Air-conditioner cooling towers
- Pathogenesis and virulence factors
  - Intracellular pathogen
  - Survive and multiply within macrophages
- Laboratory diagnosis
  - Specimens
    - Respiratory specimens are preferred
    - Urine for antigen testing
  - Growth requirements
    - Cysteine and iron
    - Buffered charcoal yeast extract (BCYE) media
    - 35° C, CO_2
    - Slow grower—hold for 2 weeks
  - Identification confirmation
    - Serology testing
    - DNA probes
    - Reference laboratory

FAMILY BRUCELLACEAE

Brucella

- Zoonotic disease with worldwide distribution
  - Acquired from animals or animal sources; most likely to contract are farmers, butchers, veterinarians, laboratory workers
- Epidemiology
  - Ingestion of contaminated dairy
- Clinical disease
  - Undulant fever, Mediterranean fever, Malta fever
  - Lymph nodes, blood, and reticuloendothelial system affected
  - Fever, chills, headache, hepatosplenomegaly
- Laboratory diagnosis
  - Safety: BSL III cabinet
  - Specimens
    - Blood, bone marrow, tissue
    - Transport blood and bone marrow in Isolator tube
    - Inoculate solid media and blood culture bottles
    - Tape plates
  - Will grow on blood and chocolate agar
  - MacConkey negative
  - Requires extended incubation for 7 to 10 days
  - Automated blood culture systems will detect in 2 weeks
  - Small gram-negative coccobacilli
  - Colonies
    - Small, translucent, moist, nonhemolytic

- All are oxidase and catalase positive
- Urea and H_2S results vary by species
- *Do not* put suspected *Brucella* in an automated system for identification
- Additional tests
  - Serology
  - Polymerase chain reaction (PCR)

FAMILY FRANCISELLACEAE

Francisella tularensis

- Epidemiology
  - Transmission: Handling animals or carcasses
  - Contaminated food or water
  - Highly contagious and invasive
- Clinical disease
  - Tularemia
  - Multiple forms of the disease
- Laboratory diagnosis
  - Specimens
    - Safety: BSL III cabinet
    - Ulcer swabs
    - Lymph node biopsy
    - Sputum
    - Bone marrow
    - Rarely isolated from blood
  - Growth requirements
    - Cysteine and iron
    - Grows on chocolate agar
    - Increased CO_2, 35° C
    - Slow growth: 2 to 5 days
  - Faint staining, gram-negative coccobacilli
  - Small, greenish, droplike colonies
  - Biochemically inert
    - Catalase positive
  - Serologic tests
  - Molecular tests

FAMILY PSEUDOMONADACEAE

- More than 150 species listed
- Based on genetic analysis (16S rRNA sequence) *Chryseomonas* and *Flavimonas* are *Pseudomonas* spp.
  - *Flavimonas oryzihabitans*
  - *Chryseomonas luteola, Chryseomonas polytricha*
- Genus previously included most glucose nonfermenting gram-negative bacilli
- *Pseudomonas*
- *Pseudo*: Greek for "false"
- *Monas*: Greek for "a single unit"
- Used early in the history of microbiology to refer to all germs
  - *Aeruginosa*: Latin for oxidized copper
- Compares to *P. aeruginosa* pigments in the laboratory
  - Most common isolates in the clinical laboratory
    - *P. aeruginosa*
    - *Pseudomonas putida*

- *Pseudomonas fluorescens*
- *Pseudomonas stutzeri*
- *Pseudomonas alcaligenes*
- General characteristics
  - Oxidase positive
  - Aerobic gram-negative bacilli
  - Water and soil—ubiquitous in environment
  - Uses numerous substrates as energy
  - Identification and differentiating beyond *P. aeruginosa* and common species can be time consuming

Pseudomonas aeruginosa

- Clinical disease
  - Wide range of diseases
  - Septicemia
  - UTI
  - Pneumonia
  - Chronic lung infections
    - Cystic fibrosis
  - Skin and soft tissue infections
- Chronic lung infections: Cystic fibrosis
  - Pulmonary infections a major cause of death
  - Repeat episodes of airway disease
  - Chronic colonization/infections
  - Exacerbations
  - Chronic therapy
- Skin and soft tissue infections
  - Intact skin is not a good medium for *Pseudomonas*
  - Water is usually associated with infections
  - Immunocompromised patients are at risk for infections
  - *Pseudomonas* folliculitis
- Laboratory diagnosis
  - Presumptive identification
    - Large colonies
    - Grapelike odor
    - Oxidase positive
    - Pyocyanin
  - For further confirmation
    - Growth at 42° C
    - Glucose oxidation
    - Pyoverdin (fluorescein)

Other Pseudomonas Species

- *P. fluorescens*
- *P. putida*
- *P. stutzeri*
- *Pseudomonas oryzihabitans*
  - Water and soil: Ubiquitous in environment
  - Uses numerous substrates as energy
  - Identification and differentiating beyond *P. aeruginosa* difficult
    - Molecular methods replacing traditional biochemical testing
  - Inherently more resistant to antimicrobial agents than common gram-negative bacilli

FAMILY MORAXELLACEAE

Moraxella Species

- 19 species in the genus
- Only a few important in human medicine
  - *M. catarrhalis*
  - *M. bovis*
  - *M. osloensis*
- Nonmotile, gram-negative coccobacilli

Moraxella catarrhalis

- Commensals of the upper respiratory tract
  - Isolated only from humans
  - Not associated with disease in healthy people
- Clinical disease
  - Causes mostly opportunistic infections
  - Can be isolated from patients with
    - Ear infections
    - Bronchitis
    - Sinusitis
    - Pneumonia
    - Predisposing pulmonary conditions (e.g., chronic obstructive pulmonary disease)
- Laboratory diagnosis
  - Grow on simple nutrient agar
    - Blood agar at 35° C
    - Chocolate agar
    - No growth on Thayer-Martin
      - Differentiates it from *N. gonorrhoeae* because of colistin
  - Opaque, gray, smooth and dry colonies
  - Gram-negative coccobacilli
  - Oxidase positive
  - CTA sugar oxidation
    - Glucose: Negative
    - Maltose: Negative
    - Lactose: Negative
    - Sucrose: Negative

Other *Moraxella* Species

- Normal flora and uncommon pathogens of human and other mammals' upper respiratory tract
- Speciation is beyond the scope of a routine laboratory
- Most susceptible to penicillins, cephalosporins, tetracyclines, and aminoglycosides
- *Psychrobacter phenylpyruvicus* formerly *Moraxella phenylpyruvicus*

Acinetobacter Species

- More than 10 species and multiple genomavars
- May be as many as 30 species
- Some are important in human medicine
  - *Acinetobacter baumannii*
  - *Acinetobacter lwoffii*
  - *Acinetobacter haemolyticus*

- General characteristics
  - Aerobic nonfermentative gram-negative bacilli
  - Most strains grow well on MacConkey agar
  - Oxidase negative
  - Nonmotile
- Epidemiology
  - Widely distributed in nature
  - Survive on various surfaces (both moist and dry) in the hospital environment
  - Strains have been isolated from food
  - Isolated from healthy human skin
- Clinical disease
  - Considered nonpathogenic to healthy individuals
  - Most infections in immunocompromised individuals
  - Frequently isolated in nosocomial infections
    - Especially intensive care units
  - *A. baumannii* is a cause of nosocomial pneumonia
    - Late-onset ventilator-associated pneumonia
  - Other infections include
    - Skin and wound infections
    - Bacteremia
    - Meningitis
- Laboratory diagnosis
  - Coccobacilli
  - Oxidase negative
  - Unable to reduce nitrate
  - Difficult to identify some species
  - Commercial systems appropriate for *A. baumannii*, but questionable for other species
  - Most strains grow well on MacConkey agar
    - Except some *A. lwoffii*
  - Non–lactose fermenting
    - May appear partially lactose fermenting on MacConkey agar

FAMILY BURKHOLDERIACEAE

Burkholderia Species

Burkholderia cepacia

- Epidemiology and clinical disease
  - Opportunistic and nosocomial pathogen
    - Major pathogen of patients with cystic fibrosis
  - Resistant to decontaminating agents
    - Has been isolated from alcohol and iodine bottles
- Laboratory diagnosis
  - Aerobic gram-negative bacilli
  - Growth on blood, chocolate, and MacConkey agar
    - Selective media usually used in patients with cystic fibrosis
  - Oxidase weakly positive
    - Routine laboratory test may be negative
  - Commercial systems may identify complex
  - Highly resistant antibiotic susceptibility pattern

Burkholderia pseudomallei
- Melioidosis
  - Aggressive granulomatous pulmonary disease
  - Seen in Vietnam veterans
- Rarely seen in the United States
- Automated systems may or may not identify correctly
- Clinical history and communication with physician critical

Burkholderia mallei
- Glanders
  - Primarily in horses, mules, and donkeys
- Usually by ingestion of contaminated food or water
- Nodular lesions in the lungs and ulceration of the mucous membranes
- Endemic in Africa, Asia, the Middle East, Central and South America
- Not to be identified in a routine clinical laboratory

Stenotrophomonas maltophilia

- Aerobic
- Nonfermentative
- Gram-negative bacillus
- They are motile by polar flagella
- Clinical disease
  - Opportunistic pathogen
  - Serious infections in immunocompromised host
  - Nosocomial infections
  - Respiratory isolates are common
  - Other sites
    - Wounds
    - Urine
    - Blood
  - The major risk factor for infection in hospitalized patients is the implantation of medical devices
    - Central venous catheters
    - Urinary tract catheters
    - Prosthetic heart valves
    - Intraocular and contact lenses
- Laboratory diagnosis
  - Growth on blood agar and chocolate agar: Green-lavender or yellow pigment
  - Non–lactose fermenter on MacConkey agar
  - Oxidase negative
  - Catalase and esculin positive
  - Strongly oxidizes maltose
    - Weak oxidation of glucose

FAMILY ALCALIGENACEAE

Achromobacter Species

- Six species
- Achromobacter xylosoxidans most common in clinical microbiology
- Achromobacter denitrificans

- Environmental organisms
  - Water
  - Soil
- Opportunistic and nosocomial infections
  - Cystic fibrosis
  - Burns
  - Immunocompromised
- Pathogenesis and virulence factors
  - Opportunistic
  - Multiple extracellular enzymes used for survival in the environment
  - Often resistant to multiple antimicrobial agents
- Laboratory diagnosis
  - Aerobic gram-negative bacilli
  - Grows on blood, chocolate, and MacConkey agar
  - Nonfermenters on MacConkey (lactose)
  - Oxidase positive
  - Motile

Alcaligenes Species

- *Alcaligenes faecalis*
  - Environmental organisms
    - Water
    - Soil
  - Opportunistic and nosocomial infections
    - Cystic fibrosis
    - Burns
    - Immunocompromised
- Pathogenesis and virulence factors
  - Opportunistic
  - Multiple extracellular enzymes used for survival in the environment
  - Often resistant to multiple antimicrobial agents
- Laboratory diagnosis
  - Grow on blood, chocolate, and MacConkey agar
  - Gram-negative bacilli
  - Nonfermenters on MacConkey (lactose)
  - Oxidase positive
  - Motile

FAMILY CHLAMYDIACEAE

Chlamydia and Chlamydophila

- Three species in *Chlamydia*
- Six species in *Chlamydophila*
  - *Chlamydophila* was recognized in 1999
  - *Chlamydia*
    - *Chlamydia muridarum*
    - *Chlamydia suis*
    - *Chlamydia trachomatis*
  - *Chlamydophila*
    - *Chlamydophila pneumoniae*
    - *Chlamydophila pecorum*
    - *Chlamydophila psittaci*

- o *Chlamydophila abortus*
- o *Chlamydophila felis*
- o *Chlamydophila caviae*
- Obligate intracellular pathogens
- Three disease-causing species in humans
  - *Chlamydia trachomatis*
    - o STDs, eye infections
  - *Chlamydophila pneumoniae*
    - o Respiratory disease in humans, horses, koalas, and other animals
  - *Chlamydophila psittaci*
    - o Respiratory disease: Humans, birds
- Life cycle
  - Elementary bodies are the small (0.3-0.4 μm) infectious form of the chlamydia
    - o They possess a rigid outer membrane that is extensively cross-linked by disulfide bonds
    - o Because of their rigid outer membrane the elementary bodies are resistant to harsh environmental conditions encountered when the *Chlamydia* organisms are outside of their eukaryotic host cells
    - o The elementary bodies bind to receptors on host cells and initiate infection
    - o Most *Chlamydia* organisms infect columnar epithelial cells, but some can also infect macrophages
  - Reticulate bodies are the noninfectious intracellular form of the *Chlamydia* organism
    - o They are the metabolically active replicating form of the *Chlamydia* organism
    - o They possess a fragile membrane lacking the extensive disulfide bonds characteristic of the elementary bodies

Chlamydia trachomatis

- General characteristics
  - Only found in humans
  - Most common bacterial STD pathogen
  - Infections may be symptomatic or asymptomatic
  - Ocular infections: Biovar trachoma
    - o 500 million people are infected worldwide
    - o 7 to 9 million people are blinded
    - o Endemic in Africa, the Middle East, India, and Southeast Asia
    - o Infections occur mostly in children
    - o Transmitted by droplets, hands, contaminated clothing, flies, and by passage through an infected birth canal
  - Genital tract infections: Biovar trachoma
    - o May be the most common bacterial STD in the United States
    - o 50 million new cases occur yearly worldwide
    - o In the United States, the highest infection rates occur in Native and African Americans
  - Genital tract infections
    - o STD that occurs sporadically in the United States
    - o Prevalent in Africa, Asia, and South America

- o Humans are the only natural host
- o Incidence is 300 to 500 cases per year in the United States
- o Male homosexuals are major reservoir of the disease
- Clinical disease
  - Urethritis, cervicitis, epididymitis
  - Pelvic inflammatory disease
  - STD: Lymphogranuloma venereum
  - Trachoma
    - o Not an STD, chronic conjunctivitis, blindness
  - Inclusion conjunctivitis
    - o Spread to infant from mother
    - o No blindness
- Pathogenesis
  - Infects nonciliated columnar epithelial cells
  - Infiltration of PMNs
  - Lymphoid follicle formation and fibrosis
  - Clinical diseases from destruction of the cells and the host inflammatory response
  - Does not stimulate long-lasting immunity

Chlamydophila pneumoniae

- Formerly classified as *Chlamydia*
- Humans only source of disease
- Atypical pneumonia
- Epidemiology
  - Affects all age groups
    - o Most common among older age groups
  - Reinfection is common after a short period of immunity
  - Causes 10% of community-acquired pneumonias treated without hospitalization
- Clinical disease
  - Commonly causes mild-to-moderate respiratory illness
    - o Pneumonia, bronchitis, sinusitis, flulike illness
  - Pneumonia symptoms indistinguishable from other causes of pneumonia
    - o Cough, fever, and difficulties breathing
  - Incidence of asymptomatic appears high
  - May be severe in immunocompromised
- Laboratory diagnosis
  - Tissue culture: historical gold standard
    - o Cultured on McCoy cells
      - Other cell lines will support the growth of *C. trachomatis*
    - o Stain 2 to 6 days after inoculation (iodine or fluorescent antibody)
  - DFA
    - o Detects outer membrane of elemental bodies
    - o Can be as sensitive as culture
  - Molecular techniques
    - o Nucleic acid amplification
      - PCR, ligase chain reaction, strand displacement
    - o DNA probes

Chlamydophila psittaci

- Epidemiology
  - Causative agent of psittacosis: Parrot fever
  - Natural reservoir can be any species of bird
  - Present in tissues, feces, and feathers of symptomatic or asymptomatic birds
  - Veterinarians, zoo keepers, pet shop employees at increased risk
- Clinical disease
  - Incubation time of 7 to 15 days
  - Symptoms include fever, chills, headache, nonproductive cough, mild lung inflammation
  - Disease usually subsides in 5 to 6 weeks
  - Asymptomatic infections are common
  - Seizure, coma, and death (5% mortality rate) can occur
- Laboratory diagnosis and treatment and prevention
  - Diagnosis is through serology
    - Fourfold rise in titer in paired sera

FAMILY MYCOPLASMATACEAE

- Class Mollicutes: Meaning "soft skin"
  - Mycoplasmataceae

Mollicutes of Humans

- Approximately 120 species of the genus *Mycoplasma*
- Seven species of the genus *Ureaplasma*
- Lack cell walls
- Very small size
- 0.2 to 0.8 µm in diameter
- Very small genome
- Require sterols for growth
- Linked to respiratory infections by Roux and Nocard in 1898
- Isolated organism from bovine pleuropneumonia
- Probably evolved from gram-positive bacteria such as *Lactobacillus, Bacillus, Streptococcus, Clostridium* spp.
- Not found growing freely as living organisms
- Depend on host for fatty acids, amino acids, nucleic acid precursor, and cholesterol
- Epidemiology
  - At least 16 species have been isolated from humans
  - More than half are considered nonpathogenic
  - Mostly *Mycoplasma* and *Ureaplasma* spp.
  - Associated with mucous membranes
    - Respiratory
    - Urogenital
- Clinical disease
  - Clinical disease: *M. pneumoniae*
    - Common cause of mild pneumonia in people younger than 40 years of age
      - 15% to 50% of all pneumonia in adults and an even higher percentage of pneumonia in school-aged children

- Clinical disease: *M. hominis*
  - Colonize male and female genital tract
  - Role in genital tract diseases unclear
  - Associated with adverse pregnancy outcomes
- Clinical disease—*U. urealyticum*
- STD
  - Urethritis in males
  - Infertility, low birth weight, premature delivery
- Others
  - Pneumonia, meningitis, bacteremia in newborns
  - Bacteremia, abscesses, arthritis in immunocompromised patients
- Laboratory diagnosis
  - Mollicutes grow slowly by binary fission and produce "fried egg" colonies on agar plates
  - Colonies of *M. pneumoniae* have a granular appearance
  - Because of slow growth, colonies may take up to 3 weeks to develop
- *Ureaplasma* split urea

FAMILY BARTONELLACEAE

- *Bartonella*
- *Grahmella*
- *Rochalimaea*
- Grahamella and *Rochalimaea* may not have valid taxonomic status

Bartonella Species

- Approximately 19 described species
  - Three subspecies of *Bartonella vinsonii*
  - Small (0.6 × 1.0 mm) gram-negative bacilli
  - Fastidious

Bartonella henselae

- Cat scratch disease
  - Acquired after exposure to cats
    - Scratches, bites
  - Disease usually benign
    - Chronic regional lymphadenopathy
- Laboratory diagnosis
  - Warthin-Starry silver staining
  - DNA amplification
  - Cultures not recommended
    - Blood or tissue transported in Isolator
    - Chocolate agar
    - Prolonged incubation with increased CO_2
  - Serology main testing
  - Cross-reactions with *Coxiella burnetii*, *Chlamydia* spp., and other *Bartonella* spp.
  - IgG/IgM EIA
    - Sensitivity 85% and specificity >98%
- Laboratory diagnosis, other than cat scratch disease
  - Serology
    - Reference or research laboratory
    - CDC

FAMILY RICKETTSIACEAE

Orientia

- *Orientia tsutsugamushi*
  - *Orientia* were formerly classified as *Rickettsia*

Rickettsia

- Approximately 26 species
- General characteristics
  - Small intracellular bacteria
    - 0.3 to 0.5 × 1 to 2 μm
  - Gram-negative–like cell wall
    - Contains LPS
  - Independent ATP and host ATP can be used
  - No apparent genes for sugar metabolism, lipid synthesis, and amino acid synthesis
- Divided into groups based on antigens
  - Spotted fever group
  - Typhus group
  - Scrub typhus group
- Epidemiology: Rocky Mountain Spotted Fever (RMSF)
  - Most common rickettsial disease in the United States
  - Approximately 500 to 700 cases per year
  - Originally described in Rocky Mountain area, but more common in South Central states
  - Transmitted by the bite of an infected tick
  - Highest incidence from April through September
  - Principal reservoir for *R. rickettsii* is hard tick
    - Transovarian passage occurs
- Clinical disease: RMSF
  - Abrupt onset of fever, chills, headache, and myalgia
  - 5 to 10 days after the tick bite
  - Rash common (~90%)
    - 2 to 3 days after fever
    - Begins on the hands and feet and spreads toward the trunk
    - Palms and soles is common
  - Complications from vasculitis
    - Respiratory failure, seizures, acute renal failure
  - Mortality rate in untreated patients is 20%
- Laboratory diagnosis
  - Clinical
  - Fluorescent or PCR for antigen in skin biopsies
    - Reference laboratories
  - Serology is the major laboratory test
    - Weil-Felix test
    - Immunoflurorescent antibody (IFA) reagent is available

FAMILY LEPTOSPIRACEAE

- Human disease
  - *Leptospira interrogans:* Leptospirosis

- *Borrelia*
  - *Borrelia burgdorferi:* Lyme disease
  - *Borrelia hermsii:* Relapsing fever
- *Treponema pallidum:* Syphilis
  - Other treponemas: Yaws, pinta, bejel
- General characteristics
  - Long, thin, spiral

Leptospira interrogans and Leptospira biflexa

- 14 species
- 6- to 20-μm coiled rods with hook
- Obligate aerobes
- Fastidious
- Epidemiology
  - Endemic worldwide
  - Most common zoonotic infection worldwide
  - Most prevalent in the tropics and subtropics
  - Contact: Animal urine
    - Directly
    - Contaminated fresh water
- Clinical disease
  - Leptospirosis
  - Severity of disease varies with serovar
  - 90% of patients mild disease
    - Low fever
    - Meningitis
    - Rash
  - 10%: Severe with hepatitis, general organ involvement
- Laboratory diagnosis
  - Clinical presentation
  - Culture
    - Blood early
    - Urine late (>2 weeks)
  - Molecular: PCR
  - Serology: Enzyme immunoassay (EIA)

Borrelia

- Approximately 30 species of *Borrelia*
- Microaerophilic
- Temperature optima 28° to 30° C
- Generation time approximately 18 hr
- Flagella determines helical shape
  - Flagella-negative mutants are straight bacilli
- Lyme borreliosis
  - Most common vector-borne disease in the United States
  - Caused by *B. burgdorferi*
  - Transmitted by the hard ticks *Ixodes* spp.
- Vector
  - *Ixodes scapularis*
    - Deer tick or black-legged tick
  - *Ixodes pacificus*

- Clinical disease
  - Stage 1 (3-30 days)
    - 75% develop erythema chronicum migrans
    - May be other symptoms
  - Stage 2 (1-7 months)
    - Cardiac and neurologic problems
  - Stage 3 (months to years)
    - Arthritis
- Laboratory diagnosis
  - Diagnosis of Lyme borreliosis is clinical diagnosis
  - Laboratory tests should not be used alone, can help support a clinical diagnosis
  - Laboratory tests
    - Serology (enzyme immunoassay)
    - Western blot
      - POS IgM = 2 of 3 protein bands
      - POS IgG = 5 of 10 protein bands

Treponema pallidum

- Syphilis
  - STD (90%)
    - Caused by direct contact with lesions that contain *T. pallidum*
  - *T. pallidum* enters cracks in mucous membranes of genitals, anus, lips, and rectum during vaginal, oral, and anal sex
  - Four untreated stages: 1 > 2 > latent > 3
  - Congenital infection possible
- Primary syphilis
  - Single primary lesion on any cutaneous or mucous membrane surface
  - Base hard but painless: Hard chancre
  - Appears in 3 weeks and disappears in 4 to 12 weeks
  - Only diagnostic test is dark-field microscopy
- Secondary syphilis
  - 6 weeks to several months
  - Cutaneous and mucous membrane lesions
  - Rough red skin rash
  - Infectious, live treponemes
- Latent syphilis
  - Early latent period; 2 yrs or less
    - Infectious lesions may reappear
  - Late latent period; over 2 yrs

- Noninfectious stage
- May last a lifetime or result in tertiary syphilis
- Tertiary or late syphilis; noninfectious stage
  - Gummas
    - Granulomas
    - No treponemes
    - Causes host response
  - Skin, subcutaneous tissue, deep tissue, bone
  - Neurosyphilis
- Congenital syphilis
  - Caused by infection in utero with *T. pallidum*
  - A wide spectrum of severity exists
- Laboratory diagnosis
  - Non-treponemal tests include RPR and VDRL
  - Treponemal tests include TP-PA and EIA

ANAEROBIC BACTERIA MOST COMMONLY ISOLATED FROM INFECTION (BOX 1-4)

- Bacteria: Relation to O_2
  - Spectrum of sensitivity to O_2
    - Strict anaerobes (<5% O_2)
    - Aerotolerant anaerobes (>5% O_2)
    - Facultative anaerobes (aerobes)
    - Strict aerobes
- Strict anaerobic bacteria
  - Superoxide (SO) anion lethal to bacteria
  - Facultative and aerobic bacteria handle SO by producing the enzyme superoxide dismutase (SOD)
  - SO converted to H_2O_2 and O_2
  - Catalase and peroxidase production assist in breaking down H_2O_2
  - Strict anaerobes lack significant levels of SOD
  - Largely intolerant of O_2 in environment
  - Lack appropriate cytochrome system to use O_2 as terminal electron acceptor
  - Energy solely by fermentation
  - Gram morphology no different from that in aerobic organisms
  - Many anaerobic bacterial species found among the normal microbial flora of humans and animals

---

BOX 1-4 Identification of Anaerobic Bacteria

- Specimen selection: what not to culture
  - Any specimen likely to be contaminated with normal or colonizing flora (nasopharyngeal, gingival, bronchial washings, expectorated sputum, vaginal or cervical samples, voided urine, surface swabs)
  - Minor wounds that are likely to respond to simple drainage
  - Specimens from acute infections where anaerobes are unlikely to play a role (bacterial meningitis, routine urinary tract infection)
- Appropriate specimens
  - Blood
  - Other normally sterile sites (like pleural fluid)
  - Dental/sinus—aspiration of abscess or biopsy
  - Lung—aspirate or biopsy, thoracentesis
  - Abdomen—aspirate of abscess, peritoneal fluid, otherwise sterile tissue
  - Female genital tract—laparoscopy, surgical biopsy, aspirate of abscess

Continued

BOX 1-4	Identification of Anaerobic Bacteria—cont'd

- Bone—aspirate, biopsy
- Soft tissue—surgical biopsy, aspiration of abscess
- Transport of Specimens
  - Tissue specimens—anaerobic pouch or anaerobic transport tube with medium
  - Fluid or aspirated pus
    - Express into anaerobic transport vials OR
    - Leave in syringe, discard needle & cover with sterile cap
  - Transport of Specimens
  - Swabs are strongly discouraged as aspirates or biopsy tissues are far better specimens
  - If swab is unavoidable, it must be collected in a sterile surgical field and transported in a special anaerobic swab device to lab
- Primary Media
  - Primary specimens should be plated on non-selective, selective, and differential media
  - All media should be supplemented with vitamin K and hemin
  - Media should be fresh
  - Routinely used:
    - Anaerobic SBA, LKV, BBE, CNA or PEA
    - Routine aerobic SBA, MAC, CNA
  - Media has reducing agents to keep O_2 levels low
  - Laked kanamycin-vancomycin (LKV) blood agar
    - Selects for gram anaerobic negative bacilli
  - Bacteroides bile esculin agar (BBE)
    - Selective/differential for *Bacteroides fragilis* grp.
  - CCFA Selective differential media for recognition of *C. difficile*
    - Cycloserine will inhibit gram-negative bacteria, while cefoxitin will inhibit both gram-positive and gram-negative organisms. *C. difficile* ferments the fructose in the medium resulting in yellow colonies
  - Phenylethyl alcohol (PEA)—selects for GPC
    - Selects for gram-positive bacilli and cocci
  - Egg Yolk Agar (EYA)—nonselective, differential medium
    - Egg yolk suspension allows detection of lecithinase and lipase
    - Lecithin breakdown results in an opaque precipitate
    - Lipase enzyme hydrolyzes results in an iridescent sheen on the colony surface
  - Thioglycolate broth
- Nonselective, reduced liquid media
- Incubation of plates
  - Anaerobes are most sensitive to oxygen during log phase of growth

- Incubate at 35° C-37° C
- Use GasPak jars, bags, or anaerobic chambers
- Use methylene blue or resazurin indicator to validate anaerobic conditions
- Do not expose plates to air for more than ½ hr
- Routine media for the interpretation of aerobic growth should be incubated in room air or low CO_2 tension if available
- Incubation time
  - Inspect at 24 h for rapid growers, 48-72 h for others, 4-5 days total
    - Organisms grow more slowly than aerobes
    - Exceptions—incubate >7 days if *Actinomyces* is suspected as it grows very slowly
    - Dissection microscope is helpful to look at tiny colonies
- Approach to Identification
  - Complete ID of anaerobes may be complicated, time consuming, and expensive
  - General current approach includes:
    - Focus on *Bacteriodes fragilis* recognition
    - Determination of mixed bacterial flora, both aerobes and anaerobes
    - Look for toxins of *C. difficile*
    - Tetanus, botulism, gas gangrene present as characteristic clinical pictures—seek *Clostridium*
    - Use simple tests to presumptively group most commonly encountered anaerobic organisms
    - Let the Gram stain guide the work up
    - Differential media and resistance to key antibiotics
- Few key biochemical tests—Common anaerobic bacilli
- Bile—growth in the presence of 20% bile
  - Incorporated in BBE agar
  - Inhibits most anaerobes other than *Bacteroides* and *Bilophilia*
- Kanamycin, vancomycin, colisitin susceptibility by disk
  - Antibiotics disks can be placed on blood agar for all three agents
  - Growth or inhibition in the presence of specific concentrations of antibiotic can be used for presumptive identification
- Catalase
  - 15% hydrogen peroxide is used to test for the production of catase by anaerobes
- Spot Indole
  - Ability to metabolize tryptophan by testing for indole in either tubes or a spot test

	Bile	Kanamycin	Vancomycin	Colistin	Catalase	Indole
Prevotella	S	R	R	V	-	-
Porphyromonas	S	R	S	R	-	+
B. fragilis grp	R	R	R	R	+	V
Fusobacterium	V	S	R	S	-	V
Bilophila	R	S	R	S	+	-

- Few key biochemical tests—anaerobic gram-negative bacilli
- Lecithinase—see egg yolk agar

	Lecithinase	Double zone of hemolysis	CCFA yellow colonies	Catalase	Indole
Clostridium perfringens	+	+	-	-	-
Clostridium difficile	-	-	+	-	-
Clostridium septicum	-	-	-	-	-
Propionibacterium	-	-	-	+	+

Peptostreptococcus

- General characteristics
  - Gram-positive anaerobic cocci in chains
  - Common member of the normal gut flora and respiratory tract
  - Almost always found, when clinically significant, in coinfections with other anaerobes and facultative anaerobes
  - Basically the only genus of the gram-positive anaerobic cocci involved in disease

Veillonella

- General characteristics
  - Gram-negative anaerobic cocci (counterpart of the aerobic *Neisseria*)
  - Common member of the mouth and intestinal flora of humans
  - Low incidence of pathogenicity
    - If clinically significant, found in coinfections with other anaerobes and facultative anaerobes

Propionibacterium

- General characteristics
  - Gram-positive, non–spore forming, anaerobic bacillus
  - Resembles *Corynebacterium* in morphology and cell arrangement
  - Some strains are aerotolerant, yet yield better growth under strictly anaerobic conditions
  - Produces propionic acid
  - Widely distributed as normal flora on skin and other body sites, including the respiratory tract, and may act as opportunistic pathogen with other copathogens

Propionibacterium acnes

- General characteristics
  - Most common gram-positive, non–spore forming, anaerobic rod encountered in clinical specimens
  - Slowly growing in culture
  - Common resident of the pilosebaceous glands of the human skin
  - Causative agent of acne vulgaris (pimples)
  - In addition to acne, *P. acnes* has been implicated in other infectionss
    - Corneal ulcers
    - Heart valves
    - Prosthetic devices
    - CNS shunts
  - Opportunistic mixed infections with other flora
  - Highly susceptible to various β-lactam antimicrobial agents such as penicillin G

Actinomyces israelii

- General characteristics
  - Most common human pathogenic species
  - Gram-positive bacillus that tends to form branches, sometimes with a beaded appearance
  - Common member of the mouth flora of humans
  - Aerotolerant anaerobe
  - Very slow growing and difficult to recover in culture
  - Responds well to long-term therapy with penicillin class of antibiotics
- Clinical syndromes
  - Cervical-facial
    - Most common, causes "lumpy jaw"
    - Slowly developing abscess, chronic infection may erupt into sinus tracts on face or neck
    - Dental surgery or facial trauma predisposition
  - Pulmonary
    - Aspiration of mouth flora to lower respiratory tract
    - Primary pneumonia may result
    - Radiography not specific to *Actinomyces*
    - Chronic infection in which abscess is formed
      - Abscess, which can bore its way to surface and produce sinus tracts
      - Sulfur granules can be seen in the fluid
      - Granules are actually aggregated microcolonies
      - Gram smear reveals the long filamentous *Actinomyces*
  - Abdominal
    - Infection follows ingestion of organism
    - GI lesions can occur, not unlike those seen in pulmonary infection
    - Abscess can rupture through musculature and skin to form tracts
  - Genitourinary
    - *A. israelii* may colonize the female genital tract as normal flora
    - Associated with long-term use of intrauterine devices
    - Indistinguishable from pelvic inflammatory disease
      - Vaginal discharge, abdominal pain, fever, urinary discomfort, etc.
    - Treated with antibiotics and removal of the device

GRAM-POSITIVE BACILLUS: CLOSTRIDIUM

- General characteristics
  - Gram-positive bacillus
    - Usually large bacilli
  - Produce endospores
    - May appear terminal or central
    - Excellent survival in environment
  - Are strictly anaerobic in metabolism
  - Produce variety of potent toxins
- *Clostridium* spp. of clinical importance
  - *Clostridium perfringens*
    - Gas gangrene
    - Food poisoning

- *Clostridium tetani*
  - ○ Tetanus
- *Clostridium botulinum*
  - ○ Botulism
- *Clostridium difficile*
  - ○ Antibiotic associated diarrhea and colitis

Clostridium perfringens

- Nonmotile gram-positive anaerobic bacillus
- Part of human intestinal flora
  - Minor opportunistic pathogen
  - Appears in mixed flora infection
- Found universally in soil
  - Potential to cause major myonecrosis called gas gangrene in wounds
- Gas gangrene
  - Results from contaminated wounds
  - Lesions progress from redness and swelling to greenish blackish decoloration
  - Toxin destroys muscle tissue
  - Gas bubbles present in blisters and under skin
  - Fatal within 48 hours without antibiotics
  - Treatment is surgical (debridement), antibiotics, and hyperbaric O_2 chamber

Clostridium tetani

- Environmental bacteria: Soil
- Motile gram-positive anaerobic bacillus
- Endospores contaminate puncture wounds, grow anaerobically, and produce toxin to cause the disease tetanus (lockjaw)
- Tetanus
  - Painful and rapidly fatal syndrome
  - Toxin binds to target nerve cells
    - ○ Inhibitory interneurons that regulate muscle contraction are blocked
    - ○ Patients undergo single, constant muscle contraction
    - ○ Infection can lead to respiratory failure
  - Treatment can include use of antitoxin
  - Protection is afforded by vaccination with toxoid to raise antibody against the toxin

Clostridium botulinum

- Environmental bacteria: Soil
- Motile gram-positive anaerobic bacillus
- Endospores may become airborne and contaminate food preparation followed by anaerobic storage (non-heated soups, canning of preserves)
- Spores germinate to produce one of the most lethal toxins in the world and result in the disease botulism

- Food or wound botulism
  - ○ Toxin: Botulism neurotoxin (BoTN)
    - Preformed in food source or made by organism contaminating a wound
    - Blocks acetylcholine release at the neuromuscular junction and causes an inhibition of muscle contraction
  - ○ Symptoms
    - Blurred vision, dizziness, muscle weakness, and flaccid paralysis
  - ○ Boiling food destroys the toxin
- Infant botulism
  - ○ Acquired by ingestion of food containing spores
  - ○ Ranges from mild to fatal disease
  - ○ Honey is the most common source of spores, which then germinate in the child's intestinal tract (contraindicated in children younger than 1 year of age)
  - ○ Toxin production causes symptoms of few days duration and then often subside
  - ○ Rare need for use of antitoxin
  - ○ Symptoms
    - Inability to suckle, constipation, flaccid paralysis, muscle weakness

Clostridium difficile

- Motile gram-positive anaerobic bacillus
- Source
  - ○ Soil, air, water, human and animal feces
- Use of broad-spectrum antibiotics lowers relative amount of other normal gut flora and allows *C. difficile* to proliferate and infect large intestine
- Disease
  - *C. difficile* releases two enterotoxins (A and B)
    - ○ Can cause diarrhea, but often causes pseudomembranous colitis with destruction of intestinal lining (also called antibiotic associate colitis)
  - Symptoms
    - ○ Watery diarrhea, abdominal cramps, fever, bloody stools, nausea, dehydration
  - Treatment: Oral metronidazole or vancomycin
  - Either or both of the following tests will confirm the disorder
    - ○ Immunoassay of stool extract for *C. difficile* toxins
    - ○ Colonoscopy showing pathologic findings of pseudomembranous colitis

ANAEROBIC GRAM-NEGATIVE BACILLI

Bacteroides fragilis

- General characteristics
  - Gram-negative anaerobic bacillus
  - Common member of the normal gut flora

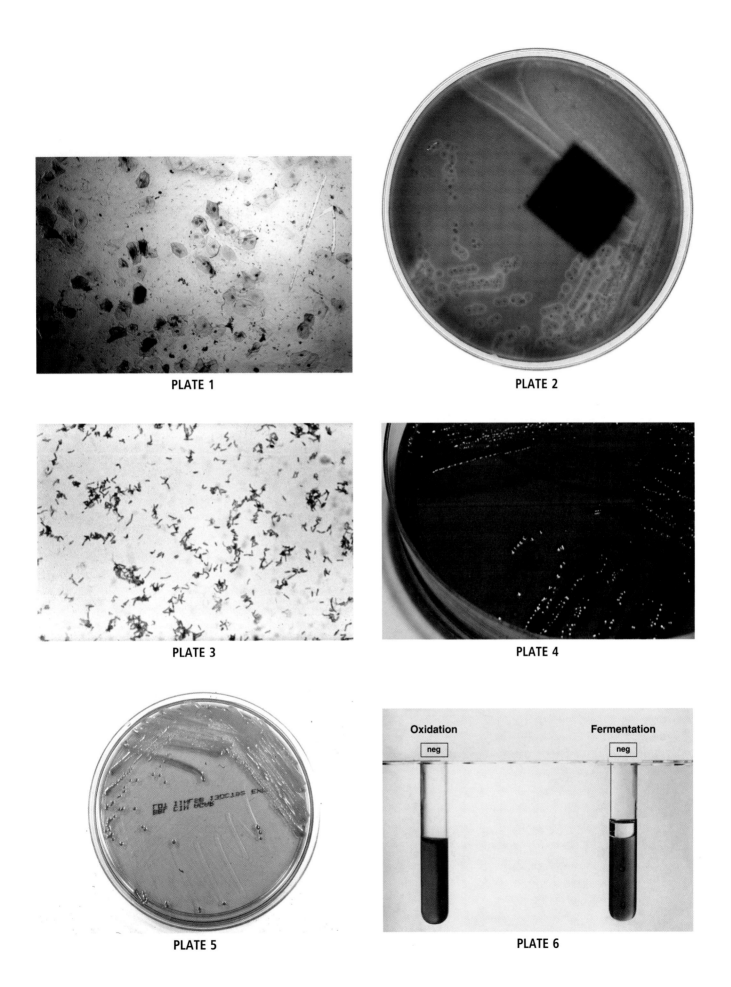

PLATE 1

PLATE 2

PLATE 3

PLATE 4

PLATE 5

Oxidation neg **Fermentation** neg

PLATE 6

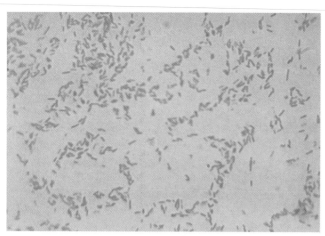

PLATE 7

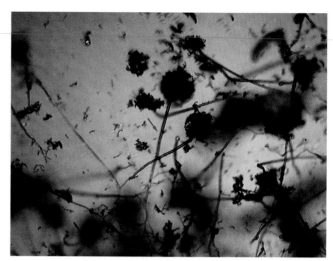

PLATE 8

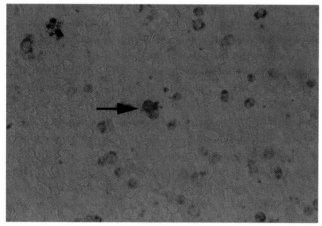

PLATE 9

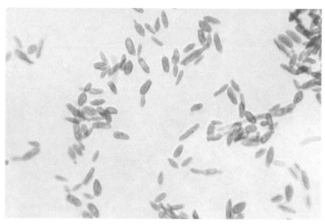

PLATE 10

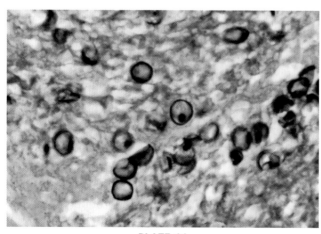

PLATE 11

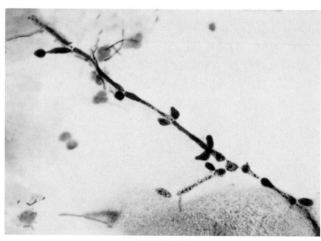

PLATE 12

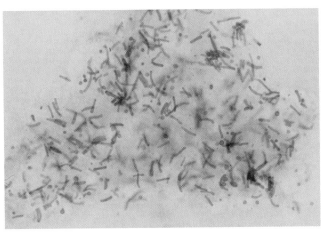

PLATE 13

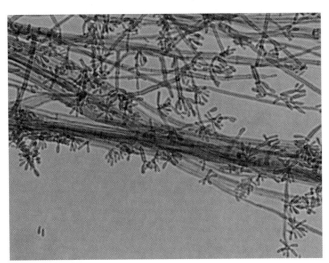

PLATE 14

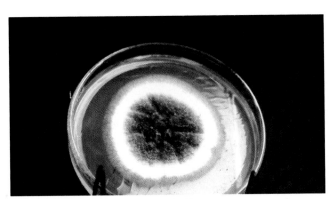

PLATE 15

PLATE 16

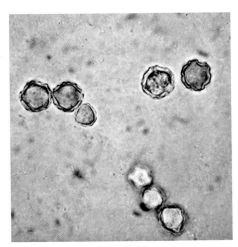

PLATE 17

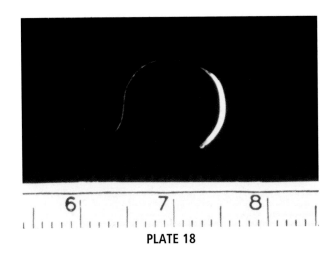

PLATE 18

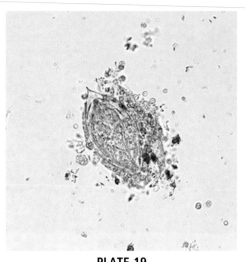

PLATE 19

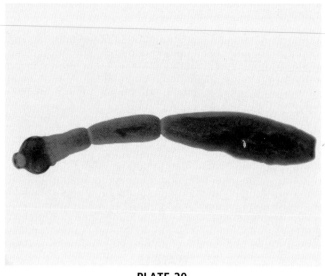

PLATE 20

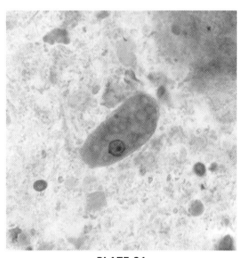

PLATE 21

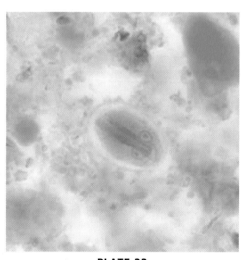

PLATE 22

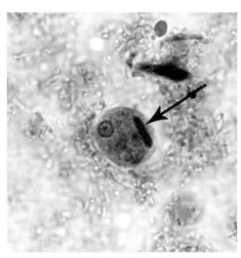

PLATE 23

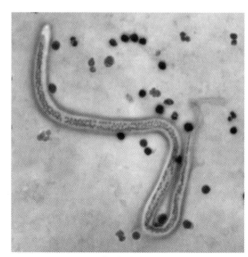

PLATE 24

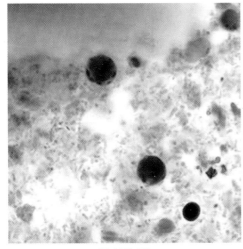

PLATE 25

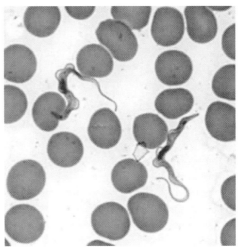

PLATE 26

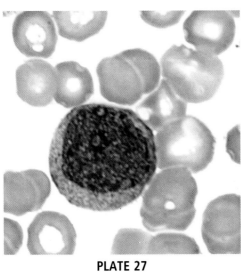

PLATE 27

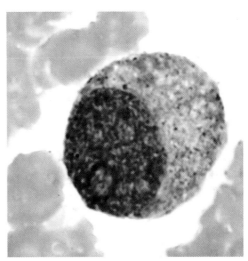

PLATE 28

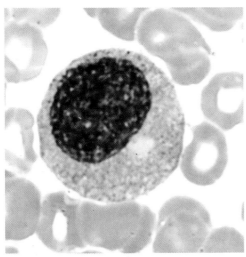

PLATE 29

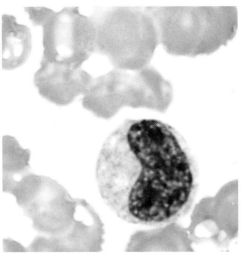

PLATE 30

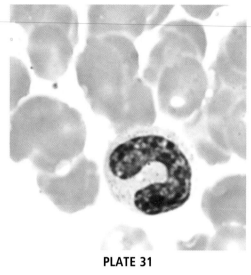

PLATE 31

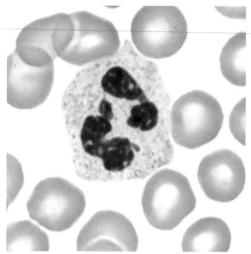

PLATE 32

- Cause of serious infections if the normal GI mucosal barrier is breached
- Can be carried to virtually any organ of the body via bloodstream
- Often found in coinfections with facultative anaerobes
- The organism does *not* have a characteristic gram-negative endotoxin

Other Gram-Negative Anaerobic Bacilli

Fusobacterium Species
- Has spindle-shaped morphology
- Found in respiratory and GI tracts
- Found in mixed infections

Prevotella melaninogenica
- Regular bacillus morphology
- Found in respiratory and GI tracts
- Cause of lung and dental infections
- Grows a black-pigmented colony

Porphyromonas Species
- Regular bacillus morphology
- Purple-pigmented bacilli on agar
- Mouth and genitourinary tract
- Head, neck, and pleuropulmonary infections and periodontal disease

ANTIMICROBIAL SUSCEPTIBILITY TESTING METHODS

- Definitions
  - Minimal inhibitory concentration (MIC)
    - Quantitative measure of the susceptibility of a bacterial isolate to an antimicrobial agent
    - The lowest concentration observed to inhibit growth of the isolate in vitro
  - Minimal bactericidal concentration (MBC)
    - Not commonly performed
    - The lowest concentration of that antibiotic to kill the bacterial isolate in vitro
- Definitions: breakpoints
  - Susceptible
    - Organism can be inhibited by achievable serum or tissue levels at the dosage of antimicrobial agent recommended for that type of infection
    - Favorable outcome
  - Intermediate
    - MICs approach usually attainable blood or tissue levels
    - Strains may be inhibited by certain antimicrobial agents in body sites where drugs may be concentrated
      - Macrolides and respiratory tract
    - Provides a buffer zone that prevents technical factors from causing discrepancies in interpretations

- Resistant
  - Strains are not inhibited by the usually achievable systemic concentrations of the agent with normal dosage schedules
  - Clinical efficacy is unlikely
- Standard for all methods
  - All testing is performed from a pure culture
  - Bacterial suspensions are made in comparison to a turbidity standard
    - 5×10^5 CFU/mL broth dilution
    - 1×10^4 CFU/mL agar dilution
    - 1×10^8 CFU/mL diffusion

ANTIMICROBIAL AGENTS

- Definitions
  - Antibiotic: A chemical substance produced by a microorganism that has the capacity to inhibit the growth of or kill other microorganisms
  - Antimicrobial: An agent that kills or suppresses growth of microorganisms
- Antimicrobial effects
  - Bacteriostatic agents prevent replication but do not kill their target
    - Tetracyclines, macrolides, sulfonamides
  - Bacteriocidal agents result in cell death
    - β-Lactams, vancomycin, fluoroquinolones
- Mechanisms of antimicrobial action
  - Cell wall inhibitors
  - Cell membrane inhibitors
  - Protein synthesis inhibitors
    - Ribosomes
  - Other metabolic pathway inhibitors
    - Folate metabolism
- Cell wall synthesis inhibitors
  - The β-lactams
    - Penicillin
    - Cephalosporins
  - Carbapenems and monobactams
    - Imipenem and meropenem
    - Aztreonam
  - Vancomycin
- Penicillins: Mechanism of action
  - Binds to penicillin-binding proteins
  - Stops transpeptidation (cell wall cross-linking)
  - Cell wall develops weak spots and bursts
  - Bactericidal, synergistic with aminoglycosides
  - Works only on growing cells
- Cephalosporins: Generation determined by the spectrum of activity
- Carbapenems
  - Imipenem/cilastatin, meropenem, doripenem
  - Broad spectrum, low MICs, but expensive
  - Problem with CNS toxicity in imipenem if overdosed
  - Mechanism of action
    - Same as other β-lactams
    - Stable to many β-lactamases

- Except metallo–β-lactamases (e.g., *S. malto-philia* and *B. cepacia*)
- Vancomycin: Mechanism of action
  - Stops gram-positive cell wall peptidoglycan chain formation
  - Bactericidal for staphylococci and streptococci
  - Bacteriostatic for enterococci
  - Mechanism of resistance
    - Gram-negative organisms are usually resistant
    - Enterococci modify the target site
      - VRE
    - Staphylococci have shown resistance
- Cell membrane inhibitors
  - Polymyxin
  - Colistin
  - Amphotericin
- Polymyxin B, Colistin
  - Hydrophobic proteins that disrupt the gram-negative cell membrane
  - Active only against gram-negative bacteria
  - Highly toxic: Renal, neurologic, nausea, vomiting, diarrhea
  - Rarely used
  - Useful for *P. aeruginosa* and other resistant gram-negative organisms
- DNA/RNA inhibitors
  - Fluoroquinolones
  - Metronidazole
  - Nitrofurantoin
  - Rifampin
- Fluoroquinolones
  - Ciprofloxacin, levofloxacin
- Fluoroquinolones: Mechanism of action
  - Inhibit DNA gyrase and/or topoisomerase
    - Prevents DNA unwinding and blocks DNA synthesis
  - Bactericidal and concentration dependent
  - Not synergistic with other antibiotics
- Metronidazole: Mechanism of action
  - Damages DNA and other molecules directly
  - Resistance
    - Reduced uptake and metabolism, increasing in anaerobes
- Rifampin: Mechanism of action
  - Prevents RNA synthesis
    - Inhibits the DNA-dependent RNA polymerase
  - Bactericidal
  - Intracellular activity
  - Active gram-positive organisms
    - Mutation rate of this enzyme is high
- Protein-synthesis inhibitors
  - Macrolides
    - Erythromycin, clarithromycin, azithromycin, dirithromycin
  - Aminoglycosides
    - Gentamicin, tobramycin, amikacin, neomycin
  - Tetracyclines
    - Tetracycline, doxycycline, minocycline
- Clindamycin
- Quinupristin/dalfopristin
- Linezolid
- Inhibitors of intermediate metabolism
  - Trimethoprim
  - Sulfa compounds
  - Trimethoprim/sulfamethoxazole
  - Mechanism of action
    - Stops folate synthesis

MICROBIOLOGY LABORATORY SAFETY: STANDARD PRECAUTIONS

- Assume all patients are infectious for HIV, HBV, or other blood-borne pathogens
- Limit access to the laboratory to trained personnel only
- Use barrier precautions at all times
  - Gloves, masks, goggles, coats or gowns where indicated
  - Leave personal protective equipment in laboratory and out of public areas
- Thoroughly wash hands and other skin surfaces after gloves are removed and immediately after any contamination
- Use particular care with handling and disposal of sharps
- Rigorously follow needle stick policies
- Refrain from
  - Eating, drinking, smoking, application of cosmetics
  - Insertion or removal of contact lenses
  - Nail biting or pen or pencil chewing
  - Mouth-pipetting
- General laboratory safety
  - Threat: Chemicals; Defense: Active chemical hygiene plan, labeling and storage standards, training, material data safety sheets (MSDS), disposal, use of fume hoods, spill kits and procedures, barrier protection, eye wash stations
  - Threat: Fire—Defense: Training, extinguishers, escape plan, elimination of open flames
  - Threat: Electrical—Defense: Active program of checks and maintenance
  - Threat: Gas cylinders—Defense: Chaining into position in well-ventilated area, transport with secure dollies
  - Threat: Radiation—Defense: Radiation safety programs, monitoring exposure among operators

CERTIFICATION PREPARATION QUESTIONS

For answers and rationales, please see Appendix A.

1. Spores are found in select groups of bacteria. Which of the following statements describes the major advantage to the bacteria that possess these structures?
   a. Spores are resistant to heat, cold, drying, most chemicals, and boiling

b. Spores allow an organism to better control its local environment

c. Spores allow bacteria to attach or adhere to host tissues

d. Organisms with spores have a more efficient exchange of genetic material

2. Choose the binomial name that is correctly written.
   a. *Staphylococcus Aureus*
   b. *Staphylococcus* species *aureus*
   c. *Staphylococcus aureus*
   d. *Staphylococcus* aureus

3. Fermentation end-products are often used to aid in the identification of bacteria. Fermentation results in which of the following?
   a. Conversion of glucose to pyruvate
   b. Lactic acid, mixed acids, alcohols, CO_2 production
   c. CO_2 and water
   d. Specific teichoic acids

4. The exchange of cellular DNA between two living bacterial cells that involves an intercellular bridge is which of the following processes?
   a. Transformation
   b. Transduction
   c. Plasmidization
   d. Conjugation

5. Transduction is defined as which of the following?
   a. The change of the bacterial genotypes through the exchange of DNA from one cell to another
   b. An internal change in the original nucleotide sequence of a gene or genes within an organism's genome
   c. The process by which genetic elements such as plasmids and transposons excise from one genomic location and insert into another
   d. A mechanism that is mediated by viruses, by which DNA from two bacteria may come together in one cell, thus allowing for recombination

6. A mordant that is applied after the primary stain to chemically bond the alkaline dye to the bacterial cell wall is which of the following?
   a. Safranin
   b. Crystal violet
   c. Gram's iodine
   d. Gram's decolorizer

7. Which of the following bacteria should be considered important pathogens when reading gram-stained smears of soft tissue abscess?
   a. *Streptococcus pneumoniae*
   b. *Neisseria gonorrhoeae*
   c. *Pseudomonas aeruginosa*
   d. *Staphylococcus aureus*

8. The most appropriate interpretation of a gram-stained smear of a sputum specimen would be which of the following? (gram-stained smear, 400×.)
   a. Few epithelial cells, many PMNs
   b. Inadequate specimen, do not culture for anaerobes

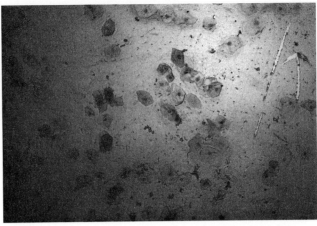

FIGURE 1-1 *(Courtesy Joel Mortensen, PhD. See also color plate 1.)*

c. Many cells, many gram-positive cocci in pairs and chains

d. More than 25 epithelial cells, probable oral contamination, suggest recollect

9. 85% N_2, 10% H_2, 5% CO_2 is the environmental condition that best suits which type of organism?
   a. Aerobes
   b. Anaerobes
   c. Capnophiles
   d. Microaerophiles

10. Which medium can be described as containing bile salts and dyes (bromothymol blue and acid fuchsin) to selectively slow the growth of most nonpathogenic gram-negative bacilli found in the gastrointestinal tract and allow *Salmonella* spp. and *Shigella* spp. to grow?
    a. Thayer-Martin
    b. MacConkey
    c. PEA (phenylethyl alcohol)
    d. Hektoen

11. Choose the group of bacteria that is described as catalase-positive, gram-positive cocci that grow facultatively anaerobic and that form grapelike clusters.
    a. *Neisseria* spp.
    b. *Rothia (Stomatococcus)* spp.
    c. *Staphylococcus* spp.
    d. *Micrococcus* spp.

12. The slide coagulase test is a rapid screening test for the production of which of the following?
    a. Clumping factor
    b. Free coagulase
    c. Extracellular coagulase
    d. Catalase

13. The first identification test performed on a clinical isolate of gram-positive, catalase-positive cocci should be which of the following?
    a. Penicillin test
    b. Gram stain
    c. Oxidase test
    d. Coagulase test

14. The *Staphylococcus* sp. that is more likely to cause uncomplicated urinary tract infections in

nonhospitalized hosts, especially sexually active young women, is which of the following?
   a. *Staphylococcus saprophyticus*
   b. *Staphylococcus aureus*
   c. *Staphylococcus epidermidis*
   d. *Staphylococcus intermedius*

15. The toxic shock syndrome toxin-1 is an important virulence factor in staphylococcal disease. This toxin is classified into which of the following groups of toxins?
   a. Cytolytic toxin
   b. Leukocidin
   c. Phospholipase
   d. Enterotoxin

16. Mannitol salt agar is selective and differential for which group of organisms?
   a. *Staphylococcus* spp.
   b. *Enterococcus* spp.
   c. Gram-positive cocci
   d. *Streptococcus* spp.

17. Within 5 hours of returning home from lunch at your most favorite fast food restaurant you feel very sick and are vomiting. Which of the following is the most likely causative organism?
   a. *Staphylococcus aureus*
   b. *Vibrio parahaemolyticus*
   c. *Shigella sonnei*
   d. *Escherichia coli*

18. The bacterial species that can be described as susceptible to bile and optochin, α-hemolytic, a major cause of bacterial meningitis, and often carrying an antiphagocytic capsule is which of the following?
   a. *Enterococcus faecalis*
   b. *Streptococcus pneumoniae*
   c. *Streptococcus pyogenes*
   d. *Streptococcus agalactiae*

19. The bacterial species that can be described as susceptible to penicillin and bacitracin, β-hemolytic, a major cause of bacterial pharyngitis, and often carrying an antiphagocytic M protein is which of the following?
   a. *Enterococcus faecalis*
   b. *Streptococcus pyogenes*
   c. *Streptococcus agalactiae*
   d. Viridans streptococci

20. The bacterial species that can be described as able to hydrolyze hippurate, β-hemolytic, a major cause of neonatal meningitis and sepsis, and producer of the CAMP factor is which of the following?
   a. *Streptococcus pneumoniae*
   b. *Streptococcus pyogenes*
   c. *Streptococcus agalactiae*
   d. Viridans streptococci

21. The rapid antigen detection methods for throat swabs used for screening patients for streptococcal pharyngitis can be best described by which of the following statements?
   a. They can be useful in quickly identifying most cases of streptococcal pharyngitis

   b. They are a quick way to rule out streptococcal pharyngitis and avoid giving antibiotics when not needed
   c. They are always very sensitive and specific for streptococcal pharyngitis
   d. They are a quick and accurate way to diagnose bacterial and viral pharyngitis

22. The hemolysis of this *Streptococcus* spp. would best be described as which of the following?

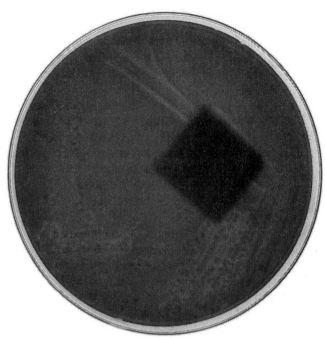

FIGURE 1-2   *(Courtesy Joel Mortensen, PhD. See also color plate 2.)*

   a. β-Hemolysis
   b. γ-Hemolysis
   c. α-Hemolysis
   d. κ-Hemolysis

23. *Enterococcus* spp. can be differentiated from most *Streptococcus* spp. by which of the following tests?
   a. Growth in presence of 6.5% salt
   b. Production of catalase
   c. Production of coagulase
   d. Growth on PEA medium

24. A pure culture of a β-hemolytic *Streptococcus* sp. recovered from a leg ulcer gave the following reactions:

CAMP test = Negative	Hippurate hydrolysis = Negative
Bile esculin slant = No growth	6.5% Salt = No growth
PYR = Negative	Bacitracin = Resistant
Optochin = Resistant	SXT = Sensitive

Which of the following is the most likely identification of this organism?
   a. *Streptococcus pyogenes*
   b. *Streptococcus agalactiae*

c. *Enterococcus faecalis*
d. *Streptococcus* sp., not groups A, B, or D

25. The ability to grow well at refrigerator temperatures is a characteristic of which of the following organisms?
    a. *Mycobacterium gordonae*
    b. *Listeria monocytogenes*
    c. *Erysipelothrix*
    d. *Bacillus cereus*

26. A catalase-positive, gram-positive bacillus that is not acid-fast, does not branch, and does not form spores could possibly belong to which group of bacteria?
    a. *Corynebacterium*
    b. *Bacillus*
    c. *Nocardia*
    d. *Mycobacterium*

27. A throat culture was taken from a 6-year-old boy with a gray pseudomembrane covering his oropharynx. A catalase-positive organism was isolated on cysteine-tellurite medium and subcultured to Tinsdale medium, where it grew as black colonies with brown halos. A Gram stain was performed on these colonies. Which of the following cellular morphologies was most likely seen?
    a. Gram-positive branching bacilli
    b. Gram-positive cocci in short chains
    c. Gram-positive bacilli in irregular clublike shape
    d. Gram-positive cocci in grapelike clusters

28. A blood culture is positive for gram-positive bacilli that gave the following growth characteristics and biochemical reactions:

    MacConkey agar: No growth | Catalase: Positive
    H$_2$S on TSI: negative | Growth of blood agar, nonhemolytic
    Nonmotile | No spores

    These reactions are consistent with which of the following organisms?
    a. *Listeria* spp.
    b. Group B β *Streptococcus*
    c. *Erysipelothrix* spp.
    d. *Corynebacterium* spp.

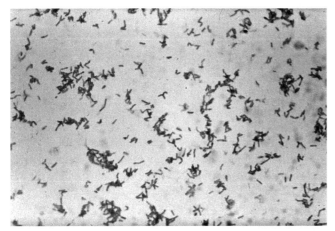

FIGURE 1-3 *(Courtesy Joel Mortensen, PhD. See also color plate 3.)*

29. A skin lesion was opened and drained in surgery. The culture was positive for a gram-positive bacillus, which gave the following growth characteristics and biochemical reactions:

    MacConkey agar: No growth | Catalase: Negative
    H$_2$S on TSI: Positive | Growth of blood agar, nonhemolytic
    Nonmotile | No spores

    These reactions are consistent with which of the following organisms?
    a. *Listeria* spp.
    b. Group B β *Streptococcus*
    c. *Erysipelothrix* spp.
    d. *Corynebacterium* spp.

30. Which of the following sets of tests provide the best differentiation of *Erysipelothrix* from *Listeria monocytogenes*?
    a. Gram-stained smear, oxidase, and optochin
    b. Gram-stained smear, catalase, and motility
    c. CAMP test, hydrogen sulfide production, esculin hydrolysis
    d. Reverse CAMP, gram-stained smear, β-hemolysis

31. Neonatal meningitis is an uncommon but significant disease. Two important causes of this disease may be somewhat difficult to differentiate on preliminary observation. Which of the following sets of tests provide the best differentiation of *Streptococcus agalactiae* from *Listeria monocytogenes*?
    a. Gram-stained smear, oxidase, and optochin
    b. Gram-stained smear, catalase, and motility
    c. CAMP test, hydrogen sulfide production, β-hemolysis
    d. Reverse CAMP, gram-stained smear, β-hemolysis

32. Which of the following tests is important as a part of the genus identification or as part of a preliminary identification but is not used as a confirmatory identification of *Bacillus anthracis*?
    a. Demonstration of a capsule
    b. Demonstration of spore formation
    c. Positive PCR test
    d. Lysis of the strain by specific bacteriophages

33. *Bacillus anthracis* and *Bacillus cereus* can be differentiated in the laboratory by a variety of different test results. Which of the following sets of tests best differentiate these two species?
    a. Catalase and glucose fermentation
    b. Motility and lecithinase production
    c. Oxidase and β-hemolysis on 5% sheep blood agar
    d. Motility and β-hemolysis on 5% sheep blood agar

34. Which of the following specimens would be best for identifying *Bacillus cereus* as the cause of an outbreak of food poisoning?
    a. Blood
    b. Rectal swabs
    c. Stool samples
    d. Food

35. A first morning sputum sample is received for acid-fast culture. The specimen is centrifuged, and the sediment is inoculated on two Lowenstein-Jensen slants that are incubated at 35° C with 5% to 10% CO_2. After 1 week, the slants show abundant growth over the entire surface. Stains reveal gram-negative bacilli. Which of the following should be done to avoid this problem?
   a. Use a medium specifically designed for the growth of AFB
   b. Dilute out the sediment before inoculation with saline
   c. Decontaminate the specimen with NALC–sodium hydroxide mixture
   d. Incubate the tubes at room temperature to retard bacterial growth

36. A patient recently arrived in the United States from Africa presents with a long-standing cutaneous lesion, which is cultured for bacteria, fungi, and AFB. An AFB smear is made and is reported as positive for AFB. After 8 weeks of culture on both non-selective and selective AFB media, no colonies appear. Which of the following organisms should be suspected?
   a. *M. kansasii*
   b. *M. tuberculosis*
   c. *M. leprae*
   d. *M. avium-intracellulare* complex

37. The mycobacterial species that occur in humans and belong to the *M. tuberculosis* complex include which of the following?
   a. *M. tuberculosis*, nontuberculous *Mycobacteria*, *M. bovis*, and *M. africanum*
   b. *M. tuberculosis*, *M. gordonae*, *M. bovis* BCG, and *M. africanum*
   c. *M. tuberculosis*, *M. bovis*, *M. avium*, and *M. intracellulare*
   d. *M. tuberculosis*, *M. bovis*, *M. bovis* BCG, and *M. africanum*

38. The Runyon system of classification is based on which of the following?
   a. Colony and microscopic morphology
   b. Biochemical characteristics
   c. Growth rate and colonial pigmentation
   d. All of the above are correct

39. In identification of mycobacterial isolates, the Tween 80 test involves which of the following?
   a. An enzyme that is able to produce Tween 80 from certain ingredients found in the medium
   b. Lipase that is able to hydrolyze polyoxyethylene sorbitan monooleate into oleic acid and polyoxyethylated sorbitol
   c. The metabolism of niacin to nicotinic acid by enzymatic action
   d. Testing the isolate for susceptibility to Tween 80

40. The gram-negative bacillus that can be described as oxidase-negative, nitrate-positive, indole-negative, citrate-positive, methyl red–positive, urease-negative, and H_2S-positive is most likely which of the following?
   a. *Klebsiella pneumoniae*
   b. *Salmonella enteritidis*
   c. *Escherichia coli*
   d. *Shigella sonnei*

41. The swarming gram-negative bacillus that can be described as oxidase-negative, nitrate-positive, indole-negative, and H_2S-positive is mostly likely which of the following?
   a. *Proteus aerogenes*
   b. *Proteus vulgaris*
   c. *Proteus mirabilis*
   d. *Escherichia coli*

42. Profuse watery diarrhea ("rice water stools"), leading to dramatic fluid loss, severe dehydration, and hypotension that frequently leads to death, is the hallmark of which toxin activity?
   a. Cholera toxin
   b. Enteric endotoxin
   c. Shiga toxin
   d. Toxin A

43. The selective medium thiosulfate citrate bile salts sucrose (TCBS) agar is especially formulated for isolating which pathogen from stool cultures?
   a. *Vibrio* spp.
   b. *Salmonella* spp.
   c. *Shigella* spp.
   d. *Plesiomonas* spp.

44. The majority of human infections with *Campylobacter* spp. are caused by which of the following?
   a. Direct contact with carriers of the bacterium
   b. Contamination of food, milk, or water with animal feces
   c. Multiplication of the organism in food products
   d. Direct contact with persons infected with the bacterium

45. In the test for urease production, the presence of the enzyme hydrolyzes urea to which of the following?
   a. Ammonia and CO_2
   b. Putrescine
   c. Amines and CO_2
   d. Amines and water

46. The bacterial isolate on XLD agar shown in the image was isolated from a routine stool culture. Which of the following genera and species is the most likely identification for this organism?
   a. *Klebsiella pneumoniae*
   b. *Salmonella enteritidis*
   c. *Shigella sonnei*
   d. *Serratia marcescens*

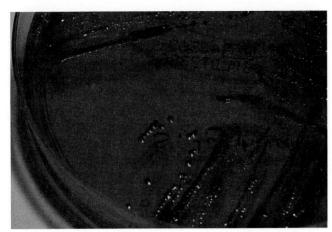

FIGURE 1-4 *(Courtesy Joel Mortensen, PhD. See also color plate 4.)*

47. The bacterial isolate shown below on CIN agar was isolated from a routine stool culture. Which of the following genera and species is the most likely identification for this organism?

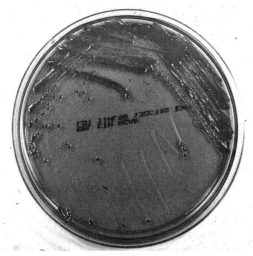

FIGURE 1-5 *(Courtesy Joel Mortensen, PhD. See also color plate 5.)*

   a. *Shigella flexneri*
   b. *Salmonella enteritidis*
   c. *Yersinia enterocolitica*
   d. *Escherichia coli*

48. Decarboxylation of the amino acids lysine, ornithine, and arginine results in the formation of which of the following products?
   a. Ammonia
   b. Urea
   c. CO_2
   d. Amines

49. An organism was inoculated into a TSI tube and gave the following reactions:

Alkaline slant
Acid butt
H_2S: Not produced
Gas: Not produced

The organism is most likely which of the following?
   a. *Klebsiella* sp.
   b. *Shigella* sp.
   c. *Salmonella* sp.
   d. *Escherichia coli*

50. The best specimen for the isolation of *Bordetella pertussis* is which of the following?
   a. Throat swabs
   b. Sputum
   c. Nasopharyngeal aspirates
   d. Anterior nose swab

51. Organisms belonging to the genus *Brucella* are best described by which of the following statements?
   a. Gram-positive diplococci
   b. Gram-positive diphtheroid bacilli
   c. Gram-negative coccobacilli
   d. Gram-negative bacilli

52. Serum samples collected on a patient with pneumonia demonstrate a rising antibody titer to *Legionella*. A bronchoalveolar lavage sample was collected and revealed a positive DFA test for *Legionella*, but no organisms were recovered from this specimen when it was cultured on the appropriate medium and incubated for 2 days at 35° C in CO_2. Which of the following is the best explanation?
   a. Culture was not incubated long enough
   b. Antibody titer
   c. Specimen was incubated at the wrong temperature
   d. Positive DFA test result is a false positive

53. Of the following media, which provides the NAD necessary for the growth of *Haemophilus* spp.?
   a. 5% sheep blood agar
   b. Brain heart infusion agar
   c. Chocolate agar
   d. Nutrient agar

54. Performing the factor requirement test for *Haemophilus* involves which of the following processes?
   a. Inoculation of unsupplemented media with a light suspension of the organism and placement of factors X and V disks on the agar surface
   b. Inoculation of liquid media, unsupplemented and supplemented with factors X and V
   c. Detecting the presence of enzymes that convert α-aminolevulinic acid (ALA) into porphyrins
   d. Growth of the organism in the presence of bacterial species that produce X and V factors as metabolic by-products

55. Of the asaccharolytic, oxidase-positive bacilli that do not grow on MacConkey agar, which one is among the HACEK group of bacteria known to cause subacute bacterial endocarditis?
   a. *Eikenella corrodens*
   b. *Weeksella virosa*
   c. *Pseudomonas maltophilia*
   d. *Sphingomonas paucimobilis*

56. Which of the following statements best completes the following thought: Presumptive identification of an

oxidase-positive, gram-negative diplococcus on Thayer-Martin medium from genital sites of a 6-year-old female as *Neisseria gonorrhoeae*?
- a. Provides the physician with quick and reliable results at minimal cost
- b. May sometimes be incorrect, and a repeat culture should be collected
- c. May sometimes be incorrect and should not be reported until confirmed
- d. Should be done only when venereal disease is suspected

57. The bacterial species that can be described as oxidase-positive, glucose-positive, maltose-positive, sucrose-negative, lactose-negative, and a major cause of bacterial meningitis is most likely which of the following?
- a. *Neisseria meningitidis*
- b. *Neisseria gonorrhoeae*
- c. *Streptococcus pneumoniae*
- d. Viridans group *Streptococcus*

58. The bacterial species that can be described as oxidase-positive, glucose-positive, maltose-negative, sucrose-negative, lactose-negative, and a major cause of venereal disease is most likely which of the following?
- a. *Neisseria meningitidis*
- b. *Neisseria gonorrhoeae*
- c. *Streptococcus pyogenes*
- d. Viridans group *Streptococcus*

59. Organisms belonging to the genus *Neisseria* are described as which of the following?
- a. Gram-positive diplococci
- b. Gram-negative diplococci
- c. Gram-negative coccobacilli
- d. Gram-negative bacilli

60. The following were observed when the Hugh-Leifson oxidative-fermentative test was performed on a bacterial isolate. Which of the options below best describes the organism's reaction?
- a. Oxidizer
- b. Nonoxidizer

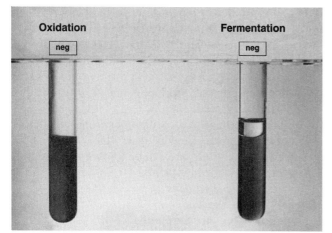

FIGURE 1-6 *(Photograph by Dr. WH Ewing, courtesy the Centers for Disease Control and Prevention, Public Health Image Library, http://phil.cdc.gov/. See also color plate 6.)*

- c. Fermenter
- d. Nonviable

61. The oxidase test is a critical test when attempting to identify nonfermenting gram-negative bacilli. This test is designed to determine the presence of which of the following?
- a. β-Galactosidase
- b. Cytochrome oxidase
- c. Glucose oxidizing enzymes
- d. Oxygen

62. The blood culture of a patient with a central venous catheter yielded a gram-negative bacillus growing on MacConkey agar with the following reactions:

Oxidase = Negative	Motility = Positive
Glucose oxidative-fermentative open = Positive (weak)	Maltose oxidative-fermentative open = Positive (strong)
Catalase = Positive	Esculin hydrolysis = Positive

Which of the following is the most likely identification of this organism?
- a. *Burkholderia cepacia*
- b. *Pseudomonas aeruginosa*
- c. *Acinetobacter baumannii*
- d. *Stenotrophomonas maltophilia*

63. Which organism is associated with the disease Melioidosis?
- a. *Burkholderia ralstonia*
- b. *Burkholderia pseudomallei*
- c. *Burkholderia mallei*
- d. *Burkholderia cepacia*

64. Differentiation of *Stenotrophomonas maltophilia* and *Burkholderia cepacia* is best accomplished by which of the following tests?
- a. Oxidase test
- b. Maltose and glucose medium
- c. Tyrosine-enriched heart infusion agar
- d. Growth at 42° C

65. The respiratory culture of a patient with cystic fibrosis yielded a gram-negative bacillus with the following reactions:

Oxidase = Positive	Motility = Positive
Glucose oxidative-fermentative open = Positive	Gelatin hydrolysis = Positive
Soluble green pigment on TSA slant	Arginine dihydrolase = Positive
Growth at 42° C = positive	

Which of the following is the most likely identification of this organism?
- a. *Burkholderia cepacia*
- b. *Pseudomonas aeruginosa*
- c. *Acinetobacter baumannii*
- d. *Stenotrophomonas xylosoxidans*

66. Which test group best differentiates *Acinetobacter baumannii* from *Pseudomonas aeruginosa*?
- a. Oxidase, motility, nitrate reduction

b. Growth on MacConkey agar, catalase, nitrate reduction

c. Growth on blood agar, oxidase, catalase

d. TSI, urea, motility

67. Which of the following sets of results represent the most common reactions for *Moraxella catarrhalis* when tested in CTA sugar tubes?
    a. Glucose: Negative; Maltose: Negative; Lactose: Negative; Sucrose: Negative
    b. Glucose: Positive; Maltose: Negative; Lactose: Negative; Sucrose: Negative
    c. Glucose: Positive; Maltose: Positive; Lactose: Negative; Sucrose: Negative
    d. Glucose: Positive; Maltose: Negative; Lactose: Positive; Sucrose: Negative

68. A soluble, bright green pigment can be produced by *Pseudomonas aeruginosa*. This pigment is known as which of the following?
    a. Pyoverdin
    b. Pyocyanin
    c. Pyorubin
    d. Pyophena

69. A small portion of a colony of a gram-negative bacilli was smeared onto a filter paper test system. One percent tetramethyl-*p*-phenylenediamine dihydrochloride was added. At 10 seconds, a dark purple color developed where the colony was added to the paper. Which of the following statements best describes the test results?
    a. Positive indole test
    b. Positive oxidase test
    c. Positive urea test
    d. Positive esculin test

70. Characteristics of *Mycoplasma* and *Ureaplasma* include which of the following?
    a. They exhibit the presence of a thin gram-positive–like cell wall with no cell membrane
    b. They demonstrate rapid growth on MacConkey agar, slow growth on basic nutrient agar
    c. The have only a cell membrane with no cell wall
    d. They exhibit rapid growth on MacConkey medium and routine blood agar plates

71. Which of the following is a cause of nongonococcal urethritis?
    a. *Mycoplasma hominis*
    b. *Mycoplasma pneumoniae*
    c. *Ureaplasma urealyticum*
    d. *Mycoplasma orale*

72. Which of the following is the most sensitive method for the diagnosis of *Chlamydia trachomatis*?
    a. Cytology
    b. Culture
    c. Nucleic acid amplification
    d. Serologic testing

73. An 8-year-old boy from Oklahoma presents with a 3-day history of fever, headache, and muscle aches. A rash first noted this morning on his ankles and wrists has now spread to include his trunk. The medical team has identified a list of possible organisms. Which of the following is the most likely cause of this infection?
    a. Q Fever
    b. Ehrlichiosis
    c. Rocky Mountain spotted fever
    d. Cat scratch disease

74. Which of the following is a stage of venereal syphilis that is characterized by the appearance of a chancre?
    a. Primary syphilis
    b. Secondary syphilis
    c. Late syphilis
    d. Tertiary syphilis

75. Which of the following is a nontreponemal serologic test in which soluble antigen particles are coalesced to form larger particles that are visible as clumps when they are aggregated by antibody?
    a. Nontreponemal flocculation (NTF)
    b. Fluorescent treponemal antibody absorption (FTA-ABS) test
    c. Venereal Disease Research Laboratory (VDRL) test
    d. *T. pallidum* particle agglutination (TP-PA) test

76. A patient in a rural area of Massachusetts had a 5-cm red rash with an expanding margin on his back. The lesion was obvious for approximately a month and then resolved. Several weeks later, the patient experienced episodes of partial facial paralysis and painful joints. Which of the following is the most likely infectious agent in this case?
    a. *Borrelia hermsii*
    b. *Borrelia burgdorferi*
    c. *Leptospira interrogans*
    d. *Spirillum minor*

77. A 16-year-old, sexually active patient comes to his physician's office because of a circular, 1-cm lesion in the groin area which is ulcerated but not painful. A rapid plasma reagin test is performed and is reactive with a titer of 1:16. Culture and gram-stain smear results from an exudate of the lesion are negative. Which of the following is the most likely cause of this lesion?
    a. *Chlamydia trachomatis*
    b. *Neisseria gonorrhoeae*
    c. *Treponema pallidum*
    d. *Haemophilus ducreyi*

78. The gram-stained smear shows an organism isolated from a blood culture after bowel surgery. Under anaerobic incubation conditions, it grew as smooth, white, nonhemolytic colonies. The organism was not inhibited by colistin, kanamycin, or vancomycin and hydrolyzed esculin. The most likely identification of this isolate is which of the following?
    a. *Fusobacterium nucleatum*
    b. *Fusobacterium varium*
    c. *Bacteroides fragilis*
    d. *Prevotella melaninogenica*

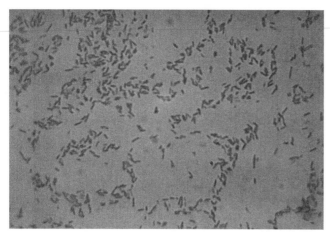

FIGURE 1-7   *(Photograph by Dr. VR Dowell, Jr, courtesy the Centers for Disease Control and Prevention, Public Health Image Library, http://phil.cdc.gov/. See also color plate 7.)*

79. Pseudomembranous colitis caused by *Clostridium difficile* is best confirmed by which of the following laboratory findings?
    a. Presence of the toxin in stool
    b. Isolation of *C. difficile* from stool
    c. Gas production in thioglycolate media
    d. Gram stain of stool showing many gram-positive bacilli

80. Lecithinase production, double zone hemolysis on sheep blood agar, and gram-stained morphology are all useful criteria in the identification of which of the following?
    a. *Clostridium perfringens*
    b. *Streptococcus agalactiae*
    c. *Escherichia coli*
    d. *Clostridium tetani*

81. When activating a hydrogen and carbon dioxide generator system used for creating an anaerobic atmosphere, which of the following is an indication that the catalyst and generator envelope are functioning properly?
    a. A decrease in temperature of the jar
    b. Bubble formation on the surface of the plates
    c. A change in color of the methylene blue indicator
    d. The formation of a visible cloud of gas

82. In a clinical specimen, the presence of sulfur granules strongly indicates the presence of which anaerobic bacterium?
    a. *Bacteroides fragilis*
    b. *Actinomyces* spp.
    c. *Fusobacterium nucleatum*
    d. *Clostridium tetani*

83. Which of the following are a common element between using the E test and agar disk diffusion (Kirby-Bauer) for antimicrobial susceptibility testing?
    a. Both establish an antibiotic gradient in agar
    b. Both create a circular zone of bacterial inhibition

c. Expression of results is by MIC for both
d. The cost of the test is similar per drug

84. Which of the following clinical indications would most benefit from having quantitative (MIC) testing rather than qualitative (Sensitive, Intermediate, Resistant catagories) data from the laboratory?
    a. Urinary tract infection
    b. Bacterial meningitis
    c. Pneumonia caused by *Mycoplasma*
    d. Streptococcal pharyngitis

85. When performing antimicrobial susceptibility testing, the following definition of the minimum inhibitory concentration (MIC) is correct:
    a. The highest concentration of an antibiotic in a dilution series that inhibits growth
    b. The lowest concentration of an antibiotic in a dilution series that inhibits growth
    c. The lowest concentration of an antibiotic in a dilution series that kills the bacteria
    d. The lowest concentration of the antibiotic obtainable in the patient without toxicity

86. In comparing quantitative MIC dilution testing to qualitative agar disk diffusion testing, the higher the MIC of the drug for that organism:
    a. The smaller is the zone of inhibition
    b. The more susceptible the organism will appear on disk diffusion
    c. The larger is the zone of inhibition
    d. The more toxic is the drug to the patient

87. In a quality control (QC) procedure on a new batch of Mueller-Hinton plates using a standard QC stock strain of *Staphylococcus aureus*, the disk inhibition zone sizes for three of the drugs tested were too small and fell below the expected QC range. Which of the following is the most likely reason for this observation?
    a. These three antibiotic disks were outdated and had lost potency
    b. These three disks were faulty in that the antibiotic content was too high
    c. Bacterial suspension of *Staphylococcus* was probably contaminated with another organism
    d. The plates received insufficient incubation time

88. Which of the following definitions best fit the term urethritis?
    a. Infection and or inflammation of the terminal portion of the lower urinary tract
    b. The isolation of a specified quantitative count of bacteria in an appropriately collected urine specimen obtained from a person without symptoms or signs of urinary infection
    c. Dysuria, frequency, and urgency but yielding fewer organisms than 10^5 colony-forming units of bacteria per milliliter (CFU/mL) urine on culture
    d. Inflammation of the kidney parenchyma, calices (cup-shaped division of the renal pelvis), and pelvis

89. The organism most commonly associated with otitis media infections is associated with which of the following positive test results?
    a. Coagulase
    b. VP
    c. Optochin
    d. Bacitracin
90. Which organism is most often responsible for impetigo?
    a. *Staphylococcus epidermidis*
    b. *Streptococcus pyogenes*
    c. *Enterococcus faecalis*
    d. *Streptococcus agalactiae*
91. How do staphylococci spread so easily when infecting the skin?
    a. They produce hyaluronidase, which hydrolyzes hyaluronic acid present in the intracellular ground substance that makes up connective tissue
    b. They produce lipase, which melts the fat under the skin, making it easier to spread
    c. The hemolysins kill the white and red blood cells; then the protease liquefies the skin protein, allowing easy penetration for the bacteria
    d. All of the above
92. Routine culture media for use with a specimen of cerebrospinal fluid should include which of the following sets of media?
    a. 5% sheep blood agar, Lowenstein Jensen agar, 7H9 agar
    b. 5% sheep blood agar, thioglycolate broth
    c. 5% sheep blood agar, MacConkey agar, Sabourad dextrose agar
    d. 5% sheep blood agar, chocolate agar, thioglycolate broth
93. A college student is examined at the emergency department; he is disoriented with a fever, intense headache, stiff neck, vomiting, and sensitivity to light. His friends say that he has been sick for about 2 days and that his condition worsened over the last 3 hours. The physician does a complete blood count (CBC) and electrolytes. The electrolytes are normal, but the patient's white blood count (WBC) is 12,000 cells/L. What test should the doctor order next?
    a. Urine culture
    b. Stool culture
    c. Cerebrospinal fluid Gram stain and culture
    d. Blood culture
94. What cells are found in bacterial vaginosis?
    a. Clue cells
    b. Lymphocytes
    c. Macrophages
    d. Squamous epithelial cells
95. Which of the following terms is used to describe an increase of lymphocytes and other mononuclear cells (pleocytosis) in the cerebrospinal fluid and negative bacterial and fungal cultures?
    a. Meningoencephalitis
    b. Aseptic meningitis
    c. Encephalitis
    d. Meningitis
96. The culture of which sample routinely uses quantitation or the counting of bacterial cells present to assist in the interpretation?
    a. Blood
    b. Sputum
    c. Urine
    d. Abscess
97. Gram staining and reading a glass slide with a mixed smear of *Staphylococcus* and *Escherichia coli* along with each Gram staining run of specimens examined within the microbiology laboratory that day is an example of which of the following?
    a. Quality assurance (QA) activity
    b. Quality control (QC) activity
    c. National regulatory activity
    d. Office of Safety and Health Administration activity
98. Tracking the rate of skin organism contamination among a laboratory's blood culture results on a monthly basis and introducing specific training to phlebotomists when rates exceed the norm would be an example of which of the following?
    a. Good laboratory practice
    b. Quality control
    c. Universal standards
    d. Quality assurance
99. Which of the following statements best defines "infectious substances"?
    a. Articles or substances capable of posing a risk to safety
    b. Substances known or reasonably expected to contain pathogens
    c. Patient samples containing bacteria
    d. Samples with class 3 pathogens
100. Which of the following is an example of an inappropriate specimen or condition that would warrant rejection for microbiology culture?
    a. A nonsterile container for a stool culture
    b. A swab of a skin and soft tissue infection
    c. A tissue sample for anaerobic culture
    d. A 24-hour urine sample for bacteriology culture

SELF-ASSESSMENT

Content Area: _____

Score on Practice Questions: _____

List the specific topics covered in the missed questions:

List the specific topics covered in the correct questions:

NOTES

Mycology, Virology, and Parasitology

Linda J. Graeter and Joel E. Mortensen

MYCOLOGY

The Fungal Organism

- A group of nonmotile eukaryotic organisms that have definite cell walls, are devoid of chlorophyll, and reproduce by means of spores (and conidia)
- Heterotrophic
  - *Hetero* means "different," and *troph* means "nourishment"
- Eukaryotic (fungi) versus Prokaryotic (bacteria)
- Capsule
  - Polysaccharide
    - Much larger than bacterial capsule
  - Antiphagocytic, virulence
  - Mostly in yeast
    - *Cryptococcus neoformans:* Encapsulated yeast
- Fungal cell wall
  - Antigenic
  - Multilayered
    - Polysaccharides (90%)
    - Chitin
    - Proteins and glycoproteins (10%)
  - Provides shape and rigidity to cell
    - Osmotic protection
- Cell membrane
  - Bilayered phospholipids
  - Sterols (ergosterol versus cholesterol)
  - Functions
    - Protects cytoplasm
    - Regulates intake of nutrients
    - Facilitates capsule and cell wall synthesis
- Cytoplasm
  - Nucleus, nucleolus, nuclear membrane, endoplasmic reticulum, mitochondria, vacuoles
- Mycology terms
  - Hypha (plural: hyphae): Filamentous, tubular growth
    - True hyphae versus pseudohyphae
  - Septate (aseptate): Cross walls in hyphae
  - Mycelium (plural: Mycelia)
    - Vegetative
    - Aerial
- Molds: Obligate hyphae
- Yeasts: Unicellular, budding
- Dimorphic: Two bodies or forms
- Mycology terms
- Perfect fungi
  - Sexual stage is known
- Fungi imperfecti
  - No known sexual stage
- Conidia
  - Reproductive structures produced by an asexual mode
- Spore
  - Reproductive structures produced sexually, and the asexual reproductive cells of the zygomycetes
- Conidiophore: Structure that supports conidia
  - Annelloconidia: Produced by annellids
  - Phialoconidia: Produced by phialide
  - Poroconidia: Produced from pores
- Sporangium: Saclike structure where sporangiospores are formed (Zygomycetes)
- Asexual reproduction
  - Arthroconidia: Directly from hyphae by modification of cell wall (barrels)
  - Blastoconidia: Budding of cell (mother and daughter)
  - Chlamydoconidia: Directly from hyphae (swelling)
- Sexual reproduction
  - Ascospore
    - Sexual spore formed in a saclike structure after meiosis
  - Zygospore
    - Round, thick-walled spore produced in a saclike structure by fusion of two hyphal tips
  - Basidiospore
    - Spore formed in a club-shaped reproductive structure after meiosis
- Mycosis (mycoses)
  - Invasive treatments
  - Immunosuppressive therapy
  - Immunocompromising infections
    - Human immune deficiency virus/acquired immunodeficiency virus (HIV/AIDS)

- Rise in common and uncommon mycoses
  - Organisms and tissue infected
- Five broad categories of fungal infections
- Opportunistic fungi
  - Immunocompromised patients
  - Many different tissues
  - Ubiquitous: Environmental saprobes
  - Monomorphs
    - Same structural characteristics under all conditions
  - *Aspergillus, Candida, Mucor, Rhizopus*
- Superficial mycoses
  - Infections of outer, "dead" layers
  - No host defense stimulation
  - No pain or discomfort
  - Usually treated because the infection is "unsightly"
  - *Exophiala, Malassezia, Piedraia, Trichosporon*
- Dermatophytic mycoses
  - Skin, hair, nails
    - Deeper than the superficial
    - Still no living skin penetration
  - Produce secondary metabolites that irritate
  - Host defense causes itching
  - Sometimes cutaneous and superficial grouped
  - *Epidermophyton, Microsporum, Trichophyton*
- Subcutaneous mycoses
  - Muscle, bone, connective tissues
  - Traumatic inoculation
    - Thorns, scratch
  - Usually remain localized
  - *Cladosporium, Exophiala, Pseudallescheria, Phialophora, Sporothrix*

- Systemic mycoses
  - Any tissue
  - Four organisms
    - "True" or "primary" pathogens
  - Endemic to specific geographic areas
    - Must travel through the area to become infected
  - Thermal dimorphs and yeasts
    - "Two bodies" based on temperature
  - *Blastomyces, Coccidioides, Histoplasma, Paracoccidioides*

BASIC CLINICAL MYCOLOGY

- Specimen collection
- Important factors in isolating and identifying a fungal pathogen
  - Correct type of specimen
  - Quality of specimen
  - Rapid transport
  - Use of appropriate culture media
- Processed within 2 hours
- Specimen transport
- Sterile, leak-proof container
  - Dermatologic requires dry container
  - No transport media
- Processed within a few hours
- Specimens can be refrigerated at 4° C
  - Only if processing is delayed
  - Blood and cerebrospinal fluid (CSF): 30° to 37° C
  - Dermatologic: 15° to 30° C
- Safety in the mycology laboratory
- Standard precautions
  - No smoking, eating, drinking, or applying cosmetics
  - Contact lenses (no removing or cleaning)
  - No mouth pipetting
- Universal precautions
- Class 2 or 3 biosafety hoods
- Disinfectant – Phenol based
- Biohazard containers
- Specimen processing: Methods
- Direct inoculation
  - Adding several drops of specimen to media
  - For solid media, the specimen can be streaked
  - Specimen types: Bronchial brush/wash, aspirates, CSF, swabs, body fluids, hairs, scrapings
- Concentration
  - Large volumes can be concentrated by centrifugation
  - Specimen types: Body fluids, CSF, urines
- Minced (homogenized)
  - Some solid specimens must be "destroyed" to expose a buried pathogen to the media
  - Specimen types: Nails, tissues, biopsies
- Culture of fungi
- Petri dishes or tubes
  - Oxygen requirements

TABLE 2-1	Major Medically Important Fungi
Category	**Genus**
Opportunistic fungi	*Aspergillus*
	Candida
	Mucor
	Rhizopus
Superficial mycoses	*Exophiala*
	Malassezia
	Piedraia
	Trichosporon
Dermatophytic mycoses	*Epidermophyton*
	Microsporum
	Trichophyton
Subcutaneous mycoses	*Cladosporium*
	Exophiala
	Pseudallescheria
	Phialophora
	Sporothrix
Systemic mycoses	*Blastomyces*
	Coccidioides
	Histoplasma
	Paracoccidioides

- Humidity
- Subculture sometimes necessary
  - Temperature range
  - Dimorphism
  - Sexual and asexual developmental structures
  - Get rid of bacterial contamination
- Teasing needles
  - Used more than bacteriologic loop
- Electric incinerator
  - Flame causes aerosols
- Culture is very important
  - Can be main identification
  - No or few biochemicals
    - Yeasts are the exception
- Culture media
  - Options
    - Test tubes for primary
      - Less likely to become contaminated, less drying
    - Petri dishes for subculture
      - Larger surface area for growth
  - Use of inhibitory substances may be required
    - Chloramphenicol, gentamicin, cycloheximide
    - May encounter some fungal inhibition
- Common media
  - Sabouraud dextrose agar (SDA)
    - Most common, many fungi grow
    - Emmon's modification: Less glucose
      - *Blastomyces dermatitidis*
  - Mycosel and mycobiotic
    - SDA + chloramphenicol + cycloheximide
    - Selective recovery of dimorphs and dermatophytes
  - Brain heart infusion (BHI) agar
    - Enriched to enhance recovery *C. neoformans* of and dimorphic transitions in *Sporothrix* and *Paracoccidioides*
    - Plates or tubes
    - Broth + penicillin for *Zygomycetes*
  - BHI + gentamicin + chloramphenicol
    - *C. neoformans* from contaminated specimen
  - Sabouraud dextrose + BHI (SABHI)
    - Strengths of both
    - Enriched medium for *Cryptococcus* spp., thermally dimorphic fungi, etc.
  - CHROMagar *Candida*
    - Selective and differential for presumptive identification of genus *Candida* from primary plates
    - Morphology and colors of the yeast colonies vary by species
    - *Candida albicans*—light to medium green; *Candida tropicalis*—light blue to metallic-blue; *Candida krusei*—light rose with a whitish border
  - Inhibitory mold agar (IMA)
    - Inorganic salts, chloramphenicol, gentamicin
    - Inhibits bacteria

- Dermatophyte test medium (DTM)
  - Dermatophytes from heavily contaminated specimens (pink-to-red color change)
  - Commonly used in office practices
- Media for subculture
  - Potato dextrose agar (PDA)
  - Potato flake agar (PFA)
  - Incubation
    - Obligate filamentous: 25° or 37° C
    - Dimorphics: 25° and 37° C
    - Yeast: 25° or 37° C
  - Aerobic
  - 3 to 4 weeks
  - Cornmeal agar for yeast morphology
    - Recommended for promoting sporulation
- Pathogen versus contaminant
  - The clinical picture
    - Are patients' symptoms consistent with fungal infection?
    - Does this fungus normally cause these symptoms?
  - Laboratory findings
    - Fungal elements in tissue or other specimen
    - Fungus grown in culture
    - More than one culture positive
- Quality control
  - Assessing quality of specimens
  - Monitoring performance
    - Tests, reagents, media, instruments
    - Quality control culture collections
  - Personnel
    - Performance evaluation
    - Proficiency testing
- Laboratory identification
  - Direct examination of clinical specimens
    - Laboratory methods and tissue stains
  - Macroscopic/microscopic evaluation
    - Colony features and hyphae/conidia morphology
  - Advanced methods
    - Exoantigen, DNA probes, DNA sequencing
  - Microscopic examination
    - Direct examination can be used on several types of specimens
      - Can identify yeast and filamentous forms
      - Culture is used regardless
    - Several preparations for direct examination
      - Potassium hydroxide (KOH) preparation
      - Calcofluor white
      - India ink: Historical
  - KOH preparation
    - Examine hair, nails, skin scrapings, fluids, exudates, and biopsy specimens
    - Can see important fungal elements
      - Hyphae, yeast
      - Need reduced light or phase-contrast
    - 15% KOH added to specimen
      - Dissolves specimen quickly (fungi slowly)

- Can be modified to include calcofluor white
  - Binds to cell wall and fluoresces blue-white under ultraviolet light
- India ink
  - Historically used with CSF specimens
  - Negative stain
    - Creates black background to visualize capsular material
    - *C. neoformans*
    - More specific/sensitive tests are now available
      - Cryptococcal antigen test
- Tissue examination: Stains
  - Giemsa, Wright-Giemsa
    - *Histoplasmosis capsulatum* (intracellular)
  - Hematoxylin and eosin (H&E)
    - Pink to pinkish-blue
  - Meyer's mucicarmine
    - *C. neoformans:* Rose red
  - Gomori methenamine silver (GMS)
    - Black
  - Papanicolaou stain
    - Pink to blue
  - Periodic acid–Schiff (PAS)
    - Red or purple
- Macroscopic examination
  - Growth conditions
    - Yeasts: 2 to 3 days
    - Molds
      - Rapid: Less than 5 days
      - Intermediate: 6 to 10 days
      - Slow: More than 11 (sometimes 8 weeks)
    - Dimorphism
  - Pigment
    - Front versus back of plate
  - Texture
    - Dictated by presence and length of aerial hyphae
    - Glabrous: Leathery, waxy
    - Velvety: Suede, plush
    - Yeastlike: Looks like *Staphylococcus*
    - Cottony: Fluffy
    - Granular: Powdery
  - Topography
    - Rugose
      - Radial grooves, "folded"
    - Crateriform
      - Central depression and raised edge
    - Verrucous
      - Rough knobs
    - Cerebriform
      - Brainlike
- Examination of molds
  - Three methods
    - Tease/cut preparation
      - Organism removed directly from culture plate
      - "Teased" apart with teasing needles
    - Scotch tape preparation
      - Scotch tape pressed onto culture plate
      - Transferred to microscope slide
    - Slide culture
      - Organism subcultured to a small piece of agar
      - Covered with a coverslip
      - Organism grows onto coverslip: Remove and examine
      - Best method
- Examination of molds
  - Use one of the three methods listed previously, followed by addition of stain
    - Lactophenol cotton blue (LPCB)
- Dermatophyte identification
  - Hair perforation
    - 5- to 10-mm sterile hair floated on sterile water and yeast extract
    - Conidia or hyphae inoculated onto water surface
    - Remove hair shafts and observe in LPCB weekly for 1 month
    - *Trichophyton rubrum* negative, *Trichophyton mentagrophytes* positive
  - Urease test
    - Tubes of urease agar are lightly inoculated
    - 5 days at room temperature
    - *T. rubrum* negative or weak, *T. mentagrophytes* positive
  - *Trichophyton* agars
    - Originally numbers 1 to 4
    - Most laboratories use only 1 and 4
      - Thiamine requirement
      - *Trichophyton* agar 1 (without thiamine) and *Trichophyton* agar 4 (with thiamine)
      - 10 to 14 days, observe for growth
  - Rice grain growth
    - Sterile, nonfortified rice grain media
    - 10 days, observe for growth
    - *Microsporum canis* versus *Microsporum audouinii*
- Summary: Mold identification
- Specimen source or infection
- Growth rate to reproductive structures
- Colony color front and back on plate
- Microscopic morphology
  - Septate or aseptate hyphae
  - Conidiophore structure
  - Microconidia/macroconidia
  - Other structures
- Advanced techniques
  - Exoantigen test
    - Rapid information of immunoidentity
      - Extract soluble antigen from unknown isolate
      - Concentrate
      - React with antiserum specific to known fungi
      - Positive control necessary for definitive identification

- Test is read at 24 hours
- *Blastomyces, Coccidioides, Histoplasma*
  - DNA probe
    - Rapid kits that use nucleic acid hybridization to identify fungi in culture
    - Highly specific to each fungus, because it is based on DNA sequence
    - Needs to be performed on cultured organisms
      - Not from specimens
    - Developed for *Coccidioides, Blastomyces, Histoplasma*
    - Specialized clinical laboratories are using DNA sequencing techniques to establish fungal identifications
- Laboratory identification of yeast
  - Macroscopic morphology
    - Colony color and texture
    - Color: White, tan, pink, salmon
      - Can have dematiaceous yeasts
    - Texture: Mucoid, butterlike, velvety, wrinkled
  - Microscopic morphology: Wet preparation
    - Hyphae
    - Pseudohyphae
    - Blastoconidia
  - Cornmeal Tween 80 agar
    - Encourages development of chlamydospores
    - Relationships among hyphae, pseudohyphae, and others
    - Clear media: Can be observed under light microscope
    - Specific organisms associated with specific morphology
  - Cornmeal agar morphology
    - Used in conjunction with carbohydrate usage
    - Four main morphology types
      - Hyphae
      - Pseudohyphae
      - Arthroconidia
      - Chlamydoconidia or blastoconidia
    - Pseudohyphae and blastoconidia only
      - *C. krusei*
      - *Candida parapsilosis*
      - *Candida kefyr*
      - *C. tropicalis*
    - Blastoconidia only
      - *Candida glabrata*
      - *C. neoformans*
    - Arthroconidia
      - *Trichosporon beigelii*
  - Physiologic tests
    - Germ tube test
      - Filamentous outgrowth from blastoconidia
      - Most basic and easiest to perform
      - Requires the use of serum or plasma
        - Some commercially made broths (will last longer)
      - Overincubation and overinoculation are biggest problems

- Other agents can form germ tubes
  - Not valid if read after 2 hours
  - "True" germ tube: *C. albicans*
  - No constriction at base, where the tube attaches to the mother cell
  - A constricted base indicates *C. tropicalis*
  - Other species have germ tubes
    - *Candida stellatoidea* (Sucrose assimilation used to differentiate from *C. albicans*)
    - *Candida dubliniensis* (no growth at 45° C)
  - Positive and negative controls are necessary
  - Fermentation/Assimilation
    - Fermentation
      - Carbohydrate use in absence of oxygen
    - Assimilation
      - Which can be used as a sole carbon source?
      - Two systems (assimilation)
    - API 20C (others): Strip test
    - Vitek: Automated
  - Urea hydrolysis
    - Detected on simple urea agar
    - Rapid, easy
    - Differentiates *Cryptococcus* from *Rhodotorula*
    - Positive: Pink
    - Negative: Little to no change
  - Temperature studies
    - *Cryptococcus* spp.
      - Weak growth at 35° C and no growth at 42° C
    - *Candida* spp.
      - Several can grow well exceeding 45° C
- Order of events
  - Most yeasts
    - Wet preparation
    - Germ tube
      - Germ tube negative and from sterile site
    - Corn meal morphology
    - Physiologic/biochemical tests
    - Temperature

THE OPPORTUNISTIC MOLDS

- Most frequently isolated fungi
- Opportunistic infections
- Infect those who are injured or debilitated
- Common inhabitant of soil and organic debris
- Laboratory and environmental contaminant

Acremonium Species

- No known sexual stage: Fungi imperfecti
- Filamentous fungus in plant debris and soil
- Two more common species
  - *Acremonium falciforme*
  - *Acremonium kiliense*
- Cause onychomycosis, keratitis, endocarditis, meningitis, peritonitis, and osteomyelitis
- Macroscopic

- Rapid grower
- White, cottony colonies
- Microscopic
  - Hyaline, septate hyphae
  - Unbranched, solitary, erect phialides formed directly on the hyphal tips
  - Conidia usually in clusters or fragile chains
  - Therapy and susceptibility testing
- In vitro susceptibility
  - Limited data and minimum inhibitory concentration (MIC) breakpoints have not been defined
  - Newer azoles (voriconazole, posaconazole) exhibit good in vitro activity
  - Itraconazole MICs somewhat higher than MICs in voriconazole
  - MICs of caspofungin are relatively low

Fusarium Species

- No known sexual stage: Fungi imperfecti
- Plants and soil
  - Normal mycoflora of commodities (rice)
- More than 20 species
  - *Fusarium solani, Fusarium oxysporum, Fusarium chlamydosporum*
- Fusariosis
  - Emerging cause of opportunistic mycoses
  - Disseminated infections have high mortality
  - Trauma or inhaled conidia
- Macroscopic
  - Rapid grower, woolly to cottony, flat, spreading colonies
  - Front: White, cream, tan, salmon, cinnamon, yellow, red, violet, pink, or purple
    - Reverse: Colorless, tan, red, dark purple, or brown
- Microscopic
  - Macroconidia: Two or more cells, thick walled, smooth, and cylindrical or sickle (canoe) shaped

Geotrichum Species

- Lack known sexual stage
- Found worldwide in soil, water, air, sewage, plants, cereals, and dairy products
- Found in normal human flora
- Genus includes several species
  - More common: *Geotrichum candidum, Geotrichum clavatum, Geotrichum fici*
- May cause opportunistic infections in immunocompromised host
  - Infections acquired via ingestion or inhalation
- Macroscopic
  - Produce rapid growing, white, dry, powdery-to-cottony colonies resembling ground glass
  - Colony may be yeastlike
  - Optimal growth temperature is 25° C

- Most strains either do not grow at all or grow weakly at 37° C
- Microscopic
  - Arthroconidia and coarse true hyphae are observed
  - Blastoconidia, conidiophores, and pseudohyphae are absent
  - Undifferentiated hyphae may be present
  - Arthroconidia observed
    - Either rectangular or rounded at the ends
    - Do not alternate with normal cells

Paecilomyces Species

- Sexual stage described: Teleomorph
- Soil, decaying plants, and food products
- Several species
  - *Paecilomyces lilacinus* and *Paecilomyces variotii* most common
- Causes wide range of mycoses
  - Emerging opportunistic pathogen
  - Onychomycosis, sinusitis, otitis media, endocarditis, osteomyelitis, peritonitis, and catheter-related fungemia
- Macroscopic
  - Rapid grower
  - *P. variotii* is thermophilic
  - Colonies are flat, powdery, or velvety
    - Initially white and becomes yellow, yellow-green, yellow-brown, olive-brown, pink, or violet, depending on the species
    - Reverse is dirty white, buff, or brown
  - May resemble *Penicillium* spp. macroscopically and microscopically
- Microscopic
  - Septate, hyaline hyphae
  - Conidiophores are often branched
  - Phialides are swollen at the base and taper toward the apice
  - Usually grouped in pairs or brushlike clusters
  - Conidia are unicellular, hyaline to darkly colored, and form long chains

Penicillium Species

- Teleomorph described
- *Penicillium marneffei* is thermal dimorph (Southeast Asia)
- Numerous species
  - More common: *Penicillium chrysogenum, Penicillium citrinum*
- Particularly virulent in patients with AIDS
  - Keratitis, endophthalmitis, otomycosis, necrotizing esophagitis, pneumonia, endocarditis, peritonitis, and urinary tract infections (UTIs)
  - *P. marneffei* often fatal
- Macroscopic

- Rapid growing; velvety, woolly, or cottony
- Initially white and become blue-green, gray-green, olive-gray, yellow, or pinkish
  - Reverse is usually pale to yellowish
- Microscopic
  - Flask-shaped phialides
  - Form brushlike clusters
  - Conidia are round, unicellular, and form unbranching chains at the tips of the phialides

Scopulariopsis Species

- Soil, plant material, feathers, and insects
- Unique in that it contains both hyaline and dematiaceous species
  - *Scopulariopsis brevicaulis* (hyaline)
  - *Scopulariopsis cinerea* (dematiaceous)
- Onychomycosis, especially of the toe nails
- Disseminated infections: High mortality
- Macroscopic
  - Grow moderately rapidly, granular to powdery
  - Front color is white initially and becomes light brown or buff
  - Reverse color is usually tan with brownish center
- Microscopic
  - Septate hyphae
  - Conidiophores are hyphae-like and simple or branched

Aspergillus Species

- More than 185 species
- Approximately 20 species have been described as agents of infection in humans
- Most common: *Aspergillus fumigatus, Aspergillus flavus, Aspergillus niger*
- Less common: *Aspergillus clavatus, Aspergillus glaucus* group, *Aspergillus nidulans*
- Clinical disease
  - Three clinical settings
    - Opportunistic infections
    - Allergic states
    - Toxin production
  - Opportunistic infections
    - Local infections
    - Local colonization in previously developed lung cavity
    - Infection of every organ system has been described
    - Disseminated infections
  - Allergic reactions
    - Allergic bronchopulmonary aspergillosis
  - Toxins
    - Aflatoxin
    - Veterinary diseases
- Laboratory Identification

- Rate of growth is usually rapid
  - Usually matures in 3 days
  - Some species are slower
- Temperature
  - *A. fumigatus* grows well at 45° C
- Macroscopic
  - First white then yellow, green, brown, or black
- Microscopic
  - Hyphae are septate
  - Unbranched conidiophore from a "foot cell"
  - Vesicles
  - Phialides cover the surface of the vesicle entirely ("radiate" head) or partially only at the upper surface ("columnar" head)
  - Phialides are either uniseriate (attached to the vesicle directly) or biseriate (attached to the vesicle via a supporting cell) metula
  - Conidia form radial chains

ZYGOMYCETES

- Zygomycetes is the name of a class of fungi
- This class includes three orders: Mucorales, Mortierellales, and Entomophthorales
- Most clinically significant are in Mucorales
  - *Absidia, Cunninghamella, Mucor, Rhizomucor, Rhizopus*
- Zygomycosis
  - Sometimes incorrectly referred to as mucormycosis
  - Inhalation of sporangiospores, trauma (inoculation)
  - Can become invasive
  - Sinus infections are common
  - Typical presentation
    - Pulmonary, rhinocerebral, cutaneous, renal, or meningeal involvement
  - Risks
    - Diabetes, leukopenia, immunosuppression, AIDS, burns, intravenous drug
  - Rapid growth
    - More tissue damage, almost always fatal
    - Rapidly fill plate in culture: "Lid lifters"
  - Differentiation
    - Presence (or absence) and location of rhizoids—rootlike structures
    - Branched or unbranched nature of sporangiophore
    - Size and shape of sporangium
    - Macroscopic of similar

Mucor Species

- Several pathogenic species
  - Many do not grow at 37° C
- Rapid growth, fluffy (cotton candy), white initially and becomes grayish-brown in time
  - Reverse is white

- Aseptate or sparsely septate, broad hyphae, sporangiophores long and branched with terminal sporangia
- No rhizoids

Rhizopus Species

- Several important species
- 50% of all zygomycoses
- 90% of rhinocerebral infections
- Grow very rapidly, cotton-candy white initially and turns gray to yellowish-brown in time
  - Reverse side is white
- Pathogenic species of *Rhizopus* can grow well at 37° C
- Broad, aseptate hyphae, long unbranched sporagiophores
- Rhizoids are produced

Rhizomucor Species

- Rare cause of zygomycosis
  - Normally fatal
- Colony similar to that of *Mucor*
- Microscopic
  - Intermediate to *Mucor* and *Rhizopus*
  - Short rhizoids and branched sporangiophores

Absidia Species

- 21 species
  - *Absidia corymbifera* is the only clinically significant species
- Rapid growth, woolly to cottony, and olive-gray colonies
  - Reverse side uncolored
- Broad aseptate hyphae, sporangiophores branched and arise in groups of two to five
- Sporangiospores are one-celled and round to oval

Cunninghamella Species

- Seven species
  - *Cunninghamella bertholletiae* is the only known human and animal pathogen
  - Rapid growing, cottony, and white to tannish-gray
    - Reverse is pale
  - Aseptate or sparsely septate broad hyphae, sporangiophores long and branched
  - Vesicles
  - Sporangiophores are erect and form short lateral branches, each of which terminates in a swollen vesicle

SUPERFICIAL MYCOSES

- Among the most prevalent of human infectious diseases
- Mycotic infections of hair, skin, and nails

- Tineas: Skin
- Piedras: Hair
- Nonliving layer of the skin and extrafollicular hair
- Lack of systemic immune response
- Specimens are cultured onto SDA
  - Sometimes with antibiotics
- Diagnosis
  - Appearance of lesion
  - Skin scrapings
  - Hair shafts
- Four main infections
  - Tinea versicolor
  - Tinea nigra
  - White piedra
  - Black piedra
- Tinea versicolor
  - *Malassezia furfur*
    - Superficial infection of the keratinized layers of skin
    - Normal flora of skin (90% asymptomatic)
    - No known reason for predisposition
    - Clinical picture
      - Patches of hypopigmented or hyperpigmented lesions
      - Brown or fawn, scaling, redness
      - Chest, back, shoulders, arms, abdomen (itch, burn)
    - Specimen: Skin
      - Direct examination: KOH will show yeastlike and hyphal forms
    - Culture: Lipophilic organism
      - Add oil overlay and incubate at 37° C
    - Microscopic
      - Thick-walled hyphae and "yeast," some budding
      - Spaghetti and meatballs
- Tinea nigra
  - *Hortaea werneckii*
  - *Exophilia* and *Cladosporium werneckii* obsolete names
  - Central and North America, Southeast Asia, Africa, Europe
  - Most likely environmental
  - Clinical disease
    - Synonyms: Pityriasis nigra, tinea nigra palmaris
    - Infection of keratinized skin layers of hand
    - More common in those under 25 years of age and females
    - Dark skin on one hand (usually only one)
    - Flat, brown lesion
      - Possibility of melanoma must be ruled out
    - Direct examination: KOH preparation
    - Culture
      - Required to differentiate from melanoma
  - *H. werneckii*
    - Macroscopic

- Colonies grow slowly and mature within 21 days
- Initially pale in color, moist, shiny, and yeastlike
- Colonies become velvety, olive black, and covered with a thin layer of mycelium
  - The reverse side is black
- Does not grow at 37° C
  ○ Microscopic features
  - Septate hyphae, yeastlike conidia, and chlamydospores
  - Hyaline initially and become olive colored
  - Annellides present
    - Annelloconidia are intercalary and lateral
  - Septate, thick-walled hyphae formed
- White piedra
  - Caused by *Trichosporon* spp.
    ○ Most commonly *T. beigelii*
    ○ *T. beigelii* may not have taxonomic status
  - infection of hair of beard and mustache
  - Environmental (soil and air)
    ○ South and North America, Far East, Europe
  - Clinical disease
    ○ Soft white to tan nodules
    ○ Surround hair shaft, separated easily from hair
    ○ Hair breaks at nodule
    ○ Can become systemic in immunocompromised
  - Direct examination: KOH preparation
  - Culture
    ○ Not normally required
    ○ SDA: Yeastlike colonies
  - Microscopic
    ○ Nodule surrounding hair
  - *Trichosporon* spp.
    ○ Macroscopic
    - Colonies are rapid growing
    - Yeastlike, may be smooth, wrinkled, raised, folded
    - White to cream colored
    - Urease production characteristic
  - Microscopic
    ○ Many pseudohyphae and hyphae
    ○ Blastoconidia are unicellular and variable in shape
    ○ Arthroconidia produced
- Black piedra
  - *Piedraia hortae*
  - Fungal infection on hair (scalp)
  - Forms black, stony, hard nodules
  - Central and South America, Southern Asia, Africa
  - Swimming in rivers and stagnant waters
  - Clinical picture
    ○ Nodules firmly attached, can be microscopic to visible by naked eye, hair feels rough
  - Direct examination
    ○ KOH preparation
  - Culture

○ Not usually required
○ Slow grower (25° C)
- Does not penetrate hair shaft
- *Piedraia hortae*
  ○ Macroscopic
    - Colonies are slow growing
    - Small, folded, dark brown to black
    - May produce a reddish-brown diffusible pigment
      - Reverse side is black
  ○ Microscopic
    - Septate hyphae, asci, and ascospores
      - Asci are ellipsoid, solitary, or in clusters and contain eight ascospores
    - Hyphae pigmented

SUBCUTANEOUS MYCOSES

- Four major infections caused by several fungi
  - Mycetoma
  - Chromoblastomycosis
  - Phaeohyphomycosis
  - Sporotrichosis
- Common to all
  - Lesion develops at site of inoculation (localized)
  - Soil saprophytes that are moderately slow growers
- Most commonly accepted
  - *Cladophialophora, Exophiala, Fonsecaea, Phialophora, Wangiella, Pseudallescheira/Scedosporium, Sporothrix schenckii*
- Most infections are due to traumatic inoculation
- Common in tropics and subtropics
- Some of these fungi cause more than one type of subcutaneous infection
- Most are dematiaceous fungi
  - Dematiaceous versus hyaline
- Conidiation of dematiaceous fungi
  - *Cladosporium* type
    ○ Resembles a tree, in which conidiophore is the trunk and branched chains of conidia form the branches
  - *Phialophora* type
    ○ Short conidiophores + phialide, vase shaped, conidia extruded from phialide and then cluster
  - *Rhinocladiella* type
    ○ Stalked conidiophores that become knobby as conidia are produced, conidia produced sequentially until a *Cladosporium* type of conidiation is reached
- Laboratory identification of subcutaneous fungi
  - Specimens collected by aspiration
    ○ Large amount of material, reduces chances that specimen will dry out
  - Granules observed and noted
  - SDA with and without antibiotics
    ○ PDA for subculture
  - Biochemicals are available, but rarely done

Mycetoma

- General
  - Chronic granulomatous disease of feet (lower extremities)
    - Madura foot or maduromycosis
  - Enlarged nodules, sinus drainage, bone destruction
  - Exudate contains granules
  - No lymphatic system involvement (remain localized)
  - Two types: Eumycotic and actinomycotic
- Laboratory procedures
  - Direct examination: KOH preparation
  - Identification granules, colorless or pigmented septate hyphae
    - Actinomycotic granules: Mycelium with hyphae 1 μm in diameter
    - Eumycotic granules: Wide hyphae (2-4 μm) terminating in chlamydoconidia

Chromoblastomycosis

- General
  - Localized disease of skin and subcutaneous tissue
  - Verrucoid (wartlike) lesions on feet, legs, hands, and buttocks
  - Soil saprophytes that are introduced by trauma (worldwide), dematiaceous
  - Spreads through the body lymphatics or by autoinoculation
- Laboratory procedures
  - Direct examination: KOH exudate, crusts from lesion
  - Microscopic: Single-celled or clusters of single cells, dark pigment
  - Culture: SDA at room temperature, hold for 6 weeks
  - Looking for three types of conidiation
    - *Cladosporium* type
    - *Rhinocladiella* type
    - *Phialophora* type
- Phaeohyphomycosis
  - Infection of subcutaneous tissue
    - Classically: Infection with a dematiaceous fungus
    - The others have become distinct
      - Mycetoma
      - Chromoblastomycosis
      - Sporotrichosis
    - Miscellaneous dematiaceous fungi: Introduced through trauma
  - Systemic infection is a disease of the immunocompromised
  - KOH preparation shows pigmented hyphae

Cladophialophora carrionii
- Cause of chromoblastomycosis
  - No shoes, trauma

- *Cladisporium carrionii* obsolete name
- Very slow grower (up to 30 days)
- Colonies are gray-green to black on surface and reverse, cottony
- Pigmented, septate hyphae
- *Cladosporium* type of conidiation

Fonsecaea pedrosoi
- Causes chromoblastomycosis and phaeohyphomycosis
  - Traumatic injury
- Gray-green to black, cottony colony within 21 days
- Pigmented, septate hyphae
- All three types of conidiation
  - Phialophora, Cladosporium, Rhinocladiella

Fonsecaea compacta
- Conidial heads of *Cladosporium* type of conidiation are more compact

Phialophora verrucosa
- Causes chromoblastomycosis and phaeohyphomycosis
- Autoinoculation and lymphatic system
- Macroscopic
  - Olive-green to black, velvety
- Microscopic
  - Pigmented, septate hyphae
  - Only *Phialophora* type of conidiation

Pseudallescheria boydii
- *Scedosporium apiospermum:* Name for alternate asexual stage
- Major etiologic agent of mycetoma in the United States and Europe
- Different from other subcutaneous
  - Grows rapidly, hyaline, has a sexual form
- Macroscopic
  - White to brownish-gray, fluffy colonies
- Microscopic
  - Hyaline, septate hyphae
  - Single anelloconidia produced on an anellophore (conidiophore)

Exophiala jeanselmei
- Cause of mycetoma and phaeohyphomycosis
- Minor trauma and contaminated fomites
- Young cultures
  - Appear as black yeasts
- Mature cultures
  - Velvety colonies
- Sticklike conidiophores with clustered conidia

Wangiella dermatitidis
- Causes pheohyphomycosis
- Macroscopic
  - Initially resemble black yeast
  - Longer 10 days, olive-gray to black velvety or glabrous colony
  - *Wangiella* spp. grow better at 40° to 42° C
- Microscopic
  - Pigmented, septate hyphae
  - Conidiophores are indistinguishable from vegetative hyphae, except that conidia are clustered at ends
- Similar morphology to *E. jeanselmei*

Acremonium Species

- Etiologic agent of mycetomas, corneal infections, and nail infections
- See Opportunistic Fungi section

Dermatophytes

- Dermatophytosis: Infections of keratinized tissue (hair, skin, nails)
- Most common: Ringworm
- Three major genera
  - *Trichophyton*
  - *Microsporum*
  - *Epidermophyton*
- Intermediate to slow growers
- Worldwide distribution
- Routes of infection
  - Defined in three ways
    - Geophilic: Soil to man
    - Zoophilic: Animal to human
    - Anthropophilic: Person to person
  - Approximately 43 accepted species
  - Types of infections
    - Tinea barbae: Facial hair
    - Tinea capitis: Scalp
    - Tinea corporis: Arms, legs, and trunk
    - Tinea cruris: "Jock itch" affects the groin area
    - Tinea faciei: Face
    - Tinea manuum: Hands
    - Tinea pedis: "Athlete's foot"
    - Tinea unguinum: Fingernails and toenails
    - Hair and hair follicles
      - Favic: Hair follicle, crusty lesions
      - Ectothrix: Colonizes outside of shaft
      - Endothrix: Hair follicle first, growth inside shaft
    - Nail and nail bed
      - Onychomycosis
    - Skin
  - Laboratory diagnosis
    - Specimens: Hair, skin scraping, nail scraping or clipping
    - KOH preparation (+ calcofluor)
      - Hair infections
        - Endothrix
        - Ectothrix
      - Skin and nail infections
        - Septate hyphae
    - Wood's lamp
  - Culture
    - SDA with and without inhibitory agents
    - 30° C for 4 weeks
    - Colony morphology
    - Microconidia and macroconidia
      - Trichophyton
        - Macroconida rare, thin-walled, smooth
        - Microconida numerous

- Microsporum
  - Macroconida numerous, thick-walled, rough
  - Microconida usually present
- Epidermophyton
  - Macroconida numerous, thin and thick walled, smooth
  - Microconida not formed

Microsporum audouinii

- Anthropophilic: Person to person
  - Children
- Positive Wood's lamp fluorescence
- Rare distorted macroconidia, rare microconidia
- Light-tan front
  - Reverse salmon to colorless
- No growth on sterile rice media

Microsporum canis

- Zoophilic
- Wood's lamp fluorescence
- Skin and hair
- Bright yellow colony reverse
  - Especially on PDA
- Large spindle-shaped macroconidia
  - 3 to 15 cells, tapering ends
  - Many microconidia

Microsporum gypseum

- Geophilic
- Rapid grower
- Not commonly infective
  - Skin and hair
- Powdery/granular buff-to-brown colony
- "Rowboat"-shaped macroconidia
  - Six or fewer septa

Microsporum nanum

- Zoophilic
- Flat beige, brown, or white colony
- Small macroconidia
  - One or two septa
- Rare cause of tinea corporis in humans

Epidermophyton floccosum

- Anthropophilic
- Tinea cruris (+ pedis, + unguium)
- Does not infect hair
- No microconidia
- Smooth-walled, club-shaped, groupings of macroconidia (beaver's tail)
- Colony: Khaki-yellow

Trichophyton mentagrophytes

- Anthropophilic and zoophilic
- Infects all three keratinized tissues
- Most common cause of athlete's foot
- Buff and powdery to white, cottony colony
  - Reverse side may be yellow, brown, colorless, or red
- Spiral hyphae
- Round clustering microconidia and cigar-shaped macroconidia
- Urease positive, perforates hair

Trichophyton rubrum
- Anthropophilic: Person to person
- Ectothrix, if infect hair
- Most commonly infects skin and nails
- White fluffy colony
  - Reverse side red
- Tear-drop shaped microconidia
  - Can produce macroconidia
- Urease negative, does not perforate hair

Trichophyton tonsurans
- Anthropophilic
- Endothrix
  - Most common endothrix dermatophyte in the United States
- "Black dot" tinea capitis
- Beige-to-olive granular colony with brown rust edge
- Size and shape variation in microconidia
- Requires thiamine

Trichophyton schoenleinii
- Anthropophilic
- Slow growing
- Endothrix
- Colonies orange/brown and wrinkled when young, flat when mature
- No macroconidia, rare microconidia
- Antler-shaped hyphae

THE CLINICALLY SIGNIFICANT YEASTS

- Significant part of the normal flora
  - Skin and mucous membranes
- Infections are often endogenous
- Opportunists
- Greater immune suppression results in a greater variety of yeast infections
- Yeasts are most frequently isolated fungi

Candida Species

- Common normal flora of skin, mucosa, and digestive tract
- Can cause many infections
  - Vulvovaginitis, thrush, pulmonary infections, eye infections, meningitis, endocarditis, and disseminated infections
- Opportunist
- Causative agent of thrush
  - Indicator of immunosuppression
  - HIV, prolonged antimicrobial therapy, and chemotherapy: Can be serious and become disseminated

Candida albicans
- Most common cause of yeast infection
- Can cause disease in any site when host defense is altered
- Macroscopic
  - Creamy
- Microscopic

- Clusters of blastoconidia along pseudohyphae, terminal chlamydoconidia
- C. albicans CMT morphology
- Germ tube positive, sucrose positive
- C. stellatoidea (sucrose negative)
- Macroscopic morphology

Candida tropicalis
- Second most common Candida spp.
  - Vaginitis, intestinal disease, systemic infections, meningitis
- Infections are aggressive and very difficult to treat with traditional antifungals
- Macroscopic
  - Creamy, glabrous with mycelial fringe
- Microscopic
  - Blastoconidia are single or small random clusters along pseudohyphae
  - C. tropicalis CMT morphology

Candida parapsilosis
- Major cause of nosocomial infections
- Indwelling catheter
- Macroscopic
  - Creamy, glabrous
- Microscopic
  - Relatively short, crooked or curved pseudohyphae
- C. parapsilosis CMT morphology

Candida kreusi
- Rarely isolated as a cause of endocarditis and vaginitis
- Macroscopic
  - Creamy, flat colonies
- Microscopic
  - Pseudohyphae and elongated blastoconidia, branch like trees
  - C. krusei CMT morphology

Torulopsis glabrata
- Also referred to as Candida glabrata
- Most commonly found as fungemia
  - Endocarditis, meningitis, UTI
- Macroscopic
  - Creamy, smooth, moist
- Microscopic
  - Blastoconidia only (on CMT), no pseudohyphae

Saccharomyces cerevisiae
- The "working yeast"
  - Bread, beer, wine
- Can occasionally be normal flora
- Increasingly isolated from immunocompromised
- Macroscopic
  - Creamy, smooth, moist
- Microscopic
  - Yeast cells and short pseudohyphae

Cryptococcus Species
- Causative agent of meningitis and pulmonary disease
- C. neoformans
  - Major cause of opportunistic infection in patients with AIDS

- Found in soil contaminated with pigeon excreta
  - Meningitis: Predilection for central nervous system
- All species are surrounded by a capsule
  - Gives the mucoid colony appearance
  - India ink detects capsule: Negative stain
  - Being replaced by latex agglutination for cryptococcal antigen
    - India ink has low detection rate
- Do not produce true hyphae or pseudohyphae on cornmeal agar, blastoconidia only
- All species are urease positive
  - Nitrate variable
- Phenol oxidase
  - *C. neoformans*
  - Causes melanin production on caffeic acid agar or bird seed agar
  - Dark colony color
- Sugar assimilation also varies

Rhodotorula Species
- Bright, salmon-colored colonies
- Closely related to *Cryptococcus*
  - Capsule production
  - Urease positive
  - Some are nitrate positive
- Not common agents of disease
- Do cause some opportunistic infections

Geotrichum candidum
- Normal flora in intestinal tract
- Causes rare infections in immunocompromised
- Macroscopic
  - White, moist, yeast-like
- Microscopic
  - True hyphae, segment into arthroconidia, no blastoconidia

Trichosporon beigelii
- Cause of white piedra
  - Personal hygiene disease
- Emerging agent of disseminated infection
  - Mostly in cancer patients
- Produces arthroconidia and blastoconidia on cornmeal agar

Malassezia furfur
- Normal skin flora in 90% of humans
- Tinea versicolor
- Catheter-related infections in patients on long-term intravenous lipids
- Macroscopic
  - Cream/brown wrinkled
- Microscopic
  - Yeastlike cells

Sporobolomyces Species
- Most often recovered from environmental samples
- Rare cause of infection in immunocompromised patients
- Macroscopic
  - Salmon-colored smooth colonies
- Microscopic
  - Oval, elongate yeast cells, projectile spores

Pneumocystis jiroveci
- Group is contested
  - Yeast-protozoa-fungus
- Opportunistic
  - AIDS
  - Cellular immunity
- *Pneumocystis* pneumonia
  - Fever, nonproductive cough, shortness of breath
  - Destroys alveolar cells
- Laboratory diagnosis
  - Must demonstrate the organism in tissue, lavage, or sputum
  - Cannot culture except in animal
  - GMS commonly used stain
    - "Deflated ball"
  - Fluorescent antibody available

DIMORPHIC FUNGI

- Mycoses that involve major body systems or more than one kind of tissue
  - Some include the opportunists in this category
  - These do not need "situational" help
- Thermal dimorphism
  - *Blastomyces dermatitidis*
  - *Coccidioides immitis*
  - *Histoplasma capsulatum*
  - *Paracoccidioides brasiliensis*
  - *Sporothrix schenckii*
  - *Penicillium marneffei*
- Clinical disease
  - Cause multiple kinds of infections, varying severities
  - Primary infection is pulmonary
    - Incidence of benign infection is far greater than fatal disseminated disease
    - Immunocompetent: Asymptomatic and resolves spontaneously
    - Common cold or flu symptoms
  - Can progress to acute or chronic disease
  - "Granulomatous" lesions in lungs
    - Granuloma: Collection of macrophages, giant cells, and proteinaceous material (wall off infection)
  - Yeast forms can enter lymph through macrophage and disseminate to other organ systems
  - Disseminated infections are fast moving and normally fatal
- Specimen processing
  - Tissue specimens: Minced
  - Pleural fluid and CSF: Concentrated
  - Mucus or pus: Mucolytic agent
  - When dimorph is suspected
    - Quick transport
    - Do not hold at room temperature (bacteria may overgrow)
    - Do not refrigerate

- Microscopic
  - KOH preparation: Easiest, quickest
    - Calcofluor
  - H&E, PAS, and GMS for in situ tissue staining
  - Culture media
    - Primary isolation
      - SDA or SABHI with and without antimicrobials
    - Incubation at 30° C
    - BHI is sometimes recommended for better recovery on primary culture
      - PDA for subculture
- Laboratory
  - Risk factors
    - CAN CAUSE LABORATORY-ACQUIRED INFECTIONS
    - Extreme caution must be taken when these organisms are handled
    - Transmitted by respiratory route
      - All cultures handled in biosafety hood
      - Slide cultures should not be performed
  - Diagnosis: Immunologic methods
    - Most are not strong antigens
      - Cellular not humoral responses
    - Antibody detection
      - Positive: Exposure (not necessarily infection)
      - Those in endemic area are positive
      - Most patients with AIDS patients will be negative (no Ab)
  - Laboratory identification
    - Exoantigen test
      - Detects cell free extracts of the fungus
      - Material extracted from mold phase is reacted with known antisera
      - More definitive identification than colony morphology alone
  - Molecular methods

Blastomyces dermatitidis

- Endemic to North America
  - Mississippi River valley
  - Gilchrist's disease
- Most likely a soil saprobe
  - Found in wood, tree bark, rotting vegetation, river banks
- Biggest threat to immunocompromised
  - 12 cases of laboratory-acquired disease
- Blastomycosis
  - Chronic granulomatous disease affecting lungs, skin, and mucous membranes
  - Chronic cutaneous blastomycosis
    - Ulcerated lesions
    - Exposed or mucocutaneous tissues
  - Systemic blastomycosis
    - Involves any organ: Bone lesions and osteomyelitis are often encountered

- Laboratory identification
  - Specimen sources
    - Sputum
    - Aspirated pus from lymph node and subcutaneous tissue
    - Skin scrapings and biopsies
    - Blood, urine, CSF (systemic)
  - Collection and handling
    - Aseptic, plated promptly
  - Macroscopic morphology
    - 25° C: Slow growth of mold on SDA, white-to-beige waxy colony
    - 37° C: Yeast appears after 10 to 15 days, on enriched media
  - Microscopic morphology
    - Mold: Fine, septate, hyaline hyphae
      - Conidia directly on hyphae or on lateral conidiophores
    - Yeast: Hyaline, large cells, budding

Coccidioides immitis

- Endemic in hot, semiarid climates
  - Southwestern United States and northern Mexico
  - Valley fever
- Saprobe in mold form (desert soil)
- Small threat to immunocompetent
  - Occupational hazard
- Most virulent of all agents of human mycoses
  - Causes mild infection in everyone who inhales it
- Clinical disease
  - Primary pulmonary coccidiodomycosis
    - Asymptomatic and self-limiting
  - Disseminated rate in immunocompromised much higher than that of other fungal agents
  - Specimen sources
    - Sputum
    - Skin scraping
    - Blood, urine
- Laboratory identification
  - Macroscopic morphology
    - 3 to 5 days on SDA/SABHI
    - Arthroconidia in 7 to 10 days
    - Colonies are white and cottony (cobwebs)
    - Yeast form not found in laboratory
      - Spherules can be experimentally formed
  - Microscopic morphology
    - Septate hyaline hyphae
      - Wide arthroconidia: Barrel shaped
      - Disjuncture cells
    - Cultures are extremely hazardous because of many arthroconidia

Histoplasma capsulatum

- Worldwide
  - Endemic to Mississippi River and Ohio River valleys

- Soil saprobe with high nitrogen content (chicken, bird, and bat guano)
  - Spelunker's disease
- Mostly occupational hazard
- Clinical disease
  - Histoplasmosis
    - Chronic granulomatous lung disease
    - 5% progress to an acute fulminating, rapidly fatal disease (mostly in children)
    - Organism found in macrophages
  - Patients with AIDS are at high risk
  - First found in histiocytes (histo)
    - No actual capsule (capsulatum)
- Laboratory identification
  - Macroscopic
    - Slow growing mold
    - Tan, fluffy colonies
    - Yeast form in 10 to 15 days on enriched media
  - Microscopic
    - Fine septate hyphae, microconidia and macroconidia
    - Macroconidia become tuberculate with age
    - Yeast cells bud at narrow neck

Paracoccidioides brasiliensis

- Endemic to northwest, central, and southern South America, Central America, and southern Mexico
- Soil saprobe of acid soil
- Causes paracoccidioidomycosis
  - Asymptomatic and self-limiting
  - Can disseminate to other tissues
  - Can cause cutaneous disease
- Specimen: Same
- Laboratory identification
  - Macroscopic
    - Mold colony mature in 2 to 3 weeks
    - Flat, white colonies
    - Yeast will form on enriched media at 37° C
  - Microscopic
    - Fine, septate, hyaline hyphae
    - Conidiation absent on modified SDA
    - Yeast form: Multiple thin-necked buds (mariner wheel)

Sporothrix schenckii

- Found worldwide (soil saprobe)
- Sometimes grouped with subcutaneous mycoses
  - Organism is also a thermal dimorph
- Occupational risks
  - Gardening: "Rose gardener disease"
- Clinical disease
  - Sporotrichosis
    - Chronic cutaneous and subcutaneous mycosis characterized by ulcers and abscesses along lymphatic channels

- Laboratory identification
  - Specimen sources
    - Exudates and pus from lesions
    - Tissue biopsy
  - Macroscopic
    - Mold in 3 to 5 days at 25° C
    - Mature colonies are dark and flat
    - Yeast at 37° C (white or tan)
  - Microscopic
    - Mold: Delicate thin hyphae, septate, frequently found as ropes, conidiophores produce multiple conidia in flowerets arrangements
    - Two types of conidia
      - Small oval, unicellular conidia
      - Large, dark walled spheres
      - Yeast: Cigar shaped at 37° C

FUNGUS-LIKE BACTERIA

- Actinomycetes
- Three major genera
  - *Actinomyces, Nocardia,* and *Streptomyces*
  - Others: *Rhodococcus, Actinomadura,* and *Nocardiopsis*
- All higher bacteria:
  - Thought to be fungi for years
  - Some species form aerial mycelia in culture
- Clinical manifestations are similar to those of systemic fungal infection
- *Actinomyces* are anaerobic, *Nocardia* and *Streptomyces* are aerobic
- *Nocardia* stain partially acid-fast, *Actinomyces* and *Streptomyces* are not acid-fast
- All genera may produce granules, *Actinomyces* almost always produce granules

Actinomyces Species

- Gram-positive obligate anaerobes
- Reside in the mouth and in the intestinal tract
- Form abscesses and swelling at site of infection
- Diagnosis can be made by direct microscopy
  - Yellow sulfur granules: Bacterium and its waste
- *Actinomyces israelii* (most common), but several other bacteria in this genus are capable of causing disease

Nocardia Species

- Nocardiosis
- Ubiquitous soil saprophytes
- Route: Inhalation, direct inoculation
- *Nocardia asteroides* most common
- *Nocardia brasiliensis*
  - Most important in tropical areas
  - Cutaneous infection with normal immune function
  - 70% of cases are seen in immunocompromised
- Nocardiosis
  - Generally: Immunocompromised population

- Nocardia may colonize the respiratory tract
  - Immunocompetent individuals with compromised pulmonary function
  - Pneumonia can disseminate
    - Kidney, skin, gastrointestinal (GI) tract, and brain are common targets
- Laboratory identification
  - Gram-variable/modified acid-fast bacilli positive
  - Strictly aerobic
  - Filamentous and branching
  - May be isolated on routine media
    - Colonies usually form within 4 days
      - May require up to 2 to 4 weeks
    - *Nocardia* spp. can be difficult to isolate by culture
      - Faster growing organisms may overgrow
- Colony morphology
  - Colonies smooth and moist or have a "moldlike," gray-white, waxy or powdery appearance
  - Distinct, strong mildew odor
- Microscopic
  - Usually gram-variable or "beaded" appearance
    - Alternating gram-positive and gram-negative segments along a filament
  - *Nocardia* under suboptimal conditions appears uniformly gram-negative
  - Modified Ziehl-Neelsen or Kinyoun acid-fast stain
    - *Nocardia* organisms are acid-fast with these modified staining procedures
    - Tests based on acid-fastness alone are not reliable for differentiation
- Differentiation of *Nocardia* spp.
  - Tap water agar morphology
    - Differentiate *Nocardia* spp. and other aerobic actinomycetes
    - *Nocardia* spp. have recursively branching hyphae with aerial hyphae
  - Biochemical characteristics
    - Hydrolysis of casein, tyrosine, or xanthine
  - *N. asteroides*
    - Does not hydrolyze casein, xanthine, or tyrosine
  - *N. brasiliensis*
    - Hydrolyzes casein and tyrosine
  - Molecular identification

Rhodococcus equi

- Soil saprophyte
  - Associated with domestic farm animals
- Causes pulmonary infection that resembles tuberculosis
  - Pneumonia that spreads to brain, liver, spleen
  - Opportunistic
  - AIDS, transplants, Hodgkin's lymphoma, lymphoma, and leukemia
- Laboratory identification
  - Colony forms in 2 to 4 days
  - Glistening, smooth, pink to red
  - Gram-positive coccobacillus

- Sometimes partially acid-fast
- Does not hydrolyze
  - Casein, xanthine, tyrosine
- No branching on tap water agar

Streptomyces Species

- *Streptomyces griseus* (found in soil)
- Musty smell
- Nonpathogenic
- Forms colony in 3 to 5 days at 35°C
  - Waxy, white powdery top
- Gram-positive filamentous bacilli
- Non–acid-fast
- Aerial, tertiary branching on tap water agar
- Hydrolyzes casein, xanthine, and tyrosine

Actinomadura Species

- Eight reported species, two more common
  - *Actinomadura madurae*
  - *Actinomadura pelletieri*
- Causes mycetoma
- Found only in tropics
- Gram-positive filamentous bacilli
- Non–acid-fast
- Aerial, tertiary branching on tap water agar
- Hydrolyzes casein and tyrosine

Nocardiopsis Species

- Soil saprophyte
- Similar to *Streptomyces* and *Actinomadura*
- Thermotolerant
  - Grows at higher temperatures
- Very rare case of mycetoma

VIROLOGY

- Properties of viruses
  - Small
  - DNA or RNA, not both
  - Replicate or multiply on their own
  - Intracellular
  - Replication is directed by viral nucleic acid
  - Lack genes and enzymes necessary for energy production
  - They depend on the machinery of the host cell for protein and nucleic acid production
  - Some are capable of inducing cancerous growth in animals and culture
    - Hepatitis B: Liver cancer
- Characteristics of a typical virion
  - Either DNA or RNA, single or double stranded
    - In contrast to eukaryotes and prokaryotes, viruses do not contain both

- A capsid or protein coat
- Enveloped viruses have an outer envelope composed of lipids and polysaccharides
- Important definitions
  - Capsid: Protein shell
  - Nucleocapsid: Nucleic acid + capsid
  - Capsomeres: Structural units of capsid
  - Envelope: Lipid membrane around nucleocapsid in some viruses
    - Stolen from cell: Essential for infectivity
  - Virion: Complete virus particle
- Characteristics used to classify viruses
  - Type of genetic material (either DNA or RNA) they contain
  - Size and shape of the assembled virus
  - Presence or absence of an envelope
  - Type of host that it infects
  - Type of disease produced
- Taxonomy/nomenclature
  - International Committee on Taxonomy of Viruses divides all viruses to families (-viridae)
  - Subfamilies (-virinae)
  - Genera (-virus)
  - Species or virus name
  - Above the family level, orders (-virales) may be used
  - http://www.virustaxonomyonline.com
- Other viruslike things
  - Prion
    - Proteinaceous infectious particle
    - Structures that replicate through conversion of other host proteins
    - Exact mechanisms of action and reproduction are unknown
    - Transmissible spongiform encephalopathy
      - Scrapie
      - Kuru
      - Creutzfeldt-Jakob disease (CJD)
      - Bovine spongiform encephalopathy (BSE): Mad cow disease
- Replication of virus particles
  - Attachment
    - Specific cell receptor
    - Responsible for varying cell tropism
  - Penetration
    - Virus passing through cell membrane
    - May take cell membrane as protection
  - Uncoating
    - Removes all or part of the capsid
    - Exposes the nucleic acid
  - Biosynthesis
    - Proteins, nucleic acids, and other components
    - Some made in tremendous excess
  - Morphogenesis
    - Components assembled
    - Often uses enzymes encoded by virus
  - Release
    - Budding through membrane
    - Lysis of membrane

Clinical Virology: Culture Method

- 1937: Propagated yellow fever virus in chick embryos
- Successfully produced an attenuated vaccine
- Influenza vaccine still produced in eggs
- Growth of viruses
  - Chicken embryos: Historical
  - Tissue explants: Research use only
  - Cell culture
    - Primary cell culture
    - Diploid cell lines
    - Continuous cell lines
- Primary cell cultures
  - Derived directly from donor (animal or human)
  - Most common are kidney cells
    - Rhesus monkey, rabbit kidney
  - One or two passages
- Diploid cell line
  - Prepared from animal tissues
    - Usually fibroblasts from lung or foreskin
  - Terminally differentiated, postmitotic
  - Limited to 20 to 50 passages
- Continuous cell lines
  - Single cell type that can be propagated indefinitely
  - Do not resemble the cell of origin
  - Often abnormal in chromosome morphology and number
  - Derived from tumors or mutagenic treatment of primary cell culture
  - Unlimited passages
- Care and feeding of cells
  - Cells are usually in tubes or in shell vials
    - Flasks are used for some applications
  - In tubes, the cells are on the "down" side
  - Cells need to be fed or refed with appropriate medium
  - Tubes and vials are read using an inverted microscope
- Cytopathic effects (CPEs)
  - CPEs can take a variety of forms
    - Rounding up and detachment
    - Cell lysis
    - Swelling of nuclei
    - Formation of fused cells termed syncytia
  - Induction time varies among viral agents
- Hemadsorption
  - Certain viruses produce hemagglutinin
  - Hemagglutinin binds erythrocytes
    - Human type O
    - Chicken
    - Guinea pig
  - Hemadsorption performed on cell cultures from respiratory specimens
- Fluorescent antibody tests
  - Used for confirmation of CPEs
  - Some can be used on patient samples
  - Examples include
    - Cytomegalovirus (CMV)

- o Respiratory viruses
- o Herpes simplex virus (HSV)
- o Enterovirus groups
- Shell vial cultures
  - Cells grown on coverslips in the bottom of a vial (shell vial)
  - Patient specimens added to vial and centrifuged to "drive" the virus into the cell
  - Incubated and stained
  - Time to positive usually much less than with conventional tube cultures
  - Used for several different agents
    - o CMV
    - o Herpes simplex and varicella-zoster
    - o Respiratory viruses
    - o *Chlamydia*
  - Some systems contain mixed cell types

Clinical Virology: Nonculture Methods

- Direct examination
  - Antigen detection
    - o Immunofluorescence, enzyme-linked immunosorbent assay (ELISA), etc.
  - Electron microscopy
    - o Morphology of virus particles
    - o Immune electron microscopy
  - Light microscopy
    - o Histologic appearance
    - o Inclusion bodies
    - o Limited to pathology
- Antigen detection
  - Enzyme immunoassay (EIA)
    - o Plate-based assays
    - o Lateral flow technology
  - Nasopharyngeal aspirate
    - o Respiratory syncytial virus (RSV)
    - o Influenza
  - Stool
    - o Rotavirus
    - o Adenovirus
- Advantages and disadvantages
  - Advantages
    - o Result available quickly, point-of-care testing
  - Potential problems
    - o Reduced sensitivity compared to cell culture or PCR: 40% to 80%
    - o Labor intensive
    - o Not well suited to a core laboratory
- Electron microscopy
  - 10^6 virus particles/mL required for visualization
  - Approximately 50,000 to 60,000 magnification normally used
  - Original method to find many viruses
  - Viruses may be detected in the following specimens
    - o Feces: Rotavirus, adenovirus, noroviruses, astrovirus, calicivirus

- o Vesicle fluid
- o HSV, varicella-zoster virus (VZV)
- o Skin scrapings: Papillomavirus, molluscum contagiosum
- Disadvantages with electron microscopy
  - o Expensive equipment
  - o Expensive maintenance
  - o Require experienced observer
  - o Sensitivity often low
- Nucleic acid amplification
  - Allows the amplification of specific target DNA sequences by a factor of approximately 10^6
  - PCR is the most common method but other variations are being developed and used
  - Detection of the PCR product usually has been by agarose gel electrophoresis, probe hybridization, or DNA sequencing
  - Real-time PCR has streamlined the amplification and the detection processes
- Advantages of PCR
  - Extremely high sensitivity
  - Fast turnaround time for real-time PCR
  - Nucleic acid amplification
- Disadvantages of PCR
  - Extremely liable to contamination
  - High degree of operator skill required
  - Not easy to set up a quantitative assay
  - A positive result may be difficult to interpret
- Serologic tests for viral infections
  - Classic techniques
    - o Complement fixation tests
    - o Hemagglutination inhibition tests
    - o Immunofluorescence techniques
    - o Counter-immunoelectrophoresis
  - Older techniques
    - o Radioimmunoassay
  - Newer techniques
    - o Enzyme-linked immune assay (EIA)
    - o Particle agglutination
    - o Western blot
    - o Recombinant immunoblot assay
    - o Lateral flow "rapid" devices
- Serology
  - Primary infection
    - o Fourfold rise titer of immunoglobulin G (IgG) or total antibody between acute and convalescent sera
    - o Presence of IgM
    - o A single high titer of IgG
  - Reinfection
    - o Fourfold or greater rise in titer of IgG or total antibody between acute and convalescent sera
    - o Absence or slight increase in IgM
- Use of serologic results
  - Disease dependent
    - o Rubella and hepatitis A
      - Clinical symptoms coincide with antibodies
      - Detection of IgM or rise in IgG: Disease

- ○ Respiratory and diarrhea viruses may cause disease before antibody rise
  - RSV or influenza
  - Serologic diagnosis would be retrospective
- ○ HIV produces clinical disease months or years after seroconversion
- ○ Antibody: Definitive diagnosis
- Some infections can be detected only by serology
  - ○ *Bartonella*
- Limitations of serology
  - Long period of time required using paired sera
  - ○ Extensive antigenic cross-reactivity
    - ○ HSV and VZV
    - ○ Japanese B encephalitis and dengue
    - ○ CMV and Epstein-Barr virus
  - Immunocompromised patients often have reduced or absent immune response
    - ○ Late AIDS
  - Patients with infectious mononucleosis or diseases such as systemic lupus erythromatosus may react nonspecifically
  - Transfusion may give a false positive result because of the transfer of antibody
- Guidelines for selecting and collecting specimens for virology
  - Culture only infected sites
  - Collect and send tissue or fluid
  - Do not use swabs
  - Send fluid in its original container/syringe
  - Collect and send as much specimen as possible
- Tools of the trade
  - Swabs
    - ○ Swab for skin lesion
    - ○ Nasopharyngeal swabs from the nasopharynx
    - ○ All must go into viral transport medium
  - Viral/chlamydial culture transport media
    - ○ Supplied by the laboratory
    - ○ Usually stored refrigerated
    - ○ Inoculate and send on ice
  - Nasal wash kit
    - ○ Sterile saline included
    - ○ Use for rapid virus tests and nucleic acid amplification test
    - ○ Use for culture by transfer to vial transport medium or directly
- Specimen labeling
  - The specimen must be labeled accurately and completely
  - Indicate exactly what the specimen is

Major Groups of DNA Viruses

- Adenoviridae
- Hepadnaviridae
- Herpesviridae
- Papillomaviridae
- Parvoviridae

TABLE 2-2	Medically Important Viruses
Groups	**Virus Families**
Major groups of DNA viruses	*Adenoviridae*
	Hepadnaviridae
	Herpesviridae
	Papillomaviridae
	Parvoviridae
	Polyomaviridae
	Poxviridae
Major groups of RNA viruses	*Arenaviridae*
	Astroviridae
	Bunyaviridae
	Caliciviridae
	Coronaviridae
	Filoviridae
	Flaviviridae
	Orthomyxoviridae
	Paramyxoviridae
	Picornaviridae
	Reoviridae
	Retroviridae
	Rhabdoviridae
	Togaviridae

- Polyomaviridae
- Poxviridae

Adenoviruses
- Double-stranded DNA (dsDNA), replicate in nucleus
- Icosahedral, nonenveloped
- 51 serotypes
- Causes respiratory disease, eye infections, and GI disease
- Can cause cancer in animals

Hepadnavirus
- dsDNA with a short single-stranded region
- Icosahedral core with envelope
- Human: Hepatitis B
- Two important antigens
  - Surface Ag
  - Core Ag
- Virus not isolated in culture
- Serologic test
- Hepatitis
  - Cirrhosis
  - Hepatocelluar carcinoma
- Transmission through blood
  - Transfusion
  - Drug abuse
  - Sexual contact
- Vaccine
  - Engineered
  - Infants at birth, health care workers

Family Herpesvidae
Herpesviruses
- dsDNA, replicate in nucleus
- Icosahedral nucleocapsid, envelope

- 120- to 200-nm diameter
- Most prominent feature: Latency
- Herpes simplex virus
  - Two types
    - Cold sores
    - Genital
  - Skin and mucous membrane infections
  - Encephalitis
  - Isolated easily in culture

Varicella-Zoster Virus
- Chickenpox and shingles
  - Vaccine important in controlling outbreaks
  - Shingles return
- Tzanck stain: Giant cells
- Isolation more difficult than HSV

Cytomegalovirus
- Isolated from blood, urine, throat
- In adults: Syndrome similar to mononucleosis, may infect kidney (shed in urine)
- In immunocompromised: Kidney, eye, lung, often fatal
- Laboratory tests
  - Shell vial culture
  - Serology

Epstein-Barr Virus
- Heterophile-positive infectious mononucleosis (85%)
- Can produce tumors
- Not isolated in culture
- Serologic diagnosis
  - Early antigen
  - Viral capsid antigen: IgM and IgG
  - Nuclear antigen

Human Herpesvirus 6, 7, and 8
- Human herpesvirus–6
  - Exanthema subitum/roseola infantum
  - Sixth disease
  - Spread by respiratory route
  - Molecular assays used for detection
- Human herpesvirus–7
  - Cause a small percentage of roseola
- Human herpesvirus–8
  - Found in Kaposi's sarcoma

Papillomavirus
- dsDNA
- Over 100 types of human (HPV)
- Infect skin and mucous membranes
- Causes
  - Warts
  - Cervical cancer
  - Laryngeal carcinoma
- No culture: Molecular assays are used

Parvoviruses
- Single-stranded DNA (ssDNA), nucleus replication
- Small nonenveloped
- Human parvovirus B-19
  - Erythema infectiosum (fifth disease)
- Infects bone marrow cells (erythrocyte)
  - Causes aplastic crisis

- Transient in normal individuals
- In immunocompromised
  - Can be severe
  - Blood hemoglobin decreases and cannot recover
- Not isolated in culture
- Detected by molecular assays

Poxviruses
- dsDNA, replicate in cytoplasm of cell
- Largest viruses (400 × 250 nm)
- Complex construction
  - Brick shape, lipid envelope
- Resistant to environmental factors
- Smallpox: Variola
  - Eradicated by the World Health Organization
  - Stocks in Atlanta and Moscow
  - Good vaccine and no animal reservoir
- Vaccinia
  - Used to immunize against smallpox
  - Rare zoonotic
  - Africa
- Others

Major Groups of RNA Viruses

- Arenaviridae
- Astroviridae
- Bunyaviridae
- Caliciviridae
- Coronaviridae
- Filoviridae
- Flaviviridae
- Orthomyxoviridae
- Paramyxoviridae
- Picornaviridae
- Reoviridae
- Retroviridae
- Rhabdoviridae
- Togaviridae

Arenaviruses
- ssRNA, enveloped
  - Helical capsid symmetry
- Lymphocytic choriomeningitis virus
  - Benign aseptic meningitis
- Lassa fever virus: Africa
- Junin and Machupo viruses: South America
- Rodent reservoir, greater than 50% mortality
- Biosafety level 4 containment

Bunyaviruses
- ssRNA, enveloped
  - Helical capsid symmetry
- La Crosse encephalitis virus
  - Mouse host, mosquito vector
  - Encephalitis
- Hantaviruses
  - Mouse host
  - Respiratory infection
- Not isolated in the laboratory

Calicivirus

- ssRNA, nonenveloped
  - Icosahedral symmetry
- Family Caliciviridae
  - Sapporo
  - Norovirus
    - Prototype strain is Norwalk virus
    - Outbreaks of diarrhea
    - Genetically and antigenically diverse
    - Noncultivatable

Coronaviruses

- ssRNA, enveloped
  - Pleomorphic/spherical capsid
  - Large club-shaped spikes on surface gives "corona" effect

Filoviruses

- ssRNA
  - Helical symmetry, long and slender
- Marburg and Ebola viruses
  - Monkey reservoir but transmitted to humans
  - More than 80% mortality
  - Pan-organ effects
  - Contact with blood
- Biosafety level 4 containment

Flaviviruses

- ssRNA, enveloped
  - Icosahedral symmetry
- St. Louis encephalitis, West Nile virus, yellow fever, dengue, hepatitis C
- Not isolated by culture

Hepatitis C Virus

- Blood or sexual contact
- No other vector
- Chronic liver infection
- Serology most common diagnosis
  - Screen with EIA
  - Western blot confirmation
- Also detected in blood by molecular assays

Orthomyxoviruses

- ssRNA: Eight segments
- Helical symmetry capsid, enveloped
- Replicate in cytoplasm
- Influenza viruses
  - Two important surface Ag
    - Neuraminidase
    - Hemagglutinin
  - Segmented genomes: Heavy reassortment
    - Antigenic shift: Large
    - Antigenic drift: Small
    - Animal strains
    - Three antigenic groups
      - A, B, C
  - Severe in elderly, immunocompromised
  - Pandemics
    - 1918
    - Avian flu
    - Swine flu

- Can be isolated in culture
  - Subtle CPE
  - Hemadsorption

Paramyxoviruses

- Helical and enveloped, larger than myxoviruses
- Have only one long ssRNA genome
  - No reassortment
- Replicate in both the nucleus and cytoplasm
- Five genera: Mumps, parainfluenza 1 to 4, measles, RSV, metapneumovirus
  - Parainfluenza virus
    - Four antigenic types
    - Respiratory infections
    - Isolated from throat
    - Grow in cell culture
    - Hemadsorption for identification
  - Measles virus
    - One serologic type
    - Maculopapular rash, fever, respiratory disease
    - Can be isolated in culture
    - Hemadsorption for identification
  - Mumps virus
    - Infects parotid salivary glands
    - Can infect testis, ovaries, kidneys
    - Isolated from throat swab or urine
    - Identified by hemadsorption
  - RSV
    - Bronchiolitis, pneumonia in infants
    - Labile virus
    - Produces typical CPE
    - Monoclonal antibody to confirm
    - Rapid testing available
  - Metapneumovirus
    - Acute respiratory tract infections worldwide in children and adults
    - Annual epidemics in winter and spring months
    - Two distinct human metapneumovirus groups with subgroups
    - PCR for diagnosis, for now

Picornaviruses

- ssRNA
- Very small: Approximately 27 nm
- No envelope, icosahedral symmetry
- Replicate in cytoplasm of cell

Enteroviruses

- Fecal-oral transmission
- Polioviruses: 3 types
- Coxsackievirus A: 24 types
- Coxsackievirus B: 6 types
- Echoviruses: 34 types
- Many cultivatable

Rhinoviruses

- Common cold virus
- More than 100 serotypes
- Can be isolated in culture
- Acid-sensitive

- Limited to upper respiratory tract
- Limited growth at 37° C

Hepatitis A Virus
- 25% of hepatitis
- Usually fecal-oral transmission
  - Food
  - Water
  - Needles
- No growth in cell culture
- Serology for diagnosis

Reovirus
- *Respiratory enteric orphan*
- dsRNA, 60 to 80 nm
- Nonenveloped, icosahedral symmetry
- Replicates in the cytoplasm
- Rotaviruses
  - Fecal-oral
  - Causes infantile diarrhea
  - Not isolated in laboratory, ELISA
  - At least six serotypes

Retroviruses
- ssRNA (may have two copies)
- Enveloped, icosahedral symmetry
- All have reverse transcriptase
  - DNA made from RNA
- Integrates into genome
- Many can cause tumors in animals
- Replicate in nucleus and cytoplasm
- HIV 1 and 2, human T-lymphotropic virus 1 and 2
  - HIV
    - 100 to 400 nm, cylindrical or conical core
    - Two broad types: 1 and 2
      - Several subtypes in type 1
      - Type 1, clade (subtype) B in United States
      - Type 2 mainly in Africa
    - Does not form tumors
    - Infects CD4+ cells
      - Lymphocytes, macrophage, brain cells, and dendritic cells
      - Destroys immune system
    - Characteristic secondary diseases
      - *Pneumocystis* pneumonia, CMV, Kaposi's sarcoma
    - ELISA and Western blot analysis

Rhabdoviruses
- ssRNA, bullet shaped, enveloped
- Replicate in cytoplasm
- Vesicular stomatitis virus of horses
- Rabies virus
  - One serologic type
  - Encephalitis
    - Bite of infected animal
    - Travels up sensory nerves to the central nervous system (CNS)
    - Incubation of 2 to 16 weeks
    - Allows time for vaccine
    - 100% fatal if untreated

- Can be isolated in culture and mice
- Diagnosis by immunofluorescence of brain tissue

Togaviruses
- ssRNA
- Enveloped, icosahedral symmetry
- Family Togaviridae
- Genus alphavirus: Arboviruses
- Genus rubivirus: Rubella

Arboviruses
- Eastern and Western equine encephalitis
  - Bird reservoir
  - Mosquito vectors
  - Symptoms include fever, encephalitis, rash
- Cell culture possible, but serology most commonly used

Rubella virus
- Transmitted by droplets
- Infection in children mild
  - Congenital disease serious
  - Mother contracts rubella in first trimester
- Vaccine developed for children because of congenital disease
- Cell culture possible but serology most common

PARASITOLOGY

- Techniques
  - Specimen collection and processing
    - Stool: Routine is three specimens, every other day within 10 days
      - Clean, watertight container with a tight lid
      - 5 g, not contaminated with water, urine, barium, or other substances
      - Liquid or near-liquid specimens examined within 30 minutes of collection to preserve motile trophozoites
      - Soft specimens examined within 60 minutes of collection
      - Formed specimens processed within 24 hours, may be refrigerated
      - Fixatives: Two-vial system, usually formalin and polyvinyl alcohol (PVA) or one-vial system of sodium acetate formalin (SAF)
        - 3 parts fixative to 1 part stool
        - 5% to 10% formalin, concentration methods, and iodine-stained mounts
        - PVA, concentration methods, and trichrome and other permanent stains
        - SAF: Concentration methods and permanent stains
        - PVA contains mercury, SAF is a mercury-free alternative
    - Concentration methods
      - Fresh or preserved stools
      - Sedimentation: Formalin-ethyl acetate
      - Floatation, zinc sulfate with specific gravity of 1.18 to 1.20

- Macroscopic
  - Consistency
  - Appearance, color
  - Contaminants
  - Larva, proglottids
- Microscopic
  - Calibrated ocular micrometer
  - Direct saline wet mount for motile trophozoites
  - Iodine-stained wet mount from processed specimen
  - Permanent stains from processed specimen
- Trichrome: Cytoplasm is blue-green, purple; nuclear structures, red to pink
- Iron hematoxylin: Primarily for intestinal protozoa, cytoplasm is blue to purple, nuclear structures are blue to black
- Modified acid-fast: For coccidian protozoa, oocysts are red
- Other specimen types
  - Specimen of choice depending on organism in question and clinical situation
  - Duodenal contents
  - Sigmoidoscopy specimens
  - Enterotest
  - Blood
  - Urine
  - CSF and other fluids
  - Sputum
  - Tissue specimens

TABLE 2-3	Major Medically Important Parasites
Classification	**Genus and Species**
Nematodes: Intestinal	*Ascaris lumbricoides*
	Enterobius vermicularis
	Necator americanus
	Ancylostoma duodenale
	Strongyloides stercoralis
	Trichuris trichiura
Nematodes: Nonintestinal	*Dracunculus medinensis*
	Trichinella spiralis
Protozoa: Amoeba	*Entamoeba histolytica*
	Entamoeba coli
	Entamoeba hartmanni
	Endolimax nana
	Iodamoeba butschlii
	Acanthamoeba spp.
	Naeglaria fowleri
Protozoa: Flagellates	*Giardia lamblia*
	Trichomonas vaginalis
	Chilomastix mesnili
	Trichomonas hominis
	Dientamoeba fragilis
Protozoa: Ciliate	*Balantidium coli*

TABLE 2-3	Major Medically Important Parasites—cont'd
Classification	**Genus and Species**
Protozoa: Coccidia	*Microsporidia* spp.
	Isospora belli
	Cyclospora cayetanensis
	Cryptosporidium parvum
Protozoa: Misc	*Toxoplasma gondii*
	Blastocystis hominis
Cestodes: Tapeworms	*Diphyllobothrium latum*
	Hymenolepis nana
	Hymenolepis diminuta
	Taenia spp.
	Taenia saginata
	Taenia solium
	Dipylidium caninum
	Echinococcus granulosus
Trematodes: Flukes	*Clonorchis sinensis*
	Fasciolopsis buski
	Fasciola hepatica
	Heterophyes heterophyes
	Metagonimus yokogawa
	Paragonimus westermani
	Schistosoma haematobium
	Schistosoma japonicum
	Schistosoma mansoni
Blood parasites: Babesia	*Babesia microti* in United States
	Babesia divergens in Europe
Blood parasites: Malaria	*Plasmodium falciparum*
	Plasmodium malariae
	Plasmodium ovale
	Plasmodium vivax
	Plasmodium knowlesi
Blood parasites: Filariae	*Brugia malayi*
	Loa loa
	Wuchereria bancrofti
	Mansonella ozzardi
	Onchocerca volvulus
Blood parasites: Hemoflagellates—Leishmania	*Leishmania braziliensis*
	Leishmania donovani complex
	Leishmania tropica complex
	Leishmania mexicana complex
Blood parasites: Hemoflagellates— Trypanosomes	*Trypanosoma cruzi*
	Trypanosoma brucei rhodesiense
	Trypanosoma brucei gambiense
Arthropods	*Pediculus humanus humanus*
	Pediculus humanus capitis
	Phthirus pubis
	Ixodes scapularis
	Dermacentor andersoni
	Dermacentor variabilis
	Ornithodoros spp.
	Cimex lectularius
	Ctenocephalides canis
	Ctenocephalides felis
	Sarcoptes scabei

Continued

Nematodes

Intestinal

Ascaris lumbricoides

- Roundworm
- Worldwide; most common intestinal helminth infection
- Ova in stool
- Ova are the infective stage
- Ova are diagnostic
- Ova 85 to 95 × 38 to 45 µm. Corticated or decorticated. Unfertilized ovoid, 40 to 74 × 30 to 50 µm
- Embryonate in soil, resist environmental conditions
- Adult larva largest intestinal nematode, 22 to 35 cm in length
- Larva emerge in small intestine, migration to bloodstream, liver, lung, to pharynx; swallowed, return to intestine
- GI symptoms, fever, pulmonary or asymptomatic, eosinophilia
- 250,000 ova per day, so worm burden can be high

Enterobius vermicularis

- Pinworm
- Worldwide; most common intestinal helminth infection in the United States
- Scotch tape preparation is specimen of choice, ova or adult larva
- Ova are infective stage
- Ova and larva are the diagnostic stages
- Ova 48 to 60 × 20 to 35 µm; oval, thick shell; flat on one side; developing larva folded inside
- Adult larva female 7 to 14 mm, male 2 to 4 mm, white to light yellow
- Hatch in small intestine, adults in colon; migrate to anus to deposit ova
- Severe anal itching, inflammation
- Ova infective in 4 to 6 hours, deposit in clothes, bed linens, toys
- Highly communicable
- Retroinfection: Ova hatch in anus but migrate back into colon to reproduce
- Autoinfection: Infective ova are ingested, hand to mouth
- Human is only known host
- Ova may carry *Dientamoeba fragilis*, dual infections are seen

Necator americanus

- New World hookworm
- North and South America typically
- Ova are the diagnostic stage, larva can also be found in stool
- Infection caused by third-stage filariform larval penetration of skin, typically the foot
- Ova 60 to 75 × 40 µm, cell cleavage can be seen, thin shell
- Rhabditiform larvae 15 × 270 µm, long buccal cavity and small genital primordium, cutting plates
- Filariform larvae is third stage, short esophagus, pointed tail

- Adult larvae 9 to 12 mm, hook at end of tail; male possesses copulatory bursa
- Filariform larvae penetrate skin, lymphatic system, to bloodstream, to lung; penetrate alveoli, coughed up, swallowed; migrate to large intestine
  - Buccal cavity has cutting plates
- Asymptomatic if light infection; GI symptoms, anemia, weight loss, breathing difficulty, bloody sputum, cough; GI symptoms more severe if worm burden heavy; eosinophilia
- Repeated infection can cause dermal irritation, ground itch
- Ova considered to be indistinguishable from those of *Ancyclostoma duodenale*

Ancyclostoma duodenale

- Old World hookworm
- Europe, Far East, Asia, Africa typically
- Ova considered to be indistinguishable from those of *N. americanus*, although *A. duodenale* ova are 55 to 60 × 40 µm
- Buccal cavity has teeth
- Other details are same as for *N. americanus*

Strongyloides stercoralis

- Threadworm
- Worldwide
- Larva in stool at rhabditiform stage are the diagnostic stage, ova rarely seen
- Infection caused by third-stage filariform larval penetration of skin, typically the foot
- Ova 48 × 35 µm, advanced cleavage state, indistinguishable from hookworm
- Rhabditiform larvae 15 × 220 µm, short buccal cavity and prominent genital primordium
- Filariform larvae is third stage, long esophagus, notched tail
- Adult female 2 mm, short buccal cavity, long esophagus
- Unique lifecycle, three mechanisms
  - Direct: Same as that of hookworm
  - Indirect: Larva freely living in environment, produce infective rhabditiform larva
  - Autoinfection: Filariform larva develop in host's intestine, invade bloodstream
    - Asymptomatic if light infection; GI symptoms, malabsorption, weight loss, breathing difficulty, bloody sputum, cough, eosinophilia
    - Repeated infection can cause dermal irritation, ground itch

Trichuris trichiura

- Whipworm
- Ova in stool
- Ova are infective stage
- Ova are diagnostic
- Ova 50 to 55 × 25 µm, barrel shaped with bipolar hyaline plugs
- Adult larva 2 to 5 cm, male smaller with curled tail; posterior end is large, resembles a whip handle; anterior end is smaller, resembles whip; can be found in stool

- Larva emerge in small intestine, migrate to cecum then to colon
- Asymptomatic with light infection; heavier worm burden includes GI symptoms, weight loss, weakness, eosinophilia; children's symptoms can include GI, anemia, and, if untreated, prolapsed rectum

Nonintestinal

Trichinella spiralis
- Trichina worm
- Worldwide
- Laboratory diagnosis
  - Histologic preparation of encysted tissue, typically skeletal muscle
  - Serologic methods
  - Elevated muscle enzymes
- Ingesting undercooked contaminated meat: Pork, deer, bear, walrus
- Encysted larva $100 \times 5\,\mu m$, coil in cyst in muscle
- Ingestion of infected meat, larva excysts, and develops in intestine; adult female deposits larva, which migrate through bloodstream to skeletal muscle and encyst, which ends lifecycle
  - Asymptomatic or flulike symptoms; heavier infection includes GI symptoms, weakness, fever, pain, edema, muscular pain; can be fatal during migratory phase

Dracunculus medinensis
- Guinea worm
- Africa, India, Asia, Middle East
- Laboratory diagnosis
  - Examination of emerging larva from the skin ulcer
- Ingestion of infected copepods; larva emerge in intestine of host, develop and migrate to connective tissue and body cavities, and to subcutaneous tissues, where adult female deposits larva; ulcer forms, from which larva can emerge
- Allergic reaction, skin ulcer

Protozoa

Amoeba

Entamoeba histolytica
- Pathogenic
- Amoebic dysentery, amoebic abscess
- Worldwide, a leading cause of parasitic death
- Cysts are infective form
- Cysts or trophozoites in stool are diagnostic, or amoebic abscess fluid or sigmoidoscopy specimen
- Cysts: 10 to 20 μm, round, one to four nuclei, central karyosome, fine and even peripheral chromatin, rounded chromatoid bar; young cysts can contain glycogen vacuole
- Trophozoites: 12 to 60 μm, rapid and directional motion, one nucleus with central karyosome; ingested red blood cells (RBCs) are diagnostic

- Asymptomatic carrier state or can cause dysentery, which can be severe, and abscesses in liver, spleen, lung, brain

Entamoeba coli
- Commensal
- Cysts or trophozoites in stool are diagnostic
- Cysts: 10 to 30 μm, round, one to eight nuclei, more than four to differentiate from *Entamoeba histolytica*, eccentric karyosome, uneven peripheral chromatin, splintered end chromatoid bar
- Trophozoites: 15 to 50 μm, slow motility, one nucleus with eccentric karyosome, coarse cytoplasm

Entamoeba hartmanni
- Commensal
- Cysts or trophozoites in stool are diagnostic
- Cysts: Less than 10 μm, resemble those of *E. histolytica*
- Trophozoites: Less than 12 μm, resemble those of *E. histolytica*

Endolimax nana
- Commensal
- Cysts or trophozoites in stool are diagnostic
- Cysts: 5 to 10 μm, one to four nuclei with blot-like karyosome
- Trophozoites: 5 to 12 μm, one nucleus with blot-like karyosome

Iodamoeba butschlii
- Commensal
- Cysts or trophozoites in stool are diagnostic
- Cysts: 5 to 20 μm, one nucleus, large glycogen vacuole
- Trophozoites: 8 to 20 μm, one nucleus

Acanthamoeba Species
- Pathogen
- Granulomatous amoebic encephalitis (GAE)
- Worldwide
- Trophozoites and cysts in CSF, in brain tissue, or at autopsy
- Trophozoites: 12-45 μm, one nucleus, slow motility
- Cysts: 8-25 μm, double cell wall, one nucleus
- Environmental organism, enters nasal passages, bloodstream to CNS; swimming in ponds, lakes in warm months
  - GAE: Stiff neck, headaches, seizures, can progress rapidly
- Eye involvement, contact lens fluid contamination, keratitis
- Keratitis: Ocular pain, vision impairment

Naeglaria fowleri
- Pathogen
- Worldwide
- Primary amoebic meningoencephalitis (PAM)
  - PAM: Stiff neck, headaches, seizures, can progress rapidly
- Trophozoites in CSF, in brain tissue, or at autopsy
- Trophozoites: 8-25 μm, one nucleus, slow motility
- Cysts: No known cyst form

- Environmental organism, enters nasal passages, then bloodstream to CNS; swimming in ponds, lakes in warm months

Flagellates
Giardia lamblia
- Pathogenic
- Worldwide
- Giardiasis, traveler's diarrhea,
- Worldwide, natural water sources
- Cysts are infective form
- Cysts or trophozoites in stool are diagnostic or on sigmoidoscopy specimen, shed irregularly
  - Immunologic methods, PCR
- Cysts: 8 to 14 μm, one to four nuclei, four axonemes, four median bodies, oval
- Trophozoites: 9 to 21 μm, two nuclei, two axonemes, eight flagella, sucking disk, tear-drop shape
- Asymptomatic or GI symptoms, can be severe, light-colored stools, incubation period is 10 to 36 days, can be self-limiting

Dientamoeba fragilis
- Pathogenic
- Thought to be worldwide
- Trophozoite is infective form
- Trophozoites in stool are diagnostic
- Cysts: No known cyst form
- Trophozoites: 7 to 12 μm, one or two nuclei, 80% binucleate
- Asymptomatic or GI symptoms, mild dysentery
- Possible association with *Enterobius vermicularis* infection

Chilomastix mesnili
- Commensal
- Worldwide
- Cysts and trophozoites in stool are diagnostic
- Cysts: 5 to 10 μm, lemon shape, one nucleus, cytosome with fibrils
- Trophozoites: 10 to 20 μm, one nucleus, four flagella, cytosome with fibrils

Trichomonas hominis
- Commensal
- Thought to be worldwide
- Trophozoites in stool are diagnostic
- Cysts: No known cyst form
- Trophozoites: 7 to 15 μm, one nucleus, four flagella, undulating membrane, axostyle

Trichomonas vaginalis
- Pathogenic
- Worldwide
- Trophozoite is infective form
- Trophozoites in urine, vaginal secretions, urethral secretions are diagnostic
- Cysts: No known cyst form
- Trophozoites: 5 to 15 μm, one or two nuclei, four flagella, undulating membrane, axostyle, jerky motility in fresh specimens

- Asymptomatic in men or urethritis, vaginitis with yellow discharge

Ciliate
Balantidium coli
- Pathogen
- Worldwide
- Cysts or trophozoites in stool are diagnostic
- Cysts: 50 to 75 μm, round, two nuclei, small micronucleus, large kidney bean–shaped macronucleus, cytosome, cilia
- Trophozoites: 50 to 100 μm, round, two nuclei, small micronucleus, large kidney bean–shaped macronucleus, cytosome, cilia
- Asymptomatic or GI symptoms, mild dysentery, abscesses in intestinal mucosa, anemia

Coccidia
Cryptosporidium parvum
- Pathogen
- Worldwide
- Oocyst is infective stage
- Oocysts in stool are diagnostic, immunologic methods, modified acid-fast stain
- Oocysts: 4 to 6 μm, round, no sporocysts
- Food-borne and water-borne illness
  - Mild GI symptoms, self-limiting, in compromised patients more severe, can be fatal

Isospora belli
- Pathogen
- Worldwide
- Oocyst is infective stage
- Oocysts in stool are diagnostic, immunologic methods, modified acid-fast stain
- Oocysts: 30 × 12 μm, ovoid, one or two sporocysts, thin shell
- Human is definitive host
- Asymptomatic or GI symptoms, mild, self-limiting

Cyclospora cayetanensis
- Pathogen
- Thought to be worldwide
- Oocysts in stool are diagnostic, modified acid-fast stain
- Oocyst is infective form
- Oocysts: 7 to 10 μm, round, two sporocysts
- Linked to water-borne and food-borne illness
- Mild GI symptoms

Microsporidia Species
- Pathogen
- Thought to be worldwide
- Spores in stool are diagnostic, modified acid-fast stain, serologic methods
- Spore is infective form
- Spores: 1 to 5 μm, round, two sporocysts
- *Enterocytozoon bieneusi* is most commonly isolated species, seen in patients with HIV
- Mild GI symptoms, peritonitis, hepatitis

Miscellaneous Protozoa

Blastocystis hominis

- Pathogen although pathogenicity is unclear
- Thought to be worldwide
- Cyst is infective stage
- Cysts in stool are diagnostic, immunologic methods
- Cysts: 8 to 30 μm, round, central vacuole surrounded by several peripheral nuclei
- Mild GI symptoms

Toxoplasma gondii

- Pathogen
- Toxoplasmosis
- Worldwide, many animals harbor the organism
- Oocyst is infective stage
- Immunologic methods
- Oocysts: 10 to 15 μm, oval, two sporocysts
- Tachyzoites: 5×3 μm, crescent shape, one central nucleus
- Bradyzoites: 5×3 μm, crescent shape, one central nucleus, form a packet in host cell that contains many bradyzoites
  - Cat is definitive host, humans are accidental hosts by four mechanisms: Ingest oocyst from cat feces; ingest contaminated meat from cattle, pig, sheep; transplacental to fetus; blood transfusion
  - Asymptomatic or flulike symptoms in mild cases, but can be chronic; congenital results in fetal death, mental retardation, blindness, severe brain damage, or neonate is asymptomatic at birth

Cestodes: Tapeworms

Diphyllobothrium latum

- Broadfish tapeworm
- Great Lakes area, Alaska, South America, Asia, Africa, Scandinavia
- Ova are infective stage
- Ova in stool are diagnostic, more rarely proglottids
- Ova: 55 to 75×40 to 55 μm, operculated, abopercular knob, not a hexacanth embryo, coracidium surrounded by dark shell
- Scolex: Almond shaped with two long sucking grooves
- Proglottids wider than long, central uterine structure
- Two intermediate hosts. Infection caused by ingestion of pleurocercoid in undercooked or raw fish. Scolex emerges and attaches to intestinal mucosa. Ova passed in stool, further develops if deposited in water. Coracidium hatches, larva ingested by copepod. Develops to procercoid in copepod, which is ingested by freshwater fish; procercoid develops to pleurocercoid larva in fish
- Can be asymptomatic or GI symptoms, weight loss, abdominal pain, vitamin B_{12} deficiency, pernicious anemia

Hymenolepis nana

- Dwarf tapeworm
- Worldwide, most common tapeworm in United States

- Ova are infective stage
- Ova in stool are diagnostic
- Ova: 45×40 μm, typically round, hexacanth embryo with three pairs of hooklets, shell with bipolar thickenings and filaments in clear embryophore
- Scolex: Four suckers, short rostellum with hooks
- Proglottids: Rectangular
- Ingestion of infective ova. Cysticercoid larva develop in intestine, scolex emerges and attaches to intestinal mucosa and further develops. Ova from the adult larva can pass in feces as an infective ovum or autoreinfect the human host
- No intermediate host required
- Can be asymptomatic or GI symptoms, weight loss, abdominal pain

Hymenolepis diminuta

- Rat tapeworm
- Worldwide
- Ova are infective stage
- Ova in stool are diagnostic
- Ova: 55×85 μm, typically round, hexacanth embryo with three pairs of hooklets, shell with bipolar thickenings but no filaments in clear embryophore
- Scolex: Four suckers, small projecting rostellum without hooks
- Proglottids: Rectangular
- Human is accidental host, primary host is rat. Ingestion of infective ova. Cysticercoid larva develop in intestine, scolex emerges and attaches to intestinal mucosa and further develops. Ova from the adult larva can pass in feces as an infective ovum or autoreinfect the human host
- No intermediate host required
- Can be asymptomatic or GI symptoms, weight loss, abdominal pain

Taenia Species

- Worldwide
- Two species
- Ova indistinguishable, 35×25 μm, round, hexacanth embryo with three pairs of hooklets, surrounded by striated embryophore, sunburst appearance, nonoperculated
- Ova in stool are diagnostic, more rarely proglottids
- Infection caused by ingesting undercooked beef or pork that contains cysticercus larva, larva emerge in small intestine where scolex attaches to intestinal mucosa

Taenia saginata

- Beef tapeworm
- Scolex: 1 to 2 mm, four suckers
- Proglottids: greater than 1000, rectangular, 15 to 30 uterine branches

Taenia solium

- Pork tapeworm
- Scolex: 1 to 2 mm, four suckers, rostellum, and hooks
- Proglottids: less than 1000, square, 7 to 15 uterine branches

- Can cause cysticercosis after ingesting infective ovum. Onchosphere migrates to organs, muscle; can invade brain, potentially fatal

Dipylidium caninum
- Dog or cat tapeworm
- Worldwide
- Egg packets in stool, or proglottids are diagnostic
- Larva are infective stage
- Egg packets each containing 10 to 30 ova, ova 40 × 60 μm, oncosphere with three pairs of hooklets
- Scolex: Four suckers, small rostellum with several circles of spines
- Proglottids: Seed shaped
- Human is accidental host, primary host is dog or cat. Intermediate host is flea ingestion of larval stage, develops to adult larva. Egg packets or proglottids passed in stool. Cycle continues if these are ingested by flea
- Flea is intermediate host
- Can be asymptomatic or GI symptoms, weight loss, abdominal pain

Echinococcus granulosus
- Hydatid tapeworm, or dog tapeworm
- West and southwest United States and Alaska, South America, Africa, Asia, Australia, Middle East, areas where dogs and sheep or cattle coexist
- Laboratory diagnosis by examining hydatid cyst fluid, hydatid sand under microscope, scolices floating in fluid; serological methods
- Ova are not the diagnostic phase but are identical to ova of *Taenia* spp.
- Hydatid cyst consists of daughter cysts surrounded by a capsule. Brood capsules can form in the germinal layer of the cyst. Daughter cysts and brood capsule contain scolices, which can develop into adult larva
- Scolex: Four suckers and hooks
- Larva: 5 mm, scolex, neck, and three proglottids
- Human is accidental intermediate and end host. Ingestion of infected ova. Larvae penetrate intestinal mucosa and migrate to organs, usually lung, liver. Hydatid cyst develops in the organ. Dog is definitive host, sheep intermediate host. Cysts form in sheep, dog ingests infected sheep viscera. Cyst develops into adult larva, which reside in dog's intestine, ova passed in feces
- Symptoms depend on location and size of cyst. Asymptomatic until cyst enlarges. Pain in area. Can be fatal if cyst ruptures, because fluid can cause anaphylactic shock. New cyst can form from ruptured cyst if scolex is extruded

Trematodes: Flukes
Clonorchis sinensis
- Chinese liver fluke
- Far East
- Ingesting undercooked fish containing infective metacercariae
- Ova in stool are diagnostic

- Ova 30 × 15 μm with miracidium, shoulders are large, operculated, terminal knob
- Metacercariae mature in liver, migrate to bile duct
- Can be asymptomatic or GI symptoms, weight loss, abdominal pain

Fasciolopsis buski
- Large intestinal fluke
- Far East, India, Indonesia
- Ova in stool
- Ova are infective stage
- Ova in the stool are diagnostic
- Ova 128 to 140 × 80 μm, oval, contain miracidium, operculated
- Adult larva: 5 × 1.5 cm, ovoid
- Ingestion of infected water plants; miracidium develops, adult resides in small intestine of host
- Abdominal pain, GI symptoms, jaundice, malabsorption syndrome, intestinal obstruction in severe cases

Fasciola hepatica
- Sheep liver fluke
- Worldwide, areas cattle and sheep ranching
- Ova are infective stage
- Ova in stool are diagnostic
- Ova 128 to 150 × 80 μm, oval, contain miracidium, operculated
- Adult larva: 3 × 1 cm, ovoid, possesses shoulders that distinguish it from *F. buski*
- Human is accidental host, sheep definitive host. Ingestion of infected water plants, miracidium develops, adult resides in bile ducts of host
- Abdominal pain in liver area, GI symptoms, jaundice

Heterophyes heterophyes
- Heterophid fluke
- Africa, Far East, Near East, Egypt
- Ova are infective stage
- Ova in the stool are diagnostic
- Ova 15 to 30 μm, oval, flask shaped, contain miracidium, operculated, small shoulders, thick shell, can lack terminal knob
- Ova of *Heterophyes heterophyes*, *C. sinensis*, and *Metagonimus yokogawa* very similar
- Adult larva: 1 × 0.5 mm, pyriform, spines cover outside
- Ingestion of undercooked fish, miracidium develops, adults reside in small intestine
- Asymptomatic or heavier infections cause GI symptoms, abdominal pain, eosinophilia

Metagonimus yokogawa
- Heterophid fluke
- Far East, Europe, Siberia
- Ova are infective stage
- Ova in stool are diagnostic
- Ova 15 to 30 μm, oval, flask shaped, contain miracidium, operculated, small shoulders, thin shell, can lack terminal knob
- Adult larva: 1 × 1.5 mm, piriform, spines cover outside
- Ingestion of undercooked fish; miracidium develops, adults reside in small intestine

- Asymptomatic or heavier infections cause GI symptoms, abdominal pain, eosinophilia

Paragonimus westermanni
- Oriental lung fluke
- Asia, Africa, India, South America
- Ova are infective stage
- Ova in stool or in sputum are diagnostic
- Ova 78 to 120 × 45 to 60 μm, oval, contain undeveloped miracidium, thin shell, operculated with shoulders, thickening at terminal end
- Adult larva: 1 × 0.5 mm, oval, spines
- Ingestion of undercooked crayfish or crab. Developing larva migrate to small intestine, into peritoneal cavity, into diaphragm, then to lung tissue
- Pulmonary symptoms, cough, bloody sputum, eosinophilia, other symptoms if larvae migrate to other organs

Schistosoma haematobium
- Bladder fluke
- Africa, Middle East, Iran, Iraq, Saudi Arabia
- Ova in concentrated urine sample, immunodiagnostic methods
- Cercariae penetrate skin to infect human host
- Ova 110 to 170 × 40 to 70 μm, oblong, contain developed miracidium, large terminal spine
- Adult larva: 2 cm, oblong, male and female organisms
- Cercariae penetrate skin to infect human host, migrate to bloodstream to develop. Adult resides in blood vessels around urinary bladder. Ova from adult females are excreted in urine. If deposited in water, miracidium infects snail, where it develops into cercariae
- Snail is intermediate host
- Reservoir hosts include cattle, sheep, dog, cat, monkeys, rodents
- Asymptomatic, skin irritation at penetration site, swimmer's itch, abdominal pain, cough, fever, eosinophilia, painful urination, hematuria

Schistosoma japonicum
- Blood fluke
- Far East
- Ova in stool or rectal biopsy
- Cercariae penetrate skin to infect human host
- Ova 50 to 85 × 40 to 60 μm, slightly oblong, contain developed miracidium, small lateral spine
- Adult larva: 2 cm, oblong, male and female organisms
- Cercariae penetrate skin to infect human host, migrate to bloodstream to develop. Adult resides in blood vessels around intestinal tract. Ova from adult females are excreted in urine. If deposited in water, miracidium infects snail, where it develops into cercariae
- Snail is intermediate host
- Reservoir hosts include cattle, sheep, dog, cat, monkeys, rodents
- Asymptomatic or skin irritation at penetration site, swimmer's itch, abdominal pain, cough, fever, eosinophilia

Schistosoma mansoni
- Manson's blood fluke
- Central and South America, Puerto Rico, West Indies
- Ova in stool or rectal biopsy
- Cercariae penetrate skin to infect human host
- Ova 100 to 185 × 40 to 75 μm, oblong, contain developed miracidium, large lateral spine
- Adult larva: 2 cm, oblong, male and female organisms
- Cercariae penetrate skin to infect human host, migrate to bloodstream to develop. Adult resides in blood vessels around intestinal tract. Ova from adult females are excreted in urine. If deposited in water, miracidium infects snail where it develops into cercariae
- Snail is intermediate host
- Reservoir hosts include cattle, sheep, dog, cat, monkeys, rodents
- Asymptomatic or skin irritation at penetration site, swimmer's itch, abdominal pain, cough, fever, eosinophilia

Blood Parasites

Babesia
- Babesiosis
- *Babesia microti* in United States
- *Babesia divergens* in Europe
- Giemsa-stained thick and thin blood smears, serologic, PCR, blood smears collected at the patient's bedside
- Small delicate ring form trophozoites, 1 to 2 μm
- Rings in single, double, or classic tetrad
- Tetrad: Maltese cross
- Fever, chills, sweating, myalgias, fatigue, hepatosplenomegaly, and hemolytic anemia

Malaria
- Tropical and subtropical worldwide
- Five *Plasmodium* spp. infect humans
- Lifecycle summary
  - Sporozoites injected during mosquito feeding
  - Invade liver cells
  - Liver replication → merozoites
  - Merozoites invade RBCs
  - Repeated erythrocytic schizogony
  - Gametocytes infect mosquito
  - Fusion of gametes in gut
  - Sporogony on gut wall sporozoites invade salivary glands
- Giemsa-stained thick and thin blood smears, serologic, PCR; blood smears are collected at the patient's bedside.
- *Anopheles* mosquito is vector

Plasmodium falciparum
- RBC normal size
- Schuffner's stippling: No
- Merozoites in schizonts: 8 to 36, average 24
- Ring forms single or double chromatin dots
- Multiple ring forms: Common

- Banana-shaped gametocyte
- Accolé forms
  ### Plasmodium vivax
- RBC normal size
- Schuffner's stippling: Yes
- Merozoites in schizonts: 12 to 24, average 16
- Ring forms single chromatin dot
- Multiple ring forms: Occasional
- Ameboid trophozoites
  ### Plasmodium malariae
- RBC normal size
- Schuffner's stippling: No
- Merozoites in schizonts: 6 to 12, average 8, rosette
- Single chromatin dot
- Multiple ring forms: Rare
- Band form trophozoite
  ### Plasmodium ovale
- RBC oval
- Schuffner's stippling: Yes
- Merozoites in schizonts: 4 to 12, average 8
- Single chromatin dot
- Multiple ring forms: Occasional
  ### Plasmodium knowlesi
- Simian malaria form thought to be rarely found in humans
- Forms resemble *P. falciparum* or *P. malariae*

Filariae
  ### Brugia malayi
- Malayan filaria
- Tropical and subtropical worldwide
- Giemsa-stained blood, Knott's technique
- Nocturnal periodicity
- *Aedes, Anopheles, Mansonia* mosquitos are vectors, intermediate host
- Sheath, two nuclei in tail tip
- Asymptomatic for months, years; granulomatous lesions, fever, chills, lymphadenopathy
- Elephantiasis
  ### Loa loa
- Eyeworm
- Africa
- Giemsa-stained blood, Knott's technique
- Diurnal periodicity
- *Chrysops* fly is vector
- Sheath, continuous nuclei in tail tip
- Inflammation at bite site, Calabar swellings at any body site
  ### Wuchereria bancrofti
- Bancroft's filaria
- Tropical and subtropical worldwide
- Giemsa-stained blood, Knott's technique
- Nocturnal periodicity
- *Aedes, Anopheles, Culex* mosquito are vectors, intermediate host
- Sheath, no nuclei in tail tip
- Fever, chills, lymphadenopathy
- Elephantiasis

Onchocerca volvulus
- Blinding filaria, river blindness
- Tropical Africa and Central America
- Giemsa-stained skin snips
- No periodicity
- Simulium blackfly is vector
- No sheath, no nuclei in tail tip
- Subcutaneous fibrous nodules
- Blindness if eye is affected
  ### Mansonella ozzardi
- New World filaria
- North, Central, and South America
- Giemsa-stained blood
- No periodicity
- Simulium blackfly is vector, or *Culicoides* midge
- No sheath, nuclei in tail but not to tip
- Asymptomatic, lymphadenopathy
- Blindness if eye is affected
- Hemoflagellates

Leishmaniae
  ### Leishmania braziliensis
- Mucocutaneous leishmaniasis
- Mexico, Central and South America
- Giemsa-stained slides of the affected body sites, amastigotes
- Sandfly is vector, bite transfers promastigotes to the human host, promastigotes migrate to reticuloendothelial cells and develop to amastigotes
- Lesions in mucocutaneous tissues
- Can be self-limiting
  ### Leishmania donovani Complex
- Visceral leishmaniasis, dumdum fever, kala-azar
- Africa, India, Middle East, Far East
- Giemsa-stained slides of the affected body sites, amastigotes, serologic methods, Montenegro screening skin test
- Affects visceral tissue
- Sandfly is vector, incubation period of weeks to months
- Flulike symptoms resembling malariae, GI symptoms, abdominal pain, hepatosplenomegaly
- Darkening of the skin, black fever or kala-azar
- Can be fatal
  ### Leishmania mexicana Complex
- New World cutaneous leishmaniasis
- Central and South America, Mexico
- Giemsa-stained slides of the lesions, amastigotes
- Affects skin
- Sandfly is vector
- Skin lesion, ulcer
- Can be self-limiting
  ### Leishmania tropica Complex
- Old World cutaneous leishmaniasis, Baghdad boil, Delhi boil
- Middle East, Northern Africa
- Giemsa-stained slides of the lesions or fluid, amastigotes, serologic testing
- Affects skin

- Sandfly is vector
- Skin lesion, ulcer
- Can be self-limiting

Trypanosomes

Trypanosoma brucei gambiense
- West African sleeping sickness
- West and Central Africa
- Giemsa-stained slides blood or lymph nodes, CSF studies
- Tsetse fly is vector; bite transfers trypomastigotes to the human host, migrate to lymphatic system, eventually to CNS
- Asymptomatic for a period. Chancre develops at bite site, flulike symptoms, rash, lymphadenopathy, Winterbottom's sign in neck area. Kerandel's sign can develop, delayed sensation to pain. CNS symptoms in final stages, coma, and death

Trypanosoma brucei rhodesiense
- East African sleeping sickness
- East and Central Africa
- Giemsa-stained slides of blood, CSF studies
- Tsetse fly is vector; bite transfers trypomastigotes to the human host, which migrate to lymphatic system, eventually to CNS
- Virulent. Asymptomatic for a short period. CNS involvement early, weight loss, lethargy, confusion, Winterbottom's sign in neck area may be present. In final stages, glomerulonephritis, myocarditis, coma, and death

Trypanosoma cruzi
- Chagas disease
- Central and South America, Mexico, southern United States
- Giemsa-stained slides to blood, serologic methods
- Reduviid bug is vector; defecates near bite, transfers trypomastigotes to the human host. Amastigotes and trypomastigotes facilitate cell damage throughout body. Liver, brain, and heart muscle involved
- Can also be transmitted by blood transfusion, placenta
- Chagas can be asymptomatic, chronic, or acute. Chagoma develops at bite site, typically face. Eye area swelling is Romaña's sign. Acute flulike symptoms. Chronic disease early or years later. Myocarditis, mega colon, hepatosplenomegaly, brain damage, death
- Children most at risk
- Arthropods

Ectoparasites and Vectors of Disease

- Lice, ticks, fleas, mites, bedbugs, mosquitos
- Structures used in arthropod identification
- Body parts, legs, wings, antenna, mouth parts

Lice
- Lice occur worldwide and in all socioeconomic classes

- Vector for typhus *(Rickettsia prowazekii)*, trench fever *(Bartonella quintana)*, and relapsing fever *(Borrelia recurrentis)*
- Spread from human to human
- Body lice usually on the body and head
- Crab lice usually in pubic region, spread to the armpits, facial hair, eyebrows, and eyelashes

Pediculus humanus humanus
- Body louse

Pediculus humanus capitis
- Head louse

Phthirus pubis
- Crab or pubic louse

Ticks

Hard Ticks

Ixodes scapularis
- Deer tick
- Main vector of Lyme disease
- *Ixodes pacificus* in the U.S. West Coast states also able to transmit Lyme disease

Dermacentor andersoni
- Rocky Mountain wood tick, western United States
- Vector of many diseases, including Rocky Mountain spotted fever, tularemia, Colorado tick fever, and Q fever

Dermacentor variabilis
- American dog tick, eastern United States

Soft Ticks
- *Ornithodoros* spp.
- Parasitize mammals
- Transmit relapsing fever

Fleas
- Cat flea: *Ctenocephalides felis*
- Dog flea: *C. canis* can be found on cats and dogs
- Serve as intermediate host for tapeworms
- Feed on humans as well as pets
  - Cause a localized skin reaction

Mites
- *Sarcoptes scabei* is the cause of scabies worldwide
  - Transmitted by contact
  - Organisms burrow into the skin on the webbing side of fingers, later spreading to the wrists, elbows and beyond

Bedbugs
- True insect
- *Cimex lectularius*
  - Preferential feeding host is human
- Nocturnal blood meals
- Symptoms occur days after bite

Mosquitos
- True insect
- Blood meals
- Transmit malariae, filariasis, dengue fever, yellow fever, West Nile virus
- Species include *Culex, Anopheles, Aedes, Mansonia*

CERTIFICATION PREPARATION QUESTIONS

For answers and rationales, please see Appendix A.

1. Which of the following terms is best described as the process of reproduction in yeast that begins with a weakening and outpouching of the yeast cell wall and then formation of a cell wall septum between the mother and daughter yeast cells?
   a. Binary fission
   b. Unisexual division
   c. Budding
   d. Outpouch germing

2. The loose intertwined network of basic structural units of the molds that penetrates the substrate from which it obtains the necessary nutrients for growth is called which of the following?
   a. Hyphae
   b. Germ tubes
   c. Pseudohyphae
   d. Mycelium

3. The term hyaline molds is used to describe which of the following?
   a. Molds that have septate hyphae
   b. Molds that have septate, nonpigmented hyphae
   c. The presence of pigmentation within the hyphae or the spores
   d. Molds with intercalated hyaline chlamydoconidia

4. Large, usually multiseptate and club-shaped or spindle-shaped spores are called which of the following?
   a. Microconidia
   b. Macroconidia
   c. Conidiophores
   d. Phialides

5. A Scotch tape preparation is made from a mold growing on solid media in the mycology laboratory. The structure shown in the image is best described as which of the following?

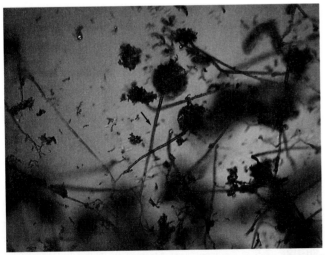

FIGURE 2-1 *(Courtesy Joel Mortensen, PhD. See also color plate 8.)*

   a. Sporangium
   b. Blastoconidia
   c. Ascospores
   d. Conidiophore

6. A patient with a Wood's lamp–positive, dermatophytic infection has a skin scraping taken for culture. The organism grows on SDA agar with a light-tan front and salmon-colored reverse. Microscopically the organism produces rare distorted macroconidia and rare microconidia. Additionally, there was no growth on sterile rice media. What is the most likely organism?
   a. *Microsporum canis*
   b. *Microsporum gypseum*
   c. *Microsporum audouinii*
   d. *Epidermophyton floccosum*

7. A KOH preparation of respiratory secretions of a 78-year-old man reveals large, spherical, thick-walled yeast cells 8 to 15 μm in diameter, usually with a single bud that is connected to the parent cell by a broad base. Which fungus will likely be isolated from the culture?
   a. *Coccidioides immitis*
   b. *Blastomyces dermatitidis*
   c. *Histoplasma capsulatum*
   d. *Paracoccidioides brasiliensis*

8. Which of the following is a key characteristic of *Coccidioides immitis*?
   a. Has a higher dissemination rate in white females
   b. Is endemic in the northeastern United States
   c. Produces endosporulating spherules in tissue
   d. Forms foot cells

9. Using PAS to stain a respiratory specimen from a patient with lung disease, the technologists observed the organisms in the image. Based on the microscopic morphology shown in the image, the most likely identification of the dimorphic fungi is which of the following?

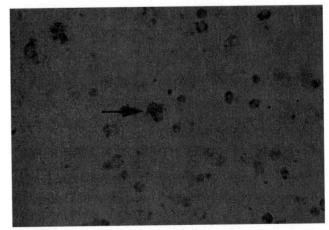

FIGURE 2-2 *(Courtesy Joel Mortensen, PhD. See also color plate 9.)*

   a. *Blastomyces dermatitidis*
   b. *Coccidioides immitis*

c. *Histoplasma capsulatum*
d. *Sporothrix schenckii*

10. A landscaper noticed a hard, unmovable lump under the skin of his index finger but decided to ignore it. A month later, the lump ulcerated to present a necrotic appearance, and two more lesions developed further up the wrist and forearm. A histologic stain of material from deep in the lesions showed elongated yeast cells resembling cigars. What disease is suspected?

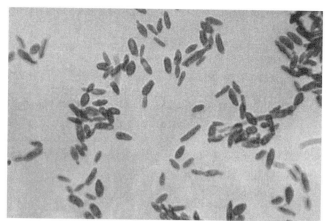

FIGURE 2-3 *(Courtesy Joel Mortensen, PhD. See also color plate 10.)*

a. Mycetoma
b. Sporotrichosis
c. Chromoblastomycosis
d. Blastomycosis

11. A germ tube–negative yeast is isolated in the laboratory. The isolate is found to be negative for urease and unable to assimilate dextrose, maltose, or sucrose. CMT agar morphology showed blastoconidia only. The organism is most likely:
a. *Candida albicans*
b. *Candida parapsilosis*
c. *Torulopsis glabrata*
d. *Geotrichum candidum*

12. Which of the following is a key characteristic by which an unknown *Cryptococcus* spp. can be identified as *Cryptococcus neoformans*?
a. Appearance of yellow colonies
b. Positive urease test
c. Presence of a capsule
d. Positive niger seed agar test

13. Which of the following statements concerning the germ tube test is true?
a. Using a heavy inoculum enhances the rapid production of germ tubes
b. Germ tubes should be read after 2 hours of incubation at 25° C
c. *Candida albicans* and *Candida tropicalis* can be used as positive and negative controls, respectively
d. Serum will be stable for 1 year if stored at room temperature

14. An immunocompromised patient exhibited fever, nonproductive cough, and shortness of breath. Routine and fungal cultures did not grow. The respiratory specimen was stained with a silver stain in anatomic pathology. Based on the microscopic morphology in the image, what is the most likely identification of this organism?

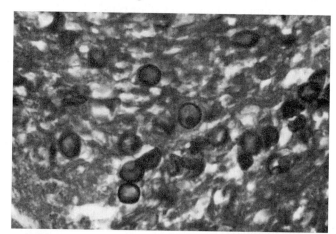

FIGURE 2-4 *(From Public Health Photo Library [PHL 960]. See also color plate 11.)*

a. *Pneumocystis jiroveci*
b. *Saccharomyces* sp.
c. *Candida albicans*
d. *Cryptococcus* sp.

15. A significant amount of yeast was isolated from a vaginal culture of a patient in the teen clinic of your hospital. It exhibited the following characteristics:
Microscopic: Clusters of blastoconidia along pseudohyphae, terminal chlamydoconidia
Positive germ tube
Positive sucrose
Which of the following is the most likely identification of this fungi? (Image from primary plate, gram-stained smear, 40×.)

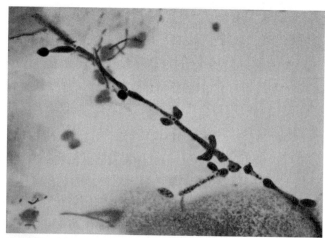

FIGURE 2-5 *(Courtesy Joel Mortensen, PhD. See also color plate 12.)*

a. *Rhodotorula rubra*
b. *Candida albicans*

c. *Geotrichum candidum*
d. *Trichosporon beigelii*

16. The pharmacy at your hospital was concerned about the hyperalimentation fluid they were preparing. The high lipid contact was a concern for contamination. A PAS stain of the suspect fluid is shown. Which of the following organism would most likely demonstrate this morphology?

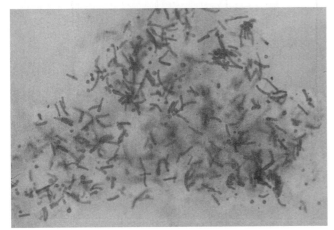

FIGURE 2-6 *(Courtesy Joel Mortensen, PhD. See also color plate 13.)*

a. *Candida albicans*
b. *Malassezia furfur*
c. *Trichosporon cutaneum*
d. *Scedosporium apiospermum*

17. Several important types of conidiation of dematiaceous fungi exist. The image is an example of which one of these forms? (Lactophenol cotton blue stain.)

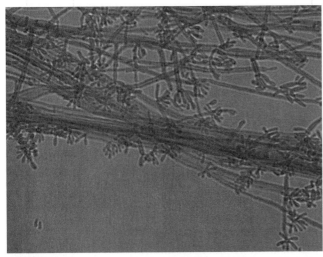

FIGURE 2-7 *(Courtesy Joel Mortensen, PhD. See also color plate 14.)*

a. *Cladosporium* type
b. *Phialophora* type
c. *Rhinocladiella* type
d. Rinderpest type

18. A mold isolated in the laboratory displays a white cottony macroscopic morphology. On microscopic evaluation, hyaline, septate hyphae, and "toothbrush"-like conidiophres are seen. The most likely organism is which of the following?
    a. *Aspergillus* sp.
    b. *Acremonium* sp.
    c. *Gliocladium* sp.
    d. *Scopulariopsis* sp.

19. A mold is isolated in the laboratory that displays a velvety, gray-green colony morphology. On microscopic evaluation, flask-shaped conidiophores arranged in a brushlike formation are seen. The most likely organism is which of the following?
    a. *Penicillium* sp.
    b. *Acremonium* sp.
    c. *Paecilomyces* sp.
    d. *Scopulariopsis* sp.

20. A patient who underwent solid organ transplant appears to have systemic fungemia. The organism that has grown from the blood cultures macroscopically had a blue-green color to the colony, matured in 3 days, and grew well at 45° C. Microscopically, foot cells were seen and the phialides were uniserate with a round vesicle and columnar conidia. Which of the following is the most likely identification of this mold?

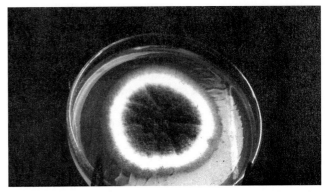

FIGURE 2-8 *(Courtesy Joel Mortensen, PhD. See also color plate 15.)*

a. *Aspergillus fumigatus*
b. *Aspergillus niger*
c. *Scopulariopsis* sp.
d. *Fusarium* sp.

21. The protein coat that surrounds the nucleic acid of a virion is called which of the following?
    a. Capsomere
    b. Capsid
    c. Capsule
    d. Nucleocapsid

22. During viral assembly, how are viral envelopes acquired?
    a. By production of envelope constituents by host cellular DNA

b. As the virion buds from a host cell membrane

c. Through replication of viral nucleic acid

d. As host cell lysis produces many membrane fragments

23. Prions are best described by which of the following?

a. Infectious viral RNA without capsid proteins

b. Infectious protein with no associated nucleic acid

c. Infectious viral DNA without capsid proteins

d. Nonenveloped virus highly resistant to heat and chemical inactivation

24. The viral nucleocapsid always contains which of the following?

a. Viral genome

b. Virus-encoded glycoprotein

c. Virus-encoded polymerase

d. Viral envelope

25. Which of the following viruses are thought to predominately cause gastroenteritis?

a. Hepadnaviruses

b. Filoviruses

c. Noroviruses

d. Arboviruses

26. Which of the following groups contains the SARS virus?

a. Calicivirus

b. Coronavirus

c. Flavivirus

d. Filovirus

27. Which of the following groups of virus is best described as:

ssRNA, enveloped,

Pleomorphic/spherical capsid

Large club-shaped spikes on surface gives "corona" effect

Causes approximately 15% of coldlike illness

a. Influenza A

b. Influenza B

c. Coronaviruses

d. Pneumovirus

28. Which of the following is the specimen of choice for detecting rotavirus?

a. Throat swab

b. Urine sample

c. Bronchoalveolar wash

d. Feces sample

29. The test of choice and most sensitive assay for use with CSF to diagnose aseptic meningitis caused by enterovirus is which of the following?

a. Cell culture

b. PCR

c. Antigenemia immunoassay

d. Shell vial assay

30. A specimen from a genital lesion was inoculated into a standard set of cells for virus isolation. On day 1 the human foreskin fibroblasts exhibited the CPE shown in the figure.

FIGURE 2-9 *(Courtesy Joel Mortensen, PhD. See also color plate 16.)*

a. Herpes simplex virus

b. Adenovirus

c. Cytomegalovirus

d. Epstein-Barr virus

31. Trophozoite forms of amoebae are found in what type of stool specimen?

a. Formed

b. Loose

c. Soft

d. Watery

32. Which preservation method is most suitable and the most widely used for subsequent fixed smear preparation?

a. Formalin-ethyl acetate

b. PVA

c. Trichrome

d. MIF

33. If the ova of this parasite are ingested by humans, the oncosphere form can migrate through the body via the bloodstream, resulting in the condition known as cysticercosis. Which of the following is correct?

a. *Taenia solium*

b. *Entamoeba histolytica*

c. *Hymenolepis nana*

d. *Clonorchis sinensis*

34. Ova recovered from the stool are routinely used to diagnose infections caused by all of the following except?

a. *Necator americanus*

b. *Ascaris lubricoides*

c. *Trichuris trichiura*

d. *Strongyloides stercoralis*

35. An MLS finds an *E. coli* cyst on a wet mount of a fresh stool specimen. Which of the following should be done?

a. Request a second specimen

b. Look for additional *E. coli* cysts

c. Examine the remaining area of the wet preparation

d. Generate a final report

36. Which of the following parasites have migration through the lungs as part of their lifecycle?
    a. *Necator americanus, Ancylostoma duodenale, Strongyloides stercoralis*
    b. *Giardia lamblia, Wuchereria bancrofti, Brugia malayi*
    c. *Enterobius vermicularis, Trichuris trichiura, Trichinella spiralis*
    d. *Toxocara canis, Toxoplasma gondii, Blastocystis hominis*

37. The image below is of a suspected parasite seen on direct examination of material taken from a corneal scraping in an ophthalmology clinic. The most likely identification of the parasite in this specimen is which of the following?

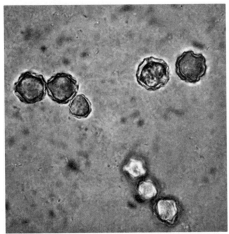

FIGURE 2-10 *(Courtesy the Centers for Disease Control and Prevention. See also color plate 17.)*

    a. *Acanthamoeba* sp.
    b. *Enterobius* sp.
    c. *Paragonimus* sp.
    d. *Naegleria* sp.

38. The organism shown below was recovered from the stool of a patient who resides in rural Texas. The most likely identification is which of the following?

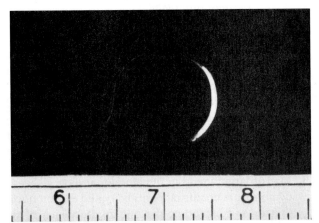

FIGURE 2-11 *(Photograph by Dr. Mae Melvin, courtesy the Centers for Disease Control and Prevention, Public Health Image Library, http://phil.cdc.gov/. See also color plate 18.)*

    a. *Ascaris lumbricoides*
    b. *Ancyclostoma duodenale*
    c. *Necator americanus*
    d. *Trichuris trichiura*

39. The eggs in the figure below were found in the urine of a Peace Corp worker who had just returned to the United State after spending 2 years in the Middle East. The eggs measured about 160 µm long × 60 µm wide. Which of the following organisms is the most likely identity?

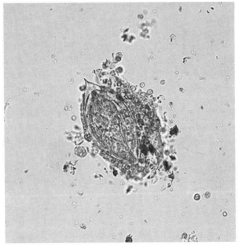

FIGURE 2-12 *(Courtesy the Centers for Disease Control and Prevention. See also color plate 19.)*

    a. *Diphyllobothrium latum*
    b. *Schistosoma haematobium*
    c. *Schistosoma japonicum*
    d. *Schistosoma mansoni*

40. A patient was diagnosed with cysts in his liver. He is originally from Australia, where he was involved in a sheep herding operation. The adult parasite shown below was passed by his pet dog. It measured 5 mm. What is the most likely identification of this organism?

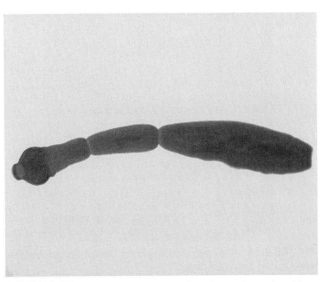

FIGURE 2-13 *(Courtesy the Centers for Disease Control and Prevention. See also color plate 20.)*

a. *Diphyllobothrium latum*
b. *Dipylidium caninum*
c. *Echinococcus granulosus*
d. *Taenia solium*

41. These trophozoites were found in a trichrome-stained slide of a stool sample, measuring an average of 25 microns in diameter. Which of the following is the most likely identity of this organism?

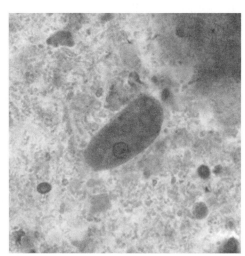

FIGURE 2-14 *(Courtesy the Centers for Disease Control and Prevention. See also color plate 21.)*

a. *Endolimax nana*
b. *Entamoeba coli*
c. *Balantidium coli*
d. *Dientamoeba fragilis*

42. The cyst in the image below was observed in a stool sample of a child at a daycare center. The ovoid cyst measures approximately 10 × 8 microns. Which organism is the most likely cause of the child's diarrhea?

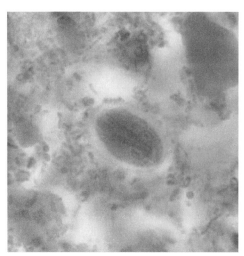

FIGURE 2-15 *(Courtesy the Centers for Disease Control and Prevention. See also color plate 22.)*

a. *Chilomastix mesnili*
b. *Cyclospora cayetanensis*
c. *Giardia lamblia*
d. *Iodamoeba butschlii*

43. The image below is a cyst found in a human fecal smear. The cyst measured about 12 μm in length and contained four nuclei and a rounded chromatoid bar. The patient had severe diarrhea and some blood in the stool. What is the most likely identification of this organism?

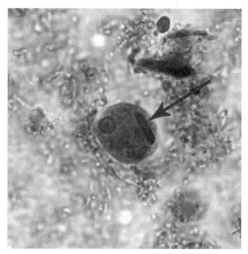

FIGURE 2-16 *(Courtesy the Centers for Disease Control and Prevention. See also color plate 23.)*

a. *Endolimax nana*
b. *Entamoeba coli*
c. *Entamoeba histolytica*
d. *Iodamoeba butschlii*

44. Match the parasite with the most appropriate description.
_____ *Plasmodium falciparum*
_____ *Plasmodium malariae*
_____ *Plasmodium ovale*
_____ *Plasmodium vivax*

a. RBC enlarged, oval, Schuffner's dots, gametocytes seen by day 4 to 18
b. Large RBC, troph irregular, multiple phases seen, gametocytes appear early
c. Delicate ring forms, multiple rings per cell, crescent-shaped gametocytes after 7 to 10 days
d. RBC normal in size and color, troph compact, band forms may be seen, gametocytes seen after weeks

45. Microfilariae found in the blood that have a sheath, demonstrate nocturnal periodicity and exhibit nuclei that do not extend to the tail tip are which of the following?

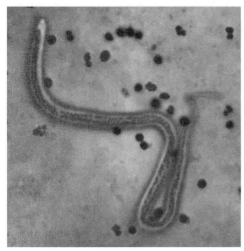

FIGURE 2-17 *(Courtesy the Centers for Disease Control and Prevention. See also color plate 24.)*

a. *Brugia malayi*
b. *Onchocerca volvulus*
c. *Loa loa*
d. *Wuchereria bancrofti*

46. *Necator americanus* rhabditiform larvae can be differentiated from *Strongyloides stercoralis* rhabditiform larvae by:
a. Length of the notched tail
b. Length of the head region
c. Segmentation
d. Size of the genital primordium

47. The image below is from a fecal smear of an individual complaining of diarrhea and intestinal discomfort. The parasites were numerous and quite variable in size, but the majority measured about 15 to 20 µm in diameter. What is the most likely identification of this organism?

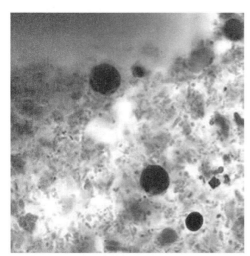

FIGURE 2-18 *(Courtesy the Centers for Disease Control and Prevention. See also color plate 25.)*

a. *Blastocystis hominis*
b. *Cyclospora cayetanensis*
c. *Isospora belli*
d. *Balantidium coli*

48. Match the scientific name with the corresponding common name.
_____ *Sarcoptes scabei*
_____ *Ixodes scapularis*
_____ *P. humanus humanus*
_____ *Cimex lectularius*
a. Body louse
b. Bedbug
c. Scabies
d. Lyme disease

49. The only known human tapeworm with an operculum is:
a. *Diphyllobothrium latum*
b. *Hymenolepis nana*
c. *Giardia lamblia*
d. *Schistosoma haematobium*

50. Identify the following organism as it appears in this peripheral blood smear.

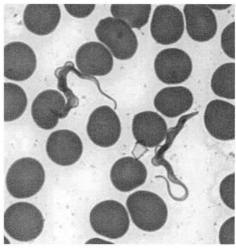

FIGURE 2-19 *(Courtesy the Centers for Disease Control and Prevention. See also color plate 26.)*

a. *Trypanosoma* sp.
b. *Leishmania* sp.
c. *Wuchereria bancrofti*
d. Loa loa

SELF-ASSESSMENT

Content Area: _____

Score on Practice Questions: _____

List the specific topics covered in the missed questions:

List the specific topics covered in the correct questions:

NOTES

3

Hematology

Sandy Cook

HEMATOPOIESIS

- Regulated process of blood cell production
  - Hematopoietic stem cells give rise to red blood cells (RBC), white blood cells (WBC), and platelets
  - Most hematopoiesis occurs in the bone marrow of adults; however, some changes in cell production occur from conception to adulthood
    - Bone marrow
      - Tissue present in the cavities of cortical bones
        - Red marrow: Hematopoietically active marrow located in most bones in early fetal and childhood development but transitions to fewer locations as an adult
        - Adults have red marrow in the proximal ends of long bones, sternum, skull, scapulae, ribs, and pelvis, with approximately equal amounts of red and yellow marrow (Figure 3-1)
      - Yellow marrow: Hematopoietically inactive marrow, consisting primarily of fat cells
  - Sites of hematopoiesis (Figure 3-2 and Table 3-1)

Cell Lines Produced

- The hematopoietic stem cells give rise to the different cell lines. Progenitor cells commit to various states of maturation, with the common lymphoid progenitor producing lymphoid cells and the common myeloid progenitor leading to the production of the neutrophil, monocyte, erythrocytic, and megakaryocytic cell lines (Figure 3-3)

RED BLOOD CELL PRODUCTION AND DESTRUCTION

- Pronormoblasts divide and progress to form mature erythrocytes
  - Production of RBCs from the multipotential stem cell
    - BFU-E: Burst-forming unit–Erythroid
    - CFU-E: Colony-forming unit–Erythroid
    - Pronormoblast dividing and progressing to become a mature erythrocyte
      - Stages from most immature to mature

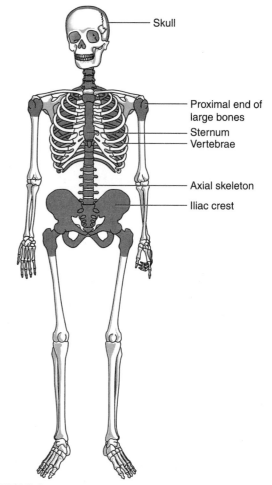

FIGURE 3-1 The adult skeleton, in which darkened areas depict active red marrow hematopoiesis. *(From Rodak BF, Fritsma GA, Keohane E: Hematology: clinical principles and applications, ed 4, St Louis, 2012, Saunders.)*

Labels: Skull, Proximal end of large bones, Sternum, Vertebrae, Axial skeleton, Iliac crest

- (1) Pronormoblast, (2) basophilic normoblast, (3) polychromatophilic normoblast, (4) orthochromic normoblast, (5) reticulocyte, (6) mature erythrocyte
  - As cells divide and mature, cell size gradually decreases and the nucleus is eventually extruded at maturity (Table 3-2)

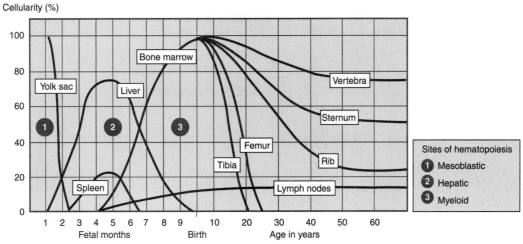

FIGURE 3-2 Sites of hematopoiesis. *(From Rodak BF, Fritsma GA, Keohane E: Hematology: clinical principles and applications, ed 4, St Louis, 2012, Saunders.)*

TABLE 3-1	Sites of Hematopoiesis		
Age	**Location**	**Product Produced**	**Other**
Embryo	Aorta-gonad-mesonephros (AGM) region/yolk sac	Hematopoietic stem cells, primitive erythroblasts, and fetal hemoglobins	
Fetal	Liver Other sites (spleen, kidney, thymus, lymph nodes) Bone marrow	Erythroblasts, granulocytes, monocytes	Liver is the primary site through first trimester Bone marrow becomes active around the fifth month of gestation
Birth through adult	Bone marrow Some involvement from lymph nodes, spleen, liver, kidney, thymus	All hematopoietic cell lines	Bone marrow is the primary site Babies and children have more red marrow activity, whereas normal adult marrow has an approximately equal composition of red and yellow marrow Thymus activity decreases after childhood

- o RBC synthesis is stimulated by erythropoietin, which is produced primarily in the kidney in response to hypoxia
- o RBCs normally have a lifespan of approximately 120 days. At the end of their life, they are removed by intravascular or extravascular hemolysis, and the contents of the cell are recycled or excreted.

HEMOGLOBIN (HGB) PRODUCTION

- Occurs from pronormoblast to reticulocyte stage of RBCs
  - Heme is synthesized in the mitochondria, so mature RBCs are unable to produce heme because of loss of mitochondria with maturation
- Normal Hgb is composed of four heme molecules nested in four globin molecules
  - Heme is composed of a protoporphyrin IX ring with Fe^{+2} at its center

- o Each heme molecule can combine reversibly with one molecule of oxygen
- The globin portion contains two pairs of globin chains, two α chains and two non-α chains
  - o α and ζ chain production is controlled by genes on chromosome 16
  - o β, γ, δ, and ε chain production is controlled by genes on chromosome 11
  - o Chain production is turned on and off through stages of development, leading to production of mainly α and β chains with maturity (Table 3-4)
- Hgb is used for the transport of gases
  - o O_2 affinity of Hgb is low at a low O_2 tension in the body and affinity is high at a high O_2 tension. This is demonstrated by the O_2 dissociation curve (Figure 3-4)
- Oxyhemoglobin is the primary Hgb for gas transport in the body, but other Hgb variants may be seen

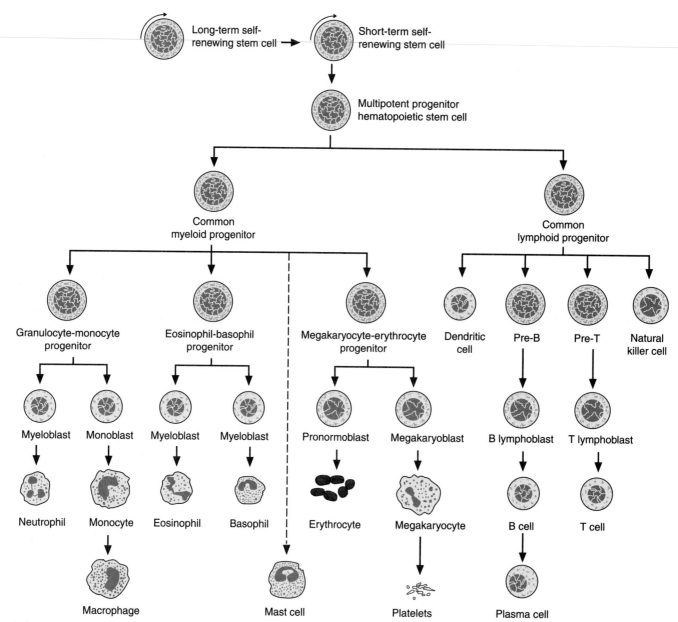

FIGURE 3-3 Diagram of hematopoiesis shows derivation of cells from the multipotent stem cell. *(From Rodak BF, Fritsma GA, Keohane E: Hematology: clinical principles and applications, ed 4, St Louis, 2012, Saunders.)*

TABLE 3-2	Red Blood Cell Maturation				
Cell or Stage	**Diameter**	**Nucleus-to-Cytoplasm Ratio**	**Nucleoli**	**% in Bone Marrow**	**Bone Marrow Transit Time (hr)**
Pronormoblast	12-20 μm	8:1	1-2	1	24
Basophilic normoblast	10-15 μm	6:1	0-1	1-4	24
Polychromatic normoblast	10-12 μm	4:1	0	10-20	30
Orthochromic normoblast	8-10 μm	1:2	0	5-10	48
Shift (stress) reticulocyte (polychromatic erythrocyte)	8-10 μm	No nucleus	0	1	48-72*
Polychromatic erythrocyte	8-8.5 μm	No nucleus	0	1	24-48*

From Rodak BF, Fritsma GA, Keohane E: Hematology: clinical principles and applications, ed 4, St Louis, 2012, Saunders.
*Transit time in peripheral blood.

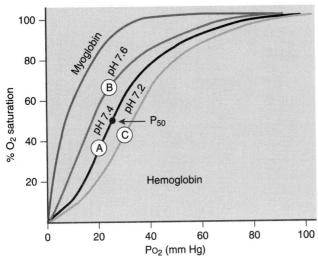

FIGURE 3-4 Oxygen dissociation curve. **A,** Normal dissociation curve. **B,** Left-shifted curve with reduced P50 caused by a decrease in 2,3-bisphosphoglycerate (2,3-BPG), partial pressure of carbon dioxide (Pco₂), temperature, and H⁺ ions (raised pH). A left-shifted curve is also seen with hemoglobin variants that have increased oxygen affinity. **C,** Right-shifted curve with increased P50 caused by an elevation in 2,3-BPG, Pco₂, temperature, and H⁺ ions (lowered pH). A right-shifted curve is also seen with hemoglobin variants that have decreased O₂ affinity. *(From Rodak BF, Fritsma GA, Keohane E: Hematology: clinical principles and applications, ed 4, St Louis, 2012, Saunders.)*

Hemoglobin Variants

Methemoglobin	Hgb containing Fe^{+3} instead of the normally reduced Fe^{+2}
	Formed normally as a result of oxidation; however, it is usually kept from overproduction because of the methemoglobin reductase pathway, an offshoot of the Embden-Meyerhof pathway
Sulfhemoglobin	Hgb formed as a result of oxidation of Hgb by materials containing sulfur
	Process is irreversible, so once Hgb has become sulfhemoglobin, it will remain for the life of the cell
	Unable to transport O_2, leading to cyanosis
Carboxyhemoglobin	Hgb resulting from heme iron-binding carbon monoxide
	CO has a high O_2 affinity and does not give up O_2 to the tissues easily
	Small amounts of carboxyhemoglobin are produced within the cells, but most problems occur as a result of environmental exposures

RED BLOOD CELL METABOLISM AND PHYSIOLOGY

- Mature RBCs have no mitochondria, so rely on anaerobic glycolysis for energy via the Embden-Meyerhof pathway
- Energy is needed for the main Embden-Meyerhof pathway
  - Maintain cation gradients
    - Keeps potassium inside and sodium outside the RBC
- Maintain the RBC membrane flexibility
- Supply offshoot pathways
  - Hexose monophosphate shunt
    - Protection of the RBC from oxidant damage by production of reduced glutathione
  - Methemoglobin reductase pathway
    - Maintaining iron in the ferrous form for Hgb to limit the production of methemoglobin
  - Rapoport-Luebering pathway
    - Regulation of O_2 delivery to tissues by the production of 2,3 bisphosphoglycerate (2,3 BPG) (Figure 3-5)

WHITE BLOOD CELLS

- Neutrophils
  - Phagocytic cells present in the peripheral circulation destroy foreign substances and microorganisms
  - Constitute the majority of circulating WBCs in adults
  - Development (Table 3-3)
    - Stages from most immature to mature include 1. myeloblast 2. promyelocyte 3. myelocyte 4. metamyelocyte 5. band 6. segmented neutrophil (Table 3-3).
  - Normal neutrophil function
    - Cells move to a site of inflammation, and granules are released to assist in travel and adhesion. Once at their target site, cells work to eliminate the foreign material by phagocytosis Granule contents and neutrophil extracellular traps are used to trap and kill microorganisms (Boxes 3-1 to 3-3)
  - Location
    - Present in a circulating pool in which neutrophils travel throughout the peripheral circulation and a marginating pool in which neutrophils line the walls of the vasculature, waiting to be called into use. In the bone marrow, before release to the peripheral vasculature, a storage pool and mitotic pool are present
- Eosinophils
  - Maturation is similar to neutrophil maturation, although granule contents are different; eosinophils have a variety of substances in their granules (see Box 3-3)
  - Normal function
    - Cells serve in immune regulation, from antigen presentation to initiation of immune response
    - Primarily increased in parasitic infection (especially helminths) and allergic disorders
- Basophils
  - Maturation is similar to eosinophil and neutrophil maturation. Basophils have several different types of granules (Box 3-4)
  - Cells have immunoglobulin E (IgE) receptors that lead to their effectiveness in allergic and hypersensitivity reactions. They also play a role in initiating the immune response

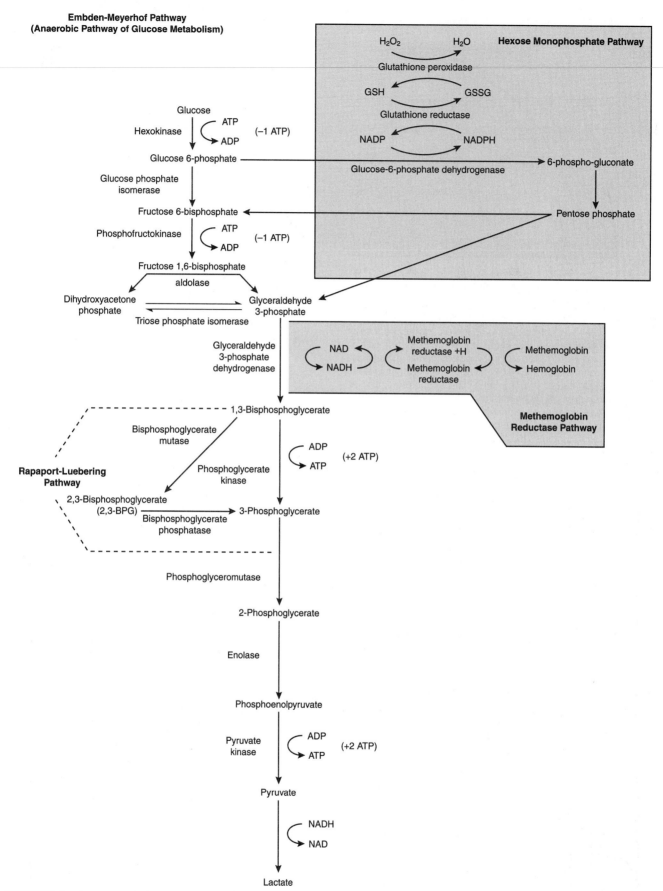

FIGURE 3-5 Glucose metabolism in the erythrocyte. *ADP,* Adenosine diphosphate; *ATP,* adenosine triphosphate; *G6PD,* glucose-6-phosphate dehydrogenase; *NAD,* nicotinamide adenine dinucleotide; *NADH,* nicotinamide adenine dinucleotide (reduced form); *NADP,* nicotinamide adenine dinucleotide phosphate (oxidized form). *(From Rodak BF, Fritsma GA, Keohane E: Hematology: clinical principles and applications, ed 4, St Louis, 2012, Saunders.)*

TABLE 3-3	Neutrophil Development	
Stage	**Description**	**Image**
Myeloblast	Earliest recognizable stage; cells are large with large nuclei and loose chromatin, some primary granules may be seen	*(From Rodak BF, Fritsma GA, Keohane E: Hematology: clinical principles and applications, ed 4, St Louis, 2012, Saunders. See Color Plate 27.)*
Promyelocyte	Cell begins to decrease in size, and chromatin begins to compact, with nucleus often appearing as eccentric; primary granules are prominent	*(From Rodak BF, Fritsma GA, Keohane E: Hematology: clinical principles and applications, ed 4, St Louis, 2012, Saunders. See Color Plate 28.)*
Myelocyte	Cell continues to decrease in size, and chromatin continues to compact into a round nucleus; last stage capable of mitosis; secondary granules are formed	*(From Rodak BF, Fritsma GA, Keohane E: Hematology: clinical principles and applications, ed 4, St Louis, 2012, Saunders. See Color Plate 29.)*

(Continued)

TABLE 3-3	Neutrophil Development—cont'd	
Stage	**Description**	**Image**
Metamyelocyte	Cell continues to decrease in size, chromatin continues to compact into a kidney bean shape; secondary and tertiary granules are formed	*(From Rodak BF, Fritsma GA, Keohane E: Hematology: clinical principles and applications, ed 4, St Louis, 2012, Saunders. See Color Plate 30.)*
Band neutrophil	Nucleus shows compact chromatin that is shaped into a horseshoe form; tertiary and secretory granules are formed	*(From Rodak BF, Fritsma GA, Keohane E: Hematology: clinical principles and applications, ed 4, St Louis, 2012, Saunders. See Color Plate 31.)*
Segmented neutrophil	Nucleus begins to segment into three to four lobes, each attached by a threadlike nuclear filament; secretory granules are formed	*(From Rodak BF, Fritsma GA, Keohane E: Hematology: clinical principles and applications, ed 4, St Louis, 2012, Saunders. See Color Plate 32.)*

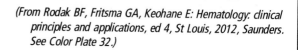

- *NOTE:* Mast cells are somewhat related to basophils; however, they are tissue cells used in allergic reactions and inflammation

- Monocytes
  - Maturation starts with a monoblast and continues to the promonocyte and mature monocyte stages
  - Cell appearance shows large cells, the largest in peripheral circulation, with finely granular cytoplasm ("ground-glass" appearance) and a nucleus with relatively loose, lacy chromatin, with the occasional presence of folding or indentation. Cytoplasm may show vacuolization
  - Functions
    o Cells are used in both innate and adaptive immunity. They can recognize and phagocytize foreign materials; in addition they can serve as antigen-presenting cells to initiate T and B cells they

TABLE 3-4	Normal Hemoglobins and Globin Chains	
Embryonic	**Fetal**	**Adult**
Gower 1: $\zeta_2\varepsilon_2$	Hgb F: $\alpha_2\gamma_2$ $\sim$50%-90%	Hgb A: $\alpha_2\beta_2$ 97%
Gower 2: $\alpha_2\varepsilon_2$	Hgb A: $\alpha_2\beta_2$ $\sim$10%-40%	Hgb A$_2$: $\alpha_2\delta_2$ $\sim$1.5%-3.5%
Portland: $\zeta_2\gamma_2$	Hgb A$_2$: $\alpha_2\delta_2 <$2%	Hgb F: $\alpha_2\gamma_2 <$2%

BOX 3-1 | Neutrophil Granules

Primary (Azurophilic) Granules
Formed during the promyelocyte stage
Last to be released (exocytosis)
Contain
  Myeloperoxidase
  Acid β-glycerophosphatase
  Cathepsins
  Defensins
  Elastase
  Proteinase-3
  Others

Secondary (Specific) Granules
Formed during myelocyte and metamyelocyte stages
Third to be released
Contain
  β_2-Microglobulin
  Collagenase
  Gelatinase
  Lactoferrin
  Neutrophil gelatinase–associated lipocalin
  Others

Tertiary Granules
Formed during metamyelocyte and band stages
Second to be released
Contain
  Gelatinase
  Collagenase
  Lysozyme
  Acetyltransferase
  β_2-Microglobulin

Secretory Granules (Secretory Vesicles)
Formed during band and segmented stages
First to be released (fuse to plasma membrane)
Contain (attached to membrane)
  CD11b/CD18
  Alkaline phosphatase
  Vesicle-associated membrane-2
  CD10, CD13, CD14, CD16
  Cytochrome b558
  Complement 1q receptor
  Complement receptor-1

From Rodak BF, Fritsma GA, Keohane E: Hematology: clinical principles and applications, ed 4, St Louis, 2012, Saunders.

BOX 3-2 | Phagocytosis

Recognition and attachment
- Phagocyte receptors recognize and bind to certain foreign molecular patterns and opsonins such as antibodies and complement components.

Ingestion
- Pseudopodia are extended around the foreign particle and enclose it within a phagosome (engulfment).
- The phagosome is pulled toward the center of the cell by polymerization of actin and myosin and by microtubules.

Killing and digestion
Oxygen dependent
- Respiratory burst through the activation of nicotine adenine diphosphate oxidase (reduced form). H_2O_2 and hypochlorite are produced.

Oxygen independent
- The pH within the phagosome becomes alkaline and then neutral, the pH at which digestive enzymes work.
- Primary and secondary lysosomes (granules) fuse to the phagosome and empty hydrolytic enzymes and other bacteriocidal molecules into the phagosome.

Formation of neutrophil extracellular traps
- Nuclear and organelle membranes dissolve, and activated cytoplasmic enzymes attach to DNA.
- The cytoplasmic membrane ruptures and DNA with attached enzymes is expelled, so that the bacteria are digested in the external environment.

From Rodak BF, Fritsma GA, Keohane E: Hematology: clinical principles and applications, ed 4, St Louis, 2012, Saunders.

BOX 3-3 **Eosinophil Granules**

Primary Granules
Formed during promyelocyte stage
Contain
    Charcot-Leyden crystal protein

Secondary Granules
Formed throughout remaining maturation
Contain
    Major basic protein (core)
    Eosinophil cationic protein (matrix)
    Eosinophil-derived neurotoxin (matrix)
    Eosinophil peroxidase (matrix)
    Lysozyme (matrix)
    Catalase (core and matrix)
    β-Glucuronidase (core and matrix)
    Cathepsin D (core and matrix)
    Interleukins-2, -4, and -5 (core)
    Interleukin-6 (matrix)
    Granulocyte-macrophage colony-stimulating factor (core)

Others
Small lysosomal granules
    Acid phosphatase
    Arylsulfatase B
    Catalase
    Cytochrome b_{558}
    Elastase
    Eosinophil cationic protein
Lipid bodies
    Cyclooxygenase
    5-Lipoxygenase
    15-Lipoxygenase
    Leukotriene C4 synthase
    Eosinophil peroxidase
    Esterase
Storage vesicles
    Carry proteins from secondary granules to be released into the extracellular medium

From Rodak BF, Fritsma GA, Keohane E: Hematology: clinical principles and applications, ed 4, St Louis, 2012, Saunders.

BOX 3-4 **Basophil Granules**

Secondary Granules
Histamine
Platelet activating factor
Leukotriene C_4
Interleukin-4
Interleukin-13
Vascular endothelial growth factor A
Vascular endothelial growth factor B
Chondroitin sulfates (e.g., heparin)

TABLE 3-5 **Normal Range Values in Adults**

	Adult Male	Adult Female
WBC ($\times 10^9$/L)	4.5-11.5	4.5-11.5
RBC ($\times 10^{12}$/L)	4.60-6.00	4.00-5.40
Hgb (g/dL)	14.0-18.0	12.0-15.0
Hct (%)	40-54	35-49
MCV (fL)	80-100	80-100
MCH (pg)	26-32	26-32
MCHC (g/dL)	32-36	32-36
RDW (%)	11.5-14.5	11.5-14.5
Platelet ($\times 10^9$/L)	150-450	150-450
MPV (fL)	6.8-10.2	6.8-10.2
Neutrophils (%)	50-70	50-70
Lymphocytes (%)	18-42	18-42
Monocytes (%)	2.0-11	2.0-11
Eosinophils (%)	1.0-3	1.0-3
Basophils (%)	0-2	0-2
Segmented neutrophils ($\times 10^9$/L)	2.3-8.1	2.3-8.1
Band neutrophils ($\times 10^9$/L)	0-0.6	0-0.6
Lymphocytes ($\times 10^9$/L)	0.8-4.8	0.8-4.8
Monocytes ($\times 10^9$/L)	0.45-1.3	0.45-1.3
Eosinophils ($\times 10^9$/L)	0-0.4	0-0.4
Basophils ($\times 10^9$/L)	0-0.1	0-0.1

Hct, Hematocrit; *Hgb*, hemoglobin; *MCH*, mean corpuscular hemoglobin; *MCV*, mean corpuscular volume; *MPV*, mean platelet volume; *RBC*, red blood cell; *RDW*, red cell distribution width; *WBC*, white blood cell.

---

are and can be used for housekeeping purposes to remove dead cells and debris

  o *NOTE:* Once monocytes migrate to tissues, they serve as tissue macrophages with similar functions

- Lymphocytes
  - The maturation stages are 1. lymphoblast 2. prolymphocyte 3. mature lymphocyte. There are three major subgroups of lymphocytes: T cells, B cells, and natural killer (NK) cells.
  - Lymphocytes can be produced in both the bone marrow and the lymphoid tissues. Cells can return from an inactive/resting form into active blasts, as needed
  - Functions
    - o B cells produce antibodies and also play a role in antigen presentation to the T cells
    - o T cells mediate the immune response

LABORATORY CONSIDERATIONS

Normal Ranges

- Patient values are compared against established normal ranges, which can vary based on age, gender, population, and geographic distribution. Although normal ranges

are relatively similar, some slight variations may occur based on a specific laboratory's population (Table 3-5)

Staining of Blood and Bone Marrow Samples

- Smears are made of blood or bone marrow to provide smears with the best possible distribution of cellular elements, leaving a "critical area" or examination area

where a single layer of cells is evenly dispersed, allowing visualization of individual cellular elements
- Wright or Wright-Giemsa stains (Romanowsky-type stains) are polychrome stains used to stain slides of peripheral blood and bone marrow, which gives elements their characteristic colors
  - Slides are fixed with a methanol fixative, followed by staining with a solution or solutions containing eosin and methylene blue to impart color to cellular elements
  - Eosin is acidic, so it will stain basic elements, such as Hgb and basic proteins found in some cell granules
  - Methylene blue is basic and will stain acidic elements, such as cell nuclei and immature cell cytoplasm
  - Stained slides can be used for counting the 100 cell count WBC differential and examining RBC and platelet morphology. In the case of bone marrow, aspirate and core biopsy slides can be stained for a bone marrow differential, myeloid-to-erythroid (M/E) ratio, or sample cellularity

Red Blood Cell Morphology

See Tables 3-6 and 3-7

Red Blood Cell Indices

- Red blood cell indices may be calculated manually or derived from automated instrumentation.

See Table 3-8

Manual and Semiautomated Techniques

- Most hematologic testing is performed using automated instrumentation; however, a few manual techniques may be used on occasion

Hemacytometer

- Counting chamber used for manual cell counting, currently most frequently used for body fluid cell counting
- Based on the use of a known counting area of nine squares each with an area of 1 mm^2 and a total volume of 0.9 mm^3 for a total area of 9 mm^3. A standard formula is used to determine a total cell count/µL (1 mm^3 = 1 µL) (Figure 3-6)

$$\text{Total cell count (cells/µL)} = \left(\frac{\text{Cells counted}}{\substack{\text{Number of squares counted} \times \\ \text{area of squares counted} \times \text{depth}}} \right) \times \text{Reciprocal dilution}$$

Manual hematocrit (Hct, also known as microhematocrit)

- Hct is the volume of packed RBCs occupying a specific volume of whole blood, expressed as a percentage or in liters per liter

- Measured by placing whole blood in capillary tubes and centrifuging to read the packed cell volume on a manual microhematocrit reading device
- Hct values are available on automated general hematology cell counters; however, values are derived by using a calculation as opposed to a physical measurement

Reticulocyte Count

- Reticulocytes are the final stage before an RBC reaches maturity. Reticulocytes may be counted manually to determine the erythrocyte production and release from the bone marrow
- Manual counts are performed by incubating ethylenediametetraacetic acid (EDTA) whole blood with a supravital stain, usually new methylene blue. If any RNA or residual organelles are present, they will take up the supravital stain and are visible microscopically
  - Various methods are used for the manual reticulocyte count, including the Miller ocular and other techniques to determine the total percentage of reticulocytes present
- Automated reticulocyte counts are now commonly performed
  - Various methods are used for automated counts, including treating RBCs with a stain or fluorescent dye to identify the reticulocyte by optical methods or flow cytometry. Automation allows for a larger number of cells to be examined.

Sickle Cell Testing

- Samples may be screened for the presence of abnormal Hgb because of the different solubility properties of various Hgb
- Hgb S exhibits decreased solubility when deoxygenated, as opposed to the more soluble Hgb A and A$_2$
  - Screening tests use a lysing agent and a dithionite solution, or other reducing agent, to induce deoxygenation of Hgb. Abnormal Hgbs have decreased solubility and will precipitate in the solution, appearing cloudy on observation
  - Positive sickle cell screens require follow-up with a more definitive test, such as Hgb electrophoresis, high-performance liquid chromatography (HPLC), or isoelectric focusing

Erythrocyte Sedimentation Rate (ESR)

- Screening test used to screen or monitor for various inflammatory states. The ESR looks at how much RBC settling will occur in a well-mixed whole blood sample over a 1-hour period
  - RBCs normally have a net negative charge, causing them to repel each other in a whole blood sample, leading to slow settling of the RBCs over time

TABLE 3-6	Description of Red Blood Cell Abnormalities and Commonly Associated Disease States

RBC Abnormality	Cell Description	Commonly Associated Disease States
Anisocytosis	Abnormal variation in RBC volume or diameter	Hemolytic, megaloblastic, iron-deficiency anemia
Macrocyte	Large RBC (>8 μm in diameter), MCV >100 fL	Megaloblastic anemia Myelodysplastic syndrome Chronic liver disease Bone marrow failure Reticulocytosis
Oval macrocyte	Large, oval RBC	Megaloblastic anemia
Poikilocytosis	Abnormal variation in RBC shape	Severe anemia Certain shapes helpful diagnostically
Spherocyte	Small, round, dense RBC with no central pallor	Hereditary spherocytosis Immune hemolytic anemia Extensive burns (along with schistocytes)
Elliptocyte, ovalocyte	Elliptical (cigar shaped), oval (egg shaped), RBC	Hereditary elliptocytosis or ovalocytosis Iron-deficiency anemia Thalassemia major Myelophthisic anemias
Stomatocyte	RBC with slitlike area of central pallor	Hereditary stomatocytosis Rh deficiency syndrome Acquired stomatocytosis (liver disease, alcoholism) Artifact
Sickle cell	Thin, dense, elongated RBC pointed at each end; may be curved	Sickle cell anemia Sickle cell–β-thalassemia
Hgb C crystal	Hexagonal crystal of dense Hgb formed within the RBC membrane	Hgb C disease
Hgb SC crystal	Fingerlike or quartzlike crystal of dense Hgb protruding from the RBC membrane	Hgb SC disease
Target cell (codocyte)	RBC with Hgb concentrated under and around the periphery resembling a target	Liver disease Hemoglobinopathies Thalassemia
Schistocyte (schizocyte)	Fragmented RBC resulting from rupture in the peripheral circulation	Microangiopathic hemolytic anemia* (along with microspherocytes) Traumatic cardiac hemolysis Extensive burns (along with microspherocytes)
Helmet cell (keratocyte)	RBC fragment in shape of a helmet	Same as schistocyte
Folded cell	RBC with membrane folded over	Hb C disease Hb SC disease
Acanthocyte (spur cell)	Small, dense RBC with few irregularly spaced projections of varying length	Severe liver disease (spur cell anemia) Neuroacanthocytosis (abetalipoproteinemia, McLeod's syndrome)
Burr cell (echinocyte)	RBC with blunt or pointed, short projections that are usually evenly spaced over the surface of cell; present in all fields of blood film but in variable numbers per field†	Uremia Pyruvate kinase deficiency
Teardrop cell (dacryocyte)	RBC with a single pointed extension resembling a teardrop or pear	Primary myelofibrosis Myelophthisic anemia Thalassemia Megaloblastic anemia

From Rodak BF, Fritsma GA, Keohane E: Hematology: clinical principles and applications, ed 4, St Louis, 2012, Saunders.
*Such as thrombotic thrombocytopenic purpura, hemolytic uremic syndrome, disseminated intravascular coagulation.
†Cells with similar morphology that are unevenly distributed in a blood film (not present in all fields) are likely the result of a drying artifact in blood film preparation; these artifacts are sometimes referred to as crenated RBCs.
Hgb, Hemoglobin; *MCV*, mean cell volume; *RBC*, red blood cell; *SC*, sickle cell.

- When a change to the charge occurs, usually resulting from increases in plasma proteins, the cells become attracted to each other, leading to increased settling speeds of the RBCs
- Tests are performed with manual Westergren and Wintrobe procedures or automated analyzers to allow for a faster reading

Hematology Instrumentation

- Cell counters
  - Automated method for performing complete blood cell counts
  - Count cells using impedance and optical measurements

TABLE 3-7	Erythrocyte Inclusions: Description, Composition, and Selected Commonly Associated Disease States			
Inclusion	Appearance in Supravital Stain	Appearance in Wright Stain	Inclusion Composition	Associated Diseases and Conditions
Diffuse basophilia	Granules and filaments	Bluish tinge throughout cytoplasm; also referred to as polychromasia	RNA	Hemolytic anemia After treatment for iron, vitamin B$_{12}$, or folate deficiency
Basophilic stippling (punctate basophilia)	Granules and filaments	Blue-purple granules distributed throughout cytoplasm	Precipitated RNA	Lead poisoning Thalassemia Hemoglobinopathies Abnormal heme synthesis
Howell Jolly body	Dense, round, granule	Dense, round, blue or purple granule; usually one per cell; occasionally multiple	DNA (nuclear fragment)	Hyposplenism After splenectomy Megaloblastic anemia Hemolytic anemia
Heinz body	Round granule attached to inner membrane	Not visible	Denatured hemoglobin	Glucose-6-phosphate dehydrogenase deficiency Unstable hemoglobins Oxidant drugs/chemicals
Pappenheimer bodies*	Clusters of small granules	Clusters of small, light blue granules, often near periphery of cell	Iron	Sideroblastic anemia Hemoglobinopathies Hyposplenism Megaloblastic anemia
Cabot ring	Rings or figure-eights	Blue rings or figure-eights	Remnant of mitotic spindle	Megaloblastic anemia Myelodysplastic syndromes
Hgb H	Fine, evenly dispersed granules	Not visible	Precipitate of β chains of hemoglobin	Hgb H disease

From Rodak BF, Fritsma GA, Keohane E: Hematology: clinical principles and applications, ed 4, St Louis, 2012, Saunders.
*Blue (siderotic) granules observed in Prussian blue stain.
Hgb, Hemoglobin.

TABLE 3-8	Red Blood Cell Indices		
	Definition	Manual Calculation	Normal Range
Mean corpuscular volume (MCV)	Average volume of an individual RBCAnalyzer: Measures directly *or*	(Hct [%]/RBC) × 10	80-100 fL
Mean corpuscular hemoglobin (MCH)	Average weight of hemoglobin in an individual RBCAnalyzer: Measures directly *or*	(Hgb [g/dL]/RBC) × 10	28-34 pg
Mean corpuscular hemoglobin concentration (MCHC)	Ratio of hemoglobin mass to the cell volume	(Hgb [g/dL]/Hct [%]) × 100	32-36 g/dL
Red cell distribution width (RDW)	Variation of RBC volume used to help identify the presence of anisocytosis Analyzer calculation = $\dfrac{\text{Standard Deviation of MCV}}{\text{Mean MCV}} \times 100$		11.5%-14.5%

o Impedance: Uses changes in electrical charge as cells, which have low conductivity, move through an electrically conductive fluid to determine cell count

▪ Pulses formed by electrical resistance are counted
　▪ The number of pulses recorded is proportional to the cell count

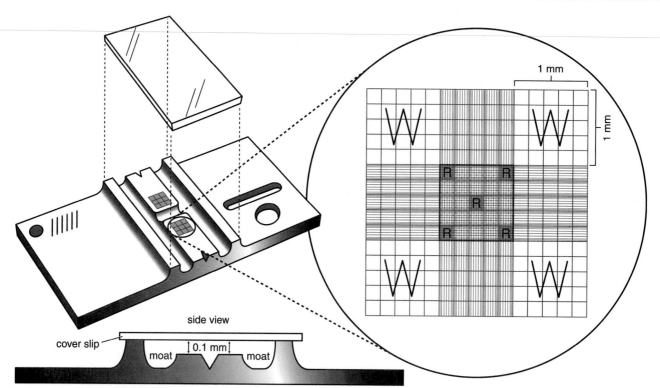

FIGURE 3-6 Hemacytometer and close-up view of the counting areas as seen under the microscope. The areas for the standard white blood cell count are labeled *W*, and the areas for the standard red blood cell count are labeled *R*. The entire center square is used for counting platelets. *(From Rodak BF, Fritsma GA, Keohane E: Hematology: clinical principles and applications, ed 4, St Louis, 2012, Saunders.)*

- Pulse size is proportional to cell size
- Can be used to count WBC, RBC, and platelets
  - Optical counts: Use of optical light scatter to determine the size and complexity of cells present as a single cell moves through a focused light source
    - Forward and side scatter are used to determine an automated differential count
- Hgb measurement
  - Determined using a cyanmethemoglobin reagent to quantitate the amount of Hgb spectrophotometrically within the instrument
- Calculations
  - Automated calculations performed from measured parameters provide values for Hct, mean corpuscular volume (MCV), mean corpuscular hemoglobin (MCH), mean corpuscular hemoglobin concentration (MCHC), and red blood cell distribution width (RDW)
- Corrected WBC count
  - In the case of elevated numbers of nucleated RBCs, the nucleated red blood cells (NRBCs) should be counted independently of the 100 cell count WBC differential. Some analyzers automatically correct for the presence of NRBCs; however, sometimes the WBC count must be corrected manually
  - Calculated WBC Correction for NRBCs
    - Corrected WBC count = Analyzer WBC count × 100/100 + number of NRBCs per 100 WBCs counted

- NOTE: If a corrected WBC count is needed, it should be lower than the original WBC count from the analyzer

Bone Marrow Collection

- Bone marrow samples may be needed for evaluation of the patient's hematologic condition. Bone marrow samples, including a core biopsy and aspirate, are collected by a physician, and the samples obtained are processed in the laboratory
- Samples are collected and analyzed for various reasons, including diagnosis and staging hematopoietic malignancies, diagnosis and evaluation of unexplained cytopenias or systemic disorders, follow-up after patients undergo various treatments (chemotherapy, radiation, transplants), determining sources of otherwise undiagnosed infections, and other miscellaneous purposes
- Bone marrow samples are collected from sites where active red marrow is more prevalent, usually the posterior superior iliac crest; however, the sternum or anterior iliac crest may be used in adult patients. Sometimes tibia samples are obtained in young children
- Aspirate samples are used to assess morphology and perform a differential count and M:E ratio
  - The M:E ratio looks at the number of myeloid cells compared to the numbers of nucleated erythroid precursors
    - Lymphocytes are not included in this ratio

- A normal M:E ratio is usually in the range of 2:1 to 4:1
- Core biopsy samples are used to determine bone marrow cellularity
  - Helps assess if the sample is normocellular, hypocellular, or hypercellular
  - Cytochemical stains, flow cytometry, and other specialized testing may be performed on bone marrow samples

Flow Cytometry

- Flow cytometry is an automated method of sorting cells. It uses a cell suspension injected into a stream sheath fluid to determine specific characteristics of the cell, including size, complexity, immunophenotype, and cytochemistry
  - Hydrodynamic focusing: Cells in suspension move through sheath fluid in a single-file line, allowing each to individually pass through a laser light
    - Allows specific characterization of each cell
      - Forward scatter for size determination
      - Side scatter for complexity of the cell
  - Gating: Electronic boundaries created to separate a specific population of interest
    - Performed during or after initial analysis
  - Fluorescently tagged antibodies can be used to determine cell lineage and aid in characterizing patient immunophenotype (Table 3-9)

Special Stains and Cytochemistry

- Special staining techniques may be performed to help differentiate cell types, particularly in cases of leukemia (Table 3-10)
  - Flow cytometry has decreased the use of cytochemistry in differentiating leukemias; however, elements are incorporated into flow cytometry or still performed as stand-alone testing to assist in a definitive diagnosis

ANEMIA AND RED BLOOD CELL DISORDERS

- Usually defined as decreased ability of blood to carry O_2 or as a decrease in RBCs/Hgb from an established reference range
- Common physical symptoms
  - Fatigue
  - Shortness of breath
  - Pallor
  - Cardiac issues
  - Other symptoms may be more related to specific causes of anemia
    - Jaundice
    - Pica

TABLE 3-9 Lineage-Associated Markets Commonly Analyzed in Routine Flow Cytometry

Lineage	Markers
Immature	CD34
	CD117
	Terminal deoxynucleotidyl transferase
Granulocytic/monocytic	CD33
	CD13
	CD15
	CD14
Erythroid	CD71
	Glycophorin A
Megakaryocytic	CD41
	CD42
	CD61
B lymphocytes	CD19
	CD20
	CD22
	κ Light chain
	λ Light chain
T lymphocytes	CD2
	CD3
	CD4
	CD5
	CD7
	CD8

  - Glossitis
  - Splenomegaly
  - Neurologic symptoms
- Common tests for initial anemia evaluation
  - Complete blood count (CBC) with peripheral smear review
    - Determines RBC, Hgb, Hct, and RBC indices

	Normal Range	Resulting Morphology (If Abnormal)
MCV	80-100 fL	<80 fL: Microcytic
		>100 fL: Macrocytic
MCH	28-34 pg	
MCHC	32-36 g/dL	<32 g/dL: Hypochromic
		36-40 g/dL: Normochromic
		>40 g/dL: Results may be invalid

    - Smear examination will reveal the appearance of RBCs (anisocytosis and poikilocytosis and inclusions)
  - Reticulocyte count
    - Shows the bone marrow response to decreases in RBCs
- Anemias may be classified by combinations of different criteria
  - Morphology
    - RBC indices are used to gauge size and hemoglobinization
      - Normocytic/normochromic

TABLE 3-10	**Staining Techniques**			
Cytochemical Stain	**Element Stained**	**Positive Reaction**	**Negative Reaction**	**Diagnostic Utility**
Myeloperoxidase (MPO)	Enzyme found in the primary granules of granulocytic cells	Myeloblasts and promyelocytes, although some weak activity may be seen in monocytes	Lymphoblasts	Differentiating AML versus ALL
Sudan black B (SBB)	Lipids found in primary and secondary granules and in lysosomal granules of monocytes	Myeloblasts and promyelocytes, although some weak activity may be seen in monocytes	Lymphoblasts	Differentiating AML versus ALL
Specific esterase (naphthol AS-D chloroacetate esterase)	Esterase enzymes found in neutrophils	Myeloblasts	Lymphoid cells	Identifying cells of myeloid origin
Nonspecific esterase (α-naphthyl acetate or butyrate esterase)	Esterase enzymes found in monocytes	Monoblasts and monocytes	Granulocytes and lymphoid cells	AML of myeloid versus monocytic origin
Tartrate-resistant acid phosphatase (TRAP)	Isoenzymes of acid phosphatase	Hairy cell lymphocytes (in hairy cells, isoenzyme 5 of acid phosphatase is not inhibited with the addition of tartrate, leaving a positive reaction)	All cells except hairy cell lymphocytes	Positive diagnosis of hairy cell leukemia
Periodic acid–Schiff (PAS)	Glycogen, mucoproteins and high-molecular-weight carbohydrates	Multiple cell types	Normal erythroblasts	AML of erythroid or megakaryoblastic origin and some cases of ALL based on staining pattern (leukemic lymphoblasts may have a coarse blocklike pattern, whereas erythroid precursors have a coarse and granular staining pattern
Leukocyte alkaline phosphatase (LAP)	Enzyme in the secondary granules of mature neutrophils	Neutrophils (activity is scored in mature bands and segmented neutrophils on a 0-4 rating scale)		Differentiation of CML (low activity) and leukemoid reaction (high activity)
Terminal deoxynucleotidyl transferase (TdT)	DNA polymerase in cell nuclei	Lymphoblasts	Myeloblasts and monoblasts	Identification of lymphoblasts in ALL

ALL, Acute lymphoblastic leukemia; *AML,* acute myelogenous leukemia; *CML,* chronic myelogenous leukemia.

- Microcytic/hypochromic
- Macrocytic/normochromic
- Function
  - Defects leading to RBC decreases
    - Proliferation: RBCs are not produced at normal rates
    - Maturation: RBCs are produced in the marrow but may not mature appropriately
    - Survival: RBCs are produced appropriately but are lost/destroyed prematurely

IRON AND HEME DISORDERS

- Iron-deficiency anemia (IDA): Lack of iron to make adequate heme
- Sideroblastic anemia: Adequate/excess iron that is not able to be effectively incorporated into heme
- Anemia of chronic disease/inflammation: Adequate iron stores that have impaired release for incorporation into heme/RBCs
- Hemochromatosis: Iron disorder that is *not* anemia, with excess iron absorption and stores

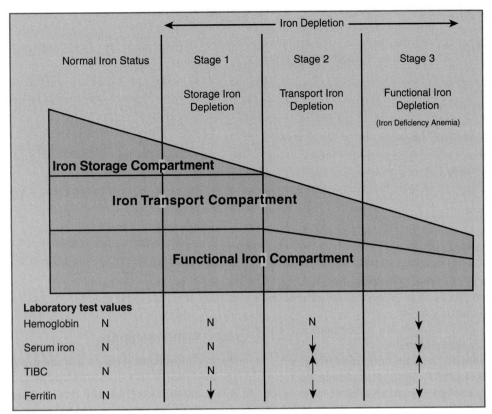

FIGURE 3-7 Development of iron deficiency anemia. ↑, Increased; ↓, decreased; *N*, normal; *TIBC*, total iron-binding capacity. (*Modified from Suominen P, Punnonen K, Rajamäki A, et al: Serum transferrin receptor and transferrin receptor–ferritin index identify healthy subjects with subclinical iron deficits, Blood 92:2934-2939, 1998; reprinted with permission.*)

Iron-Deficiency Anemia

- Iron intake and stores do not meet the body's needs for RBC production
  - Inadequate intake
    - Daily intake does not meet daily loss
    - Nutritional deficiencies
  - Increased requirements
    - Rapid growth periods
    - Menstruating women
    - Pregnancy and lactation
  - Absorption issues
    - Enterocytes are unable to absorb iron
      - Celiac disease
      - Bariatric surgeries
      - Medications
      - Other diseases impairing absorption
      - Loss of gastric absorption with age
      - Parasitic infections
- Chronic RBC loss
  - Chronic GI bleeding
  - Prolonged menorrhagia
  - Other chronic bleeds
    - Aspirin related
    - Alcohol related
    - Parasite related
- Laboratory diagnosis of IDA (Figure 3-7)
  - CBC
    - Varies with the severity of depletion
    - RBC, Hgb, Hct may be decreased
    - MCV and MCH often are decreased, resulting in microcytic/hypochromic cells
      - RBCs tend to be small with increased central pallor because of the lack of available Hgb
  - Iron studies
    - Serum iron: Decreased (may be normal in early stages)
    - Ferritin: Decreased
    - Total iron-binding capacity (TIBC): Increased
    - % Saturation: Decreased
- Treatment and follow-up
  - Determine and treat any underlying condition
  - Oral iron supplements
  - RBC transfusions only if Hgb is critically low
  - Response to therapy regimen monitored by
    - Reticulocyte counts increase within the 2 weeks of supplementation
    - CBC and Hgb increases 2 to 3 weeks after supplementation

Sideroblastic Anemia

- Anemia characterized by the presence of normal or increased iron that is not effectively incorporated into heme
- Hereditary
  - X-Linked or autosomal
- Acquired
  - Refractory anemia (as seen in myelodysplastic syndromes)
  - Drugs and toxins
    - Lead
    - Alcohol
    - Other varied drugs or toxins
- Laboratory diagnosis of sideroblastic anemia
  - CBC
    - Varies
    - RBC, Hgb, or Hct may be decreased
    - MCV and MCH may be decreased (microcytic and hypochromic cells)
      - Cells are often normocytic/normochromic in cases of lead poisoning.
      - Occasionally, siderotic granules are seen
    - Coarse basophilic stippling is seen in lead poisoning, although it can also be seen in other conditions
  - Iron studies
    - Serum iron: Increased
    - Ferritin: Increased
    - TIBC: Decreased
    - % Saturation: Decreased or normal
  - Bone marrow
    - Sometimes performed to reveal presence of increased iron/sideroblasts
- Treatment and follow-up
  - Hereditary forms may require medications to stimulate heme synthesis
  - Acquired forms may require the removal of the offending toxin or problem

Anemia of Chronic Inflammation (Disease)

- Acquired anemia characterized by abundant iron stores, yet iron cannot be readily incorporated into serum or RBCs for use
- Occurs as a result of increases in various acute phase reactants present with inflammation which slows iron release that is needed by developing cells
  - Hepcidin decreases iron release from macrophages and hepatocytes
  - Lactoferrin competes with transferrin for plasma iron, but RBCs cannot incorporate this because of lack of lactoferrin receptors
  - Ferritin binds iron, but developing RBCs lack ferritin receptors and cannot incorporate into the erythroid precursors
- Laboratory diagnosis of anemia of chronic inflammation
  - CBC
    - Anemia is usually mild
    - RBC, Hgb, Hct may be slightly decreased (Hgb 9-11 g/dL)
    - MCV and MCH are usually normal
    - Reticulocytes are normal to decreased
  - Iron studies
    - Serum iron: Increased
    - Ferritin: Increased (or may be normal)
    - TIBC: Decreased
    - % Saturation: Decreased
  - Bone marrow will show increased iron stores in macrophages
- Treatment and follow-up
  - Underlying condition may be treated
  - In some cases erythropoietin or iron may be administered for the patient

Hemochromatosis

- Iron problem that does not involve anemia
- Increased iron stores (absorption greater than loss)
  - Stored as ferritin and hemosiderin
    - Often stored around organs (heart, liver, pancreas)
- Acquired
  - Transfusion related
    - In cases of chronic transfusion, the body recycles the iron from transfused RBCs, in addition to its own senescent RBCs
  - Chronic liver disease
  - Alcoholism
  - Supplemental or dietary iron overload
- Inherited
  - Relatively high frequency in people of northern European descent (~1/200)
  - Several known mutations
    - Classic hereditary hemochromatosis, associated with the *HFE* gene
    - Hepcidin mutations, associated with the *HAMP* gene
    - Hemojuvelin mutations, associated with the *HJV* gene

MACROCYTIC ANEMIAS

- Megaloblastic anemia results from defective DNA synthesis
  - Vitamin B_{12} and folic acid deficiencies
- Nonmegaloblastic macrocytic anemia results from other causes
  - Liver disease
  - Alcoholism
  - Hypothyroidism
  - Reticulocytosis

Megaloblastic Anemia

- Impairment of DNA synthesis leads to large, abnormal cells.
  - Most commonly caused by lack of vitamin B_{12} and/or folic acid, although some other conditions may show megaloblastic changes
    - All rapidly dividing, nucleated cells, including RBCs, are affected
    - Ineffective erythropoiesis, with cells showing nuclear-cytoplasmic asynchrony as they mature
    - Vitamin B_{12} and folic acid are needed for DNA synthesis (Figure 3-8)
- Causes for folate deficiency
  - Poor dietary intake
  - Increases in need
    - Pregnancy
    - Lactation
    - Growing children
  - Impaired absorption and use
    - Intestinal diseases, including celiac disease and sprue
    - Intestinal surgery
    - Medications
  - Excessive loss
    - May occur in renal dialysis patients, so patients are often supplemented with folic acid
- Causes for vitamin B_{12} deficiency
  - Poor diet
    - Lack of dietary vitamin B_{12} or folic acid
  - Increases in need
    - Pregnancy
    - Lactation
    - Growing children
  - Impaired absorption and use
    - Inability to obtain vitamin B_{12} from food in the stomach
      - Gastric issues
        - Inability to produce hydrochloric acid, gastric bypass, drugs for lowering gastric acidity
      - Lack of intrinsic factor
        - Autoimmune disease, *Helicobacter pylori* infection, gastrectomy
      - Competition for vitamin B_{12}
        - *Diphyllobothrium latum*
        - Intestinal bacteria in blind loop syndrome
  - Excessive loss
    - May occur in renal dialysis patients, so patients are supplemented with folic acid (see Figure 3-8)
- Physical examination
  - General anemia symptoms
  - Glossitis
  - Gastrointestinal (GI) symptoms
  - Vitamin B_{12} deficiency also may result in neurologic symptoms
    - Memory loss, balance, and gait abnormalities, personality changes

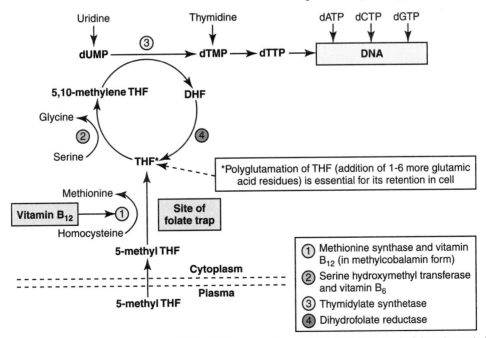

FIGURE 3-8 Role of folate and vitamin B_{12} in DNA synthesis. Folate enters the cell as 5-methyltetrahydrofolate *(5-methyl THF)*. In the cell, a methyl group is transferred from 5-methyl THF to homocysteine, converting it to methionine and generating tetrahydrofolate *(THF)*. This reaction is catalyzed by methionine synthase and requires vitamin B_{12} as a cofactor. THF is then converted to 5,10-methylene THF by the donation of a methyl group from serine. The methyl group of 5,10-methylene THF is then transferred to deoxyuridine monophosphate *(dUMP)*, which converts it to deoxythymidine monophosphate *(dTMP)* and converts 5,10-methylene THF to dihydrofolate *(DHF)*. This reaction is catalyzed by thymidylate synthetase. dTMP is a precursor of deoxythymidine triphosphate *(dTTP)*, which is used to synthesize DNA. THF is regenerated by the conversion of DHF to THF by the enzyme DHF reductase. A deficiency of vitamin B_{12} prevents the production of THF from 5-methyl THF; as a result, folate becomes metabolically trapped as 5-methyl THF. This constitutes the "folate trap." *(From Rodak BF, Fritsma GA, Keohane E: Hematology: clinical principles and applications, ed 4, St Louis, 2012, Saunders.)*

- In vitamin B_{12} deficiencies, prolonged/severe cases may have demyelination of the neurons; folic acid deficiency does not have neurologic involvement
- Laboratory diagnosis of megaloblastic anemias
  - CBC
    - Decreases in RBC count, WBC, platelet, Hgb, and Hct; elevated MCV
      - RBCs include oval macrocytes, and inclusions may be present (Howell-Jolly bodies, NRBCs, Cabot rings)
      - Neutrophils may appear hypersegmented
  - Bone marrow
    - May be used to confirm presence of megaloblastic anemia
      - Megaloblastic changes are apparent (nucleus-to-cytoplasm [N:C] asynchrony)
      - Hypercellularity with increased, abnormal RBC precursors
      - Giant bands and metamyelocytes
  - Other laboratory testing
    - Serum vitamin B_{12} and folic acid assays
      - Decreases appear with deficiencies
    - Methylmalonic acid (MMA)
      - Increased in vitamin B_{12} deficiency, because it is needed for conversion of methylmalonyl coenzyme A (CoA) in the pathway
    - Homocysteine
      - Increased in vitamin B_{12} and folic acid deficiency, because vitamin B_{12} is needed for converting homocysteine to methionine in the pathway
    - Intrinsic factor antibodies
    - Parietal cell antibodies
    - Ova and parasite examination in cases of suspected vitamin B_{12} deficiency resulting from *D. latum* infection
    - Schilling test
      - Classic two-part test used to determine if the cause of vitamin B_{12} deficiency is malabsorption, dietary deficiency, or a lack of intrinsic factor
        - Part I: Patients are dosed orally with radiolabeled vitamin B_{12}, followed by a flushing dose of unlabeled vitamin B_{12}. Excess vitamin B_{12} is filtered by the kidney, and urine is measured for radioactivity. If radiolabeled vitamin B_{12} levels are elevated, the patient is likely deficient in vitamin B_{12} and unable to absorb the vitamin
        - Part II: If the vitamin B_{12} excretion in part I is decreased, the patient receives an oral dose of radiolabeled vitamin B_{12} and a dose of intrinsic factor. If the radiolabeled vitamin B_{12} levels are increased from those in part I, the patient is lacking intrinsic factor and has pernicious anemia. If the levels are abnormal, the patient may have another defect leading to malabsorption

- Although a classic means of determining the cause of vitamin B_{12} deficiency, the Schilling test is no longer performed regularly in the United States. Homocysteine and MMA are replacing this test, because they are better indicators of the deficiency
- Treatment of megaloblastic anemia
  - Once the underlying cause is established, specific treatment can be determined
    - Remove/repair underlying problem
    - Supplement with appropriate deficient vitamin, either vitamin B_{12} or folic acid
      - In cases of intrinsic factor problems, intramuscular injection of vitamin B_{12} can be used
      - If neurologic issues occur with vitamin B_{12} deficiency, they may be irreversible based on the extent of the damage
- Follow-up testing
  - CBC and reticulocyte count
    - Reticulocyte response may be seen within a week of treatment
    - Hypersegmented neutrophils are replaced by normal neutrophils in about 2 weeks
    - CBC may return to overall normal state in 3 to 6 weeks

Nonmalignant Macrocytic Anemias

- Macrocytosis without megaloblastic changes can occur
  - Normal babies
    - After delivery, macrocytosis and reticulocytosis are normal in newborns
      - MCV may increase up to 123 fL
  - Liver disease
  - Alcoholism
  - Hypothyroidism

HYPOPROLIFERATIVE DISORDERS

- Disorders occurring as a result of decreased or absent production of hematopoietic cells in the bone marrow
  - Includes aplastic anemia, both inherited and acquired, in addition to other disorders resulting from decreases in bone marrow production
  - Other disorders resulting from decreases in bone marrow production include
    - Pure red cell aplasia
    - Congenital dyserythropoietic anemia
    - Myelophthisic anemia
    - Anemia resulting from chronic kidney disease

Aplastic Anemia

- Rare disorders characterized by pancytopenia in the peripheral circulation. Result from decreased bone

marrow production of RBC, WBC, and platelets because of deficiency or damage of hematopoietic stem cells
- Acquired aplastic anemia
  - Most cases identified are acquired, the majority of which are idiopathic
    - Cause of the marrow failure in idiopathic cases is currently unknown
    - Other acquired cases have been linked to various drugs/chemicals, radiation, viral infections, and other miscellaneous causes
- Inherited aplastic anemia
  - A smaller number of cases are inherited, including Fanconi's anemia, dyskeratosis congenita, and Shwachman-Diamond syndrome
  - Fanconi's anemia
    - Chromosomes are susceptible to breakage and the cell may not be able to repair DNA damage. Cells also show accelerated telomere shortening and apoptosis.
      - This property is used to help diagnose Fanconi's anemia
    - Genetic mutations in one of 13 genes
      - *FANCA* mutations occur most frequently. Inheritance is autosomal recessive in all of the associated genes except *FANCB*, which is an X-linked gene.
    - Appears at birth or in early childhood
      - Symptoms resulting from pancytopenia may be apparent early on or manifest later in life
    - Skeletal abnormalities may be seen in many, in addition to abnormalities in skin pigmentation, and organ problems
    - Patients may have a higher risk for malignancies, in addition to the bone marrow failure
  - Dyskeratosis congenita
    - Very rare disorder in which chromosomes have short telomeres
    - Inheritance is autosomal dominant, X-linked recessive, and autosomal recessive, with various mutations present
    - Patients may show abnormalities in skin pigmentation and nails, in addition to a variety of abnormalities
  - Shwachman-Diamond syndrome
    - Autosomal recessive disorder leading to neutropenia and/or anemia and thrombocytopenia
    - Patients have decreased pancreatic enzymes, skeletal anomalies, and increased risk of infection
- General CBC findings in aplastic anemia
  - Pancytopenia, with decreases in one or more cell lines
    - Anemia with normocytic, normochromic RBCs
    - Decreased granulocytes with normal to slightly decreased lymphocytes
    - Decreased platelets
    - Decreased reticulocyte production
  - Bone marrow

- Hypocellular with increased fat cells
  - Biopsy is needed for accurate diagnosis
- Decreased granulocytes, RBCs, and platelets
- Treatment
  - Eliminate the problem causing bone marrow failure, if it can be identified
  - Transfusions (RBCs and platelets) can be given, as needed
  - Immunotherapy may be used
  - Bone marrow/stem cell transplant can be performed for severe cases, if a suitable donor is available and the recipient meets certain criteria
  - Treatments vary based on the specific case, disorder, and suspected cause

Pure Red Cell Aplasia

- Bone marrow exhibits decreased production of RBCs and RBC precursors, whereas other cell lines are present and produced normally
- Acquired
  - Primary is idiopathic or autoimmune
  - Secondary is usually associated with tumors, infections, drugs or chemicals, other disorders
    - Transient erythroblastopenia of childhood (TEC)
    - Pure red cell aplasia (PRCA) seen in children, often related to viral infection
      - Treated by transfusion, as needed, although most patients eventually restore their ability to produce RBCs
- Congenital
  - Diamond-Blackfan anemia
    - Mutations are usually autosomal dominant; however, they also may occur sporadically
    - Many patients show symptoms before 1 year of age, although some are asymptomatic
    - Many patients have physical issues, including bone malformations
  - Congenital dyserythropoietic anemia (CDA)
    - Group of inherited rare disorders leading to ineffective erythropoiesis
      - Patients have varying degrees of refractory anemia and symptoms resulting from the ineffective erythropoiesis, in addition to variable physical effects
    - Mutations are usually autosomal recessive; however, rare cases of an autosomal dominant inheritance have been reported
    - Symptoms usually appear in childhood or adolescence
  - Anemia of chronic kidney disease
    - Individuals are unable to produce erythropoietin, leading to decreased production of RBCs
- Therapy for PRCA
  - Therapy is variable based on each specific anemia, including supportive therapy, transfusion therapy, corticosteroids, treating the underlying problem

HEMOGLOBINOPATHIES

- Disorders resulting from genetic mutations that lead to structural changes in the Hgb molecule
  - Most occur because of amino acid substitutions in the β-globin chains
  - Numerous Hgb variants exist; however, several are more common than others
- Common abnormal Hgbs
  - Hgb S
    - Usually affects African patients or patients of African descent
    - Mutation: $\beta^{6(Glu \rightarrow Val)}$
      - Hgb S polymerizes into long, thin polymers to form sickles when O_2 saturation decreases

Sickle Cell Disease

- Homozygous for Hgb S
  - Majority of Hgb present is Hgb S
- Clinical symptoms
  - Chronic hemolytic anemia, autosplenectomy, vasoocclusion, vasoocclusive crises, susceptibility to bacterial infections, acute chest syndrome, pulmonary hypertension, myocardial infarction, and numerous other complications
- Laboratory diagnosis of sickle cell disease
  - CBC
    - Normocytic, normochromic anemia
    - Various poikilocytes present
      - Drepanocytes (sickle cells)
      - Target cells, NRBC, Howell-Jolly bodies, polychromasia are commonly seen
    - WBC count usually elevated, with neutrophils predominating
  - Reticulocyte count is elevated
  - Bone marrow is not indicated
  - Other tests
    - Dithionite solubility (sickle screen) is positive
    - Hgb electrophoresis is positive for Hgb S and NO Hgb A is present
    - HPLC or isoelectric focusing may also be used to demonstrate Hgb S
- Treatment and follow-up
  - Supportive therapy and prognosis
    - Transfusions, prophylactic antibiotics, avoidance of situations leading to low O_2 saturation, and dehydration
    - Hydroxyurea to help retain Hgb F production
    - Bone marrow transplant may be an option if a matched donor is available
    - Appropriate therapy can lead to a life span of approximately 50 years

Sickle Cell Trait

- Heterozygous for Hgb S
  - Majority of Hgb present is Hgb A
    - Patients are usually normal and asymptomatic unless in extreme conditions of hypoxia
- Laboratory diagnosis
  - CBC
    - Generally normal, although some target cells may be present
  - Sickle screen
    - Positive
    - Hgb Electrophoresis and HPLC
  - Hgb A and Hgb S are present

Hemoglobin C

- Usually affects patients of West Africa or West African descent
- Mutation: $\beta^{6(Glu \rightarrow Lys)}$
  - Hgb C polymerizes into thick crystals when O_2 saturation decreases
  - RBC shape alteration is less extreme than in Hgb S
    - Crystals look like bars of gold or the Washington Monument
- Diagnosis
  - CBC
    - Mild-to-moderate anemia
    - Increased target cells and Hgb C crystals may appear
    - Some polychromasia and NRBCs may be present
  - Solubility testing is negative
  - Hgb electrophoresis and HPLC
    - Positive for Hgb C if homozygous and positive for Hgb A and C if heterozygous for the mutation
  - Treatment is usually not needed and prognosis is good
  - *NOTE:* Hgb C-Harlem is characterized by a double mutation ($\beta^{6(Glu \rightarrow Val)}$ and $\beta^{73(Asn \rightarrow Asp)}$) and is clinically significant if inherited in combination with Hgb S

Hemoglobin E

- Usually affects patients from Southeast Asian, particularly Thailand
- Mutation: $\beta^{26(Glu \rightarrow Val)}$
- Diagnosis
  - CBC
    - Mild anemia
    - Microcytes and target cells
  - Solubility testing is negative
  - Hgb electrophoresis and HPLC
    - Positive for Hgb E
  - Therapy is not usually needed and prognosis is good

Hemoglobin SC

- Combination disorder with inheritance of mutations for both Hgb S and Hgb C
  - Most common of the compound disorders
- Similar clinical picture to sickle cell disease; however, it does not usually manifest clinically until teenage years and tends to be slightly less severe than Hgb S

- Laboratory diagnosis
  - CBC
    - Mild anemia
    - Target cells and Hgb SC crystals may be present
      - Hgb SC polymerizes into crystalline structures that have features of both Hgb S and Hgb C, often described to look like birds or fingers
  - Solubility testing is positive because of the presence of Hgb S
  - Hgb electrophoresis and HPLC
    - Hgb S and Hgb C are present
  - Therapy and prognosis is similar to sickle cell disease, although expected life span is longer

Combination Disorders

- Mutations may occur in combination because of inheritance of different genetic mutations from each parent
- Each compound disorder has variable symptoms and severities
- Some examples include Hgb SC disease, Hgb S–β thalassemia, Hgb C–Harlem

THALASSEMIAS

- Disorders caused by genetic mutations that lead to quantitative changes in the amount of globin chains produced, resulting in an imbalance of globin chain synthesis
  - Types and severity of thalassemia depends on the globin gene mutated (α or β) and the number of genes affected by the mutation
  - α-Globin is coded for on chromosome 16
    - A normal genotype is designated as $\alpha\alpha/\alpha\alpha$
  - β-Globin is coded for on chromosome 11
    - A normal genotype is designated as β/β
      - β^+ Designates decreased production of β chains; β^0 shows the absence of β chains

α-Thalassemia

- Thalassemias caused by mutations or deletions in the α-globin genes
- Four main groups
  - Hydrops fetalis/Hgb Bart
    - Four gene deletion $(--/--)$ so no α chains are produced
      - Hgbs present are Bart (γ_4) with small amounts of Hgb Portland and Hgb H $(\beta 4)$
    - Not compatible with life as the blood is unable to oxygenate tissues because of high O_2 affinity of Hgb Bart
      - Fetus will either be delivered prematurely and die shortly after birth or will be delivered stillborn in the third trimester
        - Clinically exhibit severe anemia, cardiac defects, and hepatosplenomegaly

- Hgb H disease
  - Three gene deletion $(--/-\alpha)$
    - Unpaired β chains will form tetramers of Hgb H
      - Other Hgb present are Hgb A_2, some Hgb Bart
  - Clinical symptoms
    - Mild-to-moderate chronic hemolytic anemia
    - Splenomegaly
    - Other variable findings may occur
  - CBC
    - Decreased RBC and Hgb
    - Microcytic, hypochromic RBCs, target cells, and other poikilocytes may be present
    - Hgb H inclusions (precipitated Hgb H) may be seen when using a supravital stain, such as new methylene blue
- α-Thalassemia minor
  - Two gene deletion $(--/\alpha\alpha)$ or $(-\alpha/-\alpha)$
    - Asymptomatic presentation
    - Usually no therapy is needed
  - CBC
    - Mildly decreased Hgb and Hct, with microcytic, hypochromic cells
- Silent carrier
  - One gene deletion $(-\alpha/\alpha\alpha)$
  - No clinical symptoms, because globin chain ratio is almost normal
  - No therapy is needed
  - CBC
    - No hematologic abnormalities
  - Diagnosis
    - Diagnosis is by genetic analysis

β-Thalassemia

- Thalassemias caused by mutations or deletions in the β-globin genes
- Four main groups with varying clinical presentations
  - α-Thalassemia major
    - Occurs with genotypes (β^+/β^+), (β^+/β^0), (β^0/β^0)
    - Also called Cooley's anemia
    - Severe hemolytic anemia, usually diagnosed at approximately 6 months of age when Hgb F levels normally decrease (the patient cannot make Hgb A)
    - Clinical picture shows hepatosplenomegaly and distinct bone changes, if untreated, in addition to other physical issues
      - Pathologic fractures and abnormalities of the skull are frequently seen as a result of erythroid hyperplasia in the bone marrow
    - CBC
      - Severe anemia
      - RBC count is slightly elevated, but pronounced hypochromic/microcytic cells and target cells are present, in addition to other varied morphologies and NRBCs

- Bone marrow
  - Usually not performed, but would show erythroid hyperplasia and ineffective erythropoiesis
- Hgb electrophoresis and HPLC
  - Increased Hgb F, slightly increased Hgb A_2, little or no Hgb A
- Therapy and prognosis
  - Supportive therapy with regular transfusions
  - Iron chelation therapy to help avoid iron overload
  - Bone marrow transplant if a good match is available
- β-Thalassemia intermedia
  - Occurs with genotypes ($\beta^{silent}/\beta^{silent}$), ($\delta\beta^0/\delta\beta^0$), ($\beta^0/\delta\beta^0$)
    - Clinical symptoms and CBC
      - Varies because of multiple genotypic presentations
      - Usually not transfusion dependent
  - Anemia varies between that of β-thalassemia minor and β-thalassemia major
- β-Thalassemia minor
  - Occurs with genotypes (β^+/β), (β^0/β)
    - Clinical symptoms and CBC
      - Usually mild anemia
      - Normal to elevated RBC with decreased Hgb and Hct
        - Poikilocytosis (target cells and some others)
    - Hgb electrophoresis and HPLC
      - Elevated Hgb A_2 and F
  - Silent carrier
    - Occurs with genotypes (β^{silent}/β)
    - No clinical symptoms, because globin chain ratio is almost normal
    - No therapy is needed
    - CBC does not show hematologic abnormalities
      - No hematologic abnormalities
    - Diagnosis is by genetic analysis

Other Related Disorders

- Hereditary persistence of fetal hemoglobin (HPFH)
  - Deletion in the β-globin gene leading to increased production of Hgb F (γ chains)
    - Patients are usually asymptomatic; abnormalities will show up in Hgb electrophoresis/HPLC where increases in Hgb F are present
      - Hgb Lepore
        - δβ fusion gene
        - Shows anemia similar to β-thalassemia minor
      - Combination disorders
        - Hgb S–thalassemia
        - Hgb C–thalassemia
        - Hgb E–thalassemia

HEMOLYTIC ANEMIA

- Disorders of premature RBC destruction, leading to anemia
- Classified in several different ways
  - Intrinsic versus extrinsic defects
  - Acquired versus hereditary defects
  - Intravascular versus extravascular hemolysis
- General features
  - Clinical presentation
    - General anemia symptoms when hemolysis leads to anemia
    - Jaundice may be present, variable depending on cause
    - Splenomegaly in cases of extravascular hemolysis
    - Gallstones in cases of chronic hemolysis
- Laboratory testing
  - Increased bilirubin: RBCs are breaking down
  - Decreased haptoglobin: Free Hgb from intravascular hemolysis may exceed haptoglobin's binding capacity
  - Increased reticulocyte count
  - Variable anemia depending on degree and frequency of hemolysis
    - Anisocytosis and poikilocytosis on the CBC, usually including some macrocytosis and polychromasia (reticulocyte production) and spherocytes and/or schistocytes depending on the cause of the anemia

Hemolytic Anemias Resulting from Intrinsic Defects

Abnormalities in Red Blood Cell Membrane
Hereditary Spherocytosis
- Incidence is 1/3000 of northern European ancestry
- Autosomal dominant inheritance in most cases
  - Mutations affect genes coding for membrane proteins, leading to changes in the membrane skeleton and decreased survival because of decreased deformability
  - Symptoms are variable, but a symptomatic clinical picture shows anemia, jaundice, and splenomegaly
    - CBC
      - Decreased RBC, Hgb, and Hct, increased MCHC and RDW
      - Spherocytes, polychromasia
    - Other testing
      - Family history to look for evidence of inheritance
      - Direct antiglobulin test (DAT) is negative, which rules out immune-mediated cause
      - Osmotic fragility is increased because of decreased membrane deformability
      - Autohemolysis tests and membrane protein studies may be performed

- Treatment and prognosis
  - Many are asymptomatic, but those with severe hemolysis may require splenectomy or transfusion therapy

Hereditary Elliptocytosis

- Mutations in genes coding for spectrin or band 4.1, leading to disruption of the cell shape in circulation
- Incidence is 1 in 2000 to 4000, although it is more common in Africa and the Mediterranean and those descended from the area
- Several variants occur, including hereditary pyropoikilocytosis
- Many cases are asymptomatic, and disorder is discovered incidentally; however, some exhibit more pronounced hemolysis
- CBC
  - Normal (in asymptomatic cases) to decreased RBC, Hgb, and Hct (in hemolytic cases)
  - Increased elliptocytes, although morphology is more extreme in hereditary pyropoikilocytosis, which also may show schistocytes and microspherocytes
- Other testing
  - Thermal sensitivity may be increased in hereditary elliptocytosis with spectrin mutations
  - Molecular testing may be done to look for mutations
- Treatment and prognosis
  - Symptomatic cases with anemia may require transfusion therapy and sometimes splenectomy
  - Usually asymptomatic cases require no treatment and have a good prognosis

Acanthocytosis

- Spur cell anemia
  - Defects in RBC membrane lipid balance, often resulting from liver issues
  - Seen in severe liver disease as a result of excess free plasma cholesterol that accumulates on the RBC membrane, leading to deformation of the cell within the spleen, if cells are not hemolyzed
  - CBC
    - Moderate anemia with acanthocytes
  - Clinical presentation
    - Splenomegaly, jaundice
  - Therapy and prognosis
    - Prognosis is poor unless a patient can successfully undergo a liver transplant

Neuroacanthocytosis

- Rare inherited disorders with neurologic symptoms and acanthocytosis
  - Abetalipoproteinemia, McLeod's syndrome

Paroxysmal Nocturnal Hemoglobinuria

- Rare acquired disorder resulting from stem cell mutation in the *PIGA* gene
  - Defect in platelets and WBCs, as well
- Severity is variable depending on the phenotype
- Cells lack glycoslyphosphatidlyinositol-anchored proteins, including CD55 and CD59
- RBCs are susceptible to complement lysis, because CD55 and CD59 inhibit complement and are absent, cells may lyse spontaneously
- Clinical presentation
  - Usually manifests in young adults, but can occur at any age
  - Variable symptoms related to the hemolysis, thrombosis resulting from thrombophilia, and bone marrow failure may occur
- Laboratory findings
  - General signs of intravascular hemolysis, including hemoglobinuria
  - Reticulocytes show a slight increase
  - Bone marrow examination may be done to look for underlying marrow failure or cytogenetic abnormalities
  - Flow cytometry shows deficiencies of CD55 and CD59
    - CD24 and CD15 also may be deficient
- Therapy and prognosis
  - Eculizumab can be used for hemolysis to decrease complement activity
  - Supportive transfusion, prophylactic antibiotics, vitamin supplementation to counter loss through kidneys, anticoagulants are used if there are clotting complications, and stem cell transplant may be an option if a suitable donor is available

Abnormalities in Enzymes

Glucose-6-Phosphate Dehydrogenase Deficiency

- RBCs are unable to reduce glutathione, which is needed to battle oxidant damage in the cell, leading to oxidation of Hgb into Heinz bodies, which are then removed from circulation
- X-linked disorder
  - Multiple mutations and enzyme a presentation of chronic hemolytic anemia to patients with few or no abnormalities.
  - Tends to present in patients in Africa and the Mid-East, and their descendants
  - Most common RBC enzyme deficiency, with a prevalence of up to 5% worldwide
- Clinical presentation
  - Most patients are asymptomatic unless exposed to something that will trigger hemolytic episodes
  - Oxidative drugs, including antimalarial medications, infections, and fava beans are main triggers of hemolysis
    - Leads to transient hemolytic episodes within several hours of exposure and may begin the return to normal once the offending trigger is removed or resolved
    - Hemoglobinuria may be one of the first clinical clues
- Laboratory testing
  - CBC is normal unless patient has an episode

- ○ With hemolytic episodes, patients exhibit a normocytic or normochromic anemia and Hgb may drop quickly, but response can be variable
- ○ Bite and blister cells may occur on Wright's stain, and Heinz bodies are often visualized when using a Heinz body stain or other supravital stain. Other morphologic findings may be present
- Glucose-6-phosphate dehydrogenase (G6PD) enzyme activity screens and quantitative assays
  - May be used to screen or to assess the degree of severity
- Therapy and prognosis
  - Usually involves avoiding or removing the trigger for hemolysis
  - Most cases require no treatment and resolve on their own, but some severe cases may require transfusion therapy

Pyruvate Kinase Deficiency
- Autosomal recessive disorder, relatively rare
- Leads to adenosine triphosphate (ATP) depletion and increase in 2,3 BPG
- Clinical findings
  - Variable from asymptomatic to chronic hemolytic episodes
- Laboratory findings
  - CBC
    - ○ Variable RBC and Hgb
    - ○ Increased echinocytes with other variable morphologic findings
  - Pyruvate kinase enzyme activity can be measured spectrophotometrically. Activity is decreased.
- Treatment and prognosis
  - Supportive treatment with transfusions, as indicated
  - Some severe cases may require splenectomy

Hemolytic Anemias Resulting from Extrinsic Defects

- A variety of different conditions can cause mechanical destruction of the circulating RBCs; these are not immune mediated hemolytic anemias

Microangiopathic Hemolytic Anemia
- Group of disorders characterized by intravascular fragmentation of RBCs as they move through blood vessels obstructed by microclots or endothelial damage
- CBC shows decreases in Hgb and Hct with schistocytes usually appearing on the peripheral smear, in addition to possible other morphologies
- Other laboratory testing
  - Bilirubin (unconjugated) is increased
  - Haptoglobin is decreased
  - Hemostasis testing varies based on the specific disorder

Disseminated Intravascular Coagulation (DIC)
- Activation of all parts of the hemostatic systems leading to the production of fibrin clots, the consumption of platelets and coagulation proteins, and degradation of fibrin. Clotting and bleeding both occur
- Acute or chronic, both secondary to other underlying conditions
- Clinical presentation
  - Variable presentation, because patients show symptoms consistent with the underlying disorder that has prompted disseminated intravascular coagulation
  - Underlying causes may include infections, malignancies, obstetric complications, venom exposure, and chronic inflammation, among others
- CBC
  - Anemia and decreased platelet count, WBC may be elevated
  - Schistocytes and apparent thrombocytopenia
- Laboratory findings
  - Coagulation tests are abnormal
    - ○ Elevated prothrombin time (PT), activated partial thromboplastin time (aPTT)
    - ○ D-dimer/fibrin degradation products (FDPs), and decreased fibrinogen
- Therapy and prognosis
  - Underlying disorder should be treated, in addition to supportive therapies. In cases of acute DIC, therapies may be more aggressive to try to stem organ failure. Heparin can be used carefully to try to stop activation of the coagulation cascade. Blood products may also be used, including frozen plasma to replace consumed coagulation proteins and replace blood volume, platelet transfusions may be administered if thrombocytopenia is severe

Thrombotic Thrombocytopenic Purpura (TTP)
- Patients have long von Willebrand factor (vWF) multimers that bind vascular endothelium and platelets, triggering platelet aggregation. Platelets are used up in this process and microclots block small blood vessels, which leads to shearing of the RBCs in circulation
- Disorder is acquired or inherited
- Several subtypes are present
  - Most patients have a decrease or mutation in the *ADAMTS 13* gene, which is normally used to cleave long vWF multimers into smaller fractions, helping to avoid excess platelet adhesion to the endothelium
- Clinical findings
  - Usually characterized by a combination of symptoms, including microangiopathic hemolytic anemia, thrombocytopenia, neurologic symptoms, renal dysfunction, and fever
- CBC
  - Characterized by decreased Hgb (usually <10 g/dL) and platelet count ($<20 \times 10^9$/L), with schistocytes on the peripheral smear
- Laboratory testing

- Coagulation tests (PT, APTT) are usually normal
- vWF multimer analysis is abnormal
- Therapy and prognosis
  - Plasma exchange therapy to remove large vWF multimers and providing the missing ADAMTS 13 protease can lead to favorable prognosis
  - Immunosuppressive therapy may also be used

Hemolytic Uremic Syndrome (HUS)

- Microangiopathic hemolytic anemia with thrombocytopenia and renal involvement as a result of clots forming in the microvasculature of the kidney
- Acquired disorder, usually found in young children with a history of hemorrhagic *Escherichia coli* or *Shigella dysenteriae* infections, although it may be found in adults after exposure to immunosuppressive agents or chemotherapy
- Clinical presentation
  - Children often present with a bloody diarrhea, CBC abnormalities, and renal issues, whereas adults tend to present with renal issues and CBC abnormalities without bloody diarrhea
- CBC
  - Decreased RBC, Hgb (<10 g/dL), Hct, and platelets
  - Smear shows schistocytes and decreased platelets
- Laboratory testing
  - Blood urea nitrogen and creatinine are elevated
  - Culture results may be positive for *E. coli* or *S. dysenteriae*
  - Urinalysis shows elevated protein, blood, and casts
- Therapy and prognosis
  - Supportive therapy, as needed; prognosis is usually favorable

Other Causes

HELLP Syndrome

- Hemolysis, elevated liver enzymes, and low platelet count
- Relatively uncommon complication of pregnancy, although it is more likely to affect patients with preeclampsia toward the end of their pregnancy
- Vascular insufficiency in the placenta can lead to dysfunction in the maternal endothelium, causing platelet activation and fibrin deposition in the small vessels
- Laboratory testing
  - CBC shows decreased platelet count and lactate dehydrogenase is elevated
- Therapy and prognosis
  - Relatively good with supportive therapy and delivery of the fetus and placenta

Hypertensive Crisis and Malignant Hypertension

- Severe increase in blood pressure, leading to acute organ damage
- Endothelial cells are damaged, leading to activation of the hemostatic system
- Platelets return to normal once the blood pressure is controlled

Mechanical Damage

- Prosthetic heart valves
  - Mild hemolysis resulting from RBCs flowing around the implanted valves
  - Patients are often asymptomatic, but severe cases may present with noticeable anemia
  - CBC may show the presence of schistocytes
  - If anemia is severe, patients may require transfusion therapy and surgical repair of the prosthetic valve
- March hemoglobinuria (exercise induced)
  - Condition occasionally seen in long-distance runners or others who engage in intense exercise
  - Although hemolysis may occur, patients usually do not have anemia unless hemolysis is recurrent
  - Hemoglobinuria may be present, in addition to decreased haptoglobin levels
  - Therapy includes minimizing physical trauma or discontinuing the activity that leads to hemolysis

Infectious Agents

- Malaria (*Plasmodium* spp.)
  - Caused by infection with one of the major species of *Plasmodium*
  - Malarial parasites may lyse RBCs as they use Hgb, in addition to the destruction of infected cells by extravascular hemolysis; additionally, inflammatory response can lead to inhibited and ineffective erythropoiesis
  - Clinical symptoms vary but often include fever, chills, headache, and other physical manifestations
  - Organism presence can be confirmed by visualization of organism, intracellular or extracellular, on a peripheral smear
  - Treatment using chloroquine drugs is administered unless patient harbors organism from areas known for chloroquine resistance, where other drugs need to be used. Transfusion therapy may be used, too, if anemia is severe
- *Babesia*
  - *Babesia microti* is the most common cause of infection
  - Some patients are asymptomatic, whereas others show mild-to-severe anemia and generalized flulike symptoms
  - Diagnosis is confirmed by the visualization of organism (ring forms or tetrads) on peripheral smear, in addition to antibody testing for organism
- Bacteria
  - Toxin-producing microorganisms can occasionally lead to hemolysis
  - *Clostridium perfringens*
    - α-Toxin is produced and can hydrolyze membrane phospholipids, rendering changes in RBC shape and deformability
    - Hemolysis is severe and can lead to DIC and renal failure; prognosis is poor

Additional Causes of Mechanical Hemolysis

- Drugs
- Chemicals
- Venoms
- Thermal injury

Immune-Mediated Hemolytic Anemia

- RBC life span is shortened because of presence of antibodies, usually IgG or IgM, on RBC surfaces
- Autoimmune or alloimmune causes
  - IgM antibodies usually activate complement, leading to intravascular and extravascular hemolysis
  - IgG antibodies can occur with or without the presence of complement, and most removal attempts are extravascular, leading to hemolysis or the increased presence of spherocytes
- General laboratory findings in immune-mediated hemolytic anemia
  - CBC
    - Decreased RBC, Hgb, and Hct with macrocytes, spherocytes, and polychromasia; increased reticulocyte count
  - Laboratory testing
    - Increased bilirubin and lactate dehydrogenase, decreased haptoglobin
    - DAT is positive and can further be tested for IgG and C3d

Autoimmune Hemolytic Anemia

- Caused by autoantibodies that attach to the RBC surface (Table 3-11)

Warm Autoimmune Hemolytic Anemia

- Warm autoimmune hemolytic anemia is the most common autoimmune anemia (AIHA), occurring as idiopathic or secondary disease
  - Secondary particularly in B-cell lymphoid malignancies, such as chronic lymphocytic leukemia (CLL), solid tumors, autoimmune disorders, and viral infections
- Usually caused by IgG autoantibodies that react the best at 37° C
- Usually extravascular hemolysis

- CBC
  - Mild-to-severe anemia with polychromasia and spherocytes
- Laboratory testing
  - DAT is positive in majority of cases
- Treatment and prognosis
  - In symptomatic cases, prednisone therapy may be used
  - Immunosuppressive therapy may be used, but leaves the risk for side effects
  - Transfusion therapy can be used in cases with severe anemia

Cold Agglutinin Disease

- Usually caused by IgM antibodies that react best at 4° C
  - Usually do not react at temperatures above 30 ° C
- IgM antibodies bind to the RBC after exposure to colder temperatures, and they can activate the complement cascade as they move through the cooler extremities. When cells return to warmer areas, the IgM is no longer a factor; however, complement remains and is removed via extravascular hemolysis or in some cases, intravascularly
- Can occur in acute or chronic state
  - Chronic cold agglutinin disease (CAD) is rare and may be idiopathic or secondary to lymphoid malignancy
- Clinical presentation
  - Symptoms are variable, because patients have variable anemia (mild to severe). Depending on the severity, patients may show general anemia symptoms and acrocyanosis
  - Acute CAD can occur secondary to *Mycoplasma pneumoniae* and viral infections
- CBC
  - If blood has cooled before analysis, values will not occur in their normal proportions, leading to

TABLE 3-11	Characteristics of Autoimmune Hemolytic Anemias			
	Warm Autoimmune Hemolytic Anemia	**Cold Aggultinin Disease**	**Paroxysmal Cold Hemoglobinuria**	**Mixed-Type Autoimmune Hemolytic Anemia**
Immunoglobulin class	IgG (rarely IgM, IgA)	IgM	IgG	IgG, IgM
Optimum reactivity temperature of autoantibody	37° C	4° C; reactivity extends to >30° C	4° C	4°-37° C
Sensitization detected by direct antiglobulin test	IgG or IgG + C3d; only C3d uncommon	C3d	C3d	IgG and C3d
Complement activation	Variable	Yes	Yes	Yes
Hemolysis	Extravascular primarily	Extravascular; rarely intravascular	Intravascular	Extravascular and intravascular
Autoantibody specificity	Panreactive or Rh complex; rarely specific Rh or other antigen	I (most), i (some), Pr (rare)	P	Panreactive; unclear specificity

From Rodak BF, Fritsma GA, Keohane E: Hematology: clinical principles and applications, ed 4, St Louis, 2012, Saunders.
Ig, Immunoglobulin.

decreases in the RBC and Hct, with a disproportional (normal) Hgb and grossly abnormal increases in the MCV, MCH, and MCHC. The Hgb value is normal because the method of measurement requires lysis of cells before analyzing Hgb. Agglutinates may be seen on peripheral smear in high-titer cold agglutinins. Warming sample before reanalyzing may resolve the agglutination or keeping sample warm until the time of analysis may also help
- Laboratory testing
  - Cold agglutinin titer is increased
- Therapy and prognosis
  - Patients do not often require transfusions unless hemolysis leads to a severe anemia. Patients are usually instructed to avoid cold temperatures

Paroxysmal Cold Hemoglobinuria
- Acute cold AIHA associated with the Donath-Landsteiner antibody (anti-P autoantibody)
  - Donath-Landsteiner antibody is a biphasic antibody that can bind to RBCs and partially activate complement at low temperatures (optimal binding at 4°C) but full-blown complement activation and hemolysis occur at 37°C
- Clinical presentation
  - Mainly affects children, although it can occur in adults
  - Symptoms include fever, malaise, and extremity and back pain that usually manifests 1 to 2 weeks after a respiratory infection. Patients often have a rapid onset of hemolysis and hemoglobinuria, leading to a severe anemia
- CBC
  - Severe anemia after hemolytic episodes (Hgb often <5 g/dL) with morphology showing polychromasia and spherocytes, in addition to various other morphologies
- Laboratory tests
  - DAT is positive for C3d (auto–anti-P usually dissociates from RBCs at 37°C)
  - Donath-Landsteiner test is positive
- Therapy and prognosis
  - Transfusion therapy is needed with severe hemolytic episodes; however, the disorder is usually self-limiting and has a favorable prognosis

Drug-Induced Hemolytic Anemia
- Characterized by a sudden onset of anemia with hallmarks of hemolytic anemia after a patient is exposed to a medication
- Patients produce antibodies to the medication, which are either drug dependent or drug independent
- Laboratory testing
  - DAT is positive
- CBC
  - Anemia of varying severity
- Therapy and prognosis

- Drug is discontinued and should be avoided in the future
- If anemia is severe, the patient may require transfusion therapy

Alloimmune Hemolytic Anemias
- Hemolytic anemia resulting from immune incompatibility of donor and recipient (or immune incompatibility of mom and baby)
- Antibodies can be IgM or IgG with intravascular and/or extravascular hemolysis
- Onset can be immediate or delayed

Transfusion Reactions
Acute Hemolytic Reaction
- Occurs within hours of transfusion of incompatible blood products
- Most commonly caused by ABO incompatibility, because recipients produce natural IgM antibodies to the incompatible antigen, leading to complement-mediated intravascular hemolysis.
- Clinical presentation
  - Various symptoms occur, including fever, chills, urticaria, chest pain, back pain, shock, cardiac symptoms, and bleeding (if DIC is present)
- CBC
  - Hgb is decreased
- Laboratory tests
  - Hemoglobinuria, hemoglobinemia
  - DAT is usually positive on posttransfusion specimen
  - Haptoglobin is decreased
  - Coagulation tests may be abnormal if DIC occurs
- Therapy and prognosis
  - Transfused unit must be stopped as soon as possible, and treatment to minimize or correct the clinical symptoms is undertaken quickly

Delayed Hemolytic Transfusion Reaction
- Reaction may occur days to weeks after initial transfusion, because the recipient's antibody titer may take time to increase
- Antibodies implicated are usually IgG and can bind to transfused RBCs, which are then removed by extravascular hemolysis
- CBC
  - May not show adequate posttransfusion increase in Hgb
- Laboratory tests
  - DAT is positive
  - Bilirubin is usually indirect fraction may be increased

Hemolytic Disease of the Fetus and Newborn
- Rhesus (Rh) hemolytic disease of the fetus and newborn (HDFN) occurs when maternal IgG antibodies cross the placenta and enter fetal circulation, binding to fetal RBCs positive for the corresponding antigen, leading to extravascular hemolysis

- Clinical presentation
  - Fetus may show erythroid hyperplasia in the marrow and extramedullary hematopoiesis to compensate for hemolysis
- Laboratory testing
  - Maternal samples are tested for ABO and Rh to determine the need for RhIG to help prevent alloimmunization to fetal D antigen
  - Antibody titers may be used to help monitor the patient and determine if other methods are needed for monitoring the patient
- CBC (fetus)
  - Decreased Hgb with polychromasia and NRBCs on the peripheral smear
  - Reticulocyte count is increased
  - Bilirubin is usually increased
  - DAT is positive
- Therapy and prognosis
  - In severe cases, intrauterine transfusion may be indicated or exchange transfusions may be administered after delivery
  - Phototherapy can help reduce bilirubin after delivery
- NOTE: ABO HDFN also can occur and is more common than Rh HDFN; however, it is usually asymptomatic or produces mild anemia with spherocytes and polychromasia in addition to hyperbilirubinemia. IgM antibodies are unable to cross the placenta

NONMALIGNANT WHITE BLOOD CELL DISORDERS

Quantitative White Blood Cell Disorders

Neutrophilia
Causes of Neutrophilia
- Increase in relative and/or absolute numbers of cells ($>8.7 \times 10^9$/L or $>70\%$)
  - Neutrophils can move from marginating to circulating pool or increased need can lead to additional release from bone marrow into circulation
  - Physiologic neutrophilia, also known as shift or transient neutrophilia occurs when the body is under stress. Cells move from the marginating to the circulating pool. Counts will return to normal levels
  - Infections, particularly bacterial
  - Inflammation
  - Medications
  - Increases may be caused by some neoplasms, particularly myeloproliferative disorders
  - Numerous others

Neutropenia
Causes of Neutropenia
- Decrease in the absolute numbers of cells ($<2.0 \times 10^9$/L)

- Congenital neutropenia may occur in several disorders. The disorders are relatively rare
- Acquired neutropenia occurs more commonly. It is usually as a result of decreased production in the bone marrow, anti-neutrophil antibodies, chemotherapy and radiation, and severe infections. Cell production is unable to keep up with cell consumption

Eosinophilia
- Absolute counts are increased above 0.40×10^9/L
- Frequently seen in parasitic infections and allergies
- May also be increased in some myeloproliferative neoplasms, including chronic myelogenous leukemia (CML) and chronic eosinophilic leukemia

Basophilia
- Absolute counts are increased above 0.15×10^9/L
- Can be seen in some hypersensitivity reactions
- May be increased in malignancies, particularly myeloproliferative neoplasms, including CML

Monocytosis
- Absolute counts are increased above 1.1×10^9/L
- Often seen as patients are recovering from infections
- May be increased in some solid tumors and hematologic malignancies, including acute monocytic leukemia, acute myelomonocytic leukemia or chronic myelomonocytic leukemia

Lymphocytosis
- Absolute counts are increased above 10.0×10^9/L (children) or above 4.8×10^9/L (adults)
- Reactive lymphocytes are typically present in infectious mononucleosis and other viral infections
- A more normal lymphocyte morphology is seen in disorders such as *Bordetella pertussis* infection

Lymphocytopenia
- Absolute counts are decreased below 2.0×10^9/L (children) or below 1.0×10^9/L (adults)
- Decreased counts are often seen in immunodeficiencies, particularly human immunodeficiency virus infection and also during steroid treatment

Changes in White Blood Cell Morphology

- Abnormalities (changes) seen in neutrophils
  - Döhle bodies: Pale bluish inclusions in the cytoplasm composed of rough endoplasmic reticulum, usually associated with bacterial infections and inflammation
  - Toxic granulation: Large bluish-black granules appearing in the cytoplasm, usually present in inflammation
  - Vacuolization: Vacuoles within the cytoplasm that are often indicative of phagocytosis. Vacuoles can be seen in bacterial or fungal infections, but also may appear as artifact in old samples
  - Hypersegmentation: Nuclei have more than five segments, usually seen in infection. This may also

be seen as a nuclear abnormality without infection in patients with megaloblastic anemia
- Changes seen in lymphocytes
  - Reactive/variant: Mature lymphocytes showing nuclear and cytoplasmic changes after stimulation by antigens. Cells tend to be large with abundant cytoplasm with slightly less chromatin clumping than resting lymphocytes

Inherited Abnormalities of Neutrophils
- Pelger-Huet anomaly
  - Autosomal dominant mutation of the lamin B receptor
  - Neutrophils are hyposegmented, with nuclei showing mature chromatin. Nuclei shapes are round/oval, bands, or bilobed and separated by a thin filament
  - Cells function normally, as granule function is not impaired
- May-Hegglin anomaly
  - Autosomal dominant mutation of the *MYH9* gene
  - Döhle-like inclusions are found in neutrophils, eosinophils, basophils, and monocytes, in addition to the presence of thrombocytopenia and giant platelets
  - Usually asymptomatic, although patients may exhibit bleeding as a result of thrombocytopenia; WBCs function normally
- Alder-Reilly anomaly
  - Autosomal recessive disorder leading to the inability to fully degrade mucopolysaccharides
  - Cells are filled with large, prominent granules composed of mucopolysaccharides
  - WBCs function normally
- Chediak-Higashi syndrome
  - Autosomal recessive mutation of the *LYST* gene that affects all cells with lysosomal organelles
  - All WBCs may show presence of large lysosomal granules
  - Patients tend to die early in life as a result of bacterial infections, because cells do not function normally
  - Patients also may exhibit bleeding, albinism, and neurologic issues
- Chronic granulomatous disease
  - Mutations, either X-linked recessive or autosomal recessive, in the proteins coding for NADPH oxidase
  - Phagocytic cells produce superoxide, which is needed for the kill mechanism that targets many bacteria and fungi
  - Patients tend to have frequent infections
  - Cells look normal but are unable to kill many bacteria or fungi, leading to frequent infections
  - Testing for the disorder uses the nitroblue tetrazolium reduction test, in which patients with chronic granulomatous disease test negative for the ability to reduce the substance
- Leukocyte adhesion disorder (LAD)
  - Mutations in the genes needed to form cell adhesion molecules, particularly β integrins
  - Three subtypes of LAD, all affecting neutrophil adhesion
  - Patients have difficulties with recurrent infections

HEMATOPOIETIC NEOPLASMS

Myeloproliferative Neoplasms

- Clonal hematopoietic stem cell disorders that result in the overproduction and accumulation of cells in the granulocytic, RBC, and platelet cell lines, leading to chronic neoplasms
- Disorders often have an insidious onset and progress slowly through chronic stages, usually terminating in an aggressive acute stage
- Disorders can occur at any age, but most patients are over 40 years of age
- WHO has classified myeloproliferative neoplasms (MPNs) into four major categories, in addition to several less common categories
  - CML
  - Polycythemia vera
  - Primary myelofibrosis
  - Essential thrombocythemia
  - Additional, less common categories include chronic neutrophilic leukemia, chronic eosinophilic leukemia, mast cell disease, and unclassified

Chronic Myelogenous Leukemia
- Characterized by production and accumulation of neutrophils in all stages of maturation
- Chronic disorder that can lead to an acute/accelerated phase several years after onset if the disorder is not treated
- Acute phase usually terminates in an acute leukemia
- Clinical presentation
  - Anemia, bleeding, infection, sometimes splenomegaly
- CBC
  - Elevated WBC, often greater than $100 \times 10^9/L$
  - Elevations of all granulocytic cells, showing all stages of maturation
    - Left shift through the promyelocyte stage
    - Predominant WBCs tend to be segmented neutrophils, bands, metamyelocytes, and myelocytes
    - Myeloblasts and promyelocytes are present in the chronic stage, although they are less than 5% of the differential
    - Eosinophils and basophils tend to be elevated
- Bone marrow
  - Hypercellular with an elevated M:E ratio
  - Erythroid cells are often decreased
  - Megakaryocytes are present in normal to increased numbers

- Laboratory testing
  - Uric acid is increased as a result of elevated cell turnover
  - Leukocyte alkaline peroxidase (LAP) score is decreased
    - A low score can help differentiate CML from leukemoid reaction, where the LAP score is increased
- Cytogenetics and molecular testing
  - Karyotyping
    - Philadelphia chromosome is present, which is required for diagnosis
      - Formed by the translocation of the long arms of chromosomes 9 and 22, also leading to the production of the *BCR-ABL* fusion gene.
        - *BCR-ABL* codes for protein 210 (p210), which results in an increase of tyrosine kinase activity, and prognosis is more favorable if p210 is present
          - If protein 190 (p190), another protein with increased tyrosine kinase activity, is present, the prognosis is poor
  - Fluorescence in situ hybridization (FISH) testing
    - Identifies the presence of the *BCR-ABL* fusion gene used in diagnosis
  - Reverse-transcriptase polymerase chain reaction (RT-PCR)
    - Used to monitor cytogenetic and molecular remission
- Therapy and progression
  - Therapy
    - Imatinib mesylate (Gleevic) therapy has been favorable in leading to remissions
      - Tyrosine kinase inhibitor working to block the tyrosine kinase activity
      - Response can lead to complete remission
        - Relapse may occur in some patients who develop imitanib resistance
    - Previous to imatinib, various therapies were used to decrease the tumor burden, from chemotherapy to interferon-α (IFN-α)
    - Bone marrow transplant from a matched donor, particularly in younger patients, can also be used
  - Progression
    - Before the use of imitanib therapy, a chronic period of the disease would occur and then it would transition to an acute leukemia (blast phase)
      - Often, before the blast stage, the disease would transition through an accelerated stage in which clinical presentation and laboratory values would begin to deteriorate as the blast count increased
    - Blast crisis: Terminal phase of CML
      - Increased blasts in the peripheral blood and bone marrow (>20%)
        - Blast origin may be myeloid or lymphoid
      - Extramedullary hematopoiesis also may occur

- Additional chromosomal abnormalities may be present
- Patients present as they would with an acute leukemia

Polycythemia Vera

- Characterized by increased RBCs, granulocytes, and platelets in the peripheral blood, with notable increases in RBC and Hgb, while erythropoietin levels remain normal to decreased
- Patients present with a *JAK2 V617F* mutation, which affects the cellular response to erythropoietin, in addition to decreasing normal apoptosis
- Clinical presentation
  - Patients may show symptoms related to increased RBC mass, including headaches and ruddy cyanosis from the increase in circulating RBCs
- CBC
  - Elevated Hgb and Hct, with normal RBC morphology, increases in WBC and platelets
- Bone marrow
  - Hypercellular with increases in all three cell lines during the initial chronic phase
  - Some patients will progress to a "spent" phase, in which bone marrow becomes fibrotic and splenomegaly becomes prominent, often as a result of extramedullary hematopoiesis
- Laboratory testing
  - Erythropoietin level is decreased
  - RBC mass is increased
  - LAP is normal to increased
- Cytogenetics and molecular testing
  - *JAK2 V617F* mutation present in the majority of patients
  - Other *JAK2* mutations may be present
- Therapy and progression
  - Therapeutic phlebotomy is used to decrease RBC counts and provide relief from symptoms
  - Myelosuppressive therapy also may be used to control cell burden
  - Progression to an acute leukemia may occur in approximately 15% of patients

Essential Thrombocythemia

- Characterized by increased platelets and megakaryopoiesis; however, platelets may not function normally
- Clinical presentation
  - Patients may present with symptoms related to bleeding and clotting, including neurologic symptoms, myocardial infarction, headache, mucous membrane bleeds, and others
  - May be asymptomatic but incidental finding of increased platelets may lead to further workup
  - Diagnosis requires the ruling out of reactive thrombocytosis or other MPNs
- CBC
  - Increased platelet counts, $>450 \times 10^9/L$ with sustained elevations

- o Platelets may be of variable size and granularity
- Slight decreases in Hgb and Hct
- Bone marrow
  - Megakaryopoiesis without increased erythropoiesis or granulopoiesis
    - o Megakaryocytes may be larger than normal
- Laboratory testing
  - Little additional testing is currently used for diagnosis
- Cytogenetics and molecular testing
  - *JAK2 V617F* mutation may be present
- Therapy and progression
  - Prevention of bleeding and clotting episodes
  - Myelosuppression to suppress platelet production
  - Patients usually survive longer than 10 years

Primary Myelofibrosis

- Other names have been used for this disorder, including chronic idiopathic myelofibrosis and myelofibrosis with myeloid metaplasia
- Characterized by bone marrow fibrosis, extramedullary hematopoiesis, and increases in megakaryocytes
- Clinical presentation
  - Nonspecific symptoms including fatigue, weakness, shortness of breath, in addition to splenomegaly
- CBC
  - Normal to decreased Hgb and Hct with RBC and platelet abnormalities
    - o Teardrops, other morphologies, polychromasia, and NRBC
    - o Platelet counts are variable, as are platelet morphologies. Circulating micromegakaryocytes may be seen
- Bone marrow
  - Areas of fibrosis with hypercellularity of granulocytes and megakaryocytes
- Cytogenetics and molecular testing
  - JAK2 mutation may be seen
- Therapy and progression
  - Survival is approximately 5 years after diagnosis, although some patients have lived longer
  - Multiple therapies may be used, including RBC and chemotherapy and immunotherapy
  - Treatment for anemia
  - Radiation or splenectomy may be used to target splenomegaly and spleen pain or hyperfunction
  - Bone marrow transplant may be used in younger patients

Other Myeloproliferative Neoplasms
Chronic Neutrophilic Leukemia

- Chronic disorder characterized by an elevated WBC count ($>25 \times 10^9$/L) with a proportional increase in neutrophils and their precursors in the bone marrow

- Disorder similar to CML; however, the majority of the cells are mature (>90%), and fewer than 10% are immature neutrophils
- Differential diagnosis requires the absence of the Philadelphia chromosome, in addition to ruling out any other causes of reactive neutrophilia

Chronic Eosinophilic Leukemia

- Chronic disorder showing an elevated absolute eosinophil count ($>1.5 \times 10^9$/L) with no evidence of reactive eosinophilia (parasitic infections, allergic reactions, etc.) or other malignancies that feature increased eosinophils
- Abnormalities and immature forms of eosinophils are present in the peripheral circulation and bone marrow

Mastocytosis

- Group of chronic disorders with accumulations of mast cells within the organ systems. Classified into seven subcategories by the WHO
- Clinical presentation usually includes urticarial lesions and a variety of other symptoms based on the subgroup of the disorder
- Mast cells may be elevated in the bone marrow or skin lesions
- *KIT* mutations occur in many with systemic mastocytosis
- Prognosis is variable from benign to aggressive

Unclassifiable

- Catch-all group of MPNs to classify disorders that are consistent with MPN diagnosis, including those that do not meet the WHO diagnostic criteria for diagnosis or disorders that occur in conjunction with another disorder

MYELODYSPLASTIC SYNDROMES

- Group of neoplastic disorders characterized by peripheral blood cytopenias and dyspoiesis that occur in one or more cell lines
  - Cytopenias do not respond to most usual therapies
- Most cases arise de novo or related to other therapy (usually chemotherapy or radiation)
- Usually affects patients older than 50 years of age, with a median age of diagnosis of 70 years of age
- Clinical symptoms
  - Clinical symptoms parallel the dyspoietic cell line(s)
    - o RBC: Anemia symptoms
    - o Platelets: Bruising/bleeding
    - o Granulocytes: Increased infections
- CBC
  - Cytopenias may occur in one or more cell lines. Dysplasia may be present
- Bone marrow
  - Cells present are dyspoietic and have any number of abnormalities from abnormal nuclei, abnormal granulation of cytoplasm, N/C asynchrony, and other abnormalities, and they may not function normally

- ○ Examples of dyspoietic cell appearance
  - ▪ Dyserythropoieis: Oval macrocytes, multinucleate NRBCs, nuclear bridging, other abnormal nuclear shapes, inclusions (Howell-Jolly bodies, siderotic granules, basophilic stippling)
  - ▪ Dysmyelopoiesis: Abnormal granulation (lacking granules, decreased granule presence, or large granules), N/C asynchrony, abnormal nuclear shape, multinucleate WBCs
  - ▪ Dysmegakaryopoiesis: Giant platelets, agranular platelets, circulating micromegakaryocytyes, unusual nuclei
- Laboratory testing
  - Chromosomal abnormalities are present in approximately half of the cases of MDS
    - ○ Karyotyping can help determine treatments and their predicted response
  - ○ Abnormalities most frequently occur in chromosomes 5, 7, 8, 11, 13, 20
- Treatment and prognosis
  - Treatment varies between the different disorders in the group; however, supportive therapy tends to be used, often because of patient age and presence of other coexisting diseases
    - ○ Transfusion therapy, prophylactic antibiotics, growth factors to stimulate bone marrow response, or immunosuppressive therapy
    - ○ Patients <70 years of age may be candidates for stem cell transplant
  - Prognosis is variable based on subgroup, because levels of risk are based on the types of dyspoiesis, number of blasts present, and cytogenetic findings
- WHO (2008) Classification (Table 3-12)
  - Refractory Cytopenia with Unilineage Dysplasia
  - Refractory Anemia with Ringed Sideroblasts

TABLE 3-12	Peripheral Blood and Bone Marrow Findings in Myelodysplastic Syndromes	
Disease	**Blood Findings**	**Bone Marrow Findings**
Refractory cytopenia with unilineage dysplasia (RCUD), refractory anemia (RA), refractory neutropenia (RN), refractory thrombocytopenia (RT)	Unicytopenia* No or rare blasts (<1%)[†]	Unilineage dysplasia: ≥10% of cells in one myeloid lineage <5% blasts <15% of erythroid precursors are ringed sideroblasts
Refractory anemia with ringed sideroblasts (RARS)	Anemia No blasts	≥15% of erythroid precursors are ringed sideroblasts Erythroid dysplasia only <5% blasts
Refractory cytopenia with multilineage dysplasia (RCMD)	Cytopenia(s) No or rare blasts (<1%)[†] No Auer rods <1 × 10^9/L monocytes	Dysplasia in ≥10% of cells in two or more myeloid lineages (neutrophil and/or erythroid precursors and/or megakaryocytes) <5% blasts in marrow No Auer rods ±15% ringed sideroblasts
Refractory anemia with excess blasts 1 (RAEB-1)	Cytopenia(s) <5% blasts No Auer rods <1 × 109/L monocytes	Unilineage or multilineage dysplasia 5%-9% blasts[†] No Auer rods
Refractory anemia with excess blasts 2 (RAEB-2)	Cytopenia(s) 5-19% blasts ± Auer rods[‡] <1 × 109/L monocytes	Unilineage or multilineage dysplasia 10-19% blasts[†] ± Auer rods[‡]
Myelodysplastic syndrome, unclassified (MDS-U)	Cytopenia(s) ≤1% blasts[†]	Unequivocal dysplasia in <10% of cells in one or more myeloid cell lines when accompanied by a cytogenetic abnormality considered as presumptive evidence for a diagnosis of MDS <5% blasts
MDS associated with isolated del(5q)	Anemia Usually normal or increased platelet count No or rare blasts (<1%)	Normal to increased megakaryocytes with hypolobulated nuclei <5% blasts Isolated del(5q) cytogenetic abnormality No Auer rods

From Swerdlow SH, Campo E, Harris NL, et al, editors: WHO classification of tumours of haematopoietic and lymphoid tissues, ed 4, Lyon, France, 2008, IARC Press.

*Bicytopenia may occasionally be observed. Cases with pancytopenia should be classified as MDS-U.

[†]If the marrow myeloblast percentage is <5% but there are 2%-4% myeloblasts in the blood, the diagnostic classification is RAEB-1. Cases of RCUD and RCMD with 1% myeloblasts in the blood should be classified as MDS-U.

[‡]Cases with Auer rods and <5% myeloblasts in the blood and <10% myeloblasts in the marrow should be classified as RAEB-2.

- Refractory Cytopenia with Multilineage Dysplasia
- Refractory Anemia with Excess Blasts
- Myelodysplastic Syndrome with Isolated 5q Deletion
- Myelodysplastic Syndrome, Unclassifiable
- Childhood Myelodysplastic Syndromes

Refractory Cytopenia with Unilineage Dysplasia (RCUD)

- CBC
  - Dysplasia occurs in more than 10% of one cell line
  - Less than 1% blasts in peripheral blood
- Bone marrow
  - <5% blasts in bone marrow
  - Evidence of dyspoiesis
- Prognosis
  - Survival of 2 to 5 years after diagnosis

Refractory Anemia with Ringed Sideroblasts (RARS)

- CBC
  - Anemia, possibly dimorphic population of normal and hypochromic cells, dyserythropoiesis
  - No blasts in peripheral blood
- Bone marrow
  - <15% ringed sideroblasts
- Prognosis
  - Survival of 6 to 10 years after diagnosis

Refractory Cytopenia with Multilineage Dysplasia

- CBC
  - One or more cytopenias is present
  - Dysplasia in two or more lines
  - Less than 1% blasts in peripheral blood
- Bone marrow
  - Less than 5% blasts, some ringed sideroblasts may be present
- Prognosis
  - Disease course is more aggressive

Refractory Anemia with Excess Blasts (RAEB)

- Two subtypes occur: RAEB-1 and RAEB-2
- CBC
  - Cytopenias in all three cell lines, in addition to dysmyelopoiesis and/or dysmegakaryopoiesis
  - RAEB-1: 2% to 4% blasts, decreased monocytes
  - RAEB-2: 5% to 19% blasts, decreased monocytes
    - Some blasts may have Auer rods
- Bone marrow
  - RAEB-1: 5% to 9% blasts

- RAEB-2: 10% to 19% blasts, Auer rods may be present
- Prognosis
  - Disease is more aggressive because more blasts are present, leading to a higher number of cases that can transform into AML

Myelodysplastic Syndrome with Isolated 5q – Deletion (5q-Syndrome)

- CBC
  - Refractory anemia and other parameters are relatively normal
  - Other parameters are relatively normal
- Bone marrow
  - Less than 5% blasts
  - Abnormal megakaryocytes and erythroid hyperplasia
- Other testing
  - Cytogenetics showing a 5q – deletion
- Prognosis
  - Survival of approximately 12 years, disease tends to be stable

Myelodysplastic Syndrome, Unclassifiable

- Cytopenias and some marrow dysplasia are present; however, it may not meet all criteria to be classified into one of the specific groups of MDS

MYELOPROLIFERATIVE AND MYELODYSPLASTIC NEOPLASMS

- Category of disorders with features of both myeloproliferative and myelodysplastic neoplasms (MDS/MPN)

Chronic Myelomonocytic Leukemia (CMML)

- Two subgroups, CMML-1 and CMML-2, can occur in adults
- Elevated WBC count with monocytosis ($>1.5 \times 10^9$/L) and less than 20% blasts and promonocytes in the peripheral blood and bone marrow
- Dysplasia in one or more myeloid line, particularly dysgranulopoiesis
- Prognosis is variable; however, CMML-1 has fewer blasts, leading to a more favorable prognosis than CMML-2, in which more blasts are present

Juvenile Myelomonocytic Leukemia (JMML)

- Similar to CMML, but it occurs in children up to age 14
  - These patients are usually candidates for stem cell transplant

Atypical Chronic Myeloid Leukemia

- Blood picture is similar to that of CML, but cells exhibit dysplasia, particularly in the granulocyte line
- Philadelphia chromosome *BCR/ABL1* negative
- Prognosis is poor

Myeloproliferative and Myelodysplastic Neoplasms Unclassifiable

- Cytopenias and some marrow dysplasia is present, along with features of myeloproliferative disease; however, it may not meet all criteria to be classified into one of the specific groups of MDS/MPN

ACUTE LYMPHOBLASTIC LEUKEMIA (ALL)

- Acute leukemia characterized by the presence of more than 20% lymphoid blasts in the peripheral blood and/ or bone marrow
- Primarily affects children, but is also seen in older adults
- WHO classifies into B lymphoblastic leukemia/lymphoma (B-ALL) and T lymphoblastic leukemia/lymphoma (T-ALL). Both are divided into several subgroups based on recurrent genetic abnormalities. The subtype can influence treatment and prognosis
  - Genetic abnormalities in B cell lymphoblastic leukemia/lymphoma include
    - t(9;22)(q34;q11.2); *BCR-ABL1*
    - t(11q;23); *MLL*
    - t(12;21)   (p13;q22);   *TEL-AML1(ETV6-RUNX1)*
    - Hypodiploidy
    - Hyperdiploidy
    - t(5;14)(q31;q32); *IL3-IGH*
    - (1;19)(q23;p13.3); *E2A-PBX1 (TCF3-PBX1)*
- T-cell lymphoblastic leukemia/lymphoma may exhibit abnormal karyotypes, but they are not as defined as seen in B-cell acute lymphoblastic leukemia (B-ALL)
- Clinical presentation
  - Generalized symptoms including fatigue and fever, in addition to bleeding from mucous membranes
  - Lymphadenopathy and bone pain may be present because of leukemic cells
  - Malignant cells may also infiltrate the central nervous system (CNS), leading to blast presence in the spinal fluid
- CBC
  - Variable WBC count; counts can range from low to elevated numbers
  - Usually see anemia, thrombocytopenia, and neutropenia
  - Not all patients have circulating lymphoblasts; however, the lymphoblasts exhibit two main morphologies when they are seen
    - Small lymphoblasts, which are up to two times larger than a normal lymphocyte, with small amounts of cytoplasm
    - Nucleoli are present but may not be prominent
    - Large lymphoblasts, which are 2 to 3 times larger than a normal lymphocyte with prominent nucleoli and abnormalities in the nuclear membrane
- Other laboratory tests
  - Flow cytometry is used to determine specific precursor cells present based on CD markers present
    - Breaks ALL into subtypes
      1. Early B-cell (pro-B) ALL: TdT+, CD34+, CD19+, CD20−, CD22+
      2. Intermediate pre–B-cell ALL: TdT+, CD34 +/−, CD19+, CD20+/−, CD10+
      3. Pre–B-cell ALL: TdT+, CD19+, CD20+, CD22+, CD10+/−
      4. Pre–T-cell ALL: TdT+/−, CD34+/−, CD2+, CD3+, CD7+, CD10+/−
- Therapy
  - Treatment varies based on age and risk
    - Low risk: Children 1 to 10 years of age with a lower WBC count, no extramedullary disease
    - High risk: Adults, children younger than 1 year of age and those with extramedullary disease
  - Treatment usually begins with induction therapy, followed by consolidation therapy, and continuation therapy
    - Intrathecal therapy may be used if there is evidence of blasts infiltrating the CNS
  - For patients not responding to initial therapy or patients no longer in remission, stem cell transplants can be used if a matched donor is present
- Prognosis
  - Varies based on age, number of blasts, immunophenotype, and genetic mutations
    - Prognosis tends to be better in cases in which
      - Patient is younger
      - Blast counts are lower
      - Immunophenotype fits the regular criteria
      - Chromosomal translocations have variable prognosis
        - If patient is Philadelphia chromosome positive, they tend to have a poorer prognosis
        - Hyperdiploidy in children is favorable but not in adults
        - Hypodiploidy has a poor prognosis overall

ACUTE MYELOID LEUKEMIA (AML)

- Acute myeloid leukemia (AML) is characterized by the presence of greater than 20% blasts (WHO 2008 Classification System) in the peripheral blood and/or bone marrow
- Most common group of leukemias in adults and children younger than 1 year of age
- Clinical presentation

- Patients often present with nonspecific symptoms, related to the bone marrow takeover by the abnormal clone of malignant cells, which may crowd out normal cells
  - Anemia: The malignant clone decreases space available for erythroid precursors, leading to typical anemia symptoms, such as fatigue, pallor, etc.
  - Thrombocytopenia: The malignant clone decreases space available for megakaryocyte production, leading to symptoms of bleeding and bruising
  - Neutropenia: Fewer mature cells are present because of the hyperproliferation of immature myeloid cells. May lead to infections and fever
- CBC
  - WBC counts are variable, usually between 5 and 30×10^9/L, but can range from 1 to 200×10^9/L
  - Platelet and RBC counts may be decreased because of heavy leukemic clone involvement in the bone marrow
  - Blasts may be present on the peripheral smear
  - Specific smear abnormalities are present in each specific subtype
- Bone marrow
  - Hypercellular marrow with more than 20% blasts of myeloid origin present
  - Specific smear abnormalities are present in each specific subtype
- Other laboratory tests
  - Uric acid is increased because of high cell turnover
  - Lactate dehydrogenase is increased because of high cell turnover
  - Calcium may be decreased
  - Phosphate may be increased
  - Potassium may be decreased
- Therapy and prognosis
  - Variable, based on specific classifications
- WHO 2008 classifies acute leukemia subgroups based on molecular features and cytogenetics, in addition to traditional cell counts, morphologic appearance, and bone marrow examination. Specific molecular and cytogenetic features can influence treatment and prognosis

Acute Myeloid Leukemia with Recurrent Genetic Abnormalities

- AML with t(8;21)(q22;q22); (RUNX1-RUNX1T1)
  - Children and young adults
  - CBC and bone marrow show myeloblasts with Auer rods and some maturation; some dysplasia
  - Prognosis is usually favorable
- AML with inv(16)(p13.1q22) or t(16;16)(p13.1;q22); (CBFB-MYH11)
  - All ages, although usually seen in younger patients

- CBC and bone marrow show myeloblasts, monoblasts, and promonocytes, and may see dysplastic eosinophils in marrow
- Extramedullary involvement may be present, particularly in the CNS
- Prognosis often shows a good remission rate
- AML with t(15;17)(q22;q12); (PML/RARA); also referred to as acute promyelocytic leukemia (APL)
  - All ages, but usually seen in younger adults, often females
  - CBC and bone marrow show myeloblasts/abnormal promyelocytes, Auer rods usually present singly or in bundles
  - Complications can include DIC, because primary granules in promyelocytes can serve as procoagulants
  - Cells have a maturation block at the promyelocyte stage, and all-trans retinoic acid (ATRA) therapy can be used to make cells continue maturation
  - Remission may be achieved with ATRA therapy unless patients do not respond to ATRA.
- AML with t(9;11)(p22;q23); (MLLT3-MLL)
  - Rare, usually occurring in children
  - Clinical signs may involve gingival bleeding, DIC, and skin effects
  - CBC and bone marrow show increased monoblasts and immature monocytes
  - Prognosis is moderate to poor
- AML with t(6;9)(p23;q34); (DEK-NUP214)
  - Rare, usually in teenagers or younger adults
  - CBC often exhibits pancytopenia; blasts often are monocytic or have Auer rods
  - Prognosis is usually poor
- AML with inv(3)(q21q26.2) or t(3;3)(q21;q26.2); (RPN1-EVI1)
  - Rare, usually occurs in adults
  - CBC shows variable blast morphology, dyspoietic cells, platelet abnormalities
  - Bone marrow shows increased and abnormal megakaryoblasts
  - Prognosis is poor
- AML (megakaryoblastic) with t(1;22)(p13;q13); (RBM15-MKL1)
  - Rare, usually occurs in infants, especially those with Down syndrome
  - Clinical symptoms of organomegaly, anemia and thrombocytopenia, megakaryoblasts and micro-megakaryocytes
  - Marrow may show fibrotic areas
  - Prognosis has shown improvement with intense chemotherapy regimens

Acute Myeloid Leukemia with Myelodysplasia-Related Changes

- Usually affects older adults
- Patients have a history of MDS or other similar disorders

- More than 20% blasts, dysplastic cell morphology in one or more cell lines
- Usually has a poor prognosis

Therapy-Related Myeloid Neoplasms

- Myeloid neoplasms associated with treatment with chemotherapy and/or radiation
- Prognosis tends to be poor

Acute Myeloid Leukemia, Not Otherwise Specified

- Contains disorders that have not yet been recognized to have a common genetic abnormality
- Characterized by morphology, flow cytometry, and cytochemistry system

Acute Myeloid Leukemia with Minimal Differentiation

- Usually affects infants and older adults
- Flow cytometry is positive for CD13, CD33, CD34, CD117
- CBC and bone marrow show blasts with no evidence of maturation
- Cytochemistry is negative for myeloperoxidase and Sudan black B

Acute Myeloid Leukemia Without Maturation

- Usually affects adults but can occur at any age
- Flow cytometry is positive for CD13, CD33, CD117, and frequently CD34
- CBC and bone marrow show numerous blasts, many with Auer rods, and less than 10% of WBCs do not mature beyond promyelocyte stage
- Cytochemistry is positive for myeloperoxidase and Sudan black B

Acute Myeloid Leukemia with Maturation

- May occur in all age groups
- CBC and bone marrow show more than 20% blasts, more than 10% maturing cells are neutrophilic. Cells may show Auer rods and other dysplastic features

Acute Myelomonocytic Leukemia

- Flow cytometry is positive for CD13, CD33, CD14, CD4, CD11b, CD11c, CD64, CD36
- CBC and bone marrow show increased myeloid and monocytoid cells in the blood and bone marrow
- More than 20% of marrow cells are monocytoid

Acute Monoblastic and Monocytic Leukemia

- Usually seen in younger patients
- Clinical symptoms may include skin and gingival issues, in addition to bleeding problems
- Flow cytometry is positive for CD14, CD4, CD11b, CD11c, CD36, CD64, CD68
- CBC shows increases in monocytes, and >80% of marrow cells are of monocytic origin
- Cytochemistry is positive for nonspecific esterase positive

Acute Erythroid Leukemia

- Divided into acute erythroleukemia or pure erythroid leukemia
  - Both show more than 50% normoblastic cells in the bone marrow; however, acute erythroleukemia additionally shows more than 20% myeloblasts
- CBC and bone marrow show immature RBCs with obvious dysplastic changes
- Cytochemistry shows normoblasts staining with a diffuse or block pattern with periodic acid–Schiff (PAS) stain
- Prognosis is poor

Acute Megakaryoblastic Leukemia

- Characterized by cytopenias, with some cases showing thrombocytosis. Dysplastic cells are present in all cell lines
- CBC and bone marrow shows more than 20% blasts, with over 50% megakaryoblasts
- Flow cytometry is positive for CD41, CD42b, CD61

Acute Anemias of Ambiguous Lineage

- Some leukemias may have characteristics, both by morphology and immunophenotyping, of more than one cell type
- These may be designated as biphenotypic or bilineage acute leukemias

CHRONIC LYMPHOID NEOPLASMS

- Neoplasms of mature lymphoid cells, both B cells and T cells
- Increases in mature lymphoid cells in peripheral circulation (leukemic) or in masses in the tissues (lymphoma)
- Therapies and prognosis vary based on the specific disorders and mutations present (Table 3-13)

Chronic Lymphocytic Leukemia (CLL)/Small Lymphocytic Lymphoma

- Mature B-cell disorder with an indolent course
- CBC shows elevated WBC counts with a predominance of small lymphoid cells, usually with dense, hypermature nuclei and little cytoplasm, and smudge cell are frequently seen
- Bone marrow shows decreased M:E ratio because of elevated lymphoid cells.
- Flow cytometry is positive for CD5, CD19, CD20, CD23
- Usually affects the elderly with a slowly progressing disease
  - Survival is currently around 10 years after diagnosis

Prolymphocytic Leukemia

- Rare B-cell disorder that affects both T-cell and B-cell lines, looking similar to CLL but with the presence of prolymphocytes

- CBC shows elevated WBC counts with lymphocytosis, including prolymphocytes with prominent nucleoli
- Bone marrow
  - Increased presence of prolymphocytes
- Flow cytometry is positive for CD19, CD20, FMC7, and sometimes CD5
- Prognosis
  - Disease progression is more aggressive than in CLL
  - T-cell varieties are more aggressive than B-cell varieties

Hairy Cell Leukemia (HCL)

- Chronic B-cell neoplasm with lymphocytes showing threadlike or "hairy" projections
- Relatively rare, usually occurring in middle-aged adults, predominantly males
- Clinical presentation
  - Patients often present with massive splenomegaly
- CBC
  - The CBC is often relatively normal, although it may show pancytopenia. Neoplastic "hairy cells" may be seen, but they do not tend to circulate in large numbers
- Bone marrow
  - Often exhibits areas of fibrosis, leading to a dry tap on aspiration. Hairy cells may be visible on core biopsy
- Flow cytometry is positive for CD19, CD20, CD22, CD11c, CD25, CD103
- Cytochemistry (tissue samples, including bone marrow core biopsy)
  - Positive for tartrate-resistant acid phosphatase (TRAP) stain
    - Hairy lymphocytes may be seen
  - Annexin A1 is the most specific marker for HCL, in addition to being positive for DBA-44
- Prognosis
  - Patients may achieve long remissions with therapy, including IFN-α or purines

Plasma Cell Neoplasms

- B cell disorders leading to increases in plasma cells
- Typically affects older adults

TABLE 3-13	Morphologic and Immunophenotypic Features of Mature B-Cell Lymphomas			
Subtype	Architectural Features	Cytologic Characteristics	Immunophenotype/ Cytogenetics	Cell of Origin
Chronic lymphocytic leukemia/small lymphocytic lymphoma	Diffuse lymphocytic proliferation with growth lefts	Small lymphoid cells	CD20+, CD19+, CD5+, CD23+	Naive or memory B cells
B-cell prolymphocytic leukemia	Diffuse proliferation	Medium-sized lymphoid cells with distinct "punched-out" nucleoli and abundant cytoplasm	CD20+, CD19+, FMC7 +, CD5+/−	Unknown mature B cell
Mantle cell lymphoma	Diffuse, nodular, or mantle zone pattern	Medium-sized lymphocytes with irregular nuclei	CD20+, CD19+, CD5+, FMC7+, cyclin D1+, t(11;14)	Mantle zone cell
Follicular lymphoma	Follicular pattern	Medium-sized lymphocytes with indented nuclei and variable numbers of large lymphoid cells	CD20+, CD19+, CD10 +, BCL-6+, BCL-2+ t(14;18)	Germinal center cell
Extranodal marginal zone lymphoma of mucosa-associated lymphoid tissue	Diffuse lymphoid proliferation, occasionally marginal zone or nodular pattern	Medium-sized lymphocytes with irregular nuclei and clear abundant cytoplasm	CD20+, CD19+, CD43 +/−	Marginal zone cell
Plasma cell myeloma, plasmacytoma	Sheets or large aggregates of plasma cells	Plasma cells, frequently with cytologic atypia	CD20−, CD19+/−, CD38 +, CD138+, cytoplasmic light chain+	Plasma cell
Diffuse large B-cell lymphoma	Diffuse proliferation	Large lymphoid cells	CD20+, CD19+, CD10 +/−, BCL-6+/−, BCL-2+/−, CD5+/−	Different stages of mature B cells
Burkitt lymph ^_frp_secowid=85.4046 oma	Diffuse lymphoid proliferation with "starry sky" pattern	Medium-sized lymphocytes with evenly distributed chromatin, inconspicuous nucleoli	CD20+, CD19+, CD10 +, BCL-6+, BCL-2−, t(8;14)	Germinal center cell

From Rodak BF, Fritsma GA, Keohane E: Hematology: clinical principles and applications, ed 4, St Louis, 2012, Saunders.

Plasma Cell Myeloma

- Clinical presentation
  - Variable based on type of myeloma. Multiple myeloma is characterized by bone involvement, whereas Waldenström's macroglobulinemia does not show bone involvement. Plasma cells may infiltrate other tissues, such as the CNS
- CBC
  - WBC counts may appear normal or increased, with circulating plasma cells or plasmacytoid lymphocytes depending on disease progression
- Bone marrow
  - Sheets of plasma cells may be seen in the marrow
- Laboratory testing
  - Total protein tends to be elevated
  - Surface Ig is positive
  - Protein and immunoelectrophoresis is positive for the protein(s) present in excess
- Flow cytometry is positive for CD 19, CD20, CD138, CD38, and monoclonal cytoplasmic Ig, but is negative for surface Ig
- Prognosis
  - Variable depending on the specific plasma cell myeloma present; however, multiple myeloma is often quickly progressive

Lymphoma

Lymphoid Neoplasms Manifesting as Solid Tumors
Hodgkin Lymphoma
- Localized tumor of the lymph nodes, tumor cells do not enter the peripheral blood
- Manifests with the presence of Reed-Sternberg cells in the tumor
  - Reed-Sternberg cells are described as having the appearance of "owl eyes" or "popcorn"

Non-Hodgkin Lymphoma
- B-cell disorder is most common, although T-cell or NK-cell lymphomas may occur
- Sézary syndrome (mycosis fungoides) is an example of a T-cell lymphoma. The Sézary cells are small to medium sized lympoid cells with convoluted or cerebriform nuclei. The disorder has skin involvement and may disseminate throughout the body
- Multiple types of non-Hodgkin lymphoma exist, including follicular, mantle cell, diffuse large B cell, among many others
  - Flow cytometry for immunophenotyping is often used along with cytology for diagnosis

Circulating Lymphoma
- Some cases of non-Hodgkin lymphoma may have peripheral blood involvement when tumor cells enter the peripheral circulation

- Characterized by clefted cells (butt cells) in the peripheral circulation or cerebrospinal fluid

CERTIFICATION PREPARATION QUESTIONS

For answers and rationales, please see Appendix A.

1. A physician wants to obtain a measure of a patient's iron stores. Which of the following tests would be the most suitable?
   a. Serum iron
   b. Serum transferrin (TIBC)
   c. Serum ferritin
   d. Transferrin saturation

2. A 68-year-old woman visited her physician with reports of fatigue and weakness. A CBC was ordered, and the patient's results were as follows:

RBC 2.50×10^{12}/L	Hct 18.8%	MCH 24.8 pg
Hgb 6.2 g/dL	MCV 75.2 fL	MCHC 33%

   Which of the following would be a plausible diagnosis for this patient?
   a. Iron-deficiency anemia
   b. Vitamin B_{12} deficiency
   c. Anemia of chronic inflammation
   d. Hemochromatosis

3. A peripheral smear shows a decreased RBC count with microcytic, hypochromic cells with small grape-like inclusions in the RBCs on both Wright stain and Prussian blue stain. This is consistent with:
   a. Iron-deficiency anemia
   b. Sideroblastic anemia
   c. Pernicious anemia
   d. β-Thalassemia minor

4. Given the following results of iron studies, which disorder is the most likely?

↓ Serum iron	↑ TIBC
↓ Ferritin	↓ % Saturation

   a. Iron-deficiency anemia
   b. Sideroblastic anemia
   c. Anemia of chronic inflammation
   d. Hemochromatosis

5. Acquired sideroblastic anemia may be present in all of the following except:
   a. Alcoholism
   b. Lead poisoning
   c. Malabsorption
   d. Myelodysplastic syndromes

6. A patient has a macrocytic anemia, and the physician suspects pernicious anemia. Which test would best rule in a definitive diagnosis of pernicious anemia?
   a. Homocysteine
   b. Intrinsic factor antibodies

c. Ova and parasite examination for *D. latum*

d. Bone marrow examination

7. Megaloblastic anemias result from which of the following?

   a. Deficiencies in free erythrocyte protoporphyrin

   b. Deficiencies in Vitamin B_{12} and folic acid

   c. Increases in iron and hepcidin

   d. Decreases in liver function

8. A patient's bone marrow showed erythroid hyperplasia with signs of dysplastic maturation, particularly in the RBC precursors. This is consistent with which of the following?

   a. Sickle cell anemia

   b. β-Thalassemia major

   c. Pernicious anemia

   d. G6PD deficiency

9. The CBC for a 57-year-old man had the following results. Which tests would be best to order next?

RBC 2.50×10^{12}/L	Hct 26.0%	MCH 34 pg
Hgb 8.5 g/dL	MCV 104 fL	MCHC 33%

   a. Iron studies

   b. Vitamin B_{12} and folic acid levels

   c. Bone marrow examination

   d. Intrinsic factor antibodies

10. The majority of acquired aplastic anemia cases usually results from which of the following?

    a. Unknown causes

    b. Pregnancy

    c. Chloramphenicol exposure

    d. Radiation exposure

11. Which of the following values is the most likely to be normal in a patient with aplastic anemia?

    a. RBC count

    b. Absolute neutrophil count

    c. Absolute lymphocyte count

    d. Platelet count

12. Fanconi's anemia is an inherited aplastic anemia with mutations that lead to:

    a. Increased chromosome fragility

    b. Myelophthisic anemia

    c. Pancreatic issues

    d. RBC enzymatic defects

13. Which of the following is decreased in cases of intravascular hemolytic anemia?

    a. Bilirubin

    b. Urine hemosiderin

    c. Haptoglobin

    d. Plasma hemoglobin

14. Typical CBC findings in hemolytic anemia include:

    a. Microcytic, hypochromic cells with increased poikilocytosis

    b. Macrocytic, normochromic cells with increased polychromasia

    c. Microcytic, normochromic cells with increased poikilocytosis

    d. Macrocytic, hypochromic cells with increased polychromasia

15. Which of the following disorders does not have a hemolytic component?

    a. Sickle cell anemia

    b. Autoimmune hemolytic anemia

    c. Glucose-6-phosphate dehydrogenase deficiency

    d. Anemia of chronic disease

16. A patient presents with evidence of a hemolytic anemia. Spherocytes, polychromasia, and macrocytosis are observed. Which of the following would best help to distinguish the cause of the anemia?

    a. Osmotic fragility

    b. DAT

    c. G6PD activity assay

    d. Vitamin B_{12} level

17. Paroxysmal nocturnal hemoglobinuria is characterized by flow cytometry results that are:

    a. Negative for CD55 and CD59

    b. Positive for CD55 and CD59

    c. Negative for CD4 and CD8

    d. Positive for all normal CD markers

18. G6PD deficiency episodes are related to which of the following?

    a. Exposure to oxidant damage

    b. Defective globin chains

    c. Antibodies to RBCs

    d. Abnormal protein structures

19. Which of the following disorders is not classified as a microangiopathic hemolytic anemia?

    a. Disseminated intravascular coagulation

    b. Hemolytic uremic syndrome

    c. Traumatic cardiac hemolytic anemia

    d. Thrombotic thrombocytopenic purpura

20. A previously healthy 36-year-old woman with visited her physician because of a sudden onset of easy bruising and bleeding. Of the following, which is the most likely cause of her laboratory results?

WBC 10.5×10^9/L	RBC 3.00×10^{12}/L	Hgb 8.0 g/dL
Hct 25.0%	MCV 83 fL	MCH 26 pg
MCHC 32%	Platelets 18×10^9/L	Differential: Normal WBCs with moderate schistocytes and polychromasia
PT: 12.8 seconds	aPTT: 34 seconds	

    a. Sickle cell anemia

    b. Chronic myelogenous leukemia

    c. Disseminated intravascular coagulation

    d. Thrombotic thrombocytopenic purpura

21. Warm autoimmune hemolytic anemia is usually caused by which of the following?
    a. IgA antibodies
    b. IgG antibodies
    c. IgM antibodies
    d. Complement

22. Which of the following conditions is not associated with secondary warm autoimmune hemolytic anemia?
    a. CLL
    b. Idiopathic onset
    c. Rheumatoid arthritis
    d. Viral infections

23. The mutation seen in sickle cell anemia is:
    a. $\beta^{6Glu\rightarrow Val}$
    b. $\beta^{6Glu\rightarrow Lys}$
    c. $\beta^{26Glu\rightarrow Lys}$
    d. $\beta^{63Glu\rightarrow Arg}$

24. The majority of hospitalizations associated with sickle cell anemia are due to:
    a. Cardiomegaly
    b. Cholelithiasis
    c. Pneumonia
    d. Vasoocclusion

25. Patients with sickle cell trait usually have RBC morphology that includes which of the following?
    a. Normocytic, normochromic RBCs with occasional target cells
    b. Normocytic, normochromic RBCs with rare sickle cells
    c. Hypochromic, microcytic RBCs with moderate target cells
    d. Macrocytic, normochromic cells with occasional NRBCs

26. Which laboratory test is best used for definitive diagnosis of sickle cell anemia?
    a. Solubility testing
    b. Hemoglobin electrophoresis
    c. Peripheral smear review for sickle cells
    d. Bone marrow analysis

27. A peripheral smear review shows mildly anemic sample with target cells and oblong hexagonal crystalloids. What is a possible identity for the crystalloids?
    a. Hemoglobin S
    b. Hemoglobin C
    c. Hemoglobin SC
    d. Hemoglobin E

28. An 18-year-old man has a CBC done when visiting his physician for a persistent sore throat. He has the following results:

    WBC 12.5×10^9/L RBC 6.00×10^{12}/L Hgb 10.0 g/dL
    Hct 30.0% MCV 60 fL MCH 20 pg
    MCHC 33% Platelet 218×10^9/L

    Which of the following is most likely?
    a. This patient is normal with a slightly elevated WBC count because of his sore throat

    b. This patient has infectious mononucleosis and warm autoimmune hemolytic anemia
    c. This patient is likely to have β-thalassemia minor
    d. There is a specimen quality issue because of a cold agglutinin

29. Hemoglobin H disease is described as:
    a. $--/-\alpha$
    b. $-\alpha/-\alpha$
    c. $--/\beta\beta$
    d. $-\beta/-\beta$

30. A 3-year-old female patient is seen in the hematology clinic to investigate the cause of her persistent anemia. Hemoglobin electrophoresis was ordered, and results showed an elevation in Hgb F, with a small increase in Hgb A_2. What is the most likely disorder based on these results?
    a. α-Thalassemia major
    b. β-Thalassemia major
    c. α-Thalassemia minor
    d. Hemoglobin H disease

31. A 36-year-old male patient has a CBC performed as part of a routine work physical. The WBC count was 6.5×10^9/L with a differential count of 48% neutrophils, 40% lymphocytes, 8% monocytes, 3% eosinophils, and 1% basophils. The majority of the neutrophils were mature but hyposegmented, showing bandlike or single nuclei. What disorder would be suspected?
    a. Alder-Reilly anomaly
    b. Leukocyte adhesion deficiency
    c. Pelger-Huet anomaly
    d. Reed Sternberg syndrome

32. A 38-year-old male patient has the following CBC results:

WBC	RBC	Hgb 16.0 g/dL
32.5×10^9/L	5.50×10^{12}/L	
Hct 48.0%	Platelet	Differential: 49%
	225×10^9/L	segmented neutrophils, 9% bands, 25% lymphocytes, 9% monocytes, 1% eosinophils, 4% metamyelocytes, 3% myelocytes; RBC and platelet morphology appear normal

    Which of the following conditions is the most likely cause of these results?
    a. Bacterial infection
    b. CML
    c. Refractory anemia
    d. Viral infection

33. Which of the following cytochemical stains is best used to distinguish cells of monocytic origin?
    a. α-Naphthyl acetate esterase
    b. Naphthol AS-D chloroacetate esterase
    c. Myeloperoxidase
    d. Periodic acid–Schiff

34. A positive tartrate-resistant acid phosphatase (TRAP) stain is indicative of:
    a. Burkitt's lymphoma
    b. Chronic myelogenous leukemia
    c. Hairy cell leukemia
    d. Multiple myeloma

35. Which mutation is shared by a large percentage of patients with polycythemia vera, essential thrombocythemia, and primary myelofibrosis?
    a. *BCR/ABL*
    b. *JAK2 V617F*
    c. *PDGFR*
    d. *RUNX1*

36. A patient has a CBC and peripheral smear with an elevated WBC count and left shift, suggestive of a diagnosis of CML. Which of the following tests would be the most helpful in confirming the suspected diagnosis?
    a. Cytochemical staining for myeloperoxidase and LAP
    b. Karyotyping for the Philadelphia chromosome
    c. Flow cytometry for myeloid cell markers
    d. Lymph node biopsies for metastasis

37. A patient has a splenomegaly, and his CBC shows a left shift; bizarre RBCs, including dacryocytes; and notable platelet abnormalities. Which of the following would be the most helpful in determining the patient's diagnosis?
    a. Bone marrow biopsy
    b. LAP staining
    c. Karyotyping for the Philadelphia chromosome
    d. Spleen biopsy

38. Which of the following peripheral blood findings would not be expected in a patient with a myelodysplastic syndrome?
    a. Hypogranular neutrophils
    b. Binucleate neutrophils and NRBCs
    c. Circulating micromegakaryocytes
    d. Decreased vitamin B_{12} and folic acid

39. The WHO system classifies this disorder as a Myeloproliferative/Myelodysplastic syndrome.
    a. Refractory Anemia with Ringed Sideroblasts
    b. 5q – Syndrome
    c. Chronic Myelomonocytic Leukemia
    d. Refractory Anemia with Multilineage Dysplasia

40. A 4-year-old male patient presents with a slightly elevated WBC count, and occasional blasts are present on the differential. Flow cytometry is performed with the following results: CD10(+), CD19 (+), CD22(+), CD79a(+), TdT(+). Which of the following diagnoses is the most likely?
    a. Intermediate B-cell ALL
    b. Pre–B-cell ALL
    c. T-cell ALL
    d. Pre–T-cell ALL

41. Which of the following may predict a better prognosis in patients with ALL?
    a. The patient is a child
    b. Peripheral blood blast counts greater than 30×10^9/L
    c. The Philadelphia chromosome is present
    d. The patient is hypodiploid

42. A 28-year-old female patient presented to the emergency department with symptoms suggestive of DIC. A CBC and coagulation studies were ordered. The peripheral smear showed blasts and immature cells with heavy granulation and Auer rods. Which of the following disorders would be the most likely?
    a. AML with t(9;11)(p22;q23); *MLLT3-MLL*
    b. AML with t(15;17)(q22;q12); *PML-RARα*
    c. ALL with t(12;21)(p13;q22); *ETV6-RUNX1*
    d. ALL with t(9;22)(q34;q11.2); *BCR-ABL1*

43. A patient presents with an elevated WBC count, increased monocytes, and blasts present on the differential. Flow cytometry is performed with the following results: CD4+, CD11b+, CD11c+, CD13+, CD14+, CD33+, CD36+, CD64+. Which of the following diagnoses is the most likely?
    a. AML with minimal differentiation
    b. AML with maturation
    c. Acute myelomonocytic leukemia
    d. Acute monoblastic leukemia

44. A 75-year-old male patient visits his physician for an annual checkup. His CBC showed an elevated WBC count with numerous small lymphocytes and smudge cells, and a subsequent bone marrow biopsy and aspirate showed hypercellularity with increased lymphoid cells. What is a presumptive diagnosis based on this information?
    a. Acute lymphoblastic leukemia
    b. Chronic lymphocytic leukemia/small cell lymphocytic lymphoma
    c. Hairy cell leukemia
    d. Therapy-related acute myelogenous leukemia

45. Which of the following is not considered a disorder of plasma cells?
    a. Monoclonal gammopathy of undetermined significance
    b. Multiple myeloma
    c. Sézary syndrome
    d. Waldenström's macroglobulinemia

46. Which of the following sets of CD markers are associated with T lymphocytes?
    a. CD2, CD3, CD4
    b. CD13, CD14, CD15

c. CD19, CD20, CD22

d. CD34, CD71, CD117

47. Bone marrow cellularity is most often estimated by examining which of the following?
    a. Aspirate
    b. Buffy coat
    c. Core biopsy
    d. Crush preparations

48. A dry tap may be seen in bone marrow aspirations in all of the following conditions except:
    a. Aplastic anemia
    b. Hairy cell leukemia
    c. Multiple myeloma
    d. Primary myelofibrosis

49. The largest hematopoietic cells present in the bone marrow are:
    a. Lymphoblasts
    b. Megakaryocytes
    c. Osteoblasts
    d. Pronormoblasts

50. Hemoglobin A contains which of the following configurations of globin chains?
    a. $\alpha_2\beta_2$
    b. $\alpha_2\delta_2$
    c. $\alpha_2\gamma_2$
    d. $\alpha_2\epsilon_2$

51. Which of the following locations is not a site of extramedullary hematopoiesis?
    a. Bone marrow
    b. Liver
    c. Spleen
    d. Thymus

52. Patients with renal failure often exhibit compromised hematopoietic activity because of which of the following?
    a. Concurrent depression of thyroid hormones
    b. Decreased production of erythropoietin
    c. Decreased production of GM-CSF
    d. Bone marrow suppression caused by medications

53. Which of the following best describes the function of the Rapoport-Luebering pathway?
    a. It produces ATP to help maintain RBC membrane deformability
    b. It results in the reduction of glutathione
    c. It produces 2,3 diphosphoglycerate (2,3 DPG)
    d. It produces cytochrome b reductase

54. A 3-year-old male patient visits the pediatrician for a well-child checkup and routine CBC. He has a total WBC count of 5.0×10^9/L, RBC count of 3.8×10^{12}/L, and platelet count of 225×10^9/L. The differential showed 25% segmented neutrophils, 62% lymphocytes, 10% monocytes, and 3% eosinophils. This patient is likely:
    a. A normal child
    b. Suffering from an acute bacterial infection

c. Immunosuppressed

d. A patient with leukemia

55. Which of the following cell types exhibit IgE receptors on their surface membranes?
    a. Basophils
    b. Eosinophils
    c. Band neutrophils
    d. Monocytes

56. A 62-year-old female patient's CBC showed the following results: total WBC count of 14.0×10^9/L, RBC count of 3.95×10^{12}/L, and platelet count of 245×10^9/L. The differential showed 65% segmented neutrophils, 10% bands, 15% lymphocytes, and 10% monocytes. Toxic granulation and Döhle bodies were seen in many of the neutrophils. Which of the following is most likely?
    a. The patient had just finished running a half marathon
    b. The patient has a bacterial infection
    c. The patient is normal
    d. The patient has a helminth infection

57. A CBC on a patient with Chediak-Higashi syndrome is expected to exhibit which of the following?
    a. Giant platelets and Döhle-like inclusions in the cytoplasm of all granulocytes
    b. Large, darkly staining cytoplasmic granules in all WBCs
    c. Giant fused granules and lysosomes in WBC cytoplasm
    d. Leukocytosis and bilobed eosinophils

58. Patients with infectious mononucleosis often have the following CBC results:
    a. Lymphocytosis, including increased variant/reactive lymphocytes
    b. Lymphocytopenia with numerous small lymphocytes
    c. Neutrophilia, including a predominant shift to the left
    d. Neutropenia with a distinct predominance of toxic granulation

59. Flow cytometry for monitoring a patient with acquired immunodeficiency syndrome should include markers for which of the following?
    a. CD30 and CD42
    b. CD4 and CD8
    c. CD34 and CD33
    d. CD21 and CD22

60. Which of the following disorders is classified as a myelodysplastic/myeloproliferative disease?
    a. Acute promyelocytic leukemia
    b. Chronic lymphocytic leukemia
    c. Atypical chronic myelogenous leukemia
    d. Essential thrombocythemia

61. All of the following cells are derived from CFU-GEMM, common myeloid progenitor cells except:
    a. Basophils
    b. Lymphocytes

c. Neutrophils

d. RBCs

62. A patient's differential count shows an elevated eosinophil count. This is consistent with which of the following?

a. Aplastic anemia

b. Bacterial infection

c. Parasitic infection

d. Viral infection

63. Antibodies are produced by which of the following:

a. Macrophages

b. T lymphocytes

c. Plasma cells

d. Basophils

64. The nitroblue tetrazolium reduction test is used to assist in the diagnosis of:

a. Leukocyte adhesion disorders (LADs)

b. Chronic granulomatous disease (CGD)

c. May-Hegglin anomaly

d. Pelger-Huet anomaly

65. A newly diagnosed patient has an acute leukemia. Which of the following would initially be the most useful in determining the origin of the blasts seen?

a. Leukocyte alkaline peroxidase (LAP) and nonspecific esterase (NSE)

b. Periodic acid–Schiff (PAS) and tartrate-resistant acid phosphatase (TRAP)

c. Myeloperoxidase (MPO) and terminal dexoynucleotidyl transferase (TdT)

d. Sudan black B and brilliant cresyl blue

66. Therapy for CML often includes the use of a targeted tyrosine kinase inhibitor, such as:

a. Imatinib mesylate

b. All-*trans* retinoic acid

c. Ablative chemotherapy

d. 2-CDA/cladribine

67. A 58-year-old female was seen by her physician for increasing fatigue. Her CBC shows the following results:

WBC	RBC	Hgb 17.5 g/dL
15.5 × 10⁹/L	5.90 × 10¹²/L	
Hct 53.0%	Platelet	Differential: 55%
	425 × 10⁹/L	segmented neutrophils,

WBC 15.5 $\times$ 10^9/L Hct 53.0%

RBC 5.90 $\times$ 10^{12}/L Platelet 425 $\times$ 10^9/L

Hgb 17.5 g/dL

Differential: 55% segmented neutrophils, 3% bands, 30% lymphocytes, 9% monocytes, 1% eosinophils, 2% metamyelocytes; RBC and platelet morphology appear normal

Which of the following conditions is the most likely cause of these results?

a. Chronic myelogenous leukemia

b. Polycythemia vera

c. Acute bacterial infection

d. The patient is normal

68. Polycythemia vera can be differentiated from secondary polycythemia because of polycythemia vera presenting with which of the following?

a. Elevated hemoglobin results

b. Decreased erythropoietin levels

c. Normal to decreased WBC counts

d. Erythroid hyperplasia in the marrow

69. The genetic mutation associated with CML is:

a. t (15;17)(q22;q12)

b. t(11;14)(p15;q11)

c. t(9;22)(q34;q11.2)

d. t(8;21)(q22;q22)

70. Which of the following is not classified as a myeloproliferative neoplasm?

a. Chronic eosinophilic leukemia

b. Essential thrombocythemia

c. Mastocytosis

d. Waldenström's macroglobulinemia

71. What is the minimum percentage of ringed sideroblasts present in the bone marrow for a diagnosis of refractory anemia with ringed sideroblasts?

a. 10%

b. 15%

c. 20%

d. >25%

72. All of the following are considered to be signs of dyserythropoiesis except:

a. Multinucleate RBCs

b. Basophilic stippling

c. Döhle bodies

d. Oval macrocytes

73. Features of dysmyelopoiesis and dysmegakaryopoiesis seen on a peripheral smear or bone marrow in cases of myelodysplastic syndromes include all of the following except:

a. Pelgeroid neutrophils

b. Neutrophils showing hypogranulation

c. Giant abnormal platelets with abnormal granules

d. Siderotic granules

74. The peripheral blood and bone marrow picture sometimes will look similar in myelodysplastic syndromes and some RBC disorders. Which of the following RBC disorders tends to have a peripheral smear appearance similar to cases of myelodysplastic syndromes?

a. Iron deficiency anemia

b. α-Thalassemia minor

c. Megaloblastic anemia

d. Warm autoimmune hemolytic anemia

75. Most of the chromosome abnormalities seen in myelodysplastic syndrome involve which of the following chromosomes?

a. 5, 7, 8, 11, 13, 20

b. 2, 3, 9, 15, 16, 26

c. 3, 6, 10, 14, 21

d. 1, 4, 15, 17, 21

76. Which of the following is not one of the recurrent genetic abnormalities seen in cases of acute myeloid leukemia?
    a. AML with t(8;21)(q22;q22); *AML1(CBFα)/ETO*
    b. AML with t(15;17)(q22;q12); *(PML/RARα)*
    c. AML with inv(16)/p(13;q22); *(CBFβ/MYH11)*
    d. AML with t(1;19)(q23;q13); *(E2A/PBX1)*

77. AML with 11q23 *(MLL)* abnormalities are associated with which cell line?
    a. Eosinophil
    b. Erythrocyte
    c. Monocyte
    d. Neutrophil

78. T-cell ALL most commonly affects which of the following?
    a. Infants
    b. Teenaged males
    c. Adult females
    d. Elderly males

79. Which of the following disorders is considered to be classified by WHO as an AML, not otherwise classified?
    a. Acute erythroid leukemia
    b. Acute megakaryoblastic leukemia
    c. Acute promyelocytic leukemia
    d. AML without maturation

80. A 69-year-old female patient presented with symptoms of fatigue and easy bruising. A CBC was ordered. The peripheral smear showed a large number of blasts, anemia, and thrombocytopenia. A bone marrow examination was performed, revealing hypercellularity and a blast appearance similar to that of the peripheral smear. Flow cytometry revealed cells positive for CD 13, CD 33, CD 34, CD 38, CD 117, and HLA-DR. Cells were negative for TdT, myeloperoxidase, and nonspecific esterase. Based on this information, which of the following is most likely?
    a. AML with minimal differentiation
    b. AML without maturation
    c. B-cell ALL without maturation
    d. Acute monoblastic leukemia

81. A 3-year-old female patient was having symptoms of lethargy and bruising and reported pain in her legs. Her mother also mentioned noticing several swollen lymph nodes when bathing the child. The pediatrician ordered a CBC, which had the following results.

WBC		18.5×10^{12}/L
RBC		3.00×10^{12}/L
Hgb 9.0 g/dL		
Hct 27.0%	MCV 90 fL	MCH 30 pg
MCHC 33%	Platelet	58×10^9/L
Differential: 80%		blastocytes, 6% segmented neutrophils, 8% lymphocytes, 6% monocytes. RBC morphology was normal, and platelets were markedly decreased

What is the most likely reason that the physician ordered a lumbar puncture after receiving the CBC results?
    a. To rule out an acute case of meningitis
    b. To look for leukemia cells in the spinal fluid
    c. To rule out infectious mononucleosis
    d. To rule out multiple sclerosis

82. A 78-year-old man was previously diagnosed with chronic lymphocytic leukemia (CLL). Periodic CBCs were ordered, and several months of CBCs maintained an appearance consistent with cases of CLL.

WBC 58.5 $\times 10^{12}$/L	RBC 3.90×10^{12}/L	Hgb 12.0 g/dL
Hct 36.0%	MCV 92 fL	MCH 3 pg
MCHC 33%	Platelet 132×10^9/L	Differential: 70% lymphocytes, 8% segmented neutrophils, 2% monocytes, 20% unidentified cells with lymphoid appearance and a prominent nucleolus

Which of the following is most likely?
    a. The patient has developed Sézary syndrome
    b. The patient has developed prolymphocytic leukemia
    c. The patient has developed multiple myeloma
    d. The patient now has a concurrent case of CLL and ALL

83. Multiple myeloma exhibits laboratory features except which of the following?
    a. Occasional plasma cells in the peripheral blood
    b. Rouleaux
    c. Hypercalcemia
    d. Decreased immunoglobulin

84. The diagnostic cell type seen in Hodgkin lymphoma is:
    a. Binucleate plasma cell
    b. Reed Sternberg cell
    c. Bence Jones lymphocyte
    d. Burkitt lymphocyte

85. Which of the following appearances describes the types of cells seen in Sézary syndrome?
    a. Plasma cells containing immunoglobulin deposits
    b. Large circulating micromegakaryocytes
    c. Lymphocytes with convoluted, cerebriform nuclei
    d. Prolymphocytes with prominent azurophilic granules

86. Which of the following best describes the function of the hexose-monophosphate pathway?
    a. It produces ATP to help maintain RBC membrane deformability
    b. It results in the reduction of glutathione
    c. It produces 2,3 diphosphoglycerate (2,3 DPG)
    d. It produces cytochrome b reductase

87. A patient has a reticulocyte count of 3.5%. This shows which of the following?
    a. Bone marrow response in producing more RBCs because of increased need
    b. A normal reticulocyte count
    c. Patient transfusion of whole blood
    d. Lack of response to vitamin therapy after a diagnosis of iron-deficiency anemia

88. Which of the following cases does not warrant a bone marrow examination?
    a. Presence of blasts on the peripheral smear
    b. Postchemotherapy assessment for minimal residual disease
    c. Diagnosis of iron-deficiency anemia
    d. Diagnosis of suspected systemic fungal infection

89. A bone marrow sample for a patient with newly diagnosed chronic myelogenous leukemia would often be expected to have an M/E ratio of:
    a. 1:1
    b. 2:1
    c. 1:2
    d. 10:1

90. Which of the following is not implicated as a cause of nonmegaloblastic macrocytic anemia?
    a. Alcoholism
    b. Hemochromatosis
    c. Hypothyroidism
    d. Liver disease

91. Which of the following results is consistent with a diagnosis of aplastic anemia?
    a. Hypocellular bone marrow, absolute neutrophil count of 0.5×10^9/L, platelet count of 40×10^9/L, Hgb 8 g/dL
    b. Hypocellular bone marrow, absolute neutrophil count of 2.5×10^9/L, platelet count of 75×10^9/L, Hgb 10 g/dL
    c. Hypercellular bone marrow, absolute neutrophil count of 1.5×10^9/L, platelet count of 100×10^9/L, Hgb 14 g/dL
    d. Hypocellular bone marrow, absolute neutrophil count of 0.5×10^9/L, platelet count of 90×10^9/L, Hgb 11 g/dL

92. The following statement is true of mutations in α-thalassemia compared to those seen in β-thalassemia:
    a. Mutations in α-thalassemia occur as a result of reduced or absent expression of the globin gene
    b. Mutations in α-thalassemia occur as a result of the deletion of one or more globin genes
    c. The α-globin gene is expressed on chromosome 11
    d. The β-globin gene is expressed on chromosome 16

93. A patient's genotype is $-\alpha/-\alpha$. This patient will have a CBC that shows which of the following?
    a. Decreased RBC count with numerous target cells
    b. Decreased RBC count with microcytic/hypochromic RBCs

    c. Increased RBC count with normal RBCs
    d. Increased RBC count with microcytic/hypochromic RBCs

94. Patients with sickle cell anemia and β-thalassemia major may not show clinical symptoms until the patient is at least 6 months of age because of which of the following?
    a. The mutations are acquired after the child is born
    b. The mutations are activated by dietary and maternal factors
    c. The mutations may not manifest clinically at birth because the presence of hemoglobin F decreases
    d. The mutations lead to elevations in α genes that compensate for the decreased gene expression

95. The thymus is a site used as a maturation compartment for:
    a. B cells
    b. T cells
    c. Megakaryocytes
    d. Monocytes

96. A manual hemocytometer count was required to check a patient's total WBC count. A 1:20 dilution was made and used when the four large "W" squares were counted on both sides of the hemacytometer. A total of 105 cells were counted between the two sides. What was the patient's total WBC count?
    a. 0.33×10^9/L
    b. 2.1×10^9/L
    c. 2.6×10^9/L
    d. 5.3×10^9/L

97. Hereditary elliptocytosis results from defects in which of the following?
    a. Ankyrin
    b. Band 3 protein
    c. Spectrin
    d. Pyruvate

98. Primary neutrophil granules contain:
    a. Acetyltransferase, collagenase, gelatinase, lysozyme, β_2-microglobulin
    b. Alkaline phosphatase, cytochrome b_{558}, complement receptor 1, complement 1q receptor, vesicle-associated membrane-2
    c. β_2-Microglobulin, collagenase, gelatinase lactoferrin, neutrophil gelatinase-associated lipocalin
    d. Acid β-glycerophosphatase, cathespins, defensins, elastase, myeloperoxidase, proteinase-3

99. A 36-year-old man visited the emergency department because of alternating episodes of fever and chills that persisted over several days. The patient stated he had not felt well since returning from a mission trip to Africa. The physician ordered a CBC with the following results.

WBC	RBC	Hgb 12.0 g/dL
3.5×10^9/L	3.80×10^{12}/L	
Hct 36.0%	MCV 95 fL	MCH 32 pg

MCHC 33%   Platelet   Differential: Normal WBC
             145×10^9/L   distribution, normocytic
                                normochromic RBCs
                                with some inclusions
                                present and several
                                abnormal platelet-like
                                structures shaped like
                                boomerangs

What should be done with this sample next?
a. Rerun the sample to make sure it is not clotted
b. Clean the stainer and make another slide to examine
c. Refer the sample to the pathologist for further identification
d. Report the results, because the results are normal

100. Patients with suspected paroxysmal cold hemoglobinuria can be confirmed by performing which of the following?
a. Direct antiglobulin test (DAT)
b. Donath-Landsteiner test
c. Osmotic fragility test
d. G6PD activity assay

REFERENCE

Rodak BF, Fritsma GA, Keohane E: Hematology: clinical principles and applications, ed 4, St Louis, 2012, Saunders.

SELF-ASSESSMENT

Content Area: _____

Score on Practice Questions: _____

List the specific topics covered in the missed questions:

List the specific topics covered in the correct questions:

NOTES

4

Hemostasis

Charity E. Accurso

STEPS OF HEMOSTATIC RESPONSE

Injury to endothelium (or vessel)
↓
Primary hemostasis (formation of primary hemostatic plug, platelets have the main role)
↓
Secondary hemostasis (formation of fibrin clot, coagulation proteins are the major contributor)
↓
Fibrinolysis (removal of clot)

SYSTEMS OF HEMOSTASIS

1. Vasculature
2. Platelets
3. Clot formation
4. Fibrinolytic

ROLE OF VASCULATURE

- Hemostasis usually occurs in the arterioles and venules
  - Endothelial cells line lumen
  - Luminal side coated by glycocalyx (carbohydrates and proteins)
  - Abluminal side is attached to basement membrane (type IV collagen and proteins)
- Vessels are nonthrombotic under normal circumstances
  - Negatively charged surfaces repel (endothelium and platelets)
  - Inhibit platelet activation: Prostacyclin (PGI_2) and nitric oxide (NO) synthesis and secretion, ADPase
  - Inactivation of thrombin: Heparin sulfate, thrombomodulin
- Damaged vessels are prothrombotic
  - Exposure of subendothelium: Collagen—platelet activation
  - Secretion of platelet activating factor
  - Secretion of von Willebrand factor (vWF): Platelet adhesion
  - Release of tissue factor: Aids in secondary hemostasis activation

DISORDERS OF VASCULATURE AFFECTING HEMOSTASIS

Hereditary

- Hereditary hemorrhagic telangiectasia (also called Osler-Weber-Rendu disease): Abnormal formation of vessels in which arterial blood may flow directly into a vein without passing through a capillary. The connecting area is often fragile and ruptures easily, resulting in bleeding and bruising
- Ehlers-Danlos syndrome: Connective tissue disorder caused by mutation in collagen synthesis; resulting blood vessels are fragile and easily broken

Acquired

Type of Purpura (More Common Types)
- Decreased connective tissue
  - Senile purpura: Degeneration of skin matrix resulting in weak capillaries
  - Excess glucocorticoid: Cushing's syndrome and therapeutic glucocorticoids can result in vessel fragility
  - Vitamin C deficiency (scurvy): Vessel fragility resulting from disruption of collagen production
- Paraprotein disorders
  - Amyloidosis: Deposition of amyloid material in vessels leading to fragility; thrombosis is also possible
  - Paraproteins: Many different effects, depending on malignancy
- Vasculitis: Inflammation of blood vessels leading to complement activation; immune complex deposition also leads to activation and aggregation of platelets
  - Henoch-Schönlein purpura: Considered to be another form of vasculitis more commonly affecting children

ROLE OF PLATELETS

- Characteristics
  - Circulate as inert cell fragments
  - Repel each other and endothelial lining (nonthrombotic property)

TABLE 4-1	Platelet Components, Functions, and Structure	
Major Zones	**Location Within Platelet**	**Significant Components and Major Functions**
Peripheral zone	Glycocalyx Cytoplasmic membrane Open canalicular system Submembranous area	*Factor V:* Component of prothrombinase complex, attachment site for factor X on platelet surface *vWF:* Transports factor VIII, mediates adhesion between platelets via GPIb/IX Fibrinogen: Converted to fibrin in final clot formation stages *GPIb/IX:* Platelet receptor for vWF *GPIIb/IIIa:* Platelet receptor for fibrinogen (and others) *Others:* Glycolipids, phospholipids, proteins, mucopolysaccharides
Structural zone	Circumferential and throughout the platelet	Microtubules Microfilaments Intermediate filaments All involved in maintenance of shape and shape change on platelet activation
Organelle zone	Internally located	Granules α (50-80 per platelet): See Table 4-2 Dense (3-8 per platelet): See Table 4-2 Lysosomal granules: Hydrolytic Peroxisomes Mitochondria Glycogen particles
Membrane systems	Surface connected open canalicular system (SCCS, OCS) Dense tubular system (DTS)	*SCCS:* Interior of platelet and connects to platelet surface; allows substances to enter platelet and others to exit; important in storage and secretion; serves as source of surface membrane after activation *DTS:* Does not connect to platelet surface, primarily a source of ionized calcium, site of prostaglandin and thromboxane synthesis

GP, Glycoprotein; *vWF,* von Willebrand factor.

- Become activated after an injury
- After activation, platelets interact with other platelets and the damaged vessel wall

Platelet Ultrastructure

- The platelet is divided into arbitrary zones described by location and function (Table 4-1)

Platelet Functions

- Passive surveillance: Monitor vessel lining for small holes or gaps, platelets plug holes without activation of coagulation system
- Formation of primary hemostatic plug
- Provides phospholipid surface for secondary hemostasis
- Promotion of healing by stimulation of smooth muscle cells and fibroblasts

PRIMARY HEMOSTASIS

Platelet Adhesion

- Major interaction is the binding of platelet receptor glycoprotein Ib (GPIb)/IX to vWF, which binds to collagen (Figure 4-1)

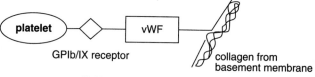

FIGURE 4-1 Platelet adhesion.

- vWF: Stored in α-granules in platelets and Weibel-Palade bodies in endothelial cells
- Important step that triggers several events leading to platelet activation

Platelet Activation

- Triggered after platelet adhesion or exposure to agonist
  - Results: Shape change, altered orientation of phospholipids, new receptor expression, changes in biochemistry
  - Platelet agonists: Collagen, adenosine diphosphate (ADP), thrombin, epinephrine, thromboxane A_2 (TXA_2), arachidonic acid
    - TXA_2: Synthesized from arachidonic acid by cyclooxygenase and thromboxane synthase, stimulates platelet granule secretion, enhances vasoconstriction; if blocked, secretion is impaired; aspirin blocks cyclooxygenase

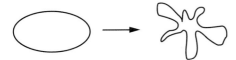

FIGURE 4-2 Shape change.

- ○ Collagen and thrombin are strong agonists
- ○ ADP and epinephrine are weak agonists
  - Required presence of TXA$_2$ and platelet aggregation

Shape Change

- Occurs after agonist stimulation, appearance of pseudopods, will convert to original shape if stimulus is not sufficient (Figure 4-2)
  - Microtubules, microfilaments, and intermediate filaments reorganize so that organelles are centrally located in the activated platelet
    - ○ Phospholipid orientation: Large surface available for biochemical reactions in secondary hemostasis
    - ○ Receptor expression: GPIb/IX on surface, increase in number of GPIIb/IIIa receptors on surface

Platelet Secretion

- Requires adenosine triphosphate (ATP); open canalicular system fuses with granular membrane, and contents of α-granules and dense bodies are released to the outside of the platelet (Table 4-2)
  - Agonists released further activate platelets
  - Calcium released for use in secondary hemostasis (Table 4-3)

Platelet Aggregation

- vWF binding to GPIb/IX activates an intracellular signaling pathway that results in the activation of GPIIb/IIIa, which then binds to fibrinogen

  vWF binding GPIb/IX
  ↓Intracellular signaling

  GPIIb/IIIa activation and binding to fibrinogen
- Fibrinogen forms bridges to other GPIIb/IIIa receptors on other activated platelets, resulting in platelet aggregates; Ca^{2+} is needed for aggregation
- Fibrinogen and Ca^{2+} are delivered locally from granules and dense tubular system
- Primary aggregation versus secondary aggregation: In vitro
  - ○ Primary: Loose aggregation, reversible if stimulus is not sufficient
  - ○ Secondary: Irreversible provided sufficient stimulus; occurs after internal ADP release, TXA$_2$ synthesis and release, further stimulation then occurs

TABLE 4-2	Major Components (and Select Functions) of Platelet Granules	
Dense Bodies	**α-Granules**	
ADP: Platelet agonist—positive feedback to enhance platelet response and recruitment	*Factor V:* Fibrin formation	
ATP: Activation of Ca^{2+} channel, agonist for other cells	*Factor XI:* Fibrin formation	
Calcium: Secondary hemostasis	*Fibrinogen:* Converted to fibrin, platelet aggregation	
Serotonin: Platelet agonist, vasoconstriction	*Protein S:* Regulation of fibrin formation via protein C pathway	
	TFPI: Regulation of fibrin formation by inhibiting factor VII/tissue factor complex	
	vWF: Binding of platelets to collagen	
	PAI-1: Inhibitor of fibrinolysis	
	PF4: Heparin neutralizing, chemoattractant	
	ß-Thromboglobulin: Chemoattractant	
	Thrombospondin: Stabilization of platelets	

ADP, Adenosine diphosphate; *ATP*, adenosine triphosphate; *PAI-1*, plasminogen activator inhibitor–1; *PF4*, platelet factor–4; *TFPI*, tissue pathway factor inhibitor; *vWF*, von Willebrand factor.

TABLE 4-3	Summary of Major Biochemical Mediators of Activation
Arachidonic pathway	*Increased cytoplasmic Ca^{2+}:* Results in phospholipase A$_2$ activation
	Phospholipase A$_2$: Hydrolyzes arachidonic acid
	Cyclooxygenase: Synthesizes thromboxane A$_2$ from arachidonic acid (thromboxane synthesis involved)
	TXA$_2$: Platelet agonist, required for secondary aggregation
	Aspirin: Inhibits cyclooxygenase (lifetime of platelet)
Ca^{2+}	*Intracellular signaling:* Required for several reactions, including secondary hemostasis, activation of some cellular enzymes
CAMP	*CAMP:* Negative regulator of platelet activation, production of CAMP inhibits protein kinase which inhibits aggregation
	ADP: Inhibits adenyl cyclase
Phospholipase C	Activation of several reactions leads to calcium mobilization, granule secretion, and fibrinogen receptor expression
G proteins	Platelet agonists bind to G protein receptors, intracellular messaging system

ADP, Adenosine diphosphate; *CAMP*, cyclic adenosine monophosphate.

SECONDARY HEMOSTASIS

- Through a series of enzymatic reactions, the primary platelet plug is reinforced by fibrin
- Secondary hemostasis is a complex system of procoagulant activities and control activities to contain and limit clot formation
- Zymogens are inactive precursors of coagulation factors
  - Zymogens serve as substrates for previous enzymatic reaction in the coagulation cascade
- Vitamin K–dependent factors: II, VII, IX, X, protein C, and protein S
- Vitamin K–dependent factors are not functional unless an additional carboxyl group (COOH) is added to the γ-carbon of the glutamic acid residues. This reaction is called γ-carboxylation and is dependent on vitamin K. The factors will be formed in the absence of Vitamin K but will not be functional because this modification is required for binding to a negative phospholipid surface
- The coagulation cascade has two pathways—intrinsic and extrinsic—and shares a common final pathway, the common pathway
- The end-point of the common pathway is the formation of a fibrin clot that reinforces the platelet plug
- The concept of the three pathways was derived from in vitro experiments; physiologically, hemostasis occurs through one pathway—the tissue factor pathway

Grouping of Coagulation Factors

See Tables 4-4 and 4-5

- Cofactors enhance activity of enzymes
  - Va is a cofactor for Xa, no enzymatic activity alone
  - VIIIa is a cofactor for IXa, no enzymatic activity alone
  - High-molecular-weight kininogen (HK) is a cofactor for XIIa and XIa
  - Protein S is a cofactor for activated protein C
  - Tissue factor is a cofactor for VIIa

- Substrate fibrinogen: Acted on by thrombin
- Enzymes: Circulate as zymogens
  - Activation: Two routes
    - Conformational change
    - Proteolytic cleavage

Intrinsic Pathway

- Activation of contact factors when they come into contact with negatively charged surfaces
  - Glass, kaolin, ellagic acid
  - Not dependent on calcium
  - Deficiency of contact factors (XII, PK, and HK) does not lead to in vivo bleeding issues. Deficiency of XI is associated with bleeding abnormalities in approximately 50% of individuals
  - Contact factors are involved in activation of fibrinolysis, complement activation, kinin formation, inflammation, and angiogenesis (Figure 4-3)

Extrinsic Pathway

- Damage to the vessel results in the exposure of tissue factor on the surface of nonvascular cells
- VII and VIIa bind to tissue factor in the presence of calcium to form the VIIa/tissue factor complex, also called extrinsic Xase, and the extrinsic pathway is thus activated. Extrinsic Xase also can activate IX in the intrinsic pathway (Figure 4-4)

Common Pathway

- Begins with the activation of X by either the intrinsic or extrinsic pathway (Figure 4-5)
- End result: Formation of fibrin clot (see Figure 4-5)
- Important notes about fibrin formation (Figure 4-6)
  - Thrombin cleaves fibrinopeptides from fibrinogen, forming a fibrin monomer. Fibrin monomers associate in half-staggered overlap pattern between the D and E domains

TABLE 4-4	Grouping of Coagulation Factors		
	Contact Group	**Fibrinogen Group**	**Prothrombin Group**
Factors	HK, PK, XII, XI	XIII, VIII, V, I	X, IX, VII, II
Consumed in clot	No	Yes	No, except for II
Molecular weight	80,000-173,000 Da	300,000-350,000 Da	50,000-100,000 Da
Critical to hemostasis	XI is essential to hemostasis XII, PK, HK do not play a major role in hemostasis (in vivo), so deficiency does not cause bleeding	Yes	Yes
Other important information	Activation of fibrinolytic, kinin, and complement systems; role in inflammation	Thrombin acts on all factors	Vitamin K dependent

HK, High-molecular-weight kininogen.

TABLE 4-5	Important Factors in Hemostasis	
Factors	**Activation and Functions**	**Important Notes**
Contact Factors		
XII (Hageman factor)	Activated to XIIa by kallikrein, plasmin, or autoactivation (from contact with negatively charged surface) XIIa cleaves PK to kallikrein XIIa (+ cofactor HK) converts XI to XIa Activates fibrinolytic and complement systems	Deficiency not associated with bleeding condition
XI	Activated by XIIa, thrombin, and XIa Activates IX in the presence of calcium	Hemophilia C Binds to surface of activated platelets
Prekallikrein (PK)	Activated to kallikrein by XIIa Cleaves HK in smaller fragments—kinin Activates plasminogen to plasmin conversion Conversion of scuPA to uPA	Majority circulates bound to HK Chemoattractant Deficiency not associated with bleeding condition
High-molecular-weight kininogen (HK)	Kinin source Accelerates XII and PK activation	Located in endothelial cells, platelets, granulocytes Deficiency not associated with bleeding condition
Prothrombin Group: Vitamin K Dependent		
II (prothrombin)	Cleaved to thrombin by prothrombinase *Thrombin:* Many functions (both procoagulant and anticoagulant; other functions described in section on regulation) Cleaves fibrinopeptides from fibrinogen to form a fibrin monomer Further activates Va, VIIIa, and XIIIa Activates platelets Stimulates release of vWF and PAI-1 from endothelial cells and expression of tissue factor	
VII	Small amount circulates as VIIa, which further activates VII after binding to tissue factor Component of extrinsic Xase (with tissue factor and Ca^{2+}) Activates X and IX as part of complex	
IX	Activated by XIa in the presence of Ca^{2+} Additional activation by VIIa/tissue factor complex Component of intrinsic Xase (with VIIIa and Ca^{2+}) Activates X (as part of Xase)	Binds to activated platelets Hemophilia B X-Linked inheritance
X	Activated by extrinsic Xase (VIIa, VIIIa, tissue factor, Ca^{2+}) or intrinsic Xase (IXa, VIIIa, Ca^{2+}) Complexes with Va, Ca^{2+} and phospholipids to form prothrombinase	
Fibrinogen Group		
VIII	Activated by Xa or thrombin Cofactor for IXa Component of intrinsic Xase (with IXa and Ca^{2+})	Circulates associated with vWF Hemophilia A X-Linked inheritance
V	Activated by thrombin and Xa Binds to activated platelet Component of prothrombinase (with Xa, Ca^{2+}, platelet)	25% in α-granules of platelets
Fibrinogen	Converted to fibrin by cleavage of fibrinopeptides A and B from fibrinogen Fibrin monomers polymerize in half-staggered overlap with other monomers forming fibrin polymer (see Figure 4-6)	Glycoprotein in plasma and platelet α-granules Most abundant coagulation protein
XIII	Stabilizes fibrin monomer by cross-linking D-domains	Transglutaminase
Others		
vWF	Mediates adhesion to vessel wall Binds to GPIb/IX on platelets Binds to collagen and elastin in subendothelium Promotes platelet aggregation by binding to GPIIb/IIIa on platelets Circulates as vWF/VIII complex in plasma, stabilizes and protects VIII	Synthesized and stored in endothelial cells and megakaryocytes
Tissue factor	Cofactor for VII and VIIa Attracts Ca^{2+} and facilitates procoagulant complex formation	Lipoprotein not normally expressed on vessel surfaces Expressed under variety of conditions (e.g., site of injury, toxins, immune complexes, interleukin-1)

GP, Glycoprotein; *PAI-1*, plasminogen activator inhibitor; *scuPA*, single-chain plasminogen activator; *uPAa*, urokinase plasminogen activator; *vWF*, von Willebrand factor.

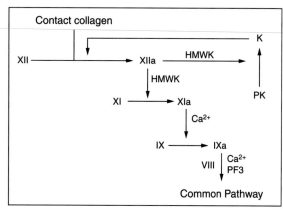

FIGURE 4-3 Intrinsic pathway. *HMWK,* High molecular weight kininogen; *K,* kallikrein; *PF3,* Platelet factor 3; *PK,* Pre-kallikrein.

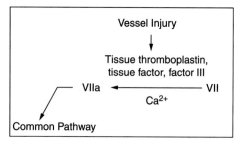

FIGURE 4-4 Extrinsic pathway.

- Factor XIII covalently cross-links D domains to form urea-insoluble fibrin clot
  - If factor XIII is deficient, clot will form but will be soluble in urea

Fibrinolysis

- Process of breaking down fibrin clot through hydrolysis of fibrin
- Activation of system occurs when the intrinsic pathway is activated
- Components
  - Plasminogen: Zymogen for plasmin
    - Contains lysine-binding sites (kringle domains)
    - Transported in eosinophils
    - Incorporated into fibrin clot
- Plasmin
  - Serine protease with broad specificity
    - Degrades proteins susceptible to trypsin degradation
    - Relevant hemostatic targets: Fibrin, fibrinogen, factors V and VIII
- Activation of plasminogen to plasmin conversion
  - Physiologic plasminogen activators
    - Tissue type plasminogen activator (tPA)
      - Produced by vascular endothelial cells, circulates in active form
      - Increased activation ability when plasminogen is bound to fibrin
      - Stimuli: Thrombin, bradykinin, histamine, venous stasis, desmopressin (DDAVP) administration
    - Urokinase type plasminogen activator (uPA)
    - Produced by renal tubular and vascular epithelium, circulates as a single-chain molecular plasminogen activator (scuPA) with little activity, converted by plasmin, factor XIIa, and kallikrein to two-chain form
    - Found in plasma and urine
    - Digests extracellular matrix
    - uPA receptor localizes
      - Exogenous plasminogen activators
  - Streptokinase
    - Causes conformational change to plasminogen when bound, allowing conversion to plasmin
    - Not localized to fibrin
  - Staphylokinase
    - Fibrin required for activation of plasminogen (Figure 4-7)
- Outcomes: Fibrin degradation products (FDPs) and D-dimers
- FDPs
  - Fragment X: Limited binding to thrombin

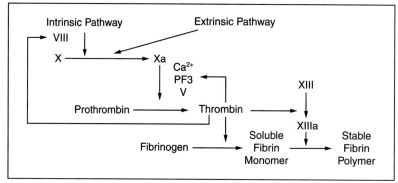

FIGURE 4-5 Common pathway. *PF3,* Platelet factor 3.

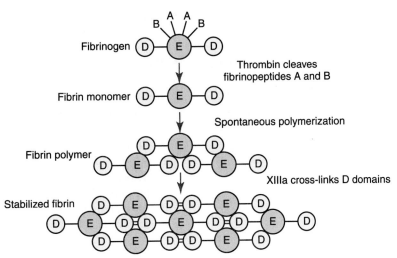

FIGURE 4-6 Formation of stabilized fibrin clot. Thrombin cleaves fibrinopeptides A and B to form fibrin monomer. Fibrin monomers polymerize because of the affinity of thrombin-cleaved positively charged E domains for negatively charged D domains of other monomers. Factor XIIIa catalyzes the covalent cross-linking of γ chains of adjacent D domains to form a urea-insoluble stable fibrin clot. *(From McKenzie SB, Clinical Laboratory Hematology, ed 2, 2010. Printed and electronically reproduced by permission of Pearson Education, Inc, Upper Saddle River, New Jersey.)*

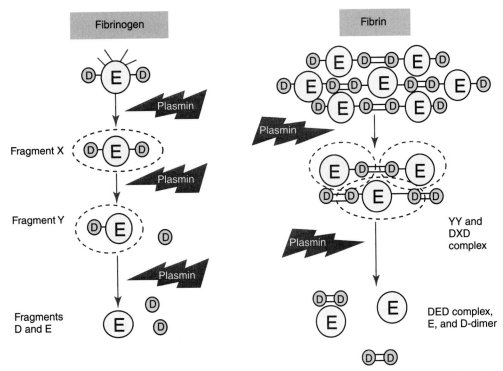

FIGURE 4-7 Degradation of fibrinogen and fibrin by plasmin. Plasmin systematically degrades fibrinogen and fibrin by digestion of small peptides and cleavage of DE domains. Fragment X consists of a central E domain with two D domains (D-E-D); further cleavage produces fragment Y (D-E), with eventual degradation to D and E domains. From cross-linked fibrin, plasmin digestion produces fragment complexes from one or more monomers. D-Dimer consists of two D domains from adjacent monomers that have been cross-linked by XIIa in the process of fibrin formation (thrombosis). *(From Rodak B, Fritsma G, Keohane E: Hematology: clinical principles and applications, ed, Philadelphia, 2012, Saunders.)*

- ○ Fragments Y, D, and E: Inhibit fibrin polymerization and platelet aggregation
- • D-Dimers
  - ○ Two D domains linked through factor XIII action
  - ○ Significance: Indicative of clot formation
- • Fibrinolysis inhibitors

- • Plasminogen activator inhibitors (PAIs)
  - ○ PAI-1: Significant role in plasminogen activation inhibition inhibits tPA, scuPA, uPA
    - ▪ Produced by endothelial cells and several other cell types
    - ▪ 70% of tPA circulates bound to PAI-1, incorporated into fibrin matrix

- Acute phase reactant
  - Deficiency: Excessive, unregulated fibrinolysis results in bleeding
  - PAI-2: Located in placenta and macrophages, inhibits tPA and uPA
- Thrombin-activatable fibrinolysis inhibitor (TFPI)
  - Inhibits binding and activation of plasminogen
  - Short half-life
- α_2-Antiplasmin
  - Inhibitor of circulating plasmin, limiting systemic fibrinolysis
  - Located in α-granules of platelets
  - Small amount incorporated into clot
- α_2-Macroglobulin
  - Wide specificity against many proteases
  - Useful after α_2-antiplasmin exhausted

CONTROL OF HEMOSTASIS

Blood Flow

- Vasoconstriction to slow blood flow for accumulation of coagulation factors and platelets, allow time for clot formation
- Return to normal blood flow limits clot formation and removes excess activated factors

Liver Clearance

- Production site for many coagulation proteins
- Removal of activated factors, factors bound to inhibitors, FDPs

Positive Feedback Amplification

- Thrombin: Activator of platelets, promotes release of platelet factor Va, exposure of negatively charged surface, activation of factors Va and VIIIa
- Factor Xa: Feedback to further activate factor VII, small amount of factor VIII activation

Negative Feedback Amplification

- Thrombin: Involved in activated protein C pathway
- TFPI inactivated factor Xa
- Fibrin binding to thrombin limits further conversion
- FDPs interfere in fibrin formation and polymerization

Biochemical Mediators

- Antithrombin: Serine protease inhibitor
  - Produced by hepatocytes and endothelial cells
  - Major inhibitor to thrombin and factor Xa, also inhibits factors XIIa, XIa, IXa, kallikrein, and plasmin
  - Heparin significantly accelerates activity

- Heparin cofactor II
  - Similar to antithrombin
  - Inhibits thrombin: Faster when bound to heparin
- Proteins C and S: Major anticoagulant system, other involved components include thrombin and thrombomodulin
  - Protein C: Vitamin K dependent, activated by thrombin
  - Protein S: Vitamin K dependent, cofactor for protein C, circulate bound to C4 binding protein
  - Thrombomodulin: Endothelial cell protein; when bound to thrombin, activates protein C with protein S
  - Activated protein C (APC) inactivates factors Va and VIIIa in the presence of protein S and calcium

Disorders of Primary Hemostasis

- Quantitative disorders: Relates to number of platelets (increase versus decrease) (Table 4-6)
- Qualitative disorders: Relates to function of platelets (Table 4-7)

Other Causes of Thrombocytopenia

- Conditions that result in decreased production or ineffective thrombopoiesis
- Hereditary thrombocytopenia: Bernard-Soulier syndrome, May-Hegglin anomaly, Wiskott-Aldrich syndrome (described later in more detail)
- Increase sequestration by the spleen resulting from other conditions
- Dilutional thrombocytopenia

Acquired Platelet Function Disorders

- Aspirin: Irreversibly inactivates cyclooxygenase; nonfunctional platelets
- Alcohol: May eventually lead to platelet dysfunction, possibly as a result of prostaglandin synthesis
- Antibiotics: Penicillins and cephalosporins, antibiotic coats platelet receptors for ADP and epinephrine, may be serious
- Cardiopulmonary bypass surgery: Activation of platelets
- Chronic renal failure: Cause unknown, decreased platelet aggregation, may be severe
- Hematologic disorders: Several can affect platelets, such as multiple myeloma, macroglobulinemia, acute leukemia

Thrombocytosis

- Primary thrombocytosis: Uncontrolled/autonomous proliferation of megakaryocytes, hemorrhagic or thrombotic episodes, platelet count greater than

TABLE 4-6	Major Quantitative Disorders				
Name	Pathophysiology	Symptoms	Diagnosis	Treatment	Prognosis/Other Important Information
Neonatal alloimmunoe thrombocytopenia (NAIT)	Maternal alloantibodies against platelet antigens	Mucosal bleeding Purpura	Symptoms Identification of antibody	Self-limiting – 2-6 weeks Platelet transfusion is controversial	
Immune thrombocytopenic purpura (ITP)	Autoantibodies bind to platelets Shortened platelet lifespan	Varies Asymptomatic to severe mucosal bleeding	Of exclusion Thrombocytopenia ($<20 \times 10^9$/L)	Acute: spontaneous remission (2-6 weeks) Prevent trauma, monitor symptoms, replacement therapy if serious situation	Acute - Associated conditions: upper respiratory infections, chickenpox, rubella, CMV, viral hepatitis
Acute ITP: children; 2-4 years of age, often follows viral infection		Acute: petechiae, abrupt onset	Acute: may see increase in lymphocytes, mild eosinophilia	Chronic: spontaneous remission is rare	Chronic: may see relapses
Chronic ITP: adults; increased female incidence		Chronic: insidious onset, lasts 6-12 months		Administer components if count $<30 \times 10^9$/L, corticosteroid, splenectomy if nonresponsive to treatment, other treatments available	
Thrombotic thrombocytopenic purpura (TTP)	Ultralarge VWF multimers present in circulation which induce platelet agglutination	Petechiae, microangiopathic hemolytic anemia, renal failure	Reduced levels of ADAMTS-13	Platelet infusion of ADAMTS-13	
Heparin induced thrombocytopenia (HIT)	Heparin-dependent IgG antibodies against platelets that complex to platelets and enhance clearance	Bleeding Occasionally thrombotic complications	Continual reduction in platelet count after heparin administration	Discontinue heparin Supportive therapy	

TABLE 4-7 Major Qualitative Disorders

Name	Pathophysiology	Symptoms	Diagnosis	Prognosis/Other Important Information
Bernard-Soulier Syndrome	Disorder of adhesion Rare, autosomal recessive GPIb/IX complex: decreased or abnormal (>600 genetic mutations possible) → Affects binding of platelet to collagen via vWF	Usually no significant bleeding issues	Moderate to severe thrombocytopenia Prolonged bleeding time ADP: normal Collagen: normal Epinephrine: normal Ristocetin: abnormal Distinguish from vWD by performing ristocetin agglutination in the presence of added vWF	Sometimes called giant platelet syndrome
Glanzmann's Thrombasthenia Type I: <5% GPIIb/IIIa receptors Type II: 15% of normal number of receptors Type III: 50-100% of normal number of receptors	Disorder of aggregation Rare, autosomal recessive GPIIb/IIIa receptor deficiency → Affects binding of platelets via fibrinogen to initiate aggregation	Usually no significant bleeding issues	Prolonged bleeding time Abnormal clot retraction ADP: no response Collagen: no response Epinephrine: no response Ristocetin: normal	
Δ-Storage Pool Disease	Decreased or absence of dense granules	Moderate to mild bleeding	Prolonged bleeding time ADP: no secondary aggregation Collagen: no response Epinephrine: no secondary aggregation Ristocetin: normal	Dense granule deficiencies also in: Chediak-Higashi, Hermansky Pudlak syndrome, Wiscott-Aldrich syndrome, TAR syndrome
Gray Platelet Syndrome Also called: A-Storage Pool Disease	Decreased or absence of alpha granules	Mild bleeding	Possible prolonged bleeding time Possible thrombocytopenia Normal platelet aggregations	Similar to Δ-Storage Pool Disease
Defective TXA$_2$ Synthesis	Three possible causes: Phopholipase A$_2$ deficiency Cyclooxygenase deficiency Thromboxane synthase deficiency	Mild bleeding	Possible prolonged bleeding time ADP: no secondary aggregation Collagen: no response Epinephrine: no secondary aggregation Ristocetin: normal	
Von Willebrand Disease (VWD)	Qualitative or quantitative deficiency of von Willebrand factor	Mild to moderate bleeding Some asymptomatic	Abnormal platelet aggregation to ristocetin APTT: normal to increased VWF functional test: decreased VWF antigen: decreased	Several types and subtypes of VWD Therapy dependent on type

ADP, Adenosine diphosphate; *GP,* glycoprotein; *TAR,* thrombocytopenia with absent radius; *TXA,* thromboxane; *vWF,* von Willebrand factor.

$1000 \times 10^9/L$, abnormal epinephrine (possibly ADP and collagen) platelet aggregation
- Reactive (secondary) thrombocytosis: Result of another condition, variable causes and platelet counts

MAJOR DISORDERS OF SECONDARY HEMOSTASIS

See Table 4-8.

Acquired Disorders with Bleeding

- Vitamin K deficiency: Vitamin K needed for γ-carboxylation step to form functional factors II, VII, IX, X, proteins C and S
  - If absent, factor is formed but nonfunctional, bleeding may result if less than 30% functional
  - Causes: Dietary deficiency, decreased gastrointestinal flora needed to synthesize vitamin K because of antibiotic therapy, immaturity of the liver
  - Expected laboratory results: Increased prothrombin time (PT), normal activated thromboplastin time (aPTT) (increases with severity of deficiency), decreased proteins C and S

- Liver disease: Site of synthesis for most hemostatic proteins
  - Expected laboratory results: Increased PT and aPTT, decreased fibrinogen, antithrombin, proteins C and S
- Disseminated intravascular coagulation (DIC): Uncontrolled bleeding and clotting, coagulation occurs systemically; condition results in a consumptive process in which hemostatic proteins, platelets, and regulatory factors are consumed at an increased rate, resulting in deficiencies
  - Causes: Infections, pregnancy complications, neoplasms, trauma or massive injury, snake bites, heat strokes
  - Diagnosis made by reviewing several different laboratory tests and patient history
    - Increased PT, aPTT, and D-dimer and decreased fibrinogen and platelet count
- Fibrinogenolysis: Plasminogen active without thrombin generation, results in degradation of fibrinogen and several coagulation hemostatic factors
  - Differentiate from DIC by negative D-dimer and normal platelet count

TABLE 4-8	Major Disorders of Secondary Hemostasis	
Disorder	**Diagnosis**	**Prognosis/Other Important Information**
Factor VIII deficiency Hemophilia A	APTT → ↑ Factor VIII activity → ↓	X-linked recessive Severity and risk of bleeding dependent on severity of deficiency Some patients (5%-20% of affected individuals) develop inhibitors to FVIII due to treatment
Factor IX deficiency Hemophilia B Christmas disease	APTT → ↑ Factor IX activity → ↓	X-linked recessive Some patients (1%-3% of affected individuals) develop inhibitors to FIX due to treatment
Factor XI deficiency Hemophilia C	APTT → ↑ (may be normal in mild deficiency) Factor XI activity → ↓	Increased frequency in the Ashkenazi Jewish population
Afibrinogenemia	PT → ↑ APTT → ↑ TT → ↑ Fibrinogen → absent	Complete absence of fibrinogen—homozygous mutation Some have severe bleeding; most have milder challenges than hemophiliacs
Hypofibrinogenemia	PT → Normal APTT → Normal TT → ↑ Fibrinogen → Normal	50% of normal plasma levels—heterozygous mutation Mild bleeding
Dysfibrinogenemia – structural abnormality	PT → Normal APTT → Normal TT → ↑ Fibrinogen → Variable	Structural abnormality—usually heterozygous Complications: 50% of affected have no clinical bleeding; 25% of affected have clinical bleeding; 25% of affected have thrombosis
Other factor deficiencies	Bleeding deficiencies → factor deficiencies of factors II, V, and X have also been reported. Diagnosis is made by observing prolongation of PT and/or APTT, and measurement using a specific factor assay. Factor XIII deficiency → Rare disorder associated with delayed wound healing as factor XIII's actions occur after fibrin formation. Non-bleeding deficiencies → factor deficiencies of factors XII, pre-kallikrein, and high molecular weight kininogen have been reported. Clinical bleeding is not observed, however the APTT is prolonged.	

aPPT, Activated partial thromboplastin time; *PT*, prothrombin time; *TT*, thrombin time.

Thrombotic Conditions

- Thrombotic conditions can occur when balance between procoagulation and anticoagulation is tilted toward procoagulation
  - Major causes
    - Factor V Leiden: Mutation in factor V causes inability to inactivate factor Va in the presence of APC
    - Deficiency of regulatory factors
      - Protein C
      - Protein S
      - Antithrombin
      - Heparin cofactor II
    - Prothrombin 20210 mutation
    - Decreased fibrinolytic activity
      - Plasminogen deficiency
      - Decreased α_2-antiplasmin
      - Increased PAI
    - Antiphospholipid antibodies
    - Hyperhomocysteinemia

Anticoagulant Therapy

Coumadin → oral anticoagulant

- Action: Vitamin K antagonist – interferes with vitamin K-dependent γ-carboxylation step regulating the production of non-functional factors (II, VII, IX, X, Protein C, Protein S); therapeutic levels reached ~4-5 days after initial dose
- Monitoring: PT in combination with INR
- Complications: bleeding

Heparin → intravenous or subcutaneous administration

- Major forms
  1. UFH – unfractionated heparin – heterogenous mixture of molecules of 5000-30,000 Daltons in size
  2. LMWH – low molecular weight heparin – more homogenous mixture of molecules of 4500-5000 Daltons in size
- Action: binds to antithrombin (AT) enhancing neutralization of serine proteases
  1. UFH – enhances activity against thrombin, FXa and FIXa
  2. LMWH – enhances activity against FXa
- Monitoring: monitoring needed as individuals respond differently
  1. FH: prolongation of APTT; therapeutic dosage 1.5-2.5 times patient's baseline APTT prior to treatment
  2. LMWH: anti-Xa assay (prolongation of APTT not predictable)

- Complications: excessive bleeding; heparin induced thrombocytopenia

Thrombolytic therapy → administered after thrombotic embolism

- Major forms – classified as plasminogen activators (PA)
  1. Streptokinase (SK)
  2. Urokinase (UK)
  3. Alteplase (tPA)
- Monitoring: thrombin time, fibrin(ogen) degradation productions, D-dimers

Antiplatelet therapy → goal to reduce or block platelet function or action

1. Aspirin: inhibits cyclooxygenase (COX-1) thereby blocking prostaglandin (TXA_2) synthesis; lasts lifespan of platelet
2. ADP receptor antagonists: block ADP receptor in platelets
3. Inhibitors to GPIIb/IIIa: affect interaction of fibrinogen and vWF

MAJOR HEMOSTASIS LABORATORY TESTS

See Table 4-9.

Major Tests to Assess Thrombosis

- Antithrombin: Previously called antithrombin III
  - Chromogenic assay: Functional activity assessed in two-part assay
    - Patient plasma mixed with excess of thrombin in the presence of heparin: Antithrombin in patient will neutralize added thrombin
    - Residual thrombin is measured in assay assessing ability to convert fibrinogen to fibrin
    - Comparison to standard curve: Residual antithrombin (what was not neutralized by antithrombin) is inversely proportional to patient antithrombin level
    - Normal range: 80% to 120%
- Protein C: Functional and antigenic measurements
  - Functional: Patient plasma mixed with protein C–deficient plasma, aPTT reagent (with an activator) and calcium chloride are added, time to clot is measured
    - If functional, APC will inactivate factors Va and VIIIa causing prolongation of aPTT result; time compared to standard curve to determine percent function
    - Normal range: 60% to 150%
    - Chromogenic functional assay available
  - Antigenic measurements: Immunologic assays

TABLE 4-9 Major Hemostasis Laboratory Tests

Test	Principle	Interpretation	Additional Information
Assessment of Primary Hemostasis			
Bleeding time (BT)	A small incision is made in the arm, and the time needed for the platelets to stop bleeding is measured in minutes.	Normal range is 1-9 min. Abnormal bleeding is >9 min.	Test is rarely performed because it is affected by many factors—depth of incision, platelet count, pressure on arm.
Platelet function analyzer (PFA)	Platelet function is assessed in whole blood by passing blood through cartridge containing agonists (collagen/epinephrine and collagen/ADP). The time needed for the platelets to occlude the aperture is measured.	A longer closure time in the presence of specific agonists may indicate a platelet disorder.	Test requires special instrument.
Platelet aggregation	The ability of platelets to aggregate in the presence of specific agonists (ADP, arachidonic acid, collagen, epinephrine, ristocetin) is measured using a photooptical instrument.	Aggregation is measured by a decrease in optical density after addition of an agonist to platelet-rich plasma. Normal or abnormal aggregation in response to agonists is compared to expected results in platelet disorders.	Patients must refrain from aspirin-containing products for 7-10 days before testing. Specimen must be tested within 4 hr of collection.
Assessment of Secondary Hemostasis			
Prothrombin time (PT)	Clot formation in citrated plasma measured in seconds after addition of thromboplastin (tissue factor + calcium).	Reported with INR normalized ratio. INR = (patient PT/mean normal PT)^{ISI}. *ISI:* International sensitivity index—correction factor from WHO for each lot of reagent. Prolonged clotting time may be associated with factor deficiency, extrinsic (VII) or common (X, V, II, I) pathway, presence of inhibitor, or circulating anticoagulant.	PT is also prolonged in the presence of deficiency of vitamin K–dependent factors. Test is used to monitor oral anticoagulant therapy.
Activated partial thromboplastin time (aPTT)	Clot formation in citrated plasma measured in seconds after addition of partial thromboplastin reagent and calcium.	Prolonged clotting time may be associated with factor deficiency, intrinsic (XII, XI, IX, VIII) or common (X, V, II, I) pathway, presence of inhibitor, or circulating anticoagulant.	Test is used to monitor heparin therapy.
Fibrinogen (FGN)	*Clauss-based method:* Measurement of time to clot after addition of thrombin (bypasses rest of cascade). Patient 1:10 plasma dilution measured against standard curve.	Inverse relationship. Longer clotting time = lower fibrinogen level.	*Decreased FGN:* DIC, primary and secondary fibrinolysis, dysfibrinogenemia, afibrinogenemia, liver disease *Increased FGN:* Acute phase reactions, pregnancy, hormone therapy Measurement is affected in low FGN levels, dysfibrinogenemia, FDPs presence, heparin therapy.
Thrombin time (TT)	Excess of thrombin is added and fibrinogen to fibrin conversion is measured.	Evaluates formation of fibrin.	
Mixing studies	Equal parts patient plasma and normal pooled plasma are mixed and measured using PT or aPTT.	Correction of clotting time = suspected factor deficiency (~50% of a factor is needed for normal PT or APTT result).	Studies are useful to differentiate between factor deficiency and circulating inhibitor.

Continued

TABLE 4-9 Major Hemostasis Laboratory Tests—cont'd

Test	Principle	Interpretation	Additional Information
Specific factor assays	Patient plasma and factor-deficient plasma are mixed and measured using PT or PTT (depending on factor suspected). Results measured against factor-specific standard curve to determine percentage of factor present.	*Normal range:* 5%-150%	Tests are functional-based assays.
Factor XIII assay – Urea Solubility Test	Clot solubility is measured in the presence of urea or monochloroacetic acid in 24 hr.	Clot dissolution corresponds to factor XIII level of 1%-2%.	Symptoms of deficiency are delayed bleeding or increased bruising.
Von Willebrand factor (vWF)	*Functional test:* Platelet aggregation test assessing ability of patient's platelets to aggregate in the presence of ristocetin; slope of aggregation compared to slopes of standard curve dilutions; also called ristocetin cofactor assay (RCoF). *Antigen test:* Levels measured using antibody against vWF; methodologies include ELISA, EIA, immunoturbidimetric.	Fluctuations over time are possible, so testing is often repeated. Results assessed in conjunction with other measurements: aPTT, vWF multimers, ADAMS-13.	Important to assess functional and antigenic levels to accurately diagnose and treat.
Assessment of Fibrinolysis			
Fibrin(ogen) degradation products (FDPs)	Patient specimen is collected into special tube containing thrombin and a fibrinolytic inhibitor (prevents in vitro fibrinolysis). Patient specimen is mixed with latex beads coated with antibodies for FDPs.	*Agglutination:* Positive response Nonspecific for fibrinogen or FDPs. Confirmatory testing needed to identify FDPs.	Other conditions with positive result are liver disease, DVT, DIC, kidney disease, carcinoma.
D-Dimers	Patient plasma is mixed with latex beads coated with a monoclonal antibody for D-dimers.	Agglutination: Positive response Positive result indicates that clotting is occurring.	Elevated in DIC, emboli, thrombi.
Assessment of Inhibitors			
Bethesda titer (factor inhibitors)	Patient plasma and normal pooled plasma are mixed (several different dilutions) and incubated at 37° C for 2 hr, and factor level is measured.	Presence if inhibitor will inactivate patient factor, resulting in decreased activity.	Used to assess inhibitor levels for patients receiving factor concentrates; most often for patients with severe hemophilia (factors VIII or IX). Inhibitor suspected when patient fails to respond to treatment.
Lupus-like anticoagulants (LAs)	Diagnosis based on several tests because no single test is diagnostic: 1. aPTT 2. Mix with normal pooled plasma 3. *Dilute Russell viper venom test (DRVVT):* In the presence of lupus anticoagulant, the DRVVT result will be prolonged because of phospholipids in the reagent.	*Criteria for LAs:* 1. Prolongation of phospholipid-dependent coagulation reaction 2. Demonstration that it is an inhibitor and not a factor deficiency 3. Demonstration of inhibitor against phospholipid inhibitor (DRVVT)	Several other tests may be used to identify, but DRVVT is most common. LAs in children are often transient.

ADP, Adenosine diphosphate; *DIC,* disseminated intravascular coagulation; *DVT,* deep vein thrombosis; *EIA,* enzyme immunoassay; *ELISA,* enzyme-linked immunosorbent assay; *INR,* international normalized ratio; *WHO,* World Health Organization.

- Protein S: Functional and antigenic measurements
  - Protein S circulates in free and bound forms
  - Functional measurement: Free portion measured by functional assay—ability of protein S to serve as cofactor for protein S determined
    - Patient plasma is mixed with protein S–deficient plasma, APC, factor Va, and calcium chloride
    - Time for clot formation is compared to standard curve
  - Antigenic measurements: Immunologic assays
- Activated protein C resistance (APCR): Screening test for factor V Leiden mutation
  - Patient tested in the presence and absence of APC
    - Normal patients: Addition of APC will cleave and inactivate factors Va and VIIIa
    - Affected patients: Clotting time will be shortened because factor Va is not cleaved and will not be inactivated
    - Ratio: Partial thromboplastin time (PTT) (+APC)/PTT
      - Normal greater than 1.0
      - Less than 1.0 suggestive of factor V Leiden defect
        - Perform confirmatory testing: Molecular testing
- Prothrombin 20210 mutation: Molecular testing to identify presence of mutation

CERTIFICATION PREPARATION QUESTIONS

For answers and rationales, please see Appendix A.

1. Which of the following lists the steps of the hemostatic response in the correct order?
   a. Fibrinolysis → injury → secondary hemostasis → primary hemostasis
   b. Injury → primary hemostasis → secondary hemostasis → fibrinolysis
   c. Injury → secondary hemostasis → primary hemostasis → fibrinolysis
   d. Injury → fibrinolysis → primary hemostasis → secondary hemostasis

2. Which of the following properties renders the vessel wall prothrombotic?
   a. Negatively charged surface
   b. Production of prostacyclin and nitric oxide
   c. Release of tissue factor
   d. Inactivation of thrombin

3. Which of the following is not true regarding platelets?
   a. Platelets are not affected by aspirin
   b. Platelets have a life span of 7 to 10 days
   c. Platelets undergo shape change and develop pseudopods when activated
   d. Von Willebrand factor serves as a bridge between platelets and collagen

4. Which of the following factors binds to platelets via the glycoprotein IIb/IIIa receptor?
   a. Von Willebrand factor
   b. Factor II
   c. Fibrinogen
   d. Thrombin

5. Which of the following is not an agonist of platelet aggregation?
   a. Saline
   b. ADP
   c. Collagen
   d. Epinephrine

6. Which enzyme is blocked by the presence of aspirin?
   a. Phospholipase A_2
   b. Cyclooxygenase
   c. Protein kinase
   d. ATPase

7. Secondary hemostasis occurs when a sufficient stimulus is present to cause the release of internal ADP, synthesis and release of thromboxane A_2, and increased calcium release.
   a. True
   b. False

8. Which of the following factors is called prothrombin?
   a. Fibrinogen
   b. Factor II
   c. Factor X
   d. Factor XIII

9. Which of the following factors usually results in no clinical bleeding when deficient?
   a. Factor XII
   b. Factor IX
   c. Factor VIII
   d. Factor VII

10. The step necessary for the functionary factors II, VII, IX, and X is called the _____ step.
    a. Oxidation
    b. Hydrolysis
    c. Cleavage
    d. γ-Carboxylation

11. Monitoring of the intrinsic pathway is accomplished by performing which of the following analytical tests?
    a. PT
    b. PTT
    c. Thrombin time
    d. Fibrinogen assay

12. Monitoring of the extrinsic pathway is accomplished by performing which of the following analytical tests?
    a. PT
    b. PTT
    c. Thrombin time
    d. Fibrinogen assay

13. Which of the following cleaves the fibrinopeptides from fibrinogen?

a. Factor VIII
b. Thrombin
c. Tissue factor
d. Factor XIII

14. Activation of factor VII after the release of tissue factor initiates which of the following pathways?
    a. Intrinsic pathway
    b. Extrinsic pathway
    c. Common pathway
    d. Fibrinolytic pathway

15. Which of the following is not true?
    a. Factor VIII is a cofactor for factor IXa
    b. Factor V is a cofactor for factor Xa
    c. Protein K is a cofactor for protein C
    d. High-molecular-weight kininogen is a cofactor for factor XIIa

16. If a deficiency of this factor is present, the cross-linking of fibrin will not occur.
    a. Factor II
    b. Factor V
    c. Factor XI
    d. Factor XIII

17. Factor VIII is protected from degradation when circulating in the plasma by its carrier protein _____.
    a. Factor IX
    b. Thrombin
    c. Von Willebrand factor
    d. Glycoprotein IIb/IIIa

18. Which of the following factors is associated with hemophilia B?
    a. Factor VIII
    b. Factor IX
    c. Factor XI
    d. Fibrinogen

19. The activation of plasmin results in which of the following?
    a. The formation of a fibrin clot
    b. The formation of the bridge between platelets and the vessel wall
    c. The start of the process to break down a fibrin clot
    d. The point at which the intrinsic and extrinsic pathways feed into the common pathway

20. Which of the following proteins is degraded by plasmin?
    a. Fibrin
    b. Fibrinogen
    c. A and B
    d. None of the above

21. Streptokinase differs from urokinase plasminogen activator (uPA) in that:
    a. Streptokinase activates plasminogen to plasmin conversion, whereas uPA inhibits the conversion
    b. uPA is effective only when given as a medication
    c. Streptokinase is an exogenous activator, whereas uPA is a physiologic activator
    d. No difference exists between streptokinase and uPA

22. Which of the following are fibrin degradation products?
    a. Fragment X
    b. Fragment Y
    c. Fragment D
    d. All of the above

23. Which of the following describes the role of PAI-1 in hemostasis?
    a. Plasminogen activator inhibitor–1 limits the activation of plasminogen
    b. Plasminogen activator inhibitor–1 stimulates the activation of plasminogen
    c. Plasminogen activator inhibitor–1 is involved in limiting clot formation in vessels
    d. Plasminogen activator inhibitor–1 blocks platelet binding to the fibrin clot

24. Which of the following fibrinolytic inhibitors is useful when α_2-antiplasmin activity has been exhausted?
    a. PAI-1
    b. Thrombin-activatable fibrinolysis inhibitor
    c. α_2-Macroglobulin
    d. Plasminogen

25. Positive feedback control of the hemostatic response is accomplished by:
    a. Fibrin binding to thrombin to limit further activation
    b. Fibrin degradation products interfere with fibrin formation and polymerization
    c. Thrombin activates platelets and promotes the release of platelet factor V
    d. Thrombin initiates activation of the protein C pathway

26. Which of the following descriptions best describes the actions of protein S?
    a. Protein S inactivates factors Va and VIIIa
    b. Protein S is involved in the activation of thrombin
    c. Protein S serves as a cofactor for protein C
    d. None of above are functions of protein S

27. A child presents to the pediatrician after having recovered from a viral infection, because the child now has petechiae. The pediatrician orders laboratory testing, and the results reveal that the platelets are decreased. An increase in lymphocytes and eosinophils is also found. What is the probable diagnosis?
    a. Acute ITP
    b. Chronic ITP
    c. NAIT
    d. Medication reaction

28. Which of the following tests would help to differentiate between Bernard-Soulier syndrome and Glanzmann's thrombasthenia?
    a. Bleeding time
    b. Platelet count
    c. PT
    d. Response to ADP, collagen, and epinephrine in an aggregation assay

29. Glanzmann's thrombasthenia is best described as a:
    a. Platelet deficiency
    b. Deficiency of glycoprotein Ib/IX
    c. Deficiency of glycoprotein IIb/IIIa
    d. Deficiency of dense granules

30. The lack of a secondary wave of platelet aggregation in response to ADP is associated with which of the following disorders?
    a. Bernard-Soulier syndrome
    b. Gray platelet syndrome
    c. Glanzmann's thrombasthenia
    d. Δ-Storage pool disease

31. A young boy is taken to his pediatrician because his parents noticed that he seems to bleed easily and has swollen knees. The following test results were obtained:

    PT = Normal   aPTT = Prolonged
    Fibrinogen = Normal   aPTT with normal pooled
    Platelet count = Normal   plasma = Corrected the aPTT

    Which of the following statements best describes the next steps?
    a. The pediatrician should order factor assays for factors VIII and IX
    b. The pediatrician should order factor assays for factors X and V
    c. The pediatrician should order platelet aggregation testing
    d. The pediatrician should request a molecular test for the factor V Leiden defect

32. Which of the following results would be expected in a patient with dysfibrinogenemia?
    a. Normal PT, normal aPTT, prolonged thrombin time
    b. Abnormal PT, normal aPTT, prolonged thrombin time
    c. Abnormal PT, abnormal aPTT, normal thrombin time
    d. Normal PT, normal aPTT, normal thrombin time

33. In factor deficiencies, normal PT and aPTT results may be recorded until a factor level is _____.
    a. Less than 30%
    b. Less than 50%
    c. Less than 75%
    d. Less than 100%

34. The following results were obtained from a patient who recently underwent major surgery.

    PT = Prolonged   APTT = Prolonged
    Fibrinogen = Decreased   Platelet count = Decreased
    D-Dimer = Positive

    Which of the following conditions is likely?
    a. Fibrinogenolysis
    b. Fibrinogen deficiency
    c. Disseminated intravascular coagulation
    d. Vitamin K deficiency

35. Which of the following conditions is not usually associated with thrombosis?
    a. Protein C deficiency
    b. Antithrombin deficiency
    c. Factor V Leiden mutation
    d. Factor V deficiency

36. Which of the following accelerates the activity of antithrombin?
    a. Coumadin
    b. Aspirin
    c. Heparin
    d. tPA

37. Which of the following tests is helpful in differentiating fibrinogenolysis from DIC?
    a. PT
    b. aPTT
    c. Fibrinogen
    d. D-Dimer

38. A patient who has been receiving a broad-spectrum antibiotic is found to have a prolonged PT. After running a couple of factor assays, you conclude that both the factor X and factor VII levels are decreased. The PT corrected when mixed with normal pooled plasma. What is a possible cause?
    a. Inherited factor deficiency
    b. Circulating anticoagulant
    c. Vitamin K deficiency
    d. Effect resulting from antibiotic presence in plasma

39. Which of the following descriptions best describes the principle of platelet aggregation?
    a. The decrease in optical density is observed after the addition of an agonist in platelet-poor plasma
    b. The increase in optical density is observed after the addition of an agonist in platelet-rich plasma
    c. The decrease in optical density is observed after the addition of an agonist in platelet-rich plasma
    d. The increase in optical density is observed after the addition of an agonist in platelet-poor plasma

40. When performing platelet aggregation assays, which of the following is an important preanalytical factor?
    a. The patient should have fasted overnight
    b. The patient must refrain from aspirin-containing products for 7 days before testing
    c. After collection, the specimen can be frozen before transport to the laboratory
    d. All of the above are important

41. Which of the following conditions will cause an increase in fibrinogen levels?
    a. DIC
    b. Afibrinogenemia
    c. Acute phase reactions
    d. Liver disease

42. Which of the following describes the principle of the thrombin time test?
    a. After the addition of thromboplastin, the time needed for plasma to form a clot is measured

b. Patient plasma is mixed with thrombin-deficient plasma, and the time to clot is measured

c. An excess of thrombin is added to patient plasma, and the time to clot is measured

d. Clot solubility is assessed using 5 M urea

43. When performing a factor assay for factor VIII, the MLS accidentally added factor IX–deficient plasma to the patient specimens. Which of the following best describes the expected results?

a. The test will not be affected because the correct factor-deficient plasma was added

b. The test will not be affected because factor-deficient plasma is not needed in a factor assay

c. The test results will not be an assessment of factor VIII levels because factor VIII is present in the factor IX–deficient plasma

d. The test results will be an assessment of factor IX levels and can be calculated using the factor VIII standard curve

44. What are the reagents needed to perform the aPTT test?

a. Calcium chloride

b. Partial thromboplastin

c. A and B

d. None of the above

45. Which of the following tests is reported in conjunction with the INR?

a. PT

b. APTT

c. Thrombin time

d. Fibrinogen assay

46. The following test results were obtained on a patient who is being seen for easy bruising.

Bleeding time = Increased	PT = Normal
aPTT = Prolonged (mix with normal pooled plasma corrected aPTT)	Platelet count = Normal
ADP, collagen, epinephrine platelet aggregation = Normal	Ristocetin platelet aggregation = Absent

Which of the following conditions is expected?

a. Hemophilia A

b. Hemophilia B

c. Von Willebrand's disease

d. Factor XII deficiency

47. During a lengthy overseas trip, a 60-year-old man went to a laboratory in Italy to have PT measured to assess his dosage of Coumadin. Typically, in the United States, his results are in the range of 17 to 18 seconds, with an average INR of 1.75. In the laboratory in Italy, his PT was 20.2 seconds and his INR was 1.74. Which of the following descriptions best describes the situation?

a. The patient is taking excessive anticoagulation medication, causing his PT to be prolonged

b. An error is expected in the results from the laboratory in Italy

c. The result is not concerning because the INR results are essentially the same

d. He should immediately return to the United States for further assessment

48. During presurgical testing, the aPTT for a patient was longer than 120 seconds. The patient's history for bleeding is negative. The result was corrected after mixing with normal pooled plasma. The surgery is delayed because the surgeon is concerned about bleeding. Which of the following descriptions best describes this situation?

a. The patient is at risk for a bleeding incident if the surgery proceeds

b. The patient likely has a circulating inhibitor

c. The patient likely has a deficiency of a contact factor that is not associated with bleeding

d. The sample was likely contaminated with heparin

49. A 30-year-old woman with a history of miscarriages is being seen by an obstetrician/gynecologist. Which of the following tests would be included in a panel to assess her condition?

a. DRVVT

b. PT and PTT

c. PT and PTT using normal pooled plasma mix

d. All of the above

50. A patient presents to the emergency department with symptoms consistent with a DVT. Which of the following tests is helpful as a screening test for the factor V Leiden mutation?

a. Protein S assay

b. Antithrombin assay

c. Prothrombin 20210 molecular test

d. APCR test

BIBLIOGRAPHY

Marder VJ, Aird WC, Bennett JS, Schulman S, White GC: Hemostasis and thrombosis: basic principles and clinical practice, ed 6, Philadelphia, 2012, Lippincott Williams & Wilkins.

McKenzie SB, Williams JL: Clinical laboratory hematology, ed 2, Upper Saddle River, NJ, 2010, Pearson Education.

Rodak BF, Fritsma GA, Keohane EM: Hematology: clinical principles and applications, ed 4, St. Louis, 2012, Saunders.

SELF-ASSESSMENT

Content Area: _____

Score on Practice Questions: _____

List the specific topics covered in the missed questions:

List the specific topics covered in the correct questions:

NOTES

Clinical Fluid Analysis

Sue King Strasinger

URINALYSIS

Types of Common Urine Specimens

- Random
  - Routine screening
  - May require confirmatory testing based on diet and exercise
- First morning
  - Collected immediately on arising
  - Routine screening/confirmatory testing
  - Orthostatic proteinuria
  - Pregnancy tests
- Midstream clean catch
  - Requires patient to cleanse the genital area
  - Void first into the toilet, then collect specimen and finish voiding into the toilet
  - Bacterial cultures
- Catheterized
  - Collected from a catheter passed into the bladder
  - Bacterial cultures
  - NOTE: When a routine urinalysis and a culture are both ordered, perform the culture first
- 24-Hour (timed)
  - Patient voids into the toilet and then begins timing
  - Collects all urine during the designated period
  - Voids and collects urine at the end of the period
  - Specimens can provide quantitative results
- Drug screening
  - Strictly follow chain-of-custody form requirements
- Preservation of urine specimens
  - Test specimens within 2 hours of collection
  - Refrigerate specimens that cannot be tested within 2 hours

Changes in Unpreserved Urine

- Increased results
  - pH
  - Nitrite
  - Bacteria
- Decreased results
  - Glucose: Glycolysis
  - Ketones: Oxidation

- Bilirubin: Oxidation to biliverdin
- Urobilinogen: Oxidation to urobilin

Urine Volume

- Normal: 600 to 2000 mL/day
- Oliguria: Decreased output, less than 400 mL/day
- Anuria: No urine output
- Nocturia: Increased urine output at night
- Polyuria: Increased urine output greater than 2.5 L/day
  - Diabetes mellitus: Increased urine output to excrete excess urine glucose
  - Diabetes insipidus: Increased urine output caused by lack of dysfunction of antidiuretic hormone (ADH)
  - Results in polydipsia

PHYSICAL EXAMINATION OF URINE

Urine Color

- Normal urine is yellow. Shades of yellow are based on fluid consumption and vary from pale yellow (dilute) to dark yellow (concentrated) (Table 5-1)

Urine Clarity

- Terminology: Clear, hazy, cloudy, turbid, milky
- Freshly voided normal urine is clear
- Refrigerated normal urine
  - White turbidity in urine with an alkaline pH from amorphous phosphates and carbonates
  - Pink turbidity in urine with an acid pH from amorphous urates
- Nonpathologic turbidity
  - Squamous epithelial cells
  - Mucus
  - Amorphous phosphates, carbonates, and urates
  - Semen
  - Feces
  - Radiographic contrast media
  - Powder and creams

TABLE 5-1	**Clinical Correlation of Urine Color**	
Color	**Cause**	**Correlation**
Orange	Bilirubin	Produces yellow foam when shaken, abnormal liver function
	Pyridium	Produces thick orange pigment that can interfere with reagent strip tests
Red	RBCs	Cloudy urine, positive test for blood, microscopic RBCs
	Hemoglobin	Clear urine, positive test for blood
	Myoglobin	Clear urine, positive test for blood, needs further testing
	Porphyrins	Negative test for blood, needs further testing
Black	Oxidized RBCs, denatured hemoglobin	Clear urine, positive test for blood
	Melanin	Clear urine, darkens on standing

RBCs, Red blood cells.

- Pathologic turbidity
  - Red blood cells (RBCs)
  - White blood cells (WBCs)
  - Yeast
  - Urothelial and renal tubular epithelial cells
  - Abnormal crystals
  - Lipids (milky)

Specific Gravity

- Screening test for renal tubular reabsorption of essential elements filtered by the glomerulus
- Based on the fact that the glomerular filtrate has a specific gravity of 1.010
- Comparison of the density of urine to the density of distilled water (1.000)
- Urine contains dissolved substances that produce density by their size and number

Tests

Reagent strip

- Primary test for routine urinalysis is the reagent strip test
- Principle is based on the number of hydrogen ions (H^+) released from a polyelectrolyte (pK_a) is proportional to the number of ions in the urine
- Increased urine concentration = increased H^+ released = low pH
- The indicator on the strip is bromothymol blue
- Reaction = yellow-green (acid) → green-blue (alkaline) (Figure 5-1)

Refractometer

- Principle: The concentration of dissolved particles in a solution determines the velocity and angle of light passing through a solution

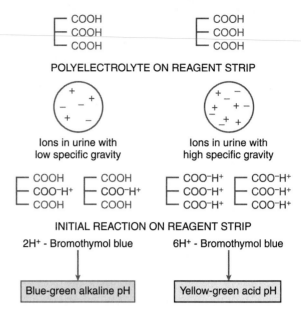

FIGURE 5-1 Reagent strip specific gravity reaction. *(From Strasinger SK, Di Lorenzo MS: Urinalysis and body fluids, ed 5, Philadelphia, 2008, FA Davis).*

- The refractometer uses a prism to direct a wave length of light through the urine; the angle of the light can be read on a scale calibrated with distilled water (1.000)

Osmolarity

- Considered more representative of renal concentrating ability than specific gravity because it measures only the number of particles and their size is not relevant
- Measurement is the number of particles into which 1 g molecular weight of a substance dissociates. Example: Nonionizing urea (molecular weight [MW] 60) = 1 particle, ionizing NaCl (MW 58.5) = 2 particles
- Reported in milliosmoles (mOsm)
- Colligative properties measured in the clinical laboratory
  - Freezing point depression
    - One mole of a nonionizing substance will lower the freezing point 1.86° C
    - Volatile substances such as alcohol can interfere
  - Vapor pressure depression
    - Actual measurement is the dew point (temperature at which vapor condenses to a liquid) of the urine sample
    - Uses microsamples on filter paper discs. Care must be taken to avoid evaporation
    - No interference from volatile substances

Clinical Significance

- Normal serum osmolarity: 275 to 300 mOsm
- Fluid intake influences urine osmolarity
- Random serum-to-urine ratio is 1:1
- Controlled fluid intake should reach 3:1
- Used to determine ADH production or tubular response to ADH for diabetes insipidus
- Harmonic oscillation density

- Automated instrumentation passes a sound wave through the urine and records the change in frequency of the sound wave, which is proportional to the urine density

CHEMICAL EXAMINATION OF URINE

Reagent Strips

Care and Quality Control
- Store in tightly closed opaque bottles
- Remove immediately before use
- Do not refrigerate (room temperature below 30° C)
- Run positive and negative controls every 24 hours
- Run controls when a new bottle is opened
- Observe expiration dates
- Observe discolored reagent pads

Technique
- Thoroughly mix specimens (detection of RBCs and WBCs)
- Warm refrigerated specimens (enzyme reactions)
- Briefly dip reagent strips (prevent leaching of reagents from strip)
- Blot strip while removing from urine (prevent runover)
- Observe manufacturer timing instructions (reaction color changes)
- Relate chemical with physical and microscopic results (Table 5-2)

KEY POINTS

pH
- The pH of fresh urine does not reach 9.0
- A reading of 9.0 indicates an old specimen that should be recollected; the normal value is 4.5 to 8.0
- Reagent strip principle: Double indicator (methyl red and bromothymol blue)

TABLE 5-2	Reagent Strip Sources of Error and Correlations	
Test	**Sources of Error**	**Test Correlations**
pH	Runover from adjacent strips Old specimens +	Nitrites Leukocyte esterase Microscopic
Protein	Highly buffered alkaline urine + Detergents + Pyridium + Chlorhexidine + High specific gravity + Microalbuminuria −	Blood Nitrites Leukocyte esterase Microscopic

Continued

TABLE 5-2	Reagent Strip Sources of Error and Correlations—cont'd	
Test	**Sources of Error**	**Test Correlations**
Glucose	Oxidizing agents + Detergents + Increased ascorbic acid − Low temperature − Old specimens −	Ketones Protein
Ketones	Red urine + Sulfhydryl medications + Levodopa + Old specimens −	Glucose
Blood	Oxidizing agents + Bacterial peroxidases + Menstrual contamination + Crenated red blood cells − Increased ascorbic acid − Increased nitrite − Unmixed specimens −	Color Microscopic
Bilirubin	Pyridium + Indican + Lodine + Specimen exposed to light − Increased ascorbic acid − Increased nitrite −	Urobilinogen Color
Urobilinogen	Multistix Porphobilinogen + Ehrlich's reactive compounds + Highly pigmented urine + Old specimens − Preservation in formalin − Chemstrip Highly pigmented urine + Preservation in formalin − Increased nitrates −	Bilirubin
Nitrite	Old specimens + Highly pigmented urine + Non–reductase-containing bacteria − Early infection − No urinary nitrate − Increased bacteria converting nitrite to nitrogen − Antibiotics − Increased ascorbic acid − High specific gravity	Protein Leukocytes Microscopic
Leukocyte esterase	Oxidizing agents + Formalin + Highly pigmented urine + Nitrofuration + Increased ascorbic acid − High protein and glucose − Antibiotics − Inaccurate timing −	Protein Nitrite Microscopic
Specific gravity	Increased protein + Highly alkaline urine − Add 0.005 to any urine with a pH of 6.5 or higher	

- Clinical significance
  - Detection of systemic acid-base disorders
- Identification of urinary crystals

Protein

- Reagent strips measure primarily albumin
- The normal value is less than 10 mg/dL
- A result of 30 mg/dL or greater is considered clinical proteinuria
- Reagent strip principle: The protein error of indicators
- Clinical significance
  - Clinically significant proteinuria is primarily caused by glomerular or tubular disorders
  - Benign orthostatic proteinuria testing requires a first morning specimen and a specimen after the patient has been active for 2 hours. The first specimen should be negative and the second specimen positive

Microalbuminuria

- Requires a different reagent strip capable of testing for only albumin at levels below 10 mg/dL
- Provides early detection of renal disease, particularly in patients with diabetes
- The Mulitsix PRO 11 reagent strip tests for microalbumin and creatinine, along with all other routine strip tests, except urobilinogen
- Albumin-to-creatinine ratio corrects for hydration in a random sample to provide an estimate of the 24-hour microalbumin level

Glucose

- Principle: Glucose oxidase test (specific for glucose)
- The renal threshold for glucose is 160 to 180 mg/dL
- Clinical significance
  - Diabetes mellitus, gestational diabetes (placental hormones blocking insulin)
  - Hormonal disorders and stress block insulin production and actions
  - Renal tubular disorders prevent tubular reabsorption of glucose
- Clinitest
  - Principle: Reducing substances including glucose and other sugars can reduce copper sulfate (blue-green) to cuprous oxide (orange-red)
  - May be used to test newborn urine for galactose
  - High levels will pass through the reaction and go from blue-green to orange-red to blue-green
  - Carefully observe the reaction

Ketones

- Intermediate metabolites of fat, acetoacetic acid, acetone, and β-hydroxybutyric acid
- Principle: Reaction of acetoacetic acid or acetone (with glycine) with sodium nitroprusside/ferricyanide

- Clinical significance: Diabetes mellitus, monitoring of insulin therapy, starvation, malabsorption, and loss of carbohydrates (vomiting)

Blood

- Positive reactions are seen with hematuria, hemoglobinuria, and myoglobinuria
- Principle: Pseudoperoxidase activity of hemoglobin
- Clinical significance: Both hemoglobinuria and myoglobinuria can cause acute renal failure
- Hematuria: Bleeding within the genitourinary system, including renal calculi, trauma, anticoagulants, glomerulonephritis, and pyelonephritis
- Hemoglobinuria: Intravascular hemolysis/transfusion reactions, lysis of old RBCs by dilute alkaline urine
- Myoglobinuria: Rhabdomyolysis caused by muscle-wasting disorders, crush injuries, prolonged coma, and cholesterol statin drugs

Bilirubin

- Both bilirubin and urobilinogen are products of hemoglobin degradation (Figure 5-2)
- Principle: Diazo reaction
- Clinical significance: Conjugated bilirubin enters the urine as a result of leakage from a damaged liver or blocked bile duct
  - The kidneys cannot filter unconjugated bilirubin
  - Patients will appear jaundiced

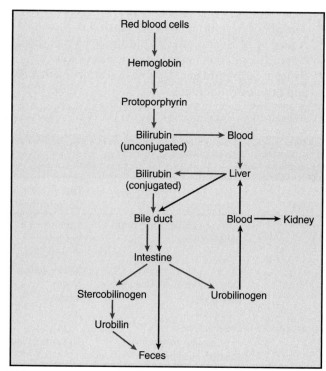

FIGURE 5-2 Processing of bilirubin and urobilinogen in hemoglobin degradation. *(From Strasinger SK, Di Lorenzo MS: Urinalysis and body fluids, ed 5, Philadelphia, 2008, FA Davis).*

Urobilinogen

- Some of the conjugated bilirubin is converted to urobilinogen in the intestine
- Then it circulates in the blood to the liver and passes through the kidneys
- A small amount of urobilinogen (1 mg/dL) is found in normal urine
- Principle: Multistix = Ehrlich's reaction, Chemstrip = diazo reaction
- Clinical significance: Early detection of liver disease and hemolytic disorders, constipation

Nitrite

- Detects the presence of reductase-producing bacteria that can convert urinary nitrate to nitrite
- Principle: Diazo reaction
- Clinical significance: Early detection of urinary tract infection
  - A positive nitrite test should be accompanied by a positive leukocyte esterase test
  - May be used to screen specimens for microbiology testing

Leukocyte Esterase

- Detects the presence of granulocytic WBCs, including lysed WBCs
- Principle: Diazo reaction; the leukocyte esterase reagent strip reaction should be read 2 minutes after urine exposure
- Clinical significance: Urinary tract infections, including with non–reductase-containing bacteria and parasitic and fungal organisms that would have a negative nitrite test
- NOTE: Specific gravity is covered in the discussion of physical examination of urine

MICROSCOPIC EXAMINATION OF URINE

Casts

See (Table 5-3).

- Composed of Tamm-Horsfall (uromodulin) protein excreted by renal tubular epithelial cells
- When other urinary constituents are present they become enmeshed in the cast matrix or attached to the matrix
- Formed in the distal convoluted tubule and collecting ducts (wider casts)
- Reported as the number per low-power field

Cells

Red Blood Cells

- Appearance
  - Small, nonnucleated discs
  - Appear crenated in concentrated urine
  - Appear as larger empty cells in dilute urine (ghost cells)
  - Regular (dysmorphic) shapes indicate glomerular bleeding
- Sources of error
  - Oil droplets
  - Air bubbles
  - Yeast cells (look for budding)
- Clinical significance
  - Glomerular membrane damage
  - Bleeding in the urinary tract
  - Renal calculi
  - Malignancy
- Urinalysis correlations
  - A clear red urine with a positive reagent strip RBC and no RBCs in the microscopic analysis indicates hemoglobinuria or myoglobinuria

TABLE 5-3	Summary of Urinary Casts		
Type	**Appearance**	**Sources of Error**	**Clinical Significance**
Hyaline	Colorless	Mucus, fibers, increased light	Glomerulonephritis, pyelonephritis, congestive heart failure, stress, exercise
RBC	Orange/red–containing RBCs	RBC clumps (look for cast matrix)	Glomerulonephritis, strenuous exercise
WBC	WBCs in cast matrix	WBC clumps (look for cast matrix)	Pyelonephritis, acute interstitial nephritis
Epithelial cell	RTE cells attached to cast matrix	WBC casts	Renal tubular damage
Bacterial	Bacteria attached to cast matrix	Granular casts	Pyelonephritis
Granular	Coarse or fine granules in the matrix	Clumps of small crystals, columnar RTE cells	Glomerulonephritis, pyelonephritis, stress, exercise
Waxy	Highly refractile, jagged edges and notches	Fibers, fecal material	Stasis of urine flow, chronic renal failure
Fatty	Fat droplets and oval fat bodies attached to cast matrix	Fecal material	Nephrotic syndrome, diabetes mellitus, crush injuries
Broad	Wider than normal	Fecal material, fibers	Extreme urine stasis, renal failure

RBCs, Red blood cells; *RTE,* renal tubular endothelial (cells); *WBCs,* white blood cells.

White Blood Cells

- Appearance
  - Larger than RBCs and contain a nucleus
  - Neutrophils have multilobed nuclei and granules
  - Eosinophils have red granules when stained with Wright or Hansel stains
  - Glitter cells are neutrophils that have swollen in dilute urine, resulting in Brownian movement of the granules in the cytoplasm
- Sources of error
  - Renal tubular epithelial cells, mononuclear lymphocytes, and monocytes
- Urinalysis correlations
  - Leukocyte esterase, nitrite, pH, and specific gravity (glitter cells)
- Clinical significance
  - Urinary tract infection (neutrophils)
  - Drug-induced interstitial nephritis (eosinophils)
  - Malignancy (mononuclear cells)

Epithelial Cells

Squamous Cells

- Largest cells in the urine sediment
- Represent normal sloughing of old lower genitourinary tract cells
- Folded squamous cells may resemble urinary casts (look for a centrally located nucleus)
- Clue cells are squamous epithelial cells covered with *Gardnerella vaginalis* bacteria, indicating a vaginal infection

Transitional (Urothelial) Cells

- Found in the renal pelvis, ureters, bladder, and male urethra
- Normally seen after catheterization procedures (often seen in clumps)
- Three different forms: Spherical, caudate, and polyhedral
- Spherical cells resemble renal tubular cells, except they have a centrally located nucleus
- Increased transitional cells may indicate malignancy

Renal Tubular Epithelial Cells

- Found in the renal tubules and collecting duct
- Cell shape varies with location
- Convoluted tubule cells are rectangular with coarse granules and may resemble a cast (look for a nucleus)
- Distal convoluted tubule cells are small and round, may resemble spherical transitional cells but have an eccentric nucleus
- Cells from the collecting duct are cuboidal with at least one straight edge and are frequently seen in clumps
- More than two renal tubular epithelial cells per high-power field is significant
- Clinical significance
  - Tubular necrosis, often from poisoning or viral infections
- Renal tubular epithelial cells absorb filtrate and may be bilirubin stained (liver damage), contain hemosiderin granules (hemoglobin) or lipids

- Oval fat bodies
  - Renal tubular epithelial cells that have absorbed lipids
  - Highly refractile
  - Seen in conjunction with free-floating lipids
  - Confirm by staining with oil red O, Sudan III, or polarized microscopy
  - Clinical significance: Nephrotic syndrome, diabetes mellitus, and crush injuries

Bacteria

- Small spheres (cocci) and rod-shaped organisms
- Should be accompanied by WBCs
- Sources of error: Amorphous urates, phosphates, and old specimens with a high pH
- Clinical significance
  - Urinary tract infection

Yeast

- Oval structures with buds or mycelia
- Should be accompanied by WBCs
- Associated with acidic urine from patients with diabetes mellitus
- Sources of error
  - RBCs
- Clinical significance
  - Diabetes mellitus, immunocompromised patients, vaginal infections

Parasites

- Most common is *Trichomonas vaginalis,* which exhibits rapid flagellar movement in wet preparations
- Sources of error
  - WBCs and renal tubular epithelial cells
- Clinical significance
  - Sexually transmitted disease that is asymptomatic in males and causes a vaginal infection in females
- Other parasites
  - *Schistosoma haematobium* (urine parasite) and *Enterobius vermicularis* (fecal contamination)

Mucus

- Strands of protein secreted by glands and renal tubular epithelial cells
- Major protein is Tamm-Horsfall (uromodulin) protein
- Sources of error
  - Clumps may resemble hyaline casts (look for the consistent shape of a cast)
- Mucus is of no clinical significance

Crystals

- Precipitation of urine solutes affected by temperature, solute concentration, and pH

- Crystals are more abundant in refrigerated urine samples
- Polarized microscopy aids in their identification
- Abnormal crystals are found only in acidic or normal urine

Normal Crystals Seen in Acidic Urine

- Uric acid crystals
  - Appearance
    - Yellow-brown, flat-sided rhombic plates, wedges, and rosettes
  - Sources of error
    - Cystine crystals (uric acid crystals polarize and cystine crystals do not polarize)
  - Clinical significance
    - Patients receiving chemotherapy
    - Lesch-Nyhan disease
- Amorphous urates
  - Appearance
    - Small spheres producing brick-dust (uroerythrin) or yellow-brown sediment
- Calcium oxalate crystals
  - May also be seen in alkaline urine
  - The dihydrate form is envelope shaped; clumps in fresh urine may indicate renal calculi
  - The monohydrate form is oval or dumbbell shaped; presence of this form indicates ethylene glycol (antifreeze) ingestion

Normal Crystals Seen in Alkaline Urine

- Triple phosphate crystals
  - Coffin-lid shaped
  - Associated with a very high pH and bacteria found in old specimens
- Amorphous phosphate crystals
  - Produce a white precipitate after refrigeration
- Calcium carbonate crystals
  - Dumbbell and spherical shapes
  - Produce gas with acetic acid
- Ammonium biurate crystals
  - Yellow-brown thorny apple-shaped crystals
  - Associated with old specimens with bacteria

Abnormal Crystals

- Cystine crystals
  - Appearance
    - Hexagonal flat plates
  - Clinical significance

- An inherited disorder that inhibits the reabsorption of cystine by the renal tubules (cystinuria); renal calculi form at an early age
- Cholesterol crystals
  - Appearance
    - Rectangular plates with notched corners, highly birefringent under polarized light
  - Seen in refrigerated urine and accompanied by fatty casts and oval fat bodies
  - Clinical significance
    - Nephrotic syndrome
- Tyrosine crystals
  - Appearance
    - Yellow needle-shaped forms in clusters or rosettes
  - Clinical significance
    - Severe liver disease
- Leucine crystals
  - Appearance
    - Yellow-brown spheres with concentric circles
  - Seen in conjunction with tyrosine crystals
  - Clinical significance
    - Severe liver disease
- Bilirubin crystals
  - Appearance
    - Bright yellow clumped needles and granules
  - Clinical significance
    - Liver damage often from viral infections that damage the renal tubules, preventing reabsorption of bilirubin
- Sulfonamide crystals
  - Appearance
    - Needle, rosette, and rhombic shapes
  - Clinical significance
    - Inadequately hydrated patients taking sulfonamide medications
- Ampicillin crystals
  - Appearance
    - Colorless needles that form clumps after refrigeration
  - Clinical significance
    - Inadequately hydrated patients taking ampicillin

Artifacts

See (Table 5-4).

TABLE 5-4	Artifacts			
Artifact	**Appearance**	**Sources of Error**	**Comments**	
Starch granules	Refractile spheres with concentric circles	RBCs	Negative reagent strip for blood	
Oil droplets	Refractile spheres	RBCs	Negative reagent strip for blood	
Air bubbles	Refractile spheres	RBCs	Negative reagent strip for blood	
Pollen grains	Spheres with concentric circles	Red blood cells	Large size often makes them out of focus	
Fibers	Elongated strips	Casts	Check with polarized light, because only fatty casts polarize light	

RBCs, Red blood cells.

RENAL PHYSIOLOGY

Nephrons

- Controls the ability of the kidney to clear waste products and maintain the body's water and electrolyte balance
- Types of nephrons
  - Cortical nephrons are located in the cortex of the kidney and remove waste products and reabsorb nutrients
  - Juxtaglomerular nephrons extend into the medulla of the kidney and concentrate the urine

Nephron Functions in the Production of Urine

- Renal blood flow
  - Renal artery → afferent arteriole → efferent arteriole → proximal convoluted tubule capillaries → vasa recta/loop of Henle → distal convoluted tubule capillaries → renal vein
  - Normal renal blood flow is approximately 1200 mL/min
  - Normal plasma flow is approximately 600 to 700 mL/min
- Glomerular filtration
  - Nonselective filtration of plasma substances with MWs less than 70,000 (MW of albumin is 67.000)
  - Filtration pressure is controlled by the renin-angiotensin-aldosterone system (RAAS) (Figure 5-3)
- Renal tubular reabsorption
  - Passive transport reabsorbs water and urea
  - Active transport reabsorbs glucose, amino acids, chloride, and sodium

- Renal tubular concentration
  - Takes place in the ascending and descending loops of Henle (Figure 5-4)
- Renal tubular secretion
  - Removes nonfiltered waste products from the blood to the filtrate and maintains the acid-base balance in the body
  - Substances such as medications are bound to plasma carrier proteins and are too large to be filtered
  - In the tubules they disassociate from the carrier protein and are then secreted into the filtrate
  - Small hydrogen molecules (H⁺) are easily filtered and must be returned to the blood. In the filtrate they combine with phosphate ions or ammonia secreted by the renal tubular cells and are secreted back to the blood
  - Small bicarbonate ions (HCO_3^-) needed for the acid-base buffering system are also easily filtered. They combine with the hydrogen molecules, producing bicarbonate (H_2CO_3) that can be secreted back into the blood

Renal Function Tests

- Glomerular filtration rate (GFR)
  - Normal value is approximately 120 mL/min, with some variance for body size
  - Classic test is creatinine clearance, which requires a timed urine specimen (usually 24 hours)
  - Formula

$$C = \frac{U\,V}{P}$$

  - Calculated GFR estimates (eGFR) do not require a timed urine specimen

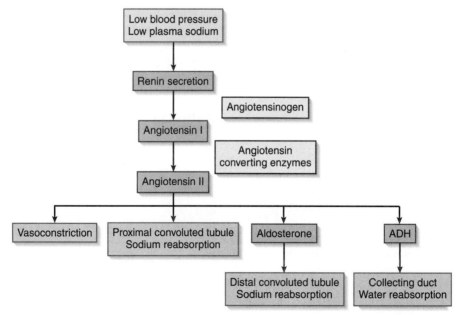

FIGURE 5-3 The renin-angiotensin-aldosterone system. *ADH*, Antidiuretic hormone. *(From Strasinger SK, Di Lorenzo MS: Urinalysis and body fluids, ed 5, Philadelphia, 2008, FA Davis).*

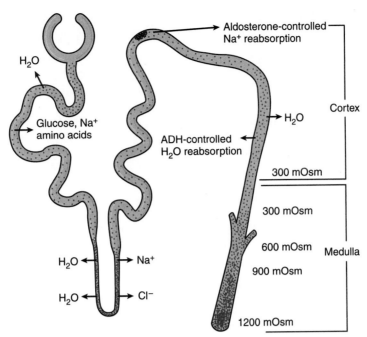

FIGURE 5-4 Renal concentration. *ADH, Antidiuretic hormone. (From Strasinger SK, Di Lorenzo MS: Urinalysis and body fluids, ed 5, Philadelphia, 2008, FA Davis).*

- Formulas may use serum creatinine and combinations of age, sex, ethnicity, blood urea nitrogen (BUN), and serum albumin
- Measurement of serum markers
  - Cystatin C is a small molecule produced at a constant rate by all nucleated cells
  - It is completely filtered, reabsorbed, and then broken down by the renal tubular cells. Serum level remains constant unless the GFR decreases causing the serum level to rise
- Renal tubular reabsorption
  - Primary tests are serum and urine osmolarity (see discussion of specific gravity)

- The free water clearance test measures the ability of the kidney to respond to body hydration
- Formula

$$C_{osm} = \frac{U_{osm} \times V}{P_{osm}}$$

- Tubular secretion tests
  - Titratable acidity detects the inability of the proximal convoluted tubule to secrete hydrogen molecules
  - Urinary ammonia detects the inability to produce ammonia in the proximal and distal convoluted tubules (Table 5-5)

TABLE 5-5	Renal Disease and Urinalysis Correlations	
Disorder	**Urinalysis Results**	**Comments**
Glomerular Disorders		
Acute glomerulonephritis	Macroscopic hematuria, proteinuria, RBC casts	Poststreptococcal infection
Goodpasture's syndrome	Macroscopic hematuria, proteinuria, RBC casts	Anti–glomerular basement membrane antibodies
Wegner's granulomatosis	Macroscopic hematuria, proteinuria, RBC casts	Antineutrophil cytoplasmic antibody
Henoch-Schönlein purpura	Macroscopic hematuria, proteinuria, RBC casts	Primarily seen in children after respiratory infections
Membranous glomerulonephritis	Microscopic hematuria, proteinuria	Autoimmune disorders
Chronic glomerulonephritis	Hematuria, proteinuria, glycosuria, cellular, waxy and broad casts	Progression of previous disorders
IgA nephropathy	Hematuria, proteinuria, glycosuria, cellular, waxy, broad casts	Immune IgA complexes deposited on the glomerular membrane
Nephrotic syndrome	Heavy proteinuria, hematuria, RTE cells, oval fat bodies, fatty and waxy casts	Circulatory disruption decreasing blood flow to the kidney, increased serum lipids
Minimal change disease	Heavy proteinuria, light hematuria fat droplets	Seen in children after allergic reactions, heavy edema, good prognosis

Continued

TABLE 5-5	Renal Disease and Urinalysis Correlations—cont'd	
Disorder	**Urinalysis Results**	**Comments**
Focal segmental glomerulosclerosis	Hematuria, proteinuria	Drugs of abuse and HIV
Tubular Disorders		
Acute tubular necrosis	RTE cells and casts, positive blood reagent strip	Hemoglobinuria, myoglobinuria, and antibiotics
Fanconi's syndrome	Glycosuria, proteinuria	General failure of tubular reabsorption
Renal glycosuria	Glucose	Failure of active transport of only glucose
Tubulointerstitial Disorders		
Cystitis	Positive LE, nitrite, elevated pH, WBCs, bacteria	Bladder infection
Acute pyelonephritis	Positive LE, nitrite, and WBC casts	Tubular infection indicated by WBC casts
Chronic pyelonephritis	Positive LE, nitrite, WBCs, granular, waxy and broad casts	Structural abnormalities that affect normal tubular emptying, often in children
Acute interstitial nephritis	Hematuria, proteinuria, and WBC casts	Urine eosinophils, no bacteria, reaction to toxic medications
Renal lithiasis (calculi)	Microscopic RBCs, high specific gravity	Patient with severe back pain; pH varies with type of calculi

HIV, Human immune deficiency virus; *IgA*, immunoglobulin A; *LE*, leukocyte esterase; *RBC*, red blood cell; *WBC*, white blood cell.

BODY FLUIDS

Cerebrospinal Fluid

Physiology

- Cerebrospinal fluid (CSF) is formed in the choroid plexuses
- Circulates through the arachnoid space of the meninges lining the brain and spinal cord and is reabsorbed in the arachnoid granules of the brain
- The tight-fitting endothelial cells in the choroid plexuses make the blood-brain barrier that protects the brain from toxic substances

Collection and Distribution of Cerebrospinal Fluid Specimens

- CSF is collected in three or four sterile tubes numbered in the order of collection
- Three tube distribution
  - Tube 1: Chemistry/immunology—least affected by blood or bacteria contamination from the spinal tap
  - Tube 2: Microbiology
  - Tube 3: Hematology—less contamination of cell count from the puncture
- Four tube distribution
  - Tube 1: Hematology—provides a comparison between the cells from the puncture with the cells in the fourth tube collected
  - Tube 2: Chemistry
  - Tube 3: Microbiology—less chance of outside contamination
  - Tube 4: Hematology—results compared with those of tube 1 for possible outside interference from the tap (Table 5-6)

TABLE 5-6	Cerebrospinal Fluid Appearance and Clinical Significance	
Appearance	**Cause**	**Clinical Significance**
Crystal clear		Normal
Hazy, cloudy	WBCs	Meningitis
	Microorganisms	Blood-brain barrier disorders
	Protein	IgG production in the CNS
Bloody	RBCs	Hemorrhage
		Traumatic tap
Xanthochromia	Hemoglobin	Old hemorrhage
	Bilirubin	Elevated serum bilirubin
	Protein	Blood-brain barrier disorders
	Carotene	Elevated serum levels
Pellicle	Clotting factors	Refrigerated tuberculosis meningitis specimens

CNS, Central nervous system; *IgG*, immunoglobulin G; *RBCs*, red blood cells; *WBCs*, white blood cells.

Hematology Tests

Cell Counts

- Perform counts immediately because RBCs and granulocytes lyse within 1 hour
- The adult normal CSF WBC count is 0 to 5/μL
- Newborns and children may have slightly higher counts and more monocytes
- Cell counts are performed using a Neubauer counting chamber
  - Formula

$$\frac{\text{Number of cells counted} \times \text{dilution}}{\text{Number of squares counted} \times \text{volume of 1 square}} = \text{cells}/\mu\text{L}$$

TABLE 5-7	Appearance and Significance of Cerebrospinal Fluid Cells	
Cell	**Clinical Significance**	**Appearance**
Lymphocytes	Normal, viral, tubercular, fungal meningitis, multiple sclerosis	All developmental stages
Neutrophils	Bacterial meningitis, early stages of other types of meningitis, cerebral hemorrhage	Granules may be less prominent
Monocytes	The same as lymphocytes	Seen mixed with lymphocytes
Macrophages	RBCs in the CSF	May contain phagocytized RBCs, hemosiderin granules, hematoidin crystals
Blast forms	Acute leukemias	Myeloblasts, lymphoblasts, monoblasts
Plasma cells	Multiple sclerosis	Traditional forms
Ependymal, choroidal, spindle-shaped cell	Diagnostic procedures	Seen in clusters with distinct nuclei and cell walls
Malignant cells	Metastatic cancers, primary CNS carcinomas	Seen in clusters with fusing nuclei and cell walls

CSF, Cerebrospinal fluid; *RBCs*, red blood cells.

- WBC counts require lysis of RBCs using percent glacial acetic acid
- Differential
  - Concentration by cytocentrifugation is recommended to ensure an adequate number of cells for evaluation (Table 5-7)

Chemistry Tests

- Normal values differ from plasma values because of the selective filtration by the blood-brain barrier

Cerebrospinal Fluid Protein

- Normal value: 15 to 45 mg/dL (plasma protein is measured in grams per deciliter)
- The τ transferrin protein is found only in CSF
- Clinical significance
  - Elevated results: Damage to the blood-brain barrier (meningitis, tumors, hemorrhage), multiple sclerosis (increased immunoglobulin G [IgG] produced in the central nervous system [CNS])
  - Decreased results: CSF leakage and trauma
  - CSF serum/albumin index
    - Detects damage to the blood-brain barrier
    - An index value less than 9 is normal
    - Formula

$$\text{CSF/serum albumin index} = \frac{\text{CSF albumin (mg/dL)}}{\text{Serum albumin (g/dL)}}$$

  - CSF IgG index
    - Detects production of IgG within the CNS
    - Normal values are approximately 0.70 or lower
    - Formula

$$\text{IgG index} = \frac{\text{CSF IgG (mg/dL)/serum IgG (g/dL)}}{\text{CSF albumin (mg/dL)/serum albumin (g/dL)}}$$

- CSF electrophoresis
  - Detects oligoclonal bands that represent inflammation in the CNS
  - Primary testing is for multiple sclerosis. Two or more bands are seen in the CSF and no bands in the serum; Other disorders have banding in the serum

- Detection of the τ transferrin protein identifies a fluid as CSF
- Myelin basic protein
  - The presence of myelin basic protein indicates destruction of the myelin sheath that protects the axons of the neurons
  - Monitors the course of multiple sclerosis
- CSF glucose
  - Normal values: 60% to 70% of the blood glucose
  - Compare with a blood glucose drawn approximately 2 hours before the spinal tap
  - Elevated CSF levels occur when the serum level is elevated
  - Clinical significance
    - Helpful in the differentiation of types of meningitis. Decreased levels indicate damage to transport of glucose across the blood-brain barrier and increased use of glucose by the brain cells
- CSF lactate
  - Increased by tissue destruction caused by lack of oxygen
  - Normal value: Less than 25 mg/dL
  - Clinical significance
    - Aids in the differentiation of meningitis organisms
- CSF glutamine
  - The normal CSF value is 8 to 18 mg/dL
  - Increased glutamine indicates increased ammonia in the CNS
  - Values greater than 35 mg/dL disrupt consciousness
  - Elevated values are seen in children with Reye's syndrome that affects the liver (Table 5-8)

Microbiology Tests

- Gram stains are routinely performed on concentrated specimens
- *Cryptococcus neoformans* produces a starburst Gram stain pattern. India ink preparations and latex agglutination tests may be performed
- Immunologic tests are available for bacterial antigens

TABLE 5-8	**Differential Diagnosis of Meningitis**		
Bacterial	**Viral**	**Tubercular**	**Fungal**
Elevated WBCs	Elevated WBCs	Elevated WBCs	Elevated WBCs
Neutrophils	Lymphocytes	Lymphocytes and monocytes	Lymphocytes and monocytes
Markedly decreased glucose	Normal glucose	Decreased glucose	Normal to decreased glucose
Marked protein elevation	Moderate protein elevation	Moderate-to-marked protein elevation	Moderate-to-marked protein elevation
Lactate >35 mg/dL	Lactate <25 mg/dL	Lactate >25 mg/dL	Lactate >25 mg/dL

WBCs, White blood cells.

SEMINAL FLUID

Physiology

- Semen consists of four components
  - Spermatozoa: Germ cells
  - Seminal fluid: Provides nutrients and fructose for sperm energy
  - Prostate fluid: Provides substances for coagulation and liquifaction
  - Bulbourethral gland fluid: Provides alkaline mucus to neutralize the acidity of prostate fluid and the vagina

Specimen Collection

- The majority of the sperm are in the first part of the ejaculate, so a complete collection is essential
- Collect after 2 to 3 days but not more than 5 days of abstinance
- Collect in warm glass or plastic containers (no routine condoms)
- Keep the specimen at room temperature and deliver to the laboratory within 1 hour
- Record the time of collecton and delivery at the laboratory

Semen Analysis

- Appearance
  - Normal: Gray-white, translucent
  - White turbidity: WBCs, infection
  - Red: RBCs
  - Yellow: Urine contamination (urine is toxic to sperm)
- Liquifaction
  - Fresh semen is clotted
  - Normal liquifacton takes place within 30 to 60 minutes
  - Abnormal liquifaction indictes a deficiency of prostate enzymes
- Volume
  - Normal: 2 to 5 mL
- Viscosity
  - Normal: Ability to form discrete droplets from a pipette
  - Increased viscosity and delayed liquifaction impede sperm motility

- pH
  - Normal: 7.2 to 8.0
  - Increased pH indicates infection
  - Decreased pH indicates increased prostatic fluid
- Sperm concentration and count
  - Sperm concentration
    - Normal: Greater than 20 million/mL
    - Test is performed in a counting chamber
    - Fluid must be diluted with specified diluting fluid to immobilize the sperm
    - Counts must be corrected from microliters to milliliters
    - Spermatids and WBCs are counted separately; more than 1 million spermatids indicates disrupted spermatogenesis, more than 1 million WBCs indicates infection
  - Sperm count
    - The number of sperm per milliliter times the specimen volume = the sperm count
  - Sperm motility
    - Evaluated by the speed and direction of the sperm movement
    - Criteria: Rapid, straight line; slower speed, some lateral movement; slow forward movement, noticeable lateral movement; no forward movement; no movement
  - Sperm morphology
    - Head: Contains the acrosome with enzymes for ovum penetration; double and irregularly shaped heads interfere with penetration
    - Neck piece: Attaches the head to the midpiece; a neckpiece too long causes a bent head that interferes with motility
    - Midpiece: Contains mitochondria to provide energy for the tail
    - Tail: Acts as a flagella to propel the sperm, double and coiled tails interfere with motility
    - Normal values: Greater than 30% normal sperm using routine criteria and greater than 14% using strict criteria
  - Sperm viability
    - Stain smears with eosin-nigrosin, nonviable sperm absorb the stain and appear red
    - Viable sperm do not stain
    - Normal value: 75% normal sperm per 100 cells counted

Postvasectomy Semen Analysis

- Carefully evaluate a wet preparation for viable and nonviable sperm
- Report any sperm seen
- Negative specimens may be centrifuged and reexamined

SYNOVIAL FLUID

Physiology

- Synovial fluid is located in the cavities between the moveable joints
- Synoviocytes secrete hyaluronic acid, a large molecule that produces the viscosity of the fluid
- Damage to the joints produces arthritis (Table 5-9)

Laboratory Testing

- Color
  - Normal is colorless to pale yellow
- Viscosity
  - The mucin clot test detects and measures hyaluronic acid
  - Addition of acetic acid to normal synovial fluid will form a firm mucin clot surrounded by clear liquid; clots become less firm as the viscosity decreases
  - Addition of acetic acid to a questionable fluid identifies it as synovial fluid if a clot forms
- Cell counts
  - Do not use normal WBC diluting fluid (acetic acid), use normal saline
  - Normal WBC count is less than 200 cells/μL
- Differential
  - Incubate fluid with hyaluronidase before slide preparation
  - Primary cells are monocytes and macrophages, followed by neutrophils at less than 25% and lymphocytes at less than 15% and occasional synoviocytes
- Crystal identification
  - Primary crystals are monosodium, urate seen in gout, and calcium pyrophosphate dihydrate, seen in pseudogout
  - Identify using polarized and compensated polarized light
  - Monosodium urate crystals
    - Needle-shaped, strongly birefringent under polarized light
    - Yellow when aligned with the slow vibration of compensated polarized light and blue when vertical to the slow vibration
    - Elevated serum uric acid levels aid in the identification
  - Calcium pyrophosphate dihydrate crystals
    - Rhombic, often seen intracellularly in neutrophil vacuoles (phagocytized monosodium urate crystals puncture the cell membrane)
    - Blue when aligned with the slow vibration of compensated polarized light and yellow when vertical to the slow vibration

Microbiology

- Gram stains and cultures are routinely run on synovial fluid specimens
- Cultures require enriched agar (chocolate) for detection of possible *Haemophilus* sp. and *Neisseria gonorrhea*

SEROUS FLUID

Physiology

- Serous fluid is located between the parietal and visceral membranes that line the closed body cavities, mesothelial cells line the membranes
- Cavities: Pleural, pericardial, and peritoneal
- Serous fluid is normally produced and reabsorbed at a constant rate; disruption of this process produces an effusion

Transudates and Exudates. (See Table 5-10)

- Effusions caused by systemic disorders are transudates
- Effusions caused by membrane disorders are exudates

TABLE 5-9	Classification of Arthritis	
Class	**Pathology**	**Laboratory Results**
Noninflammatory	Osteoarthritis	Clear, yellow, good viscosity WBCs <1000/μL, neutrophils <30%
Inflammatory/ immunologic	Autoimmune disorders	Cloudy, yellow, poor viscosity WBCs 2000 to 75,000/μL, neutrophils >50%
Inflammatory/ crystals	Gout, pseudogout	Clear or milky, low viscosity, WBCs up to 100,000/μL, neutrophils <75%
Septic	Infection	Cloudy, yellow-green, low viscosity, WBCs 50,000-100,000/μL, neutrophils >75%
Hemorrhagic	Trauma, coagulation disorders	Cloudy, red, low viscosity, WBCs and neutrophils equal to blood values

WBCs, White blood cells.

TABLE 5-10	Differentiation Between Transudates and Exudates	
Test	**Transudates**	**Exudates**
Appearance	Clear	Cloudy
Fluid-to–serum protein ratio	<0.5	>0.5
Fluid-to–serum LD ratio	<0.6	>0.6
White blood cell count	<1000/μL	>1000/μL
Spontaneous clotting	No	Yes

LD, Lactate dehydrogenase.

Pleural Fluid

- Collected by thorocentesis
- Appearance
  - Milky: Thoracic duct leakage (chylous effusion), chronic infection (pseudochylous effusion)
  - Bloody: Hemothorax, hemorrhagic effusion (embolus, tuberculosis, malignancy)
  - Viscous: Malignant mesothelioma producing hyaluronic acid
- Hematology: Differential count
  - Neutrophils: Pneumonia, pancreatitis
  - Lymphocytes: Tuberculosis, viral infections
  - Eosinophils: Pneumothorax
  - Mesothelial cells: Normal, decreased with tuberculosis
  - Plasma cells: Tuberculosis
  - Malignant cells: Small cell and adenocarcinoma, metastatic carcinoma cells
- Chemistry
  - pH less than 7.0 indicates the need for chest tube drainage
  - pH less than 6.0 indicates esophageal rupture
  - Pleural fluid cholesterol: equal to or less than 45 to 60 mg/dL (transudate), higher (exudate)
  - Pleural fluid: Serum cholesterol ratio: Less than 0.3 (transudate), higher (exudate)
  - Pleural fluid: Serum bilirubin ratio: Less than 0.6 (transudate), higher (exudate)
- Microbiology
  - Acid-fast stains

Pericardial Fluid

- Collected by pericardiocentesis
- Appearance
  - Cloudy, blood-streaked: Infection, malignancy
  - Grossly bloody: Cardiac puncture, anticoagulant medications
- Hematology
  - Increased neutrophils are seen in bacterial endocarditis
  - Refer metastatic malignant cells for cytologic examination
- Microbiology
  - Gram stains and cultures are performed on concentrated specimens
  - Acid-fast stains for tuberculosis are associated with acquired immunodeficiency syndrome

Peritoneal Fluid

- Often called ascitic fluid, effusion is ascites
- Effusions are caused by liver disorders (cirrhosis), intestinal infection (peritonitis), and malignancy

Transudates and Exudates

- The serum-ascites albumin gradient is the recommended method for differentiation
- Measure serum and ascites albumin levels
  - Serum albumin − fluid albumin = 1.1 or higher is a transudate
  - Serum albumin − fluid albumin = 1.1 or lower is an exudate
- Appearance
  - Turbid: Infection
  - Green: Gallbladder or pancreas disorder
  - Blood-streaked: Trauma, infection, malignancy
  - Milky: Lymphatic trauma or blockage
- Hematology
  - Normal WBC count: Less than 350/μL
  - Absolute neutrophil count distinguishes between cirrhosis and peritonitis
  - More than 250 neutrophils/μL or 50% of the differential indicates peritonitis
- Differential count
  - Additional cells seen include abundant mesothelial cells, lipophages, yeast, *Toxoplasma gondii,* and malignant colon, prostate, and ovarian cells
- Chemistry
  - Glucose: Decreased in infection and malignancy
  - Amylase: Elevated in pancreatitis and gastrointestinal (GI) perforations
  - Alkaline phosphatase: Elevated in intestinal perforation
  - BUN and creatinine: Bladder rupture or puncture
  - Tumor markers: Carcinoembryonic antigen and CA125
- Microbiology
  - Gram stains and cultures for both aerobic and anaerobic organisms
  - Blood cultures aid in the detection of anaerobic organisms

AMNIOTIC FLUID

Specimens

- Collected by amniocentesis
- Hemolytic disease of the newborn (HDN) specimens must be protected from light
- Specimens for fetal lung maturity (FLM) are delivered on ice and refrigerated or frozen
- Specimens for cytogenic testing are kept at room temperature and delivered immediately
- **Appearance**
  - Colorless: Normal
  - Blood-streaked: Trauma, traumatic tap
  - Yellow: Bilirubin, HDN
  - Dark green: Meconium
  - Dark red-brown: Fetal death

Tests for Fetal Distress

- HDN: Spectrophotometric analysis at optical densities between 365 and 550 nm (Figure 5-5)
- Neural tube defects
  - Detected first by increased maternal serum α-fetoprotein
  - Amniotic fluid levels are measured first between gestational weeks 12 to 15 and compared to maternal serum levels
  - Report both serum and fluid levels in multiples of the mean (MOM)
  - Abnormal value: Two times the laboratory median value in both serum and fluid
  - Positive tests are followed by measuring amniotic acetylcholinesterase

Tests for Fetal Maturity

- Respiratory distress syndrome is caused by decreased lung surfactant
- Primary lung surfactants are lecithin, sphingomyelin, and phosphatidylglycerol
- Aminostat-FLM
  - Immunologic agglutination test for phosphatidylglycerol
  - Not affected by meconium and blood contamination
- Lamellar bodies
  - The storage form of phospholipids in the lungs. Secreted by the type II pneumocytes and enter the amniotic fluid at 26 weeks of gestation
  - Fluid can be run through the platelet counting channel of automated cell counters
  - Normal values are 32,000 to 35,400 based on the instrument
  - An optical density measurement of the fluid at 650 nm of 0.150 is also normal

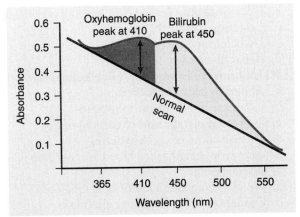

FIGURE 5-5 Spectrophotometric scan of fetal bilirubin. *(From Strasinger SK, Di Lorenzo MS: Urinalysis and body fluids, ed 5, Philadelphia, 2008, FA Davis).*

FECAL ANALYSIS

Physiology

- Final digestion and reabsorption of food takes place in the small intestine with the aid of enzymes from the pancreas and bile salts from the liver
- The large intestine receives the digestive products and water from the digestive process
- Much of the water is reabsorbed
- Additonal water results in diarrhea, and too little water produces constipation
- Types of diarrhea
  - Secretory caused primarily by bacterial, viral, or protozoan infection; fecal WBCs are seen in the stool
  - Osmotic caused by incomplete breakdown or reabsorption in the small intestine and retention of water in the large intestine

Laboratory Tests

- Color and appearance
  - Normal: Color is brown, caused by urobilin
  - Black: Upper GI bleeding, iron therapy, and antacids
  - Red: Lower GI bleeding, food coloring
  - Pale yellow/white: Bile duct obstruction, barium tests
  - Bulky/frothy: Bile duct obstruction, steatorrrhea
  - Blood-streaked mucus: Colitis, dysentry, malignancy
- Microscopic tests
  - Fecal leukocytes: Detects invasive non–toxin-producing microorganisms
  - Muscle fibers: Detects undigested striated fibers seen with pancreatic insufficiency
  - Only undigested fibers are counted; fiber classification
    - Digested fibers: No visible striations
    - Partially digested fibers: Striations are in only one direction
    - Undigested fibers: Vertical and horizontal fibers visible
  - Qualitative fecal fats: Monitoring of malabsorption disorders
  - Neutral fats (triglycerides) stain easily with Sudan III in alcohol
  - Soaps, fatty acids and cholesterol require application of heat to the slide
- Chemical tests
  - Occult blood: Screening for colorectal cancer
    - Classic test (fecal occult blood test [FOBT]) uses the pseudoperoxidase activity of hemoglobin with gum guiac as the indicator (Figure 5-6)

Hemoglobin $\longrightarrow$ H_2O_2 $\longrightarrow$ Guaiac $\longrightarrow$ Oxidized guaiac + H_2O
                                    Peroxidase   (Blue color)

FIGURE 5-6 Measurement of hemoglobin using pseudoperoxidase and guiac.

- Patients must follow dietary instructions avoiding meat, fish, vegetables that contain pseudoperoxidase, aspirin, and vitamin C
- Immunologic FOBTs (iFOBTs) use antihuman hemoglobin antibodies that are specific for the globin portion of hemoglobin
- Advantages: Do not require dietary and medication restrictions. Detects lower GI bleeding, which is more indicative of colorectal cancer. Blood from upper GI bleeding degrades before reaching the large intestine
- Procedure: Stool samples should be taken from the center of the stool to avoid contamination. Two samples from negative samples from three different stools confirms a negative
- Quantitative fecal fats
  - Confirmatory test for fecal fats
  - Requires collection of a timed 3-day specimen and maintenance of a 100 g/day fat diet
  - Testing methods: Titration, acid steatocrit test, and near-infrared reflectance spectrophotometry
- Fecal enzymes
  - Elastase I is pancreatic-specific enzyme measured by immunoassay using monoclonal antibodies against human pancreatic elastase I
  - This differentiates pancreatic steatorrhea from non-pancreatic causes of steatorrhea
- Fecal carbohydrates
  - Increased fecal carbohydrates are caused by failure to reabsorb carbohydrates (celiac disease) or lack of digestive enzymes (lactose intolerance)
  - Clinitest is the common screening test, followed by carbohydrate intolerance tests
  - Measuring stool pH can be used to test infant diarrhea. Normal stool pH is 7 to 8, pH levels below 5.5 indicate carbohydrate disorders

CERTIFICATION PREPARATION QUESTIONS

For answers and rationales, please see Appendix A.

1. The specific gravity of the glomerular ultrafiltrate is _____.

   a. 1.000
   b. 1.010
   c. 1.025
   d. 1.040

2. In an unpreserved urine specimen left at room temperature overnight, which of the following will have increased?
   a. Bacteria and nitrite
   b. Specific gravity and bilirubin
   c. Glucose and ketones
   d. Urobilinogen and protein

3. A first morning specimen would be requested to confirm which of the following?
   a. Diabetes insipidus
   b. Fanconi's syndrome
   c. Urinary tract infection
   d. Orthostatic proteinuria

4. Failure to collect the last specimen of a timed urine collection will:
   a. Cause falsely increased results
   b. Affect the preservation of glucose
   c. Cause falsely decreased results
   d. Adversely affect reagent strip results

5. Which of the following is the principle of the reagent strip test for pH?
   a. A double indicator reaction
   b. The protein error of indicators
   c. The diazo reaction
   d. A dye-binding reaction

6. Which of the following best describes the chemical principle of the protein reagent strip?
   a. Protein reacts with an immunocomplex on the pad
   b. Protein causes a pH change on the reagent strip pad
   c. Protein accepts hydrogen ions from an indicator dye
   d. Protein causes protons to be released from a polyelectrolyte

7. Which of the following is the principle of the reagent strip test for glucose?
   a. A double sequential enzyme reaction
   b. Copper reduction
   c. The peroxidase activity of glucose
   d. Buffered reactions of mixed enzyme indicators

8. Glucosuria not accompanied by hyperglycemia can be seen with which of the following?
   a. Hormonal disorders
   b. Gestational diabetes
   c. Diabetes mellitus
   d. Renal disease

9. Which of the following will cause ketonuria?
   a. Ability to use carbohydrates
   b. Adequate intake of carbohydrates
   c. Decreased metabolism of carbohydrates
   d. Excessive loss of carbohydrates

10. Reagent strip reactions for blood are based on which of the following?
   a. Pseudoperoxidase activity of hemoglobin
   b. Oxidation of hemoglobin peroxidase
   c. Reaction of hemoglobin with bromothymol blue
   d. Reduction of a chromogen by hemoglobin

11. Myoglobinuria may be caused by which of the following?
   a. Decreased glomerular filtration
   b. Incompatible blood transfusions
   c. Strenuous exercise
   d. Biliary obstruction

12. A patient with severe back pain comes to the emergency department. A urine specimen has a 1 + reagent strip reading for blood and a specific gravity of 1.030. This can aid in confirming a diagnosis of

   _____.
   a. Pyelonephritis
   b. Appendicitis
   c. Renal calculi
   d. Multiple myeloma

13. When a reagent strip is positive for bilirubin, it can be assumed that the bilirubin:
   a. Is conjugated
   b. Has passed through the small intestine
   c. Is attached to protein
   d. Is unconjugated

14. Which of the following results would be seen in urine from a patient with autoimmune hemolytic anemia?
   a. Bilirubin=negative, urobilinogen=negative
   b. Bilirubin=positive, urobilinogen=positive
   c. Bilirubin=positive, urobilinogen=negative
   d. Bilirubin=negative, urobilinogen=positive

15. Which of the following is the principle of the reagent strip test for specific gravity?
   a. Disassociation of the indicator bromothymol blue, producing a pH change
   b. Ionization of a polyelectrolyte, producing a pH change detected by bromothymol blue
   c. Disassociation of polyelectrolyte, producing a pH change detected by bromothymol blue
   d. Change in the pK of bromothymol blue to produce a pH change

16. These constituents are primarily seen in urine with an:

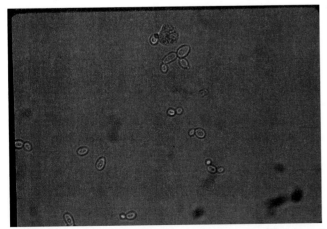

FIGURE 5-7   *(From Strasinger SK, Di Lorenzo MS: Urinalysis and body fluids, ed 4, Philadelphia, 2001, FA Davis.)*

   a. Acid pH and a positive protein
   b. Alkaline pH and bacteria

   c. Acid pH and a positive glucose
   d. Alkaline pH and a positive protein

17. The presence of dysmorphic red blood cells in the urine sediment is indicative of which of the following?
   a. A coagulation disorder
   b. Menstrual contamination
   c. Urinary tract infection
   d. Glomerular bleeding

18. The location of epithelial cells in the urinary tract in descending order is:
   a. Squamous, transitional, renal tubular
   b. Transitional, renal tubular, squamous
   c. Renal tubular, transitional, squamous
   d. Squamous, renal tubular, urothelial

19. Urinary casts are formed in which of the following?
   a. Distal tubules and collecting ducts
   b. Distal tubules and loops of Henle
   c. Proximal and distal tubules
   d. Proximal tubules and loops of Henle

20. These crystals were seen in the urine of a child who had ingested antifreeze. They are:

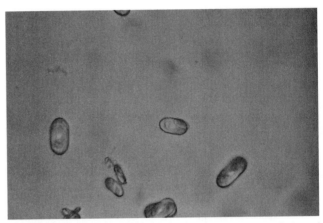

FIGURE 5-8   *(From Strasinger SK, Di Lorenzo MS: Urinalysis and body fluids, ed 5, Philadelphia, 2008, FA Davis.)*

   a. Triple phosphate
   b. Calcium oxalate dihydrate
   c. Calcium oxalate monohydrate
   d. Calcium phosphate

21. The test for which of the following results should be repeated?
   a. Positive blood and protein
   b. pH 7.0 with ammonium biurate crystals
   c. Positive nitrite and leukocyte esterase
   d. pH 5.0, WBCs, and triple phosphate crystals

22. Anti–glomerular basement antibody is seen with:
   a. Wegener's granulomatosis
   b. IgA nephropathy
   c. Goodpasture's syndrome
   d. Diabetic nephropathy

23. The most common composition of renal calculi is:
   a. Calcium oxalate
   b. Magnesium ammonium phosphate

　　c. Cystine
　　d. Uric acid

24. Pyelonephritis can be differentiated from cystitis by the presence of _____.
　　a. Eosinophils
　　b. Hyaline casts
　　c. White blood cell casts
　　d. Bacteriuria

25. Children develop a form of nephrotic syndrome called:
　　a. IgA nephropathy
　　b. Henoch-Schönlein purpura
　　c. Minimal change disease
　　d. Acute glomerulonephritis

26. Focal segmental glomerular nephritis is associated with which of the following?
　　a. Untreated streptococcal infections
　　b. Heroin abuse
　　c. Diabetes mellitus
　　d. Autoimmune disorders

27. Which of the following would be most characteristic of chronic glomerulonephritis versus acute glomerular nephritis?
　　a. Red blood cells and red blood cell casts
　　b. Hyaline casts and mucus
　　c. Waxy and broad casts
　　d. Proteinuria

28. Which of the following results is not consistent with cystitis?

Color: Yellow	Protein: 1+	Blood: Trace
Clarity: Hazy	Glucose: Negative	Urobilinogen: 1.0 EU
Specific gravity: 1.015	Ketones: Negative	Nitrite: Positive
pH: 7.0	Bilirubin: Negative	Leukocyte esterase: ++
80-100 WBC/hpf 10-15 renal tubular epithelial cells/hpf	5-10 red blood cells/hpf	Many bacteria

　　a. pH
　　b. Protein
　　c. 5 to 10 RBC/hpf
　　d. 10 to 15 renal tubular epithelial cells/hpf

29. Cerebrospinal fluid is produced primarily by which of the following?
　　a. Secretion by the choroid plexus cells
　　b. Diffusion from the plasma into the central nervous system
　　c. Ultrafiltration of plasma in the choroid plexuses
　　d. Excretions from the ependymal cells lining the central nervous system

30. Three tubes of cerebrospinal fluid are submitted to the laboratory. They are numbered l, 2, and 3 and show blood in all tubes but decreasing in amount in tubes l through 3. This observation should be interpreted as:
　　a. The tubes were numbered in wrong sequence, because an increasing amount of blood would be expected

　　b. A traumatic or bloody tap and in all likelihood of no pathogenic significance
　　c. The pathologic presence of RBCs and reported to your supervisor immediately
　　d. A pathologic presence of RBCs, but because the RBC morphology is normal, the importance is minimal

31. An IgG index greater than 0.80 is indicative of which of the following?
　　a. Synthesis of IgG within the CNS
　　b. Alterations in the blood-brain barrier
　　c. Active demyelination of neural tissue
　　d. Increased reabsorption of IgG from the peripheral blood

32. Which of the following can decrease CSF protein?
　　a. Fluid leakage
　　b. Meningitis
　　c. Multiple sclerosis
　　d. Hemorrhage

33. CSF lactate is used to verify cases of which of the following?
　　a. Multiple sclerosis
　　b. Bacterial meningitis
　　c. Reye's syndrome
　　d. Tertiary syphilis

34. Which of the following can be used to identify a fluid as CSF?
　　a. Oligoclonal bands
　　b. Xanthochromia
　　c. Transferrin τ protein
　　d. Absence of glucose

35. Oligoclonal bands are significant in the diagnosis of multiple sclerosis when:
　　a. They are seen in both the serum and CSF
　　b. At least five bands are seen in the CSF
　　c. They are seen in the CSF and not in the serum
　　d. They appear in both the albumin and globulin fractions of serum and the CSF

36. Calculate the sperm count on a 3-mL semen specimen with a concentration of 12,000/μL.
　　a. 4000/mL
　　b. 12,000/μL
　　c. 20,000/μL
　　d. 36,000/mL

37. The most important sugar found in semen is _____.
　　a. Sucrose
　　b. Maltose
　　c. Fructose
　　d. Lactose

38. The mucin clot test determines the presence of synovial fluid _____.
　　a. Protein
　　b. Glucose
　　c. Fibrinogen
　　d. Hyaluronic acid

39. What is added to synovial fluid to determine the viscosity?
   a. Sodium hydroxide
   b. Acetic acid
   c. Hydrochloric acid
   d. Hyaluronic acid

40. Crystals that appear needle-shaped under polarized light and are yellow when aligned with the slow vibration of compensated polarized light are _____.
   a. Monosodium urate
   b. Calcium pyrophosphate
   c. Hydroxyapatite
   d. Corticosteroid

41. The fluid that builds up between the serous membranes is _____.
   a. A transudate
   b. An abscess
   c. An exudate
   d. An effusion

42. Which of the following sets of results most closely indicates a transudate?
   a. Clear, fluid-to–serum LD ratio: 0.8, fluid-to–serum protein ratio: 0.7, WBC count: 1000/μL
   b. Cloudy, fluid-to–serum LD ratio: 0.5, fluid-to–serum protein ratio: 0.6, WBC count: 1200/μL
   c. Cloudy, fluid-to–serum LD ratio: 0.8, fluid-to–serum protein ratio: 0.7, WBC count: 2500/μL
   d. Clear, fluid-to–serum LD ratio: 0.45, fluid-to–serum protein ratio: 0.40, WBC count: 800/μL

43. The most likely cause of increased neutrophils is a pericardial fluid exudate is _____.
   a. Tuberculosis
   b. Bacterial endocarditis
   c. Cardiac puncture
   d. Pneumonia

44. Pleural fluid is obtained by which of the following?
   a. Paracentesis
   b. Pneumocentesis
   c. Thoracentesis
   d. Pulmonary puncture

45. Which of the following tests is used to differentiate between an effusion caused by cirrhosis and one caused by peritonitis?
   a. Absolute neutrophil count
   b. Fluid-to–serum bilirubin ratio
   c. Serum-ascites gradient
   d. Serum to LD ratio

46. Amniotic fluid for fetal lung maturity testing should be preserved _____.
   a. In the refrigerator
   b. At room temperature
   c. In a dark container
   d. At 37° C

47. Which of the following results of a test on the mother would suggest a possible neural tube defect in the fetus?
   a. A positive antibody screen
   b. A glucose value of 140 mg/dL
   c. An α-fetoprotein result of 0.1 MOM
   d. An α-fetoprotein result of 3.0 MOM

48. A pale, frothy stool is indicative of which of the following?
   a. Barium testing
   b. Osmotic diarrhea
   c. Steatorrhea
   d. Excess carbohydrates

49. The acid steatocrit test is performed to analyze which of the following?
   a. Grossly bloody stools
   b. Qualitative fecal fats
   c. Carbohydrate reabsorption
   d. Quantitative fecal fats

50. The most sensitive fecal enzyme test for the diagnosis of pancreatic insufficiency measures _____.
   a. Lipase
   b. Trypsin
   c. Elastase I
   d. Chymotrypsin

SELF-ASSESSMENT

Content Area: _____

Score on Practice Questions: _____

List the specific topics covered in the missed questions:

List the specific topics covered in the correct questions:

NOTES

Immunology and Serology

Elizabeth G. Hertenstein

INNATE IMMUNITY

The Natural Barriers of Immunity

- Mucous membranes
- Skin
- Cough reflex
- Cilia
- pH of secretions
- Enzymes in saliva and tears
- Normal flora competes for space and nutrients

Cells of the Innate Immune System

- Neutrophils: Early responders to foreign particles, particularly bacteria, and move through vessel walls by diapedesis to site of injury; response is phagocytosis and inflammation enhanced by cytokines
- Eosinophils: Responder/effector cells in allergic and parasitic infections; can be involved in phagocytosis but not to large degree because the numbers of eosinophils in response is low
- Basophils: Effector cells in immediate hypersensitivity reactions also can be involved in phagocytosis, but to a small degree because the number of circulating basophils is low
- Mast cells: Similar to basophils but have a longer life span, play a role in hypersensitivity reactions, bind immunoglobulin E (IgE)
- Dendritic cells: Have long membranous extensions, are antigen-presenting cells and phagocytic, present to T cells in bloodstream or lymphoid tissue
- Monocytes: Large lobular phagocytic cells, in tissues are called macrophages
- Tissue macrophages: In tissue, macrophages are named by their location
  - Liver: Kupffer cells
  - Lung: Alveolar macrophage
  - Spleen: Splenic macrophage
  - Brain and central nervous system (CNS): Microglial cells
- Monocyte-macrophage: Important regulators
  - Phagocytosis of bacteria and parasites
  - Secret mediators such as cytokines

- Turmoricidal effects
- Antigen presentation
- Toll-like receptors: Also known as pattern-recognition receptors; the receptors recognize patterns in microbial cell walls or membranes and enhance recognition by phagocytic neutrophils and monocytes

Humoral Components of the Innate System

- C-Reactive protein
  - Increases rapidly after infection or trauma, with a rapid decline
  - Can act as an opsonin and activate the classical complement pathway
- Complement
  - A series of proteins that mediate lysis of bacteria and foreign particles via the mannose-binding lectin (MBL) pathway of complement activation (see later discussion)

Innate System Processes

- Phagocytosis: Stages of phagocytosis
  - Chemotaxis: Phagocytic cell is attracted to the invading organism by chemical mediators secreted by other immune system cells
  - Physical contact: Phagocytic cell and invading organism attach
  - Engulfment: Phagocytic cells engulf the particle
  - Phagosome formation: Organism is enclosed in a vacuole
  - Formation of phagolysosome: Vacuole fuses with granules in the cytoplasm to release contents
  - Digestion: Enzymes break down contents of phagolysosome
  - Excretion: By-products of digestion are transported to cell membrane and released outside the cell
- Inflammation
  - Both cellular and humoral response aids healing, but can also cause damage to tissue around the site of inflammation
  - Effectors
    - Neutrophils and macrophages are attracted to the site

- Secretion of chemoattractants and chemical mediators
- Complement acts as opsonin
- Physical hallmarks of inflammation are redness, pain, swelling, and fever and are due to increased blood supply to site, increased capillary permeation, migration of white blood cells (WBCs) to inflamed area
  - Localized inflammation: At site of injury
  - Systemic inflammation: System-wide; if persists, adaptive immunity is activated
  - Chronic: Infection cannot be eradicated, inflammatory process remains activated

ADAPTIVE IMMUNITY

Organs of the Lymphatic System

- Primary: Maturation sites
  - Bone marrow: B-lymphocyte maturation site
  - Thymus: T-lymphocyte maturation site
- Secondary: Activation sites
  - Spleen
  - Lymph nodes
- Outer cortex: B cells in primary and secondary follicles (or germinal center), few plasma cells
- Paracortex: Area of T cells
- Inner medulla: Plasma cells with few T cells
  - Tonsils
  - Peyer's patches: Cluster of lymphocytes found around the small intestine

Cells of Adaptive Immunity

B-Lymphocyte Maturation: Antigen-Independent Phase

- Pro–B cell
  - Shows first rearrangement of immunoglobulin genes
  - Expresses CD 19 (acts as a coreceptor), 10, 45 (signaling)
  - Successful rearrangement of immunoglobulin heavy chains leads to next stage or pre–B cell
- Pre–B cell
  - μ is first heavy chain produced
  - CD10 and CD19 expressed on surface
  - Pre–B-cell receptor (pre-BCR) on surface of B cell is made of μ chain, surrogate light chains, and two transmembrane molecules
  - A functional pre-BCR does not bind antigen, but rather signals the cell nucleus for further maturation
- Immature B cell
  - Expresses IgM on surface (different from previous stages)
  - B-cell receptor (BCR) on surface is IgM plus two transmembrane molecules
  - BCR is capable of binding antigen

- Recognition of self-antigens, negative signals sent to nucleus will stop maturation, and cell dies by apoptosis
- CD 21, CD 40, and major histocompatibility complex (MHC) molecules appear
- CD20 found on surface, marker for later stages of B-cell development
- Mature B cell
  - Loss of CD10 on cell surface (marker for early stages of B-cell development)
  - Leaves the bone marrow, travels to secondary organs to await activation
  - IgM and IgD on cell surface, thought to act as activating signalers for antigen contact

B-Lymphocyte Maturation: Antigen-Dependent Phase

- Plasma cells
  - Immature B cells are activated to plasma or memory cells
  - Produce and secrete antibody
  - No further maturation, these cells die within days of producing antibody
- Memory cells
  - Antigen-stimulated B cells waiting activation from second exposure of specific antigen

T-Lymphocyte Maturation

- Precursors released from bone marrow and mature in the thymus
- Two main subsets of T cells to mature: CD4+ and CD8+
  - CD4+: Helper T cells that indirectly protect from fungi and bacteria by secretion of cytokines to activate B cells to maturity and produce antibody
  - CD8+: Cytotoxic T cells that directly protect from viral infection by cell lysis
- Double-negative stage of T-cell maturation
  - CD4 and CD8 are not present on cell
  - Cells possess pre–T-cell receptor (pre-TCR), which is made of CD3 plus functional β chains
  - Signaling by β chains enhances maturation of the cell to express both CD4 and CD8
- Double-positive stage
  - T cell expresses both CD 4 and CD8 on surface
  - T-cell receptor (TCR) is composed of CD3 plus α and β chains
  - Positive selection: Only cells with TCR, CD4, CD8 survive
  - Negative selection: T cells that react strongly with self-antigens are eliminated
- Mature T cell
  - Survivors of selection express either CD4 or CD8 on surface
  - Released from thymus to secondary lymphoid organs
  - Become activated when antigen is presented by antigen-presenting cell
  - CD4+ T cells
    - Produce cytokines helping B cells to produce antibody and stimulate hematopoiesis
    - Kill tumors
    - Involvement in graft rejection

- CD8+ T cells
  - Kill virally infected or diseased cells by cytotoxicity
- Natural killer (NK) cell
  - Considered a bridge between the innate and adaptive immune systems because it is thought to have the same precursor as a lymphocyte but can respond to diseased cells without prior exposure to antigen
  - Thought to act by recognizing a lack of MHC class I proteins on diseased or cancerous cells
  - The lack of these proteins along with signalers enhances the NK cell to cytolytic action against the damaged cell
  - Also act by way of antibody-dependent cell cytotoxicity (ADCC), or recognition and lysis of antibody-coated infected cells

Humoral Components of the Adaptive Immune System

Cytokines
- Regulate growth and differentiation of immune system effector cells
- Pleotropic, with many different effects
- Redundant: The same cytokine can be produced by different cells
- Autocrine effects: Affect the cell it was secreted from
- Paracrine effects: Affect a nearby cell
- Endocrine effects: Have a systemic affect (Table 6-1)

Complement. See (Figure 6-1)
- Series of proteins that result in lysis of foreign particles, particularly bacteria, when activated
- Proteins are found normally circulating in plasma
- Complement regulator proteins present to keep from uncontrolled activation
- Three known pathways of complement activation: Classical, alternative, and MBL pathways
- Classical pathway of complement activation
  - Activated by antigen–antibody complexes
  - The "recognition unit": C1 is made of three subunits designated as C1q, C1r, and C1s
  - C1q binds to Fc portion of antibody, two molecules of C1q needed to bind for activation
  - At this step, two IgG molecules are necessary; however, only 1 IgM is needed because of its pentameric shape
  - C1r and C1s become enzymatically active and cleave C4 and C2

TABLE 6-1	Selected Cytokines and Activity			
Cytokine Family	Cytokine	Produced By	Target	Biologic Activity
Interferon	INF-α INF-β	Virally infected dendritic cells	NK cells	Antiviral activity, mediates MHC class I and II expression
	INF-γ	T-helper cells	Macrophages, cytotoxic T cells, NK cells	
Tumor necrosis factors	TNF-α	Macrophages, gram-negative bacteria	Macrophages, mast cells	Mediates inflammation by recruiting and activating phagocytes
	TNF-β	Epithelial cells	T cells and B cells	Also known as lymphotoxin
Interleukins	IL-1 superfamily	Monocytes, macrophages	Hypothalamus, epithelial cells	Acute phase reactions, mediate cell adhesion for diapedesis
	IL-2	T-helper cells	T cells and B cells, macrophages	Growth and differentiation of T cells and B cells, activates monocytes, macrophages, and NK and cytotoxic cells
	IL-4	Naive T cells and T-helper cells	T cells	Induces growth of T-helper cells, mediates humoral immunity
	IL-5	T-helper cells	Eosinophils, B cells	Growth of eosinophils, mediator of type 1 hypersensitivity reactions
	IL-6	T cells, B cells, monocytes, macrophages, other nonimmune cells	B cells, T cells	Acute phase reactions, antibody production, stimulates B cells to plasma cells
	IL-10	Monocytes, macrophages, T cells	T-helper cells, antigen-presenting cells	Antiinflammatory and suppressive effect
Transforming growth factor	TGF-β	T-regulatory cells	T cells, B cells	Activates and inhibits proliferation, regulates inflammatory response
Colony-stimulating factors	CSFs	T cells	Bone marrow stem cells	Stimulate hematopoietic stem cell differentiation of granulocytes, macrophages

CSF, Cerebrospinal fluid; *MHC*, major histocompatibility complex; *NK*, natural killer

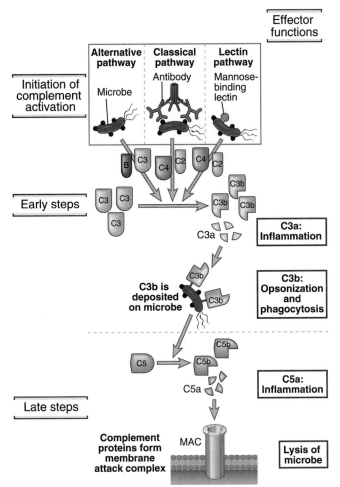

FIGURE 6-1 Pathways of complement activation. *MAC, Macrophage attack complex. (From Abbas A, Lichtman A, Pillai S: Basic immunology: functions and disorders of the immune system, ed 4, Philadelphia, 2013, Saunders.)*

- C4 is cleaved to C4a and C4b, C2 is cleaved to C2a and C2b
- C4a and C2b are released, C4a has anaphylatoxic activity
- C4b and 2a bind to antigen = C4b2a = C3 convertase enzyme
- C3 convertase cleaves C3 to C3a and C3b
- C3a released has anaphylatoxic activity
- C3b binds to complex = C4b2a3b = C5 convertase
- C5 convertase cleaves C5 to C5a and C5b
- C5b deposits on cell membrane of antigen
- C5b plus C6, C7, C8 make up the membrane attack complex (MAC); on the surface of a cell, this complex bound together causes a small pore in the membrane
- C9 binds and stabilizes complex, leading to larger pore and ultimately cell lysis
- C1 Inhibitor is a complement protein that keeps this system from uncontrolled activation
- Additional activities of complement proteins include anaphylatoxic reactions of C4a, C3a, and C5a
- Released C3b can also act as opsonin

- Alternative pathway of complement activation
  - Is triggered by polysaccharide components of bacterial cell walls, parasites, fungi, tumor cells, viruses, yeast
  - Inactive C3 in normal plasma is activated to C3b
  - C3b binds with factor B to microbial cell wall
  - Enzymatically active factor D cleaves cell-bound factor B to Ba and Bb
  - Ba is released to plasma
  - The resulting C3aBb = C3 convertase, capable of cleaving additional C3 to C3a and C3b
  - More C3b is bound to complex, forming C3bBb3b = C5 convertase
  - C5 convertase cleaves C5 to C5a and C5b
  - C5b binds to antigen and begins the first part of the MAC, same as in the classical pathway
  - Properdin is a protein of the alternative pathway that stabilizes the C3 convertase complex, allowing the complex to function properly
  - Factor H prevents the binding of C3b to factor B in the early steps of this pathway, preventing uncontrolled activation
- MBL pathway of complement activation
  - Activated when MBL binds to certain sugars found in cell walls and membranes of bacteria, yeasts, and some parasites
  - MBL is similar to C1q
  - When bound to cell surface, a series of MBL-associated serine proteases cleave C2 and C4
  - The rest is the same as in the classical pathway (Table 6-2)

Antibodies. See (Figure 6-2)
- Two heavy chains
  - Heavy chains are designated as μ (IgM), δ (IgD), γ (IgG), α (IgA), and ε (IgE)
  - Each heavy chain is made of three constant domains, C_H^1, C_H^2, C_H^3, and one variable (V) domain, V_H
- Two light chains
  - Light chains are designated as κ or λ
  - Each light chain is made of one constant domain, C_L and one variable domain, V_L
- The constant domains are unique to each class of antibody and determine the isotype—μ, γ, δ, α, or ε
- Minor variations of amino acid sequences in the constant domains of the molecule between individuals are known as allotypes
- Immunoglobulin molecule variations in the variable domains are known as idiotypes
- The constant domain is where biological activity of the molecule occurs
  - Agglutination
  - Complement fixation
  - Antigen attachment to aid opsonization
  - ADCC
  - Viral neutralization
- The variable region is unique to each antibody molecule and makes up the antigen-binding site

Complement component	**Pathway**	**Activity**	**Other information**
C1qrs	Classical	Binds antibody and cell surface	Recognition unit
C4 and C2	Classical	C4a and C2b released into plasma	Activation
C4b2a	Classical	Cleaves C3	C3 convertase enzyme
C3	Classical, alternative, and mannose binding	C3a released in plasma, C3b combines with C4b2a in classical and factor B in alternative	Activation
Factor B	Alternative	Is split into Ba and Bb, combine with C3	Activation
C3bBb	Alternative	Cleaves C3	C3 Convertase enzyme
C4b2a3b	Classical, mannose binding	Cleaves C5	C5 convertase enzyme
C3bBb3b	Alternative, mannose binding	Cleaves C5	C5 convertase enzyme
C5-C9	Classical, alternative, and mannose binding	Cell lysis	Membrane attack complex

TABLE 6-2 Complement Components, Pathways, and Related Activity

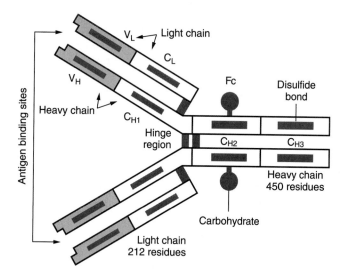

V_L and V_H = Variable regions
C_L and C_H = Constant regions

FIGURE 6-2 Basic structure of immunoglobulin G. *(Modified from Turgeon ML: Fundamentals of immunohematology, ed 2, Baltimore, 1995, Williams & Wilkins.)*

- Hinge region
  - Area that gives molecule flexibility allowing for multiple binding sites
  - Located between the C_H^1 and C_H^2 domains
  - Enzyme papain cleaves the antibody molecule above the hinge region
    - Leaves three fragments: Two Fab fragments and one Fc
  - Enzyme pepsin cleaves the antibody molecule below the hinge region
    - Leaves one $F(ab)_2$ (capable of binding antigen)
    - Fc fragment is destroyed (Table 6-3)
- IgM: Large macroglobulin, first immunoglobulin produced in the primary immune response
- IgG: Predominant immunoglobulin in the body, primary immunoglobulin in the secondary immune response

- IgA: Primary protective antibody in secretions and intestinal mucosa
- IgE: Primary antibody in allergic responses, able to bind basophils and mast cells
- IgD: Unknown function but may play a role as B-cell signaler and/or coreceptor

Antigens and Immunogens

- Antigen: Foreign particles that may elicit an immune response
- Immunogen: Any foreign particle that elicits an immune response
- All immunogens are antigens, but not all antigens are immunogens
- Traits that make good immunogens
  - Large molecular weight
  - Chemical complexity: The higher the complexity, or variety of makeup, the more immunogenic
- Foreignness
- Stability: The ability for the immunogen to be digested and processed is greater if it is less stable
- Proteins make good immunogens because of their complexity
- Carbohydrates such as glycolipids or glycoproteins are less immunogenic because they consist of fewer molecules and are of lesser complexity
- Epitopes: Sites of the antigen that can vary
  - Different epitopes of the same antigen causes polyclonal immune response
- Recognition of epitopes differs for B- or T-cell activation
  - B-cell activation: Epitopes are capable of cross-linking with immunoglobulin
  - T-cell activation: Immunogen epitope is presented to the T cell in the form of MHC proteins (see later discussion)
- Haptens
  - Small molecules considered nonimmunogenic by themselves

TABLE 6-3	Summary of Immunoglobulin Structure and Function				
Feature	IgA	IgD	IgE	IgG	IgM
Structure (monomer, dimer or pentamer, include subunits)	Monomer and dimer with J chain	Monomer	Monomer	Monomer	Pentamer with J chain
Subclasses	2 (α_1, α_2)	None	None	γ1-4	None
Found in	Secretions (saliva, tears, breast milk), intestinal fluids, and serum	On surface of B cells	Blood	Blood: Intravascular and extravascular spaces	Blood: Intravascular spaces
Summary of biologic activity	In secretions it protects against foreign antigens	Basically unknown, but thought to play a role in antigen binding in association with IgM and B-cell activation	Binds to mast cells and basophils mediating release of histamine and heparin Plays a role in helminth infections	Neutralize toxins, activates complement, crosses placenta, agglutination, opsonization	Complement activation and agglutination

- Are immunogenic when coupled with a larger molecule to produce an immune response
- Can react with specific antibody alone, but cannot produce a visible reaction such as precipitation or agglutination
- When coupled with a carrier, can react with antibody and produce a visible reaction

IMMUNE RESPONSE TO ANTIGEN

- Primary response
  - After exposure to antigen a lag phase occurs
  - IgM is typically first antibody produced
  - IgG secretion begins shortly after IgM
  - Both levels decline after antigen has been eliminated
- Secondary or anamnestic response
  - After second exposure to same antigen
  - More rapid response because of activation of memory B cells
  - Rapid rise in levels of antigen-specific IgG antibody
  - Some IgM may be produced but in lesser quantities in comparison to levels of IgG
- Antibody responses are typically polyclonal—that is, the antibody response is directed against more than one epitope of the specific antigen
- Monoclonal antibodies are produced artificially by hybrid cell lines called hybridomas. The myeloma fused cell lines produce antibody from a single clone and are used in a variety of immunologic arrays

Major Histocompatibility Complex

- Main function is to present antigen, or digested antigen molecules, to T cells for activation
- Class I MHC
  - On all nucleated cells in the body
  - Presents endogenous antigens (antigens inside infected cells) to CD8+ cytotoxic T cells
  - Endogenous antigens are those made in the infected cells, such as proteins and molecules synthesized from viruses
  - For protection against viruses and parasites
  - Tumor cells and some viruses cause a disruption to the creation of MHC class molecules from forming on the surface, decreasing the cytotoxic effect of CD8+ cells
  - These MHC class I–deficient diseased cells trigger and activate NK cells
- Class II MHC
  - Mainly on antigen-presenting cells: B cells, monocytes, macrophages, and dendritic cells
  - These cells predominantly take up exogenous antigens or antigens that exist outside the host cell and are engulfed by phagocytosis
  - Presentation is to CD4+ helper T cells for production of cytokines that enhance the production and secretion of antibody from B cells
  - For protection against bacteria, viruses, and other exogenous antigens

ANTIGEN–ANTIBODY REACTIONS AND BASIC PRINCIPLES

- Affinity: Force between a one-Fab site on the immunoglobulin and one epitope of the antigen
- Avidity: Total of all forces between the immunoglobulin and epitopes of the antigen
- Zone of equivalence: Area where antigen and antibody are approximately equal and visualization of the reaction is optimized by either precipitation or agglutination
- Lattice formation: Antigen and antibody together in approximately equal proportions, the immunoglobulin molecules cross-link with the specific antigen
- Precipitation: Visible reaction between antibody and soluble antigen
- Agglutination: Visible reaction between antibody and particulate antigen
- Prozone phenomenon: Concentration of antibody exceeds that of the antigen in solution, and lattice formation does not happen
- Postzone phenomenon: Concentration of antigen is in excess and lattice formation does not occur
- Both prozone and postzone can cause false-negative serologic reactions and erroneous titer results

PRECIPITATION TESTS AND ASSAYS

- Nephelometry: Measures the amount of light scattered in a solution containing antibody–antigen complexes
  - Can be used to measure both antibody and antigen
  - Is widely used to quantify immunoglobulins
- Turbidimetry: Measures the decrease in light intensity in a solution of antibody–antigen complexes
  - The lower the light intensity, the higher the concentration of complexes
- Radial immunodiffusion: Gel containing antibody with cut small holes as wells
  - Sample containing the antigen is placed in the well
  - Line of precipitation forms in a circle around the well
  - Diameter of the circle is proportionate to the concentration of antigen in the sample
- Ouchterlony diffusion
  - Wells are cut in gel with multivalent antibody is placed in a center well and antigen in remaining wells
  - Precipitation lines that form will identify relationship between antigens
  - No identity: Precipitation lines formed will crisscross, as an X, indicating no identity between antigens
  - Partial identity: Precipitation lines formed will appear partially crossed, as a line with a spur on the end, indicating cross reactivity between the antigens
  - Identity: Precipitation lines meet but do not cross, no spurs, indicating no relationship between the antigens
- Rocket electrophoresis
  - Antibody in gel and antigen pipetted into a cutout well
  - Electrical current is applied and resulting precipitation lines form narrow triangles, like a rocket

- The rocket lines are formed as antigen concentration decreases
- Immunoelectrophoresis: Simple, two-step assay
  - Serum, containing antigen, is placed in wells and electrophoresed to separate proteins
  - The second step involves adding antibody in troughs cut in the gel alongside the electrophoresis trail
  - The antigen and antibody are allowed to diffuse
  - The location, shape, and intensity of the precipitation lines are measured
  - Used to measure many serum proteins
- Immunofixation electrophoresis
  - Sample containing antigen is placed in a well and electrophoresed, separating proteins
  - Reagent antibody on a cellulose or agarose gel template is placed over the electrophoresed sample
  - Reactions between antibody and antigen occur and are made visible by staining
- Electrophoretic errors can occur when current is too strong or too weak, current is applied backward, buffer is not at correct pH, or time to run is too long or too short

AGGLUTINATION TESTS AND ASSAYS

- Agglutination is the visible reaction of antibody with particulate antigen
- Particulates in agglutination can be synthetic latex beads or organic red blood cells (RBCs)
- Two steps to agglutination: Sensitization and lattice formation
  - Sensitization occurs when the antibody and specific antigen (on the surface of the particulate) combine
    - The size and class of the antibody and the nature of the antigen epitope can affect this step
  - Lattice formation occurs when antibody–antigen complexes cross-link
  - The particulates must be somewhat neutral in charge for the complexes to link
  - RBCs carry a net negative charge that acts as a repellent (zeta potential)
    - Low ionic strength saline or albumin is used to lower the zeta potential (enhance the lattice formation when RBCs are used as the particulate)
  - This stage is influenced by ionic strength of solution, pH, and temperature
- Latex agglutination
  - Use latex beads (as the particulate) coated with antigen to directly agglutinate patient serum containing specific antibody
- Agglutination inhibition
  - Assays based on the principle of no agglutination as a positive result
  - Serum (containing antigen) is mixed with beads coated with antigen
  - If agglutination occurs, the antigen is *not* present

- Hemagglutination
  - Assays that use RBCs as the antigen particulate reacting with antibody
  - Reactions can occur either in vivo or in vitro depending on the test
  - Direct antiglobulin test (DAT) identifies in vivo reactions of RBC antigen with specific antibody
  - Indirect antiglobulin test (IAT) identifies reactions of reagent RBC antigen with specific antibody when the reaction occurs in vitro

OTHER IMMUNOASSAYS

- Noncompetitive assay
  - Capture or sandwich assays
  - Antibody is bound to solid phase and allowed to react with patient sample containing antigen
  - Amount of reactivity is proportional to concentration of antigen
- Competitive assays
  - Labeled antigen and patient antigen are mixed with antibody at the same time
  - Antigens compete for the limited amount of antibody binding sites
  - Concentration of bound label is inversely proportional to concentration of antigen in the sample
- Multiple detection methods for these assays
  - Use of radioisotopes (radioimmunoassay)
  - Color reaction from enzyme and substrate (enzyme immunoassay [EIA])
- Heterogeneous assays: Those that require a step to separate bound and free analyte
- Homogenous assays: Those that do not require a separation step
- Direct fluorescent assays
  - Antibody tagged with a fluorescent dye to react directly with patient specimen containing antigen
  - Typically prepared on a slide and viewed under a fluorescent microscope
- Indirect fluorescent assays (IFAs) are two-step assays
  - Patient serum is incubated with known antigen
  - Antihuman globulin tagged with fluorescent dye is added
- Chemiluminescence assays
  - Light is produced during a chemical reaction and measured
  - Used widely in immunochemical instrumentation
- Serologic assays
  - Technique called a titer to semiquantitate antibody levels in serum
    - Titers are performed using serial dilutions (see discussion of serial dilutions in Chapter 11)
    - Titer results are used to evaluate immunity in terms of exposure, acute phase, or convalescence of an organism or disease
    - When comparing initial titer results to subsequent or convalescent titer results for the same antibody and same patient, a result of more than fourfold or two-tube difference is considered diagnostic
    - Titers are generally not performed on infant samples because it is not known if the antibody was produced by the infant or is of maternal origin

INFECTIOUS DISEASES AND SEROLOGY

Bacteria

- Bacteria evade host defenses by avoiding phagocytosis and inactivating or blocking complement
- Streptococci
  - Bacteria divided into serotypes based on the M and T proteins in the cell wall
  - Some streptococci possess a hyaluronic acid capsule that helps the organism evade phagocytosis
  - Beneath the cell wall is a carbohydrate that is divided further into Lancefield groups A to H and K to V
  - The main virulence factor of group A streptococci is the M protein, which helps the organism evade phagocytosis and inactivates complement
  - Other virulence factors include exoantigens produced by the organism during the infection
  - The most common exoantigens tested for include DNase B and streptolysin O
  - Acute pharyngitis is typically detected by a throat swab and culture
  - Throat swabs chemically or enzymatically remove antigen and are tested by a rapid enzyme assay or agglutination
  - Anti–streptolysin O (ASO) titers may be performed if rheumatic fever is suspected
    - In a traditional ASO titer, the patient sample containing ASO inhibits red blood cell lysis
    - In a serial dilution, a titer is determined
    - A high titer indicates a recent infection and declines to a low titer later in the infection, but can remain positive
  - Anti–DNase B titers are useful in poststreptococcal glomerulonephritis and skin infections
- Most bacteria or bacterial infections are identified by culture, polymerase chain reaction (PCR) testing, and/or serologic tests

Rickettsia

- Suspected rickettsial infections are detected primarily by serologic test using immunofluorescence, EIAs, and molecular techniques
- Weil-Felix test
  - An agglutination test that detects antibodies in patients with rickettsial infections
  - Antibodies cross react with antigens present on certain strains of *Proteus* spp.

Parasites

- Parasites evade hosts by
  - Living within host cells to avoid the immune response
  - Can change surface antigens to confuse the host's immune response
  - Acquire host's antigens, masking themselves as self-antigens
- Immunologic response to parasites include the production of cytokines to induce
  - Migration of cytotoxic cells
  - Proliferation and concentration of neutrophils and macrophages
  - Antibody production
- IgE and mast cells activate eosinophils to release the contents of cellular granules

Spirochetes

Syphilis

- Causative organism: *Treponema pallidum*
- Four stages of syphilis
  - Primary stage
    - Characterized by a chancre
  - Secondary stage of syphilis
    - Characterized by lymphadenopathy, rash, fever, and pharyngitis
  - Latent stage
    - Characterized by *no* symptoms of the disease
  - Tertiary stage
    - Seen later in the disease with cardiac and nervous system involvement
- Nontreponemal tests for syphilis:
  - Rapid plasma reagin (RPR)
    - Reagents contain charcoal, which allows for macroscopic visualization
  - The Venereal Disease Research Laboratory (VDRL) test is viewed under a microscope and interpreted microscopically
    - A positive VDRL result obtained using spinal fluid is indicative of neurosyphilis
- Both RPR and VDRL detect reagin in patient's serum
  - Reagin is an antibody formed against material from cells damaged by the spirochete
- A positive nontreponemal result must be confirmed with a test to directly detect treponemal organisms
  - Fluorescent treponemal antibody absorption test (FTA-ABS)
  - *T. pallidum* microhemagglutination assay (MHA-TP)
  - Darkfield microscopy
  - EIAs used to detect antibodies to the treponemal spirochete
- Congenital syphilis
  - Spirochete is transmitted from mother to fetus
  - Difficult to detect serologically because when using a test that detects an IgG antibody, it is not known if the antibody is passively acquired from the mother or is from the infant
  - Best to use a test that detects IgM antibodies (EIA or Western blot)
  - Detection of IgM antibodies in an infant is an indication that the antibodies are produced by the infant's immune system

Lyme disease

- Vector-borne illness, typically carried by a tick
- Caused by the spirochete *Borrelia burgdorferi*
- Symptoms
  - Rash, initially localized known as erythema migrans (bulls' eye or target)
  - Joint involvement
  - Neurologic and heart involvement if left untreated
    - A classic sign of neurologic involvement includes facial palsy
  - Early clinical symptoms are most useful in early diagnosis of Lyme disease
- Early serologic tests are not useful
  - Antibody response to Lyme disease does not occur for approximately 3 to 6 weeks
  - IgM and IgG response in Lyme disease is somewhat atypical
    - Both antibody responses, when detected, can be detected together
  - When patient diagnosis occurs early and antibiotic treatment has begun, serologic findings may be limited
- Centers for Disease Control and Prevention recommends specific algorithm for laboratory diagnosis of Lyme disease
  - First step - test patient serum using IFA or EIA for antibodies as a screening measure
  - Second step - confirmation must be made using a Western blot test (because of cross reactivity using these tests)

Viruses

- Innate, humoral, and cell-mediated defenses protect against viruses
  - Cells infected by virus produce interferon, which enhances activity of NK cells
  - Antibodies produced and involved in
    - Viral neutralization
    - ADCC
    - Activation of complement
- Ways viruses avoid the immune system
  - Fast replication: Evolve and mutate quickly
  - Alter the function of immune system cell by inserting their genetic material into a host cell
- TORCH testing is a panel of serologic procedures used to detect a group of viruses and other organisms that cause congenital disease
  - Toxoplasma
  - Other (viruses)

- Rubella
- Cytomegalovirus (CMV)
- Herpes simplex virus

Herpesviridae Family of Viruses
Epstein-Barr Virus
- Most common infection is infectious mononucleosis (IM)
- Infects B cells that produce different types of antibodies
  - Virus-specific antibodies
    - Anti-VCA (viral capsid antigen)
    - Anti–EA-D (early antigen diffuse)
  - Both IgM anti–EA-D and anti-VCA indicates acute infection
  - IgG anti-VCA may persist for life, so may represent a past infection
  - Anti-EBNA (EBV nuclear antigens)
    - Anti-EBNA may indicate the convalescent phase of the infection
- Heterophile antibodies
  - In approximately 90% of patients with infectious mononucleosis
  - React with similar antigens from unrelated species
  - Infectious mononucleosis heterophile antibodies can react with sheep, bovine, and horse RBCs
  - Testing for heterophile antibodies is a screening test
  - Should test for specific viral antibodies if patient has clinical symptoms and negative screening test
- Autoantibodies can be produced

Cytomegalovirus (CMV)
- Population at risk
  - Transplant patients
  - Immunocompromised
  - Newborns
  - Up to 80% of people and infants with CMV are asymptomatic
  - Can be diagnosed with viral culture, PCR, and antibody tests for IgM or IgG
  - Presence of IgM indicates new or reactivation of infection

Herpes Simplex 1 and 2
- Cause sores on and around the mouth and genital areas
- Can be passed congenitally to infant
- If untreated, progresses to disseminated disease
  - Can be fatal for infant
- Serology: Currently only method approved by U.S. Food and Drug Administration for diagnosing herpes simplex virus infections

Varicella-Zoster
- Initial disease is chickenpox
- Causes a rash that blisters and forms scabs in recovery
- Severe cases can lead to varicella-zoster pneumonia
- After initial infection, virus lies dormant
  - Possible reactivation years later as shingles
- Diagnosis is made by testing for antigen (virus) by immunofluorescence
- Antibody testing: Rise in antibody titer using two specimens weeks apart is diagnostic

Rubella
- Togaviridae family
- Also known as German measles
- Causes systemic rash in children
- Severe complications if congenital
- Vaccination to rubella is important in reducing the number of infants born with congenital rubella
- Antibody titers are performed to determine immunity
  - Titers are compared to a standard provided by the manufacture of the test kit

Rubeola
- Not to be confused with rubella
- Also known as measles
- Caused by a virus in the Paramyxoviridae family
- Diagnosis is made typically by EIA for IgM antibody or rise in titer in subsequent specimens from the same patient

West Nile Virus
- A flavivirus
- Causes respiratory illness with possible encephalitis and fatality
- Fastest diagnosis is through serologic testing for IgM or IgG in the cerebrospinal fluid, if nervous system involvement is suspected

Hepatitis
- Hepatitis A (HAV)
  - Picornaviridae family
  - Contracted through the fecal-oral route
  - Is limiting
    - Does not cause reinfection
    - Does not progress to a chronic stage
  - Diagnosis is made by EIA for antibody
  - IgM anti-HAV indicates initial infection
  - HAV antigen testing performed on fecal specimens
  - Testing for IgG anti-HAV: Recovery or immunity to the virus
- Hepatitis E (HEV)
  - Hepeviridae family
  - Transmitted through fecal-oral route
  - Typically limiting, with very few cases becoming severe
  - Diagnosis is by serologic testing for anti-HEV
- Hepatitis B (HBV)
  - Hepadnaviridae virus family
  - Transmitted parenterally (through contact with blood and body fluids)
  - Diagnosis by serologic testing for the HBV antigen or antibody markers
  - Hepatitis B surface antigen (HBsAg): First marker to appear
  - Hepatitis E antigen (HBeAg): Also positive in the early stages
  - Both HBsAg and HBeAg
    - Present during the chronic/carrier state of the disease
    - Patients with chronic HBV may be asymptomatic

TABLE 6-4	Hepatitis B Serology	
Hepatitis B Infection Stage	**Marker**	**Positive or Negative**
Acute	HBsAG	Positive
Acute	Anti-HBc, IgM	Positive
Chronic	Anti-HBc, Total (IgM and IgG)	Positive
Chronic	Anti-HBs	Negative (no recovery)
Chronic	HBeAg	Positive
Recovery	HBeAg	Negative
Recovery	Anti-HBs	Positive
After vaccination	Anti-HBs	Positive
After vaccination	Anti-HBc	Negative
Carrier	HBsAG	Positive
Carrier	Anti-HBc	Positive (IgG)

HBc, Hepatitis B core (antigen); *HBs*, hepatitis B surface (antigen); *HBeAg*, hepatitis E antigen; *HBsAg*, hepatitis B surface antigen; *Ig (G, M)*, immunoglobulin.

- Presence of both indicates a highly infectious state and viral replication
- Anti-HBc, antibody to the viral core
  - First antibody to be produced and detected
  - IgM anti-HBc indicates a recent acute infection
  - Total anti-HBc, IgM, and IgG indicates a past or current infection
  - IgM levels of anti-HBc may decrease, but IgG anti-HBc remains positive for life
- Anti-HBe, antibodies to HBeAg
  - Produced after the disappearance of antibodies
  - Indicates beginning of recovery
- Anti-HBs, antibodies to HBsAg
  - Appear after the disappearance of HBsAg
  - An indicator of recovery and immunity to HBV
  - Anti-HBs is the antibody produced after vaccination (Table 6-4)
- Hepatitis D (HDV)
  - Also known as the δ virus
  - Is transmitted parenterally
  - Only present in coexistence with HBV
  - Identified serologically by testing for anti-HDV or RNA testing
- Hepatitis C (HCV)
  - Flaviviridae family
  - Transmitted through contact with contaminated blood and body fluids
  - Diagnosis: Detection of anti-HCV antibodies followed by a confirmatory test for HCV RNA

Human Immune Deficiency Virus
- Retroviridae family
- Transmitted
  - Contact with contaminated blood/body fluids
  - Sexual contact
  - Mother to infant

- Intracellular virus uses host cell machinery to replicate
- Host cells are CD4+ T-helper lymphocytes
- Serologic testing includes testing for anti-HIV, HIV antigen, and viral nucleic acid
  - Enzyme-linked immunosorbent assay (ELISA) used to detect anti-HIV
    - Positive samples are tested in triplicate
    - If two of three samples are reactive with ELISA, confirmatory testing is required
  - Confirmatory testing with Western blot
    - Positive: Two of three HIV protein bands (p24, gp41, gp120/gp160) are present
    - Indeterminate: Present protein bands do not meet the standard for positive
      - Specimens should be recollected at a later date and retested
      - These patients could be in the early stages of the disease
- CD4 cell counts are measured frequently for effectiveness of treatment
- Molecular testing: Recent and quantitative tests to determine viral load

AUTOIMMUNE DISEASES IN IMMUNOLOGY
- Autoimmunity
  - Body produces antibody to self-components, such as proteins, hormones, and cellular components such as DNA
  - Systemic
  - Organ-specific

Systemic Lupus Erythematosus
- Immune complex autoimmune disease
- Autoantibodies produced to intracellular components of dying cells
  - Cellular DNA
  - RNA
  - Other intracellular constituents
- Immune complexes are deposited in joints and major organs
- Complement deficiency is also seen
  - Complement is continuously activated and used to help clear these immune complexes
- Autoantibodies formed in response to cellular breakdown
  - Anti-dsDNA: Anti–double-stranded DNA
  - Anti-ssDNA: Anti–single-stranded DNA
  - Anti-ENA: Anti–extractable nuclear antigen
  - Antihistones
  - Anti-DNP (DNA coupled with histone)
  - Anti-Sm: Anti-Smith antibody
- Anti-dsDNA is most specific for systemic lupus erythematosus (SLE)

- Anti-Sm is seen only in SLE, but only a small percentage of patients are positive for this autoantibody
- The other autoantibodies, as well as anti–SS-A and anti–SS-B can be found in other autoimmune diseases
- Antinuclear antibody (ANA) test
  - Characteristic laboratory test for these SLE autoantibodies
  - IFA staining of cells
  - Specific staining patterns are characteristic of certain diseases
    - Homogenous or diffuse staining
      - Characteristic of SLE
      - Pattern is staining of the whole nucleus
      - Indicates presence of anti-dsDNA, anti–dinitrophenyl antibody (anti-DNP), and antihistones
      - Peripheral or rim pattern
    - Presence of anti-dsDNA
    - Suggestive of SLE
      - Speckled pattern
    - Anti-Sm, anti-ENA, anti–SS-A, and anti–SS-B
    - Associated diseases are SLE, Sjögren's syndrome, and other mixed connective tissue disease
      - Nucleolar
    - Staining of the nucleolus
    - Associated with anti–nucleolar RNA in SLE and scleroderma

Rheumatoid Arthritis

- Systemic autoimmune disease
- Immune complexes deposit in the joints, activate complement and continuous inflammation
- Characteristic rheumatoid factor (RF)
  - IgM autoantibody produced
  - Autoantibody against the FC portion of IgG
  - The majority of patients with rheumatoid arthritis (RA) are positive for RF
  - RF factor is not specific for RA
    - RF factor can be positive in other diseases
- Agglutination tests for RF are indicative of RA
- Anti–cyclic citrullinated peptides (anti-CCP) autoantibodies are also assayed in RA
  - Present in the majority of patients with RA
  - Rarely seen in patients without RA
- Monitor RA
  - C-reactive protein (CRP)
  - Complement levels
  - Both are markers of inflammation

Organ-Specific Autoimmune Diseases

Hashimoto's Thyroiditis
- Autoantibodies to thyroglobulin
- Results in hypothyroidism

Grave's Disease
- Autoantibody to the thyroid-stimulating hormone (TSH) receptor on the thyroid
- Hyperthyroid

Type I Diabetes Mellitus
- Autoantibodies to islet cells of the pancreas
- Autoantibodies to the enzyme glutamic acid decarboxylase

Other Autoimmune Diseases
- Multiple sclerosis
- Myasthenia gravis
- Goodpasture's syndrome
- Celiac disease

IMMUNOPROLIFERATIVE DISEASES

Leukemia

- Malignancy arises in the bone marrow or peripheral blood
- Classification
  - Acute
  - Chronic
  - Myeloid
  - Lymphoid

Lymphoma

- Malignancy is in the lymphoid tissue
- Classification
  - Hodgkin's: Classic Reed-Sternberg cells
  - Non-Hodgkin's: Cancerous cells are mostly B cell

Plasma Cell Dyscrasias

Multiple Myeloma
- Malignant plasma cells produce monoclonal immunoglobulin
- Serum protein electrophoresis shows increase in γ region with monoclonal spike (M spike)
- Monoclonal immunoglobulin is commonly IgG but can be IgA
- Bence Jones protein in urine: Free immunoglobulin light chains
- Testing for light chains in serum may be more sensitive
  - Light chains are rapidly absorbed by kidneys for secretion
  - Urine levels may be undetectable before serum levels
- Free light chains in disease
  - Produced during maturation of B cells and plasma cells
  - B cell tumors, diseases, and inflammatory responses yield light chains in serum
  - Aids in diagnosis and disease monitoring/progression

Waldenström's Macroglobulinemia

- Malignancy of IgM-producing lymphocytes
- Serum protein electrophoresis indicates elevated levels of γ region
- Concentration of IgM antibody is confirmed using immunofixation

Monoclonal Gammopathy of Unknown Significance

- Disorder with a monoclonal immunoglobulin in serum
- No clinical manifestations of myeloma or macroglobulinemia
- Small percent of patients progress to multiple myeloma or Waldenström's macroglobulinemia

IMMUNODEFICIENT DISEASES

Transient Hypogammaglobulinemia of Infancy

- Condition occurs during the newborn's first year
- After circulating passive maternal antibodies disappear
- Some infants' immunoglobulins are not produced early enough
- Low levels of immunoglobulin persist
- May acquire infections
- Test low for IgG antibodies initially
- Later testing shows increased levels of immunoglobulin

Common Variable Immunodeficiency

- Onset in early adulthood
- Can be either congenital or acquired
- Usually identified after recurrent severe infections
- B-cell levels appear normal but do mature to plasma cells
- No to low immunoglobulin production
- Common variable immunodeficiency remains for life, with increased risk for other immunologic diseases

X-Linked Agammaglobulinemia (Bruton's Agammaglobulinemia)

- X-linked inherited condition affecting males
- Early diagnosis as a result of recurrent infections as infants
- Genetically linked to the lack of Bruton's tyrosine kinase enzyme necessary for B-cell maturation
- B cells are not detectable, but T cells have been demonstrated to be normal

DiGeorge's Syndrome

- Genetic deletion resulting in abnormal development of the thymus
- T- cell function is normal
- T-cell levels are low to nondetectable
- Results in recurrent infections
- Associated with additional bone, facial, and cardiac abnormalities

Severe Combined Immunodeficiency

- Several genetic causes
  - Autosomal recessive
  - X-linked
- Variety of molecular defects resulting in enzyme deficiencies
- Both T-cell and B-cell development is affected
- Identified in infancy
- Patients are very susceptible to infections from all organisms
- Bone marrow transplantation is the traditional therapy
- Gene therapy has been used

Chronic Granulomatous Disease

- Inherited disease-effecting neutrophil phagocytic function
- Defective enzyme nicotinamide adenine dinucleotide phosphate (NADPH) oxidase
  - Enzyme necessary for production of cellular hydrogen peroxide
  - Hydrogen peroxide essential for the oxidative burst and microbicidal effect on catalase-positive organisms
  - No enzyme results in no production of hydrogen peroxide, with little to no oxidative burst
- Traditional test is the nitroblue tetrazolium test
  - Measures the oxidative reduction capability
  - Produces blue color if positive
  - If no enzyme, test result is negative or no color
- Flow cytometry can now be used to identify neutrophils that lack the capability of producing the oxidative burst

Leukocyte Adhesion Deficiency

- Genetic defect
- Results in a defective molecule (β-integrin)
- Necessary for the adherence of leukocytes to endothelium
- Leukocytes/phagocytes cannot move through membranes into extravascular spaces
- Prolonged wound healing and skin and respiratory infections

Complement Deficiencies

- MAC or C5-9 deficiencies are associated with recurrent *Neisseria* infections.
- Early complement-component deficiencies
  - C1qrs, C2, and C4, are associated with a lupus-like syndrome

- Immune complexes fail to be cleared and are deposited in joints and tissue
- C1-Inhibitor (C1-INH) deficiency
  - Hereditary angioedema
  - Characterized by swelling and rash

HYPERSENSITIVITY

Type 1

- Immediate hypersensitivity reactions
- Also known as anaphylactic reactions
- Immune mediator is IgE
- Cellular involvement includes basophils and mast cells
- Production of IgE that binds to basophils and mast cells
- Cross-linkage occurs between two or more IgE antibodies and the basophils and/or mast cells
- Chemical meditators are released into the bloodstream, causing the clinical symptoms
- Examples of type I hypersensitivity
  - Urticaria
  - Hay fever
  - Asthma
  - Anaphylactic reactions to bee stings, venom, peanut allergies
- Direct inoculation of small amounts of allergen subcutaneously used to determine an individual's sensitivity to certain allergens
- Laboratory testing
  - Testing for total IgE by the radioimmunosorbent test
  - Allergen-specific IgE by the radioallergosorbent test
  - Newer methods use the chemiluminescence format to test for IgE

Type II

- Cytotoxic reactions mediated by IgG and IgM and complement
- Cells destroyed by
  - Phagocytosis
  - Direct cytotoxic effects of complement triggered by antibody coating of cells
  - Macrophages, neutrophils, and NK cells contribute to cell damage
- Examples
  - Transfusion reactions
  - Hemolytic disease of the fetus and newborn
  - Hemolytic anemia
  - Goodpasture's syndrome
- Testing
  - DAT
    - Detects in vivo binding of antibody or complement to RBCs

Type III

- Immune complex destruction
  - Soluble antigen by IgG or IgM and complement

- Precipitate out of the serum
- Deposit in tissue that mediates the involvement of complement
- Examples
  - Serum sickness (systemic)
  - Arthus reaction (localized)
- Laboratory testing
  - Testing for specific disease
  - Certain autoimmune disease reactions are considered as type III
    - SLE
    - RA

Type IV

- Delayed hypersensitivity
- Involves T-helper cells and cytotoxic T cells
- Symptoms appear several days to weeks after exposure
- Cytotoxic T cells and cytokines produced by T-helper cells
  - Cause inflammation
  - Tissue damage at the site of allergen contact
- Examples
  - Contact dermatitis
    - Jewelry and latex
    - Poison ivy
    - Farmer's lung
    - Skin test for *Mycobacterium tuberculosis*
      - Exposure to *M. tuberculosis* involves a T-cell–mediated response

TUMOR IMMUNOLOGY

- Tumor immunity: Evidence that tumors are eradicated
  - Tumor-infiltrating lymphocytes
  - NK cells via loss of MHC class I molecules on defective cells
  - Antibodies
  - Cytokines
    - Tumor necrosis factor (TNF) is toxic to some tumors
- Evasion of host immunity by tumors
  - Tumor cells do not produce warning signals for innate system
    - Failure of T-cell responses
  - Certain tumor cells have decreased MHC class I molecules
  - Rapidly dividing tumor cells can acquire and share antigens with normal tissue
- Tumor antigens/markers
  - Tumor-specific antigens are produced by tumor
  - Tumor-associated antigens are surface molecules of virally infected cells
  - Used in laboratory testing
    - Aid diagnosis or staging of cancer
    - Monitor recurrence
    - Help determine prognosis and treatment
    - Screening in normal population (Table 6-5)

TABLE 6-5 Selected Tumor Markers and Associated Cancers

Tumor Markers	Disease Association
CEA (carcinoembryonic antigen)	Colorectal cancer
β-2 Microglobulin	Multiple myeloma
CA125 (carbohydrate antigen 125)	Ovarian cancer
CA15-3	Breast cancer
CA19-9	Pancreas cancer
HER2/neu	Breast cancer
PSA (prostate-specific antigen)	Prostate cancer
ER/PR (estrogen receptor/progesterone receptor)	Breast cancer
AFP (α-fetoprotein)	Liver and testicular cancers

TRANSPLANTATION IMMUNOLOGY

Major Histocompatibility Complex

- Genes on short arm of chromosome 6
- Code for proteins called human leukocyte antigens (HLAs)
  - Class I: HLA-A, HLA-B, HLA-C
    - At the same loci and are inherited together
  - Class II: HLA-DR, HLA-DQ, HLA-DP
  - Mendelian inheritance of haplotypes from each parent
  - These proteins on cell surfaces have destructive effect if transplants occur against HLAs
    - HLA proteins regulate immune response of T cells
    - Will process and present unmatched HLA as foreign
- Transplants
  - Solid organ
    - Must be ABO group compatible
      - Stem cell
      - Bone marrow
      - Autograft: Recipient receives own tissue
      - Syngeneic graft: Recipient receives transplant from identical twin
      - Allograft: Transplant between individuals of same species
      - Xenograft: Transplant between individuals of different species
- Rejection
  - Transplanted cells are recognized as foreign
    - Hyperacute rejection
      - Minutes to hours after transplant
      - Transplants across ABO group barrier
      - Mediated by ABO blood group antibodies
    - Acute
      - Days to weeks after transplant
      - Cytotoxic T-cell–mediated rejection

  - Chronic
    - Months after transplant
    - Cell mediated along with cytokine production that enhances destruction of tissue and transplant
- Graft-versus-host disease
  - Complication in bone marrow and stem cell transplants
  - T cells in transplanted product recognize host cells as foreign
  - Severity is related to HLA match of donor
- Graft-versus-leukemia effect
- Benefit of T cells in transplant: Graft-versus-leukemia effect
  - Promote cellular engraftment
  - Improve immune responses
- Recipients of transplants are
  - HLA typed
  - HLA matched with a donor
  - Cross-matched to rule out preformed antibodies to HLA from donor

CERTIFICATION PREPARATION QUESTIONS

For answers and rationales, please see Appendix A.

1. Natural barriers of the immune system include all except which of the following?
   a. pH of secretions
   b. Coughing
   c. Hair follicles
   d. Intestinal bacteria

2. The fundamental difference between primary and secondary organs of the lymphatic system is:
   a. Antibody production occurs only in the primary lymph organs
   b. Complement production occurs only in the primary lymph organs
   c. Maturation of lymphocytes occurs in secondary organs, and activation occurs in primary organs
   d. Maturation of lymphocytes occurs in primary organs, and activation occurs in secondary organs

3. Toll-like receptors act in which way?
   a. Enhance recognition of bacteria by phagocytic cells
   b. Activate B cells to produce antibody
   c. Activate helper T cells
   d. Aid in processing antigen in the form of an MHC molecule

4. Neutrophils and monocytes have receptors for which part of the immunoglobulin molecule?
   a. Fc
   b. Fab
   c. Hinge region
   d. Variable region

5. One B-cell marker of early-stage B-cell development is _____, whereas _____ is a marker for later stages of B-cell development.
   a. CD20; CD10
   b. CD21; CD10

c. CD10; CD20
d. CD19; CD10

6. A double-positive T cell would express which markers?
   a. CD4 + CD8 + CD3 +
   b. CD4 − CD8 + CD3 +
   c. CD4 − CD8 − CD3 −
   d. CD4 + CD8-CD3 +

7. Which cell is considered to be a bridge between the innate and adaptive immune systems?
   a. NK cell
   b. Mast cell
   c. Monocyte-macrophage
   d. T cell

8. _____ are involved in cell-mediated immunity, whereas _____ are involved in humoral immunity.
   a. T cells; B cells
   b. T cells; antibodies
   c. B cells; T cells
   d. A and B

9. Antigens that make very good immunogens include which of the following?
   a. Carbohydrates
   b. Proteins
   c. Both a and b
   d. Neither a or b

10. The function of the complement system include(s) which of the following?
    a. Clearance of cellular debris
    b. Chemotaxis
    c. Lysis of bacteria
    d. All of the above

11. When C3 is cleaved by C3 convertase, what is the result?
    a. C3a is released
    b. C3b is used as an opsonin
    c. C3b is combined with other complement proteins to form C5 convertase
    d. All of the above

12. Characteristics of cytokines include which of the following?
    a. They can have a pleomorphic effect
    b. Cytokines are redundant
    c. Cytokines enhance cellular differentiation of lymphocytes
    d. All of the above

13. Immunoglobulin idiotypes are antibodies with variations in the domains of which of the following?
    a. C_H^1 and C_H^2
    b. V_H and V_L
    c. V_H and C_L
    d. C_H^1, C_H^2, and C_H^3

14. Mannose-binding lectin is similar to which component of the classical pathway?
    a. C3
    b. C2
    c. C1q
    d. C5a

15. A patient with a viral infection to the ABC virus is found to have a high antibody titer to the ABC virus's RNA, or anti-ABCr. Which of the following is true?
    a. MHC class I molecules presented antigen to CD4+ T cells
    b. MHC class II molecules presented antigen to CD8+ T cells
    c. MHC class I molecules presented antigen to CD8+ T cells
    d. MHC class II molecules presented antigen to CD4+ T cells

16. What is the main difference between agglutination and precipitation reactions?
    a. Agglutination occurs between a soluble antigen and antibody
    b. Agglutination occurs when the antigen is particulate
    c. Precipitation occurs when the antigen is particulate
    d. Precipitation occurs when both antigen and antibody are particulate

17. Postzone causes false-negative reactions in antibody titers as a result of which of the following?
    a. Too much diluent added to test
    b. Excess antibody in test
    c. Excess antigen in test
    d. Incorrect diluent added to test

18. Antibodies produced against two or more epitopes of specific antigen are considered _____.
    a. Monoclonal
    b. Pleomorphic
    c. Dimorphic
    d. Polyclonal

19. In the radial immunodiffusion test, the gel contains which of the following?
    a. The antigen to be tested
    b. Antibody
    c. Patient sample
    d. None of the above; the gel is the medium to which the antibody and antigen are applied in equal proportion

20. Which statement is true regarding the radial immunodiffusion test?
    a. The area of the precipitin ring is directly proportional to the concentration of antigen in the sample
    b. The area of the precipitin ring is directly proportional to the concentration of antibody in the sample
    c. The area of the precipitin ring is directly proportional to the concentration antibody and the antigen in the sample
    d. The area of the precipitin ring indicates a partial identity to the antibody in the sample

21. The indirect antiglobulin test is for _____, whereas the direct antiglobulin test is for_____.
    a. Serum antigen; bound antigen
    b. Serum antigen; bound antibody
    c. Serum antibody; bound antigen
    d. Serum antibody; bound antibody

22. In an indirect immunofluorescent antibody test for CMV antibodies, the conjugated antibody used for visualizing is:
    a. Antihuman globulin conjugated to a fluorescent dye
    b. Anti-CMV antibody conjugated to a fluorescent dye
    c. CMV virus conjugated to a fluorescent dye
    d. Antihuman globulin conjugated to an enzyme

23. What is the difference between nephlometry and turbidimetry?
    a. There is no difference between the two assays, only in name
    b. Nephlometry is a newer example of turbidimetry
    c. Nephlometry measures light transmitted through a solution, and turbidimetry measures light scattered in a solution
    d. Nephlometry measures light scattered in a solution, and turbidimetry measures light transmitted through a solution

24. In an Ouchterlony immunodiffusion, the line of precipitation between the antibody and the antigen wells forms an X. This reaction would be described as which of the following?
    a. Nonidentity
    b. Partial identity
    c. Identity

25. An initial titer of 4 followed by a subsequent titer of 16 for the same patient, drawn 2 weeks later, is indicative of which of the following?
    a. Infection
    b. Convalescence
    c. Past exposure
    d. No exposure

26. A deficiency of T cells can result in which of the following?
    a. Low levels of complement
    b. Dysfunctional macrophages
    c. Fewer B cells maturing to plasma cells
    d. Contact dermatitis

27. A 2-week-old baby is seen for a possible infection with CMV. Which of the following statements is false?
    a. A positive anti-CMV result from baby's specimen is inconclusive
    b. An initial titer of anti-CMV IgG would need to be established
    c. A positive result for anti-CMV IgM would indicate infection
    d. All are false statements

28. What is the basic difference between the RPR and VDRL tests?
    a. The RPR detects antigen, whereas the VDRL detects antibody
    b. The RPR test is read macroscopically, whereas the VDRL is read microscopically
    c. The RPR test is a treponemal test, whereas the VDRL is nontreponemal
    d. There is no difference because they are both specific tests for syphilis

29. A patient has the following hepatitis B serology:
    HBsAg: Negative
    Anti-HBc: Positive
    Anti-HBS: Positive
    These results are consistent with which of the following?
    a. Acute hepatitis B
    b. Chronic hepatitis B
    c. Recovery from hepatitis B
    d. Acute hepatitis A

30. The HLA genes are inherited as:
    a. Diplotypes: Two diplotypes from each parent
    b. Haplotypes: One haplotype from each parent
    c. HLAs are not inherited, instead are proteins absorbed onto cells
    d. Only the HLA-A antigen is an inheritable trait

31. Agglutination and precipitation that is visible depends on antigen–antibody ratios _____.
    a. With antigen in excess
    b. With antibody in excess
    c. That are equivalent
    d. All of the above

32. Which of the following cell types is implicated in immediate hypersensitivity?
    a. Neutrophil
    b. Mast cell
    c. Macrophage
    d. Monocyte

33. Anti-dsDNA antibodies are associated with which of the following?
    a. Syphilis
    b. CMV infection
    c. Systemic lupus erythematosus
    d. Hemolytic anemia

34. Rheumatoid factor is typically an IgM autoantibody with specificity for which of the following?
    a. SS-B
    b. Double-stranded DNA
    c. Ribonucleoprotein
    d. Fc portion of IgG

35. All of the following are autoimmune diseases except:
    a. Rheumatoid arthritis
    b. Rh disease of the fetus and newborn
    c. Grave's disease
    d. Myasthenia gravis

36. In Grave's disease, one of the main autoantibodies is:
    a. Anti-CCP
    b. Antibody to islet cells of pancreas
    c. Antibody to thyroid-stimulating hormone receptor
    d. Anti-dsDNA

37. An autoantibody found in patients with Hashimoto's thyroiditis reacts with which of the following?
    a. TSH receptor
    b. Islet cells
    c. CRP
    d. Thyroglobulin

38. Skin testing for exposure to tuberculosis is an example of which type of hypersensitivity?
- a. Type I
- b. Type II
- c. Type III
- d. Type IV

39. Which of the following is a test for specific treponemal antibody?
- a. VDRL
- b. RPR
- c. FTA-ABS
- d. All of the above

40. Serum tested positive for HBsAg and anti-HBc IgM. The patient most likely has which of the following?
- a. Acute hepatitis C
- b. Chronic hepatitis B
- c. Acute hepatitis B
- d. Acute hepatitis A

41. The main difference between leukemias and lymphomas is which of the following?
- a. Leukemias are malignancies of cells in the bone marrow
- b. Lymphomas are maligniancies of cells in the bone marrow
- c. Lymphomas are classified as either acute or chronic
- d. Leukemias are malignancies in lymphoid tissue

42. A 1-year-old boy is seen for having many recurrent infections with *Streptococcus pneumoniae*. Laboratory tests revealed a normal quantity of T cells, but no B cells and no immunglobulins were seen on electrophoresis. Which of the following would most likely be the cause?
- a. Chronic granulotomatous disease
- b. Bruton's agammaglobulinemia
- c. DiGeorge's syndrome
- d. Wiskott-Aldrich syndrome

43. A patient with hereditary angiodema has which of the following deficiencies?
- a. C5-9
- b. Phagocytic cell function
- c. Mature B cells
- d. C1 Inhibitor

44. A radiograph of a 1-year-old boy indicates the lack of a thymus. Complete blood count and flow cytometry confirm a below-normal lymphocyte count and a lack of T cells. Which of the following would most likely be the cause?
- a. DiGeorge's syndrome
- b. Wiskott-Aldrich syndrome
- c. Bare lymphocyte syndrome
- d. Bruton's agammaglobulinemia

45. Severe combined immunodeficiency is characterized by which of the following?
- a. Diagnosed in infancy
- b. Shortened life span
- c. No antibody production
- d. All of the above

46. A 3-year-old boy is seen by his physican because of many recent bacterial infections. Flow cytometery indicates normal levels of T and B cells. The nitroblue tetrazolium test for oxidative reduction is negative. The most likely cause is:
- a. Wegener's syndrome
- b. Chronic granulomatous disease
- c. Bruton's agammaglobulinemia
- d. Diabetes mellitus

47. A 25-year-old man was seen by his physican for recurrent infections. Immunoelectrophoresis revealed hypogammaglobulinemia. This man most likely has which of the following?
- a. Bruton's agammaglobulinemia
- b. Common variable immunodeficiency
- c. X-linked agammaglobulinemia
- d. DiGeorge's syndrome

48. In which disease would you expect to see an IgM spike on electrophoresis?
- a. Transient hypogammaglobulinemia of infancy
- b. Wiskott-Aldrich syndrome
- c. Leukocyte adhesion disease
- d. Waldenström's macroglobulinemia

49. A person has an infected bug bite with pain, swelling, and redness. What is the cause of these physical symptoms of inflammation?
- a. Production of antibody
- b. Secondary immune response
- c. Increased blood flow and neutrophils to site
- d. Activation of NK cells

50. The type of graft rejection that occurs within minutes of a tissue transplant is _____.
- a. Acute
- b. Chronic
- c. Hyperacute
- d. Accelerated

BIBLIOGRAPHY

Abbas AK, Lichtman AH: Basic immunology: functions and disorders of the immune system, ed 3, Philadelphia, 2011, Saunders.

Brebner JA, Stockley RA: Polyclonal free light chains: a biomarker of inflammatory disease or treatment target? Retrieved June 2013 from http://f1000.com/prime/reports/m/5/4/.

Coico R, Sunshine G: Immunology: a short course, ed 6, Hoboken, NJ, 2009, John Wiley & Sons.

Male D, Brostoff J, Roth DB, Roitt I: Immunology, ed 8, Philadelphia, 2013, Saunders.

Turgeon ML: Immunology and serology in laboratory medicine, ed 4, St. Louis, 2009, Mosby.

SELF-ASSESSMENT

Content Area: _____

Score on Practice Questions: _____

List the specific topics covered in the missed questions:

List the specific topics covered in the correct questions:

NOTES

7

Immunohematology and Blood Transfusion Medicine

Brenda C. Barnes and Elizabeth G. Hertenstein

BLOOD GROUP ANTIGENS AND ANTIBODIES

- Red blood cells (RBCs) contain surface markers or antigens on their surface or as part of their membranes
- Surface markers are identified as antigens capable of initiating an immune response, which can affect RBC compatibility
- The antigens are either sugars or proteins

ABO Blood Group

See (Box 7-1)

- Described by Karl Landsteiner in 1900
- Most important blood group system: Individuals possess antibodies against antigens they lack
  - If A or B antigen is not present, person will make antibody(ies) against the missing antigen(s)
  - This complementary relationship permits ABO testing of patient sera and RBCs
  - ABO antibodies are naturally occurring, stimulated by nature
  - Production initiated at birth, but titer low until 3 to 6 months of age
- Genetics
  - Antigens in this group exhibit autosomal codominant inheritance
    - One locus on chromosome 9 occupied by one of three alleles: A, B, O
    - Each person has a pair of chromosomes that carry one allele
    - Group O: Silent allele (gene product not detectable)
  - Genes at three separate loci control the presence and location of the A, B, and H antigens: *ABO, Hh,* and *Se* (Figure 7-1)
  - *A* and *B* genes encode glycosyltransferases that produce A and B antigens
    - Genes do not directly encode for the antigen
    - Genes encode for the enzyme that transfers the immunodominant sugar that confers the specificity (see Figure 7-1)
    - *O* gene does not encode a functional enzyme (silent allele—no detectable gene product)
- *H* and *Se* genes
  - *Hh* and *Se* (secretor) are on chromosome 19 and are closely linked
  - Each locus has two recognized alleles, one allele is an amorph
    - *H*: Produces a glycosyltransferase that acts on type 2 chains—H antigen on RBCs
    - *h*: Amorph allele, does not express a detectable product—that is, no glycosyltransferase is produced
    - *Se*: Produces a glycosyltransferase that acts on type 1 chains—H antigen in secretions
    - *se*: Amorph allele
- Bombay phenotypes
  - Genotype *hh* known as Bombay phenotype
  - *hh*: Very rare, does not make transferase to form the H antigen
  - Characteristics
    - Bombay RBCs fail to react with anti-A, anti-B, or anti-H lectin
    - Bombay serum contains anti-A, anti-B, anti-A,B, and Anti-H (potent, reacts strongly at 37° C)
    - Only blood from other Bombay phenotypes can be transfused
- Para-Bombay phenotype
  - Genotype: *hh Se*
  - Normal amount of H antigen is detectable in saliva because these people are secretors
  - May produce a weak anti-H
- Subgroups
  - A subgroups
    - 80% A_1
    - 20% A_2 or weaker
    - Inheritance of A_2 gene: Small amount of H antigen conversion
    - Immunodominant sugars same
    - Differentiation of A_1 and A_2 subgroups based on reactivity with anti-A_1 (lectin *[Dolichos biflorus]* or human-based)
      - A_1 cells react with anti-A_1

H Substance
Large Amount   Least Amount
O > A2B > A2B > A1 > A1B

- A_2 cells do not react with anti-A_1
- Weak A subgroups
  - Show weaker reactivity than A_2
  - 1% population
  - A_3: Mixed-field pattern of agglutination with anti-A
  - A_x: Stronger reaction with anti-A,B than anti-A
  - Weaker subgroups detected only by elution and adsorption of anti-A
- B subgroups
  - Very rare
  - Little consistency in description
  - Usually recognized by variations in strength of reaction with anti-B and anti-A,B
- Antibodies to A and B antigens
  - People typed as A and B generally produce IgM class ABO antibodies
  - Small quantities of IgG are present
  - People typed as O produce IgG class antibodies—anti-A,B
    - Readily crosses the placenta

- Routine ABO testing (Table 7-1)
  - Forward typing or RBC typing
    - Anti-A and anti-B
    - Reagents used are generally monoclonal antibodies
      - Designed to give strong reactions
      - Should see at least a 3+ or greater reaction in the front type when using monoclonal reagents
  - Reverse typing or serum typing
    - A_1 cells and B cells: Reagent cells used for ABO typing are Rh negative
    - Expect to see a 2+ reaction: Anything weaker could be indicative of a serum problem
  - Both are required in patients and donors
    - Serve as a check for each other
  - Nonroutine reagents
    - Anti-A,B
      - Used to aid in classification of subgroups
      - Confirm group O units (retype)
    - A_2 cells
      - Discrepancy resolution
    - Lectins
      - Anti-A_1: *D. biflorus*
      - Anti-H: *Ulex europaeus*
- ABO discrepancy resolution
  - Causes of discrepancies are classified into four groups
  - Weak or missing antigen reactivity: Cell grouping tests

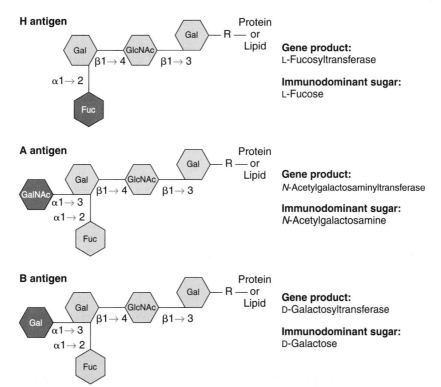

FIGURE 7-1 Biochemical structures of the H, A, and B antigens. *Gal,* D-Galactose; *GlcNAc,* N-acetylglucosamine; *Fuc,* L-fucose; *GalNAc,* N-acetylgalactosamine. *(From Funk MK, Grossman BJ, Hillyer CD, et al, editors: Technical manual, ed 18, Bethesda, MD, 2014, AABB, p 293.)*

TABLE 7-1   ABO Typing Interpretation

Forward Type (Patient Red Blood Cells)		Reverse Type (Patient Serum)		
Anti-A	Anti-B	A_1 Cells	B Cells	Interpretation
0	0	+	+	0
+	0	0	+	A
0	+	+	0	B
+	+	0	0	AB

- ○ Subgroups of A and B
  - ▪ A_3 subgroup
    - ▪ Mixed-field pattern with anti-A from group O or B donors
  - ▪ A_x subgroup
    - ▪ No agglutination with human anti-A from group B donors
    - ▪ Agglutination with anti-A,B from group O donors
    - ▪ May react with monoclonal anti-A
  - ▪ A_{el} subgroup
    - ▪ Not agglutinated by anti-A or anti-A,B of any origin
    - ▪ A antigen demonstrable only by adsorption and elution studies
  - ○ B subgroups: Rare
  - ○ Cis-AB phenotype: Rare chromosome
  - ○ Newborns: Lower number of A and/or B antigen sites
  - ○ Leukemia: Weak expression of A and/or B antigens
  - ○ Mixed-cell populations and chimeras: Review transfusion and transplant history
  - ○ Transfusions are the most common cause of chimerism
  - ○ Excessive blood group substance: Can neutralize reagents
- • Extra antigen reactivity: Cell grouping tests
  - ○ Acquired B
    - ▪ Patient types as AB, but serum contains anti-B
    - ▪ Transient condition associated with disorders of gastrointestinal tract
    - ▪ Certain clones used to make monoclonal anti-B cause strong reactions with acquired B cells
    - ▪ Strength of reactivity weakened with reduced reagent pH
    - ▪ Resolution
      - ▪ Review patient's clinical history and historical blood type
      - ▪ Associated with colonic bacterial infections
      - ▪ Test autocontrol or other acquired B cell
  - ○ Will be negative if patient has acquired B
    - ▪ Test cells with monoclonal anti-B reagent that does not detect acquired B

- ▪ Test RBCs with human anti-B acidified to pH 6.0
- ○ Positive direct antiglobulin test (DAT)
  - ▪ Strongly reactive DAT cells can spontaneously agglutinate with cell grouping reagents
  - ▪ Most often seen with Rh typing reagents
  - ▪ Can occur with ABO reagents if coating antibody is cold-reactive
  - ▪ Resolution
    - ▪ Wash cells with 37° C saline
    - ▪ Incubate patient cell suspension at 37° C and wash with warm saline
    - ▪ Or can elute antibodies from RBCs with chloroquine diphosphate or dithiothreitol (DTT)
- ○ Contaminated cord blood samples
  - ▪ Wharton's jelly is main cause
  - ▪ Resolution
    - ▪ Wash with saline 3 or 4 times, retest
    - ▪ Request heel-stick sample
- ○ Unwashed cell suspensions
  - ▪ Washing can dissipate problems caused by
    - ▪ Patient antibodies to reagent components
    - ▪ Rouleaux formation
- • Weak or missing antibody reactivity: Serum grouping tests
  - ○ Low antibody levels (newborns or older patients)
  - ○ Missing antibodies (immunocompromised patients)
  - ○ Chimeras: Persistent chimeras develop a tolerance to both cell populations—*check patient history!*
  - ○ Subgroups: Cells from A subgroup patients often typed as group O
    - ▪ Titer of anti-A is usually higher than that of anti-B in most group O individuals
    - ▪ Weak reactivity with A_1 cells in group O person should be investigated
    - ▪ Same is true for group B people
    - ▪ May be due to anti-A_1 or other alloantibodies and not by anti-A
    - ▪ Testing panel of A_1, A_2, and O cells can help determine if a discrepancy exists
- • Extra antibody reactivity: Serum grouping tests
  - ○ Rouleaux
    - ▪ Resolution is generally to try saline replacement technique
  - ○ Cold-reactive antibodies (autoantibody or alloantibody)
    - ▪ Mini–cold panel used to aid in resolution
    - ▪ Testing with A_2, O, and autologous cells, in addition to tests with A_1 and B cells can help explain serum discrepancies
  - ○ Passively acquired antibodies: *Check patient transfusion history!*
- • Suggested resolution process for ABO serologic problems
  - ○ Repeat testing on same sample

- ○ Wash patient cells
- ○ Obtain patient information
  - Diagnosis
  - Historical blood group
  - History: Transfusions, transplants, medications
- ○ Review results with group O RBCs and autocontrol
  - Alloantibodies or autoantibodies
- ○ Obtain new sample if contamination is suspected

Rh Blood System

- Genetics
  - Two closely linked genes encode Rh antigens
    - ○ *RHD*: Determines D expression (D or non-D)
    - ○ *RHCE*: Determines C, c, E, e antigens (alleles: *ce, Ce, cE, CE*)
  - Over 50 antigens define system
  - D, C, E, c, e: Most typically discussed (Figure 7-2)
  - Biochemistry
    - ○ Nonglycosylated, transmembrane, integral part of RBC membrane (Figure 7-3)
- D antigen
  - Most clinically significant non-ABO antigen
  - Highly antigenic
  - Described as a "mosaic"
    - ○ Several subparts make up the complete antigen
    - ○ D+individuals usually have all parts
    - ○ D−individuals have no parts of the antigen
  - Weak D antigen
    - ○ Weakened expression of D antigen
    - ○ D antigen reactive *only at antihuman globulin (AHG)*
    - ○ Results from an atypical inheritance at D locus
      - Partial D (mosaic)
      - Position effect (*D* gene inherited *trans* to C gene)
      - Genetic (variant *R⁰* gene in blacks)
    - ○ Testing for weak D
      - Performed at AHG phase, must include a control (must be negative for test to be valid)

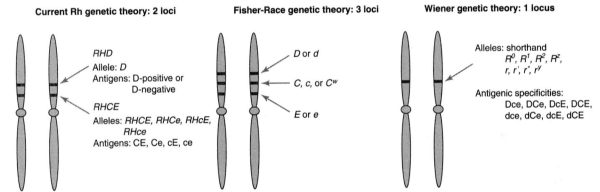

FIGURE 7-2 Comparison of Rh genetic theories. Comparison of three Rh genetic theories that have influenced the nomenclature of the Rh blood group system. Modern molecular techniques have established that the Rh blood group system antigens are determined by two genetic loci. *(From Blaney K: Basic & applied concepts of blood banking and transfusion practices, ed 3, St. Louis, 2012, Mosby.)*

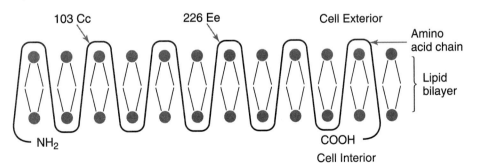

Antigen	Amino acid	Number
C	Serine	103 Cc
c	Proline	103 Cc
E	Proline	226 Ee
e	Alanine	226 Ee

FIGURE 7-3 Model of the Rh polypeptide. Model of the differences in the amino acid sequence for the antigens produced by the *RHCE* gene. The basic structure is similar. Differences in the amino acid at the residue number indicated determine the serologic typing to be C or c, E, or e. *(From Blaney K: Basic & applied concepts of blood banking and transfusion practices, ed 3, St. Louis, 2012, Mosby).*

- Donated units of blood and blood products must have weak D type determined before labeling
  - Transfusion recipients: Typing for weak D not required
  - Obstetric patients: D and weak D type determined in first trimester
  - Infants born to D-negative mothers should be tested for D antigen including weak D
- Rh antibodies
  - Clinically significant (can cause hemolytic disease of the fetus and newborn [HDFN] and hemolytic transfusion reaction [HTR])
  - Immunoglobulin G (IgG), subclass 1 or 3
  - Produced after exposure to foreign RBCs
  - Very immunogenic, especially D
  - Order of immunogenicity: D > c > E > C > e
  - Most react at 37° C and AHG
  - Enhanced by enzymes or high-protein additives
  - Usually do not bind complement
  - May show dosage with a homozygous expression of antigen
  - May occur in concert
    - Anti-c and anti-E
    - Anti-D and anti-G (anti-G reacts with all D-positive and C-positive RBCs)
  - Persist for years and remain detectable
- Rh (D) typing
  - Routine testing is for D antigen only
  - Most testing now performed with licensed monoclonal/polyclonal blend reagents
  - Rh control required if high-protein reagents used
- Unusual phenotypes
  - Rh null
    - Individuals whose RBCs lack all Rh antigens
    - Rh phenotype is −/−
    - Two mechanisms
      - Amorph gene $(r^= r^=)$ at Rh locus
      - Suppressor gene $(X^0 r\ X^0 r)$ at regulator locus
    - Form anti-Rh 29 (total Rh)
  - Rh deletions
    - Rh complexes lacking alleles at Ee or Cc locus
    - D−−/D−− individuals
      - Lack all C and c antigens
      - Lack all E and e antigens
      - Lack many high-incidence Rh antigens
      - Form anti-Rh 17 (anti-Hr$_o$) if exposed to normal RBCs
    - D−− RBCs have greatest amount of D antigen (because all Rh material is converted to D antigen)

Other Blood Group Systems

- Duffy
  - Fy^a and Fy^b: Codominant alleles
  - Most important antigens in Duffy system
  - Antigens well developed at birth

- Duffy antigens do not store well (elute)
  - Destroyed by common enzymes
  - Only moderate immunogens
  - Antibodies
    - IgG class
    - May cause HTRs, HDFN is uncommon
    - Nonreactive in enzyme tests (antigens are degraded by enzymes)
    - May show dosage
  - Miscellaneous
    - 68% of blacks are $Fy(a-b-)$
    - Whites are most commonly $Fy(a+b+)$
- Ii
  - I: High-frequency antigen expressed on adult RBCs
    - Exists on precursor A, B, and H chains
    - Associated with branched chains
  - i: Expressed on newborn or cord cells
    - Not antithetical to I
    - Expressed on linear precursor chains
    - i matures to be I as precursor chains become more branched
  - Antibodies
    - Anti-I is a common IgM autoantibody
    - Enhanced by enzymes
    - May mask clinically significant alloantibodies
- Kell
  - K and k: Codominant alleles
  - Antigens destroyed by sulfhydryl reagents (2-mercaptoethanol [2-ME], DTT, s-[2-aminoethyl] isothiuronium bromide [AET])
  - Antibodies
    - Usually IgG, reactive at AHG
    - Some examples do not react well in a low ionic strength saline (LISS) environment
    - Can show dosage
    - Can cause HTRs and HDFN
  - Miscellaneous
    - K$_o$ cells lack all antigens of the Kell system
    - McLeod phenotype: Depressed Kell system antigens
      - Inherited as X-linked trait
      - Persons have poorly defined abnormality of neuromuscular system
      - Associated with chronic granulomatous disease
- Kidd
  - Jk^a and Jk^b: Codominant alleles
  - Antigens located on RBC urea transporter
  - Antibodies
    - IgG, reactive at AHG
    - Often show dosage
    - Enhanced by enzyme-treated cells
    - May bind complement
    - Do not store well, reactivity can quickly decline in vitro
    - Can cause HDFN, but usually mild
    - HTRs and delayed HTRs because antibody titers can rise and fall quickly in patients

- Lewis
  - Le^a and Le^b: Note that these are not alleles
  - Antigens are not intrinsic to RBCs
  - Only expressed on type I precursor chains, adsorbed onto RBCs
    - Oligosaccharides intrinsic to RBC membrane are all type II
  - Not found on cord cells because Lewis antigens are poorly developed at birth
  - *Le* gene fucosyltranferase attaches fucose in $\alpha(1 \rightarrow 4)$ linkage to the subterminal GlcNAc
    - Le^a antigen
  - *Se* gene fucosyltranferase attaches fucose in $\alpha(1 \rightarrow 2)$ linkage to the terminal Gal
    - Le^b antigen
  - *Le* and *Se* gene interaction
    - *Le* without *Se*
      - Le^a on RBCs and in saliva
    - *Le* and *Se*
      - Le^b on RBCs, Le^a and Le^b in saliva
    - *lele*, secretor status irrelevant
      - Le(a−b−) on RBCs and in saliva
  - *sese*
    - No H in secretions (Figure 7-4)
  - Lewis antibodies
    - Almost always IgM: Do not cross placenta
    - Not associated with HDFN
    - May bind complement
    - Most often room temperature (RT) reactive
    - May be seen at 37° C, but at decreased strength
    - Rarely seen at AHG phase
    - Neutralization techniques may be helpful to confirm presence of Lewis antibody or determine presence of other underlying antibodies

- MNS
  - Complex system of over 40 antigens: M, N, S, s, and U are most important
    - M/N (glycophorin A [GYA]) and S/s (glycophorin B [GYB]) are both codominant alleles
    - U expressed on GYB close to RBC membrane
  - Antibodies
    - Anti-M
      - Saline reactive (RT or lower)
      - Often found in sera of persons with no history of exposure to RBCs
      - IgG or IgM
        - IgG is rarely clinically significant
      - Usually do not bind complement
      - Do not react with enzyme-treated cells
      - Acidic test system may aid detection
      - Demonstrates dosage
      - Common in children and burn patients
      - Rarely causes HTR or HDFN
    - Anti-N
      - Rarely encountered
      - IgM cold-reacting antibody
      - Usually not clinically significant
    - Anti-S and anti-s
      - Usually clinically significant IgG antibodies reactive at 37° C and at AHG phase
      - May/may not react with enzyme-treated cells
      - May bind complement
      - May cause HTR and HDFN
    - Anti-U
      - U is a high-incidence antigen
      - Suspect anti-U in patients who are black and S−s−, whose serum shows an antibody reacting to a high-incidence antigen
- P blood group
  - Contains only P$_1$ antigen
  - Globoside collection: P, P^k, LKE
  - Antigens are "built" on glycolipids, analogous to development of A, B, and H antigens
  - Phenotypes
  - P$_1$
    - RBCs have P$_1$ and P antigens
    - Analogous to A$_1$ subgroup
  - P$_2$
    - RBCs cells have P antigen
    - Analogous to A$_2$ subgroup
  - Antibodies
    - Anti-P$_1$
      - Formed by P$_2$ individuals
      - Naturally occurring
      - Optimal reactivity is at 4° C
      - Almost always IgM
      - Can be neutralized with commercially available P$_1$ substance
    - Anti-P (usually found as an autoantibody)
      - Cold reactive IgG autoantibody

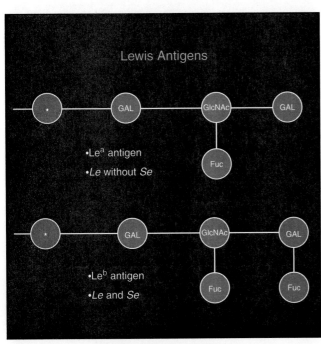

FIGURE 7-4 Lewis antigens.

- Associated with paroxysmal cold hemoglobinuria
- Biphasic antibody
  - Attaches to RBC when cold
  - Lysis occurs as RBC warms
  - Donath-Landsteiner test

ANTIBODY SCREEN AND IDENTIFICATION

- Acceptable sample to use for transfusion testing
  - Patients who have blood drawn for transfusion service requests must be properly identified by name and unique identification number
  - There must be a record of phlebotomist or person who drew the specimen
  - Date specimen was drawn must be on specimen label
  - Specimen must not be hemolyzed
  - Plasma and serum specimens are appropriate to use; often plasma is preferred

- Fibrin clots formed with serum may be present in incompletely clotted specimens, may cause false-positive reaction in gel testing
- Clotting may be incomplete in certain patients—for example, patients being treated with heparin
- Antibody screens and identification are performed to detect antibodies in
  - Patients requiring transfusion
  - Obstetric patients
  - Patients with suspected transfusion reactions
  - Blood and plasma donors
- Must include 37° C incubation and use of an antiglobulin test
- Reagents
  - Screening cells
    - Group O RBCs that provide specific antigens
    - Usually distributed in two-vial or three-vial sets (Table 7-2)
  - Enhancement media increases sensitivity of a test system (Table 7-3)
  - AHG reagents

TABLE 7-2 Representative Antibody Screen Antigen Sheet (Three-Vial Set)

D	C	c	E	e	K	k	Fy^a	Fy^b	Jk^a	Jk^b	M	N	S	s
+	+	0	0	+	0	+	+	0	+	0	+	+	0	+
+	0	+	+	0	+	+	+	+	+	+	+	0	+	0
0	0	+	0	+	0	+	0	+	0	+	0	+	0	+

NOTE: Only major antigen systems are displayed.

TABLE 7-3 Comparison of Potentiators and Methods

Potentiator	Use	Limitations
Low-ionic-strength saline (LISS)	Sensitive, economical, and allows for shorter incubation time	Enhances cold autoantibodies Some weak anti-K antibodies may be missed Equal parts of plasma/serum and LISS is important
Bovine serum albumin (BSA)	Affects second stage of agglutination Does not enhance warm autoantibodies	Needs longer incubation Not sensitive for most antibodies except in Rh blood group system
Polyethylene glycol (PEG)	Shows increased sensitivity	Enhances warm autoantibodies Recommend using anti-IgG AHG, not anti-IgG, -C3d AHG No 37° C readings May require extra wash
Enzymes: ficin, papain	Eliminates reactivity of Fy^a, Fy^b, M, and N antigens; S and s antigens are variable Enhances Rh, JK, LE, P1 antibodies	Enhances cold and warm autoantibodies Should not be used as the only method
Gel technology	Avoids cold reactive antibodies Shows increased sensitivity Can be automated	Enhances warm autoantibodies Weak anti-K may be missed owing to LISS-suspended red cells
Solid phase (SPRCA)	Avoids cold reactive antibodies Shows increased sensitivity Can be automated	Enhances warm autoantibodies Weak anti-K may be missed owing to LISS potentiators Manual method may be difficult to read

From Blaney K, Howard P: Basic & applied concepts of blood banking and transfusion practices, ed 3, St. Louis, 2012, Mosby.
AHG, Antihuman globulin.

○ Used to detect clinically significant antibodies
○ Must contain anti-IgG when used for antibody detection and compatibility testing
○ Polyspecific AHG
  ▪ Contains both anti-IgG and anti-complement (usually anti-C3d or anti-C3b)
  ▪ Used primarily in DAT testing
○ Monospecific AHG
  ▪ Used in differential DAT testing, antibody detection, and identification
  ▪ Directed against one type of globulin
    ▪ Monospecific anti-IgG
    ▪ Monospecific anti-complement (anti-C3d and/or anti-C3b)
○ Coombs control cells
  ▪ Use required for control of negative AHG tests
  ▪ Must react when added to negative AHG tests or test must be repeated
  ▪ Verifies that adequate washing was performed
  ▪ Also verifies that AHG was added and working properly

• Indirect antiglobulin test method (NOTE: This is the method for tube testing; solid phase and gel testing procedures will differ)
  • Label tubes
  • Add 2 drops patient serum to each tube
  • Add 1 drop reagent screen cells to each tube
  • Centrifuge and observe for hemolysis and agglutination
    ○ Some institutions refer to this phase as immediate spin
  • Grade and record results (some institutions may omit this step)
  • Add 2 drops of enhancement reagent to tubes (if used)
  • Incubate 15 to 20 minutes at 37° C
  • Centrifuge and observe for hemolysis and agglutination
  • Grade and record results (some institutions may omit this step)
  • Wash four times
  • Decant last wash to dry cell button
  • Add 2 drops AHG
  • Spin, read, and record results
    ○ Negative: Add 1 drop of Coombs control cells, spin, and read; must be positive
    ○ Positive at any phase: Investigate
• Negative antibody screen
  • Patient is eligible for immediate spin or electronic crossmatches, if no history of clinically significant antibodies
    ○ History of antibodies, must do indirect antiglobulin test (IAT) crossmatch
• Limitations of antibody screen
  • Antibody screen will not detect antibodies when the titer has dropped below the sensitivity level of the screening method being used

• Screen will not detect antibodies to low-frequency antigens that are not present on any of the screening cells
• Factors affecting sensitivity
  • Cell-to-serum ratio
    ○ Antibody in excess: False-negative because of prozone
    ○ Antigen in excess: False-negative because of postzone
    ○ Increasing the amount of serum in the test system can help increase sensitivity when working with weak antibodies, but potentiators usually cannot be used (check manufacturer's instructions)
  • pH
    ○ Most antibodies react best at neutral pH of 6.8 to 7.2
  • Temperature
    ○ Clinically significant antibodies generally react at 37° C or at AHG phase
    ○ Immediate spin and RT phases are often omitted to limit detection of insignificant cold antibodies
  • Length of incubation
    ○ Too little contact time, not enough cells are sensitized
    ○ Incubation time too long, bound antibody may dissociate
    ○ Time depends on media used: Follow manufacturer's instructions
• Grading agglutination reactions (tubes) (Box 7-2)
  • Reactions are graded using a qualitative standard scale
    ○ Gives information on
      ▪ Strength of reaction
      ▪ Amount of antibody available to form antigen–antibody complexes
    ○ 4+ reaction
      ▪ Solid agglutinate, clear supernatant background
      ▪ No free RBCs detected
    ○ 3+ reaction
      ▪ RBC button breaks into several large agglutinates, clear supernatant background
    ○ 2+ reaction
      ▪ RBC button breaks into many medium-sized agglutinates, clear supernatant background, no free RBCs
    ○ 1+ reaction
      ▪ RBC breaks into numerous medium-sized and small agglutinates, background is turbid with many RBCs

---

BOX 7-2 | **Grading Agglutination Reactions**

It is important for reaction grading to be standardized to maintain consistency among different technologists. Each institution will have policies in place describing their reaction grading procedure.

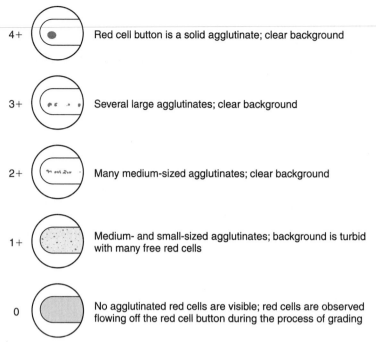

4+	Red cell button is a solid agglutinate; clear background
3+	Several large agglutinates; clear background
2+	Many medium-sized agglutinates; clear background
1+	Medium- and small-sized agglutinates; background is turbid with many free red cells
0	No agglutinated red cells are visible; red cells are observed flowing off the red cell button during the process of grading

FIGURE 7-5 Grading antigen–antibody reactions. Consistency in grading reactions allows for correct interpretation of results in the immunohematology laboratory. *(From Immucor, Inc.)*

- ○ Negative
  - ▪ No agglutinated RBCs are visible, RBCs are observed flowing off the cell button during the process of grading (Figure 7-5)
- Antibody identification
  - ▪ Clinically significant antibody: Some define as an antibody that reacts in vitro at 37° C and/or by IAT, but this is not always true
  - ▪ Better characterized as *an antibody that shortens the survival of transfused RBCs* or has been associated with HDFN
    - ○ Rely on published data to determine clinical significance
    - ○ If data are scarce or unavailable, respect the antibodies that react at 37° C and/or on IAT
  - ▪ Interpretation of the positive antibody screen can provide initial clues
  - ▪ Initial considerations
    - ○ Phase of reactivity
    - ○ Possible warm or cold autoantibody or alloantibody?
    - ○ True agglutination or rouleaux?
    - ○ Does patient have previously identified antibodies?
  - ▪ Patient history: It is helpful to find out the following before the antibody identification process
    - ○ Transfusion history
      - ▪ Recent transfusions may indicate recent antibody stimulation
      - ▪ Antigen typing considerations
    - ○ Pregnancy history
      - ▪ Recent antibody stimulation
    - ○ Recent drug therapy

- ▪ Intravenous immunoglobulin, Rh immunoglobulin (RhIG): Passive antibody transfer
  - ○ Diagnosis, age, race
    - ▪ Offer additional clues to nature of antibody problem
- Antibody panel
  - ○ Group O RBCs
  - ○ Available in sets ranging from 10 to 20 vials
  - ○ Thought of as extended antibody screens (Table 7-4)
  - ○ Best to test using same enhancement media used in the screen
  - ○ Panel antigen profiles are lot-specific—make sure you have the correct one
  - ○ Grade consistently using laboratory guidelines
  - ○ Autocontrol (Figure 7-6)
    - ▪ Patient's RBCs tested against patient's serum in the same manner as the antibody panel
    - ▪ Optional to perform
    - ▪ Not normally done with screen
    - ▪ Most workers test autocontrol (AC) with an antibody panel
    - ▪ Helps determine whether alloantibody or autoantibody specificity exists
- Panel interpretation
  - ○ Phase of reactivity
    - ▪ IgM reacts best at low temperatures (immediate spin phase)
    - ▪ IgG reacts best at AHG phase
    - ▪ Reactions at more than one phase may indicate a combination of IgM and IgG antibodies (Table 7-5)

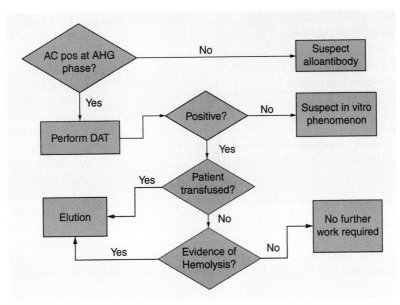

FIGURE 7-6 Suggested flowchart for interpretation of positive autocontrol.

TABLE 7-4	Representative Antibody Panel Antigen Sheet (11-vial set)														
Cell No.	D	C	c	E	e	K	k	Fyᵃ	Fyᵇ	Jkᵃ	Jkᵇ	M	N	S	s
1	+	+	0	+	+	0	+	+	0	+	+	+	+	0	+
2	+	+	0	0	+	+	+	0	+	0	+	+	0	0	+
3	+	0	+	+	0	0	+	0	+	0	+	0	+	0	+
4	+	0	+	0	+	0	+	0	+	+	+	0	+	0	0
5	0	+	+	0	+	0	+	0	+	+	+	+	0	0	+
6	0	0	+	+	+	0	+	+	0	+	+	+	0	+	+
7	0	0	+	0	+	+	+	0	+	+	+	+	+	0	+
8	0	0	+	0	+	0	+	+	0	+	0	+	+	0	+
9	+	+	0	0	+	+	+	0	+	+	+	+	+	+	0
10	+	+	0	+	+	0	+	+	0	+	+	+	0	+	+
11	+	+	0	0	+	+	+	+	0	0	+	0	+	0	+
AC															

NOTE: Only major antigen systems are displayed.

TABLE 7-5	Antibodies and Phase of Reactivity		
Phase	**Room Temperature**	**37° C**	**AHG**
Antibodies	Cold autoabs (I, H, IH), M, N, P₁, Leᵃ, Leᵇ, Luᵃ	Potent cold autoabs, D, E, K	Rh, K, Duffy, Kidd, S, s, Luᵇ, Xgᵃ
Immunoglobulin class	IgM	IgG	IgG
Clinically significant	No	Yes	Yes

- Reaction strength
  - Clue to number of antibodies present
  - Varying strengths suggest more than one antibody or dosage
- Autocontrol (see Figure 7-6)
  - If negative, suspect alloantibody
  - If positive, suspect autoantibody

- Suspect delayed transfusion reaction if patient recently has received a transfusion
- DAT should be performed
- Exclusion or ruling out – *Provisional step only*
  - Panel cells that give negative reactions in all phases can be used for exclusion
  - Begin with the first nonreactive cell

TABLE 7-6	Examples of Substances for Neutralization for Certain Antibodies
Antibodies	**Neutralization Substances**
Anti-P_1	Hydatid cyst fluid, pigeon droppings, turtledoves' egg white, commercial P_1 substance
Anti-Lewis	Plasma or serum, commercial Lewis substance
Anti-Chido, Anti-Rogers	Plasma or serum
Anti-Sd^a	Urine

- Look across the panel and place a line through the antigen specificity that is positive (+) on the panel
- Continue with each nonreactive cell
- *Provisional step only*
- Matching the pattern
  - Look at the reactions that are positive and match the pattern
  - Single antibody will match one of the antigen columns
  - If specificities remain that have not been excluded, additional testing is required
- Probability or "rule of three"
  - Used to ensure pattern of reactivity is not due to chance alone
  - Conclusive evidence derived by testing enough antigen-positive and antigen-negative cells
  - Many laboratories require a probability *(p)* value of .05 or less
    - Means a 5% chance the observed pattern happened by chance alone or you are correct 95% of the time
  - Standard approach has been to require three antigen-positive cells that react and three antigen-negative cells that fail to react
    - Required for each antibody specificity
    - *Institution's approach may differ, but this is the current academic recommendation—answer test questions accordingly*
- Phenotype the patient
  - Individuals cannot make alloantibodies to antigens they possess
  - Test patient RBCs to ensure they are negative for the antigen corresponding to the identified antibody
    - Testing complications include a positive patent DAT or recent transfusion
- Multiple antibodies
  - Serum with two or more alloantibodies may make interpretation of test results difficult

- Clues that indicate multiple antibodies
  - Observed pattern does not fit that of a single antibody
    - Determine whether pattern fits combined specificities
  - Reactivity is present at different test phases
    - Evaluate each phase separately
  - Unexpected reactions occur when trying to confirm the specificity of a suspected single antibody
    - Test selected cells
  - No discernible pattern
    - Perform exclusions to eliminate some specificities
    - Test cells with strong antigen expression or increase sensitivity of the test system
    - Phenotype the patient
    - Use of enzymes can help rule in or out
- Finding compatible blood
  - Phenotype frequency
    - Can help determine number of units compatible for a patient with antibodies
    - How many units are compatible with a patient with anti-Jk^a?
      - 77% of random population is Jk(a+)
    - Combined phenotype calculations
      - Can estimate number of units that will have to be tested to find a certain number of antigen-negative units
  - Example
    - Patient has anti-c, anti-K, anti-Jk^a
    - How many units must be tested to find four of the appropriate phenotype?
      - C negative: 20%
      - K negative: 91%
      - Jk(a) negative: 23%
    - Multiply the individual phenotypes to get the combined phenotype
      - $0.20 \times 0.91 \times 0.23 = 0.04$ or 4% of individuals will be c−K−Jk(a−)
    - 100 units will have to be tested to find 4 units
- Hardy-Weinburg law
  - Mathematical formula used to explain persistence of recessive alleles in a population
  - Based on the following assumptions
    - Population must be large, and mating must occur at random
    - Mutations must not occur
    - There must be no migration, differential fertility, or mortality of the genotype
  - Equation for a two-allele system
    - $p^2 + 2pq + q^2 = 1$
    - $p + q = 1$
  - Blood bank example
    - Kidd blood group system (Jk^a and Jk^b)

- p = frequency of Jk^a allele
- q = frequency of Jk^b allele
- p^2 = frequency of Jk^aJk^a genotype
- $2pq$ = frequency of Jk^aJk^b genotype
- q^2 = frequency of Jk^bJk^b genotype
  - 77% of population expresses Jk^a antigen
    - $p^2 + 2pq$ = frequency of persons who are Jk(a+) and carry the allele Jk^a
    - $q^2 = 1 - (p^2 + 2pq)$ = frequency of persons who are Jk(a−)
    - $q^2 = 1 - 0.77 = 0.23$
    - $q = \sqrt{0.23}$
    - $q = 0.48$ (allele frequency of Jk^b)
  - The sum of frequencies of both alleles must equal 1.00
    - $p + q = 1.00$
    - $p = 1 - q$
    - $p = 1 - 0.48$
    - $p = 0.52$ (allele frequency of Jk^a)
  - Number of Jk(b+) persons can be calculated
    - $2pq + q^2$ = frequency of Jk(b+)
    - $= 2(0.52 \times 0.48) + (0.48)^2$
    - $= 0.73$

CROSSMATCH AND SPECIAL TESTS

- Crossmatch: Performed before transfusion of donor products containing RBCs
  - Immediate spin crossmatch
    - Patient has no clinically significant antibody(ies) detected and no history of antibody(ies)
    - Checks for ABO compatibility
    - Procedure
      - Mix patient serum with donor cells
      - Spin and read
  - Antiglobulin crossmatch
    - Patient has currently reactive antibody(ies) or history of an antibody(ies) that may or may not be demonstrating
    - Procedure
      - Same as immediate spin
      - Continues to include 37° C incubation
      - Concludes with AHG phase (review IAT procedure)
      - Enhancement media can be used
      - Recommended to use same methodology as used for the antibody screen/identification
  - Electronic crossmatch
    - Computer is used to make the final check of ABO compatibility
    - Specific eligibility requirements apply
    - Patient cannot have history of or any currently reacting unexpected antibodies
- Special tests
  - DAT: One-step test to detect RBCs sensitized with antibody or complement in vivo
  - Used to diagnose certain clinical events

- Autoimmune hemolytic anemia
  - Patient autoantibody
- Hemolytic disease of the newborn
  - Maternal antibody
- Drug-related mechanism
  - Drug/antidrug complex
- Transfusion reactions
  - Recipient antibody against donor cells
- Elution is a technique used to dissociate IgG antibodies from sensitized RBCs
- The recovered antibody is called an eluate and can be tested like serum to determine antibody specificity
- Various methods
  - Temperature variation
    - Heat elution
    - Freeze–thaw elution
  - pH manipulation
    - Acid elution is most commonly performed
      - Acidic solution decreases pH and disrupts antigen–antibody bond, releasing antibody into acid solution (eluate), with buffer added at end of procedure to raise pH
  - Chemical
- Adsorption is the process of removing antibody from serum
  - Patient serum is incubated with appropriate RBCs under optimal conditions depending on the antibody to be removed
    - Warm: 37° C
    - Cold: 4° C
- Most commonly used to remove autoantibodies from serum
- Autoadsorption
  - Limited by transfusion history and amount of sample
  - Patients transfused within previous 3 months do not qualify
  - Severely anemic patients may not have enough RBCs to carry out procedure
  - Cells are usually treated with enzyme to remove bound autoantibody
    - Examples: DTT, chloroquine diphosphate (CDP), ethylenediaminetetraacetic acid (EDTA)-glycine-hydrogen chloride (HCL)
  - Alloadsorption
    - Cells phenotypically similar to those of patient are used
    - Enzyme treatment removes some antigens to aid in matching and enhances antibody uptake
- Titration studies are performed to measure the titer of an antibody (quantify amount of antibody present)
  - Twofold serial dilutions of serum are tested against antigen-positive RBCs
  - Reciprocal of the highest dilution showing visible agglutination is the antibody titer

- Most often used to monitor quantity of antibody in a woman's serum during pregnancy
  - Considered significant: Fourfold increase (i.e., 4 to 16)
- Prewarm technique is a procedure in which RBCs and serum (or plasma) are prewarmed separately to 37° C before they are combined
  - May be used when cold autoantibodies are present that may mask the presence of clinically significant antibodies
  - Should be used with caution
    - Reactivity of potentially significant antibodies can be diminished
    - Weak antibodies can be missed
- Neutralization uses soluble antigen to inhibit reactivity of certain antibodies
  - Soluble antigen added to serum sample
  - Mixture incubated at room temperature to neutralize (by occupying antigen-binding sites)
  - Neutralized serum tested against RBCs (panel cells)
  - Must have control (saline), it must be reactive to ensure neutralization occurred and reactivity was not eliminated because of dilution (see Table 7-6)
- Rosette test (Figure 7-7)
  - Principle: Demonstrates small number of D-positive cells in D-negative cell suspension
    - Cell suspension is incubated with human origin anti-D
      - Some kits use chemically modified anti-D
    - Antibody attaches to sites on D-positive cells, if present
    - Indicator D-positive cells are added
    - If antibody is present, indicator cells bind to the antibody attached to the D-positive cells in suspension
    - Visible agglutinates (rosettes) are formed
  - Limitations
    - Weak D-positive cells do not react as strongly as normal D-positive cells
    - If a newborn is weakly D-positive, must quantify fetal maternal hemorrhage with the Kleihauer-Betke stain
- Kleihauer-Betke stain identifies fetal hemoglobin F (Hgb F)

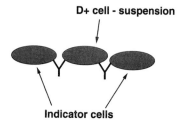

D+ cell - suspension

Indicator cells

This method will detect a 10 mL FMH.

This is considered sensitive enough for a screening test.

FIGURE 7-7 Principle of the rosette test.

---

*Mother's arbitrarily assigned blood volume.

- Principle: In slides subjected to an acid elution step, adult Hgb dissolves out of cells, whereas HbF, which is acid resistant, remains intracellular and is stained
- Procedure
  - Maternal blood smear treated with acid
  - Stained with counterstain
  - 2000 cells counted under microscope
  - Percent of fetal cells calculated
- Limitations
  - Precision and accuracy may be poor
  - Slide quality
  - Area of slide counted
  - Judgment of technologist
- Calculation
  - 300 µg dose of RhIG will protect against up to 15 mL of D-positive RBCs (approximately 30 mL of fetal whole blood)
  - Number of doses of RhIG required is determined by dividing the estimated volume of fetal blood present by 30 (Box 7-3)
- Safety margin
  - When number to the right of the decimal point is less than 5, round down and add 1 dose of RhIG
    - $2.2 = 3$ doses
  - When number to the right of the decimal point is 5 or greater, round up to the next number and add on dose of RhIG
    - $2.8 = 4$ doses

BLOOD DONATION, TRANSFUSION THERAPY, TRANSFUSION REACTIONS, AND HEMOLYTIC DISEASE OF THE FETUS AND NEWBORN

Blood Donation

- Starts the process of providing safe and adequate blood products for patients who need transfusion therapy support
- Donor requirements
  - Donor screening: Regulated by the U.S. Food and Drug Administration (FDA)
    - Registration: Donor must be fully identified according to specific requirements
    - Health history: Performed for the protection of the donor and recipient
    - Helps identify situations in which prospective donor would be deferred

- Permanent deferral: Prospective donors are ineligible to donate for a recipient other than themselves
- Indefinite deferral: Prospective donors are unable to donate for a recipient other than themselves for an unspecified period; may become eligible if current requirements change
- Temporary deferral: Prospective donors are unable to donate for a limited period
- Physical examination: Performed for the protection of the donor (Table 7-7)
- Eligibility (per FDA guidelines as reported in the *AABB Technical Manual*)
  - Whole blood: 8 weeks
  - Two-unit RBC collection: 16 weeks
  - Infrequent plasmapheresis: 4 weeks
  - Plasmapheresis, plateletpheresis, or leukapheresis: More than 2 days
- Donation types
  - Allogeneic: Intended for patient use
  - Autologous: Intended for donor use
    - Screening procedures focus
      - Medications
      - Associated medical illnesses
      - Cardiovascular risk factors
      - Presence of bacteremia
    - Unused units cannot be "crossed over" into allogeneic inventory
  - Directed: Intended for target patient from selected donors
    - Subjected to same selection and testing criteria as allogeneic donors
      - Units can be "crossed over"
      - 56-day waiting period may not apply
- Volume collected (whole blood donation) should not exceed 10.5 mL/kg
  - Donor testing: FDA required tests
    - ABO and D phenotype
    - Antibody screen
    - HBsAg
    - Anti-HCV
    - Anti-HBc
    - HCV NAT
    - Anti-HIV-1/2
    - HIV NAT
    - Anti-HTLV-I/II
    - Syphilis: Rapid plasma reagin or hemagglutination
    - West Nile virus nucleic acid testing (NAT)
    - IgG antibody to *Trypanosoma cruzi* (Chagas' disease)

Transfusion Therapy

- RBCs
  - Contain Hgb
  - Serve as primary mechanism for tissue O_2 transport
  - Provide increased O_2 carrying capacity and increased RBC mass
  - Indications:
    - Treatment of anemia in normovolemic patients
    - Based on clinical status (Table 7-8)
- Platelets
  - Essential to formation of primary hemostatic plug
  - Provide surface for fibrin formation
  - Decreased numbers result from
    - Decreased platelet production
    - Increased destruction

TABLE 7-8 ABO Compatibility for Whole Blood, Red Blood Cells, and Plasma Transfusions

Recipient	Donor		
ABO Phenotype	Whole Blood	Red Blood Cells	Plasma
A	A	A, O	A, AB
B	B	B, O	B, AB
AB	AB	AB, A, B, O	AB
O	O	O	O, A, B, AB

From Blaney K, Howard P: Basic & applied concepts of blood banking and transfusion practices, ed 3, St. Louis, 2012, Mosby.

TABLE 7-7 Physical Examination Criteria

Criteria	Acceptable Limit	
	Allogeneic	Autologous
Age	Applicable state law or ≥16	Determined by medical director
Blood pressure	Systolic, ≤180 mm Hg Diastolic, ≤100 mm Hg	Determined by medical director
Pulse	50-100 beats/min without pathologic irregularity, <50 beats/min acceptable if an otherwise healthy athlete	Determined by medical director
Temperature	≤37.5° C (99.5° F) if measured orally, or equivalent if measured by another method	Deferral for conditions presenting risk for bacteremia
Hemoglobin/ hematocrit	≥12.5 g/dL or a hematocrit value of ≥38%	≥11 g/dL or a hematocrit value of ≥33%

Data from information from the AABB Technical manual, ed 17, Bethesda, Md, 2011, American Association of Blood Banks.

- Platelet components
  - Random donor platelets
    - Prepared from a unit of whole blood
    - Suspended in 40 to 70 mL plasma
    - Contain 5.5×10^{10} platelets
  - Plateletpheresis
    - Collected by apheresis from a single donor
    - Contains 3×10^{11} or more platelets
    - Comparable to 4 to 8 platelets units
    - Volume of 100 to 500 mL (Table 7-9)
- Fresh frozen plasma (FFP)
  - Contains all clotting factors, including labile factors V and VIII
  - Only approved component for clinically significant deficiency of factors II, V, X, and XI
  - Indications
    - Used in bleeding patients with multiple coagulation factor deficiencies
    - Liver disease
  - Warfarin treatment
  - Dilutional and consumption coagulopathy
- Cryoprecipitated AHF
  - Cold-insoluble portion of FFP thawed at 1° to 6° C
  - Contains
    - 80 international units factor VIII
    - 150 mg fibrinogen (AABB quality control requirement)
    - On average, each unit contains approximately 250 mg fibrinogen
    - 20% to 30% of factor XIII of original unit
    - 40% to 70% von Willebrand factor (vWF) of original unit
  - Indications
    - Second-line therapy
      - von Willebrand's disease
      - Hemophilia A
      - Control bleeding associated with fibrinogen deficiency
      - Factor XIII deficiency
- RhIG
  - IgG anti-D derived from pools of human plasma
    - Full 300-μg dose counteracts 15 mL of D-positive RBCs
    - Equals 30 mL of fetal whole blood
  - 50-μg dose counteracts 2.5 mL of D-positive RBCs

  - Used for first-trimester miscarriages or abortions
  - Rarely used
    - Fear of miscalculating length of pregnancy
    - Cost
- Special component considerations
  - Leukocyte reduction
    - Less than 5×10^6 residual white blood cells (WBCs)
      - Cells, plateletpheresis, and pooled platelets
    - Less than 8.3×10^5 residual WBCs
      - Platelets, leukocytes reduced (prepared from whole blood)
    - May reduce risk for
      - Febrile nonhemolytic reactions
      - Cytomegalovirus (CMV) transmission (often considered "CMV safe" [not the same as CMV negative])
      - Human leukocyte antigen (HLA) alloimmunization
  - CMV negative
    - Collected from seronegative donors
  - Washed
    - RBCs
      - Removes 99% of plasma proteins, electrolytes, and antibodies
      - Can lose up to 20% of unit
      - Expiration is 24 hours
    - Platelets
      - Expiration is 4 hrs after washing
    - Irradiation
      - Only acceptable method to prevent graft-versus-host disease (GVHD)
      - Ordered for immunocompromised patients receiving components that contain viable lymphocytes
        - RBCs, platelets, granulocytes, nonfrozen plasma
      - Prevents proliferation of transfused lymphocytes
      - Some damage is done to RBCs, and viability is affected
        - Expiration is original expiration of unit or 28 days, whichever comes first
- Neonatal considerations
  - Washed or fresh cells often indicated
    - Difficulty in metabolizing citrate and potassium (washed)
    - Maximize level of 2,3-diphosphoglycerate (fresh)
  - CMV negative
    - Infection risk to preterm infants born to seronegative mothers
    - Leukocyte reduction is also recommended
  - Irradiation
    - Recommended to prevent possible transfusion-associated GVHD (TA-GVHD) in
      - Intrauterine transfusions

TABLE 7-9	Platelet ABO and Rh Compatibility					
Recipient	Donor					
	A	B	O	AB	Rh+	RH−
A	✓			✓		
B		✓		✓		
O	✓	✓	✓	✓		
AB				✓		
Rh positive					✓	✓
Rh negative						✓

- Exchange transfusions
- Transfusion to a premature (<1200 g) neonate
  o Transfusions in a full-term newborn infant do not require routine irradiation
- Hemoglobin S (Hgb S)
  o Infants who are hypoxic or acidotic should receive blood tested and negative for Hgb S
  o Hgb S–negative units are needed for exchange transfusions
- Intrauterine transfusion
  o Hematocrit (Hct) of RBCs should be greater than 70% because
    - Small volume transfused
    - Need to correct severe anemia
- Testing considerations

  o Crossmatch is not necessary as long as initial antibody screen from heel stick or maternal specimen is negative
  o Infants do not form antibodies during first 4 months of life
  o Antigen-negative blood must be provided if mother or infant possesses an RBC alloantibody
  o ABO identical or ABO compatible D negative or same type as infant can be transfused during first 4 months
  o *Group O RBCs are most generally used for intrauterine and neonatal transfusions*
  o *Rh-negative blood used for fetuses and neonates when blood type is unknown or Rh negative* (Table 7-10)
- Issuing of components

TABLE 7-10	Component Information	
Component	**Storage**	**Expiration**
Whole blood	1°-6° C If intended for room temperature components, store at 1°-6° C within 8 hr of collection	ACD/CPD/CP2D: 21 days CPDA-1: 35 days
Whole blood irradiated	1°-6° C	Original outdate or 28 days from date of irradiation, whichever is earlier
Red blood cells (RBCs)	1°-6° C	ACD/CPD/CP2D: 21 days CPDA-1: 35 days Open system: 24 hr Additive solutions: 42 days
Washed RBCs	1°-6° C	24 hr
RBCs leukocytes, reduced	1°-6° C	ACD/CPD/CP2D: 21 days CPDA-1: 35 days Open system: 24 hr Additive solutions: 42 days
Washed and rejuvenated RBCs	1°-6° C	24 hr
RBCs irradiated	1°-6° C	Original outdate or 28 days from date of irradiation, whichever is earlier
RBCs frozen, 40% glycerol	≤ −65° C	10 yr
RBCs frozen, 20% glycerol	≤ −120° C	10 yr
Deglycerolized RBCs	1°-6° C	24 hr
Platelets	20°-24° C with continuous gentle agitation	24 hr to 7 days, depending on collection system*
Pooled platelets (or open system)	20°-24° C with continuous gentle agitation	4 hr, unless otherwise specified
Platelets leukocytes, reduced	20°-24° C with continuous gentle agitation	Open system: 4 hr* Closed system: No change from original expiration date*
Platelets irradiated	20°-24° C with continuous gentle agitation	Open system: 4 hr Closed system: No change from original expiration date*
Granulocytes	20°-2° C without agitation	24 hr
Fresh frozen plasma	≤ −18° C or ≤ −65° C	12 mo (−18° C) 7 yr (−65° C, with approval of FDA)
Fresh frozen plasma (after thawing)	1°-6° C	24 hr
Cryoprecipitated AHF	≤ −18° C	12 mo
Cryoprecipitated AHF (after thawing)	20°-24° C	4 hr if open system or pooled, 6 hr if single unit or pooled

*Note: Maximum time without agitation is 24 hr.
Data from information from the AABB Technical Manual, ed 17, Bethesda, Md, 2011, American Association of Blood Banks.

- Systems should be in place to ensure the correct blood component is being issued to the correct patient
- When component is issued to an individual (as opposed to being sent to a location—e.g., surgical suite), a second check of information reviewed should occur and be documented
- Electronic or manual processes should be in place to check
  - Component's unique blood number
  - Recipient's name and another patient identifier
  - Blood type
  - Expiration date
  - Crossmatch status
  - Other serologic information (e.g., CMV negative)
  - Documentation of status of visual inspection
  - Time and date of issue
  - Person (or location) to whom it was issued

Transfusion Reactions

- A transfusion reaction is any adverse effect of transfusion therapy that occurs during or after administration of a blood component
- Transfusion of any blood component can result in a transfusion reaction
- Signs and symptoms
  - Fever
    - Generally defined as 1° C or greater rise in temperature above 37° C
  - Chills with or without rigors
  - Respiratory distress, including wheezing, coughing, and dyspnea
  - Hypertension or hypotension
  - Abdominal, chest, flank, or back pain
  - Pain at the infusion site
  - Skin manifestations, including urticaria, rash, flushing, pruritus, and localized edema
  - Jaundice or hemoglobinuria
  - Nausea/vomiting
  - Abnormal bleeding
  - Oliguria/anuria
- Clinical evaluation of suspected transfusion reaction
  - Patient-focused steps
    - Stop transfusion and maintain intravenous access with normal saline
    - Perform clerical recheck
    - Contact treating physician immediately for instructions for patient care
  - Component-focused steps
    - Contact transfusion service for directions for investigation
    - Obtain instructions for returning any remaining component, associated intravenous fluid bags, and tubing
    - Determine appropriate samples to send to laboratory

- Laboratory investigation of suspected transfusion reaction
- Clerical check of component bag, label, paperwork, and patient sample
- Repeat ABO testing on posttransfusion sample
- Visual check of pretransfusion and postransfusion sample to look for hemolysis
- Perform DAT on posttransfusion sample
- Report findings to blood bank supervisor or medical director
- Acute HTR
  - Incompatible RBCs transfused to recipient with preformed antibody
  - Misidentification most common cause of ABO incompatibility
  - Occurs within minutes of start of infusion
  - Intravascular reaction
    - IgM or complement-fixing IgG
    - Most severe reactions associated with ABO incompatible transfusions
    - Hemoglobinemia, hemoglobinuria
    - Decreased Hct, decreased haptoglobin, increased lactate dehydrogenase, increased plasma hemoglobin
    - Increased serum bilirubin 6 to 12 hours later
    - Severe clinical symptoms: Shock, hypotension, bronchospasm, disseminated intravascular coagulation (DIC)
      - Complement fragments, anaphylatoxins C3a and C5a
      - Renal ischemia, tubular necrosis, acute renal failure
      - Activation of coagulation cascade, DIC
      - Cytokines interleukin–1b (IL-1b), IL-6, IL-8, TNF-α
    - Extravascular reaction
      - Complement activation incomplete, extravascular clearance
        - Typical with non-ABO antibodies
      - Milder clinical symptoms
        - Fever, new positive DAT, falling Hct with no overt signs of bleeding
        - Hemoglobinemia, hemoglobinuria rarely seen
        - Non–immune-mediated hemolysis
  - "Abused" unit
    - Improper storage/shipping temperatures, mishandling
    - Malfunctioning blood warmers, microwave ovens, hot water baths, inadvertent freezing
  - Mechanical hemolysis
    - Roller pumps, pressure infusion pumps, small-bore needles
  - Osmotic hemolysis
    - Addition of drugs or hypotonic solutions
    - Inadequate deglycerolization of frozen RBCs

- o Bacterial growth in blood units
- o Intrinsic RBC defect such as glucose-6-phosphate dehydrogenase (G6PD) deficiency in patient or donor
- Transfusion-associated sepsis
  - o Fever, shock, hemoglobinuria, DIC, abdominal cramps, diarrhea, vomiting
  - o Mortality rates vary by component
  - o More likely to affect products stored at room temperature (platelets)
  - o Laboratory investigation: Rule out hemolytic reaction, Gram stain and culture of unit and recipient, visual inspection of blood bag
- Febrile nonhemolytic reactions
  - o Temperature increase 1° C (2° F) or more associated with transfusion (during or delayed until after transfusion)
  - o Incidence: 0.1% to 1% with universal leukocyte reduction
  - o Usually benign, may be accompanied by chills, rigors, and/or discomfort
  - o Causes
    - Interaction between preformed antibody in recipient's plasma and antigen on donor lymphocytes, granulocytes, or platelets (HLA antibodies are most notable)
    - Cytokine release in the recipient in response to antigen–antibody reactions may increase severity of reaction
    - Any unexplained, transfusion-associated rise in temperature deserves prompt attention
    - Rule out other serious causes (acute HTR, sepsis)
- Allergic reaction
  - o Hypersensitivity reaction (IgE-mediated allergic reaction)
  - o Triggered by exposure to soluble substance in donor plasma to which recipient is sensitized
  - o Ranges from rash and/or urticaria (hives) and itching to an anaphylactoid reaction
  - o Usually *not* accompanied by fever
- Transfusion-related acute lung injury (TRALI)
  - o May occur as frequently as 1 in 5000 transfusions
  - o Signs and symptoms
    - Fever, chills, dyspnea, cyanosis, hypotension, new onset of bilateral pulmonary edema
    - Symptoms arise within 6 hours of transfusion
    - Most cases evident within 1 to 2 hours after transfusion
  - o All plasma-containing components have been implicated
  - o Must distinguish TRALI reaction from
    - Anaphylactic reaction
    - Transfusion-associated circulatory overload (TACO)
    - Transfusion-related sepsis

- o Pathophysiology
  - Associated with infusion of antibodies to leukocyte antigens and infusion of biologic response modifiers (BRMs)
    - Either may initiate cellular activation and damage of basement membrane
    - Pulmonary edema occurs secondary to leakage of protein-rich fluid into alveolar space
  - HLA antibodies have been implicated in some cases
  - BRMs can accumulate during storage
- TACO
  - o Massive transfusion or single unit
    - Volume overload or rapid infusion
  - o Young children and elderly at most risk
  - o Dyspnea, cough, cyanosis, severe headache, peripheral edema, systolic hypertension, congestive heart failure
    - Must differentiate from TRALI
- Complications of massive transfusion
  - o Citrate toxicity
  - o Hyperkalemia and hypokalemia
  - o Hemostatic abnormalities
  - o Air embolism
  - o Hypothermia
- Delayed immunologic response: Alloimmunization
  - o Immune response to foreign antigens on RBC, or WBC and platelets (HLA)
  - o Primary versus secondary response
  - o Approximately 1% to 1.6% of RBC transfusions are associated with antibody formation
- TA-GVHD
  - o Immunologic transfusion complication
  - o Donor lymphocytes proliferate and attack recipient
  - o Greater than 90% mortality rate
  - o Clinical: Fever, skin rash, hepatitis, enterocolitis, pancytopenia, and immunodeficiency
  - o Symptoms usually appear within 8 to 10 days of transfusion
  - o Three requirements for GVHD to develop
    - Expressed HLA antigens different between donor and recipient
    - Graft must contain immunocompetent cells
    - Host must be incapable of rejecting immunocompetent cells
  - o Irradiation
    - Irradiation of cellular components recommended
    - Patients identified at risk for TA-GVHD
    - Transfusions of cellular components between blood relatives
    - Transfusion of HLA-selected products
- Posttransfusion purpura
  - o Uncommon, usually in women
  - o Abrupt onset of severe thrombocytopenia (<10,000/µL), 1 to 24 days after blood

transfusion in a previously pregnant or transfused patient

- 70% of posttransfusion purpura cases associated with antibodies against HPA-1a (Pl^{A1}) Ag
- Usually self-limited with full recovery, although some patients can die from intracranial bleeding

- Iron overload
  - One RBC unit contains approximately 250 mg iron
  - Chronically transfused patients at risk
  - Iron deposits interfere with heart, liver, and endocrine glands, causing cardiomyopathy, arrhythmias, and hepatic and pancreatic failure
  - Threshold for clinical damage: Lifetime exposure to more than 50 units of RBCs in a non-bleeding person
  - Treatment: Iron-chelating agents, "fresh" blood

- Transfusion fatalities
  - Fatalities resulting directly from the effects of transfusion must be reported to the FDA (Center for Biologics Evaluation and Research) within 24 hours and by written report within 7 days
  - Most deaths are unrelated to transfusion, but if there is any suggestion that transfusion contributed, initiate investigation into case

Hemolytic Disease of the Fetus and Newborn

- Fetal RBCs are coated with maternal alloantibody
- Directed against antigen inherited from the father that is absent from the mother
- IgG-coated RBCs are destroyed
- Before and after birth
- Severity ranges from intrauterine death to asymptomatic (serologic detection only)
- Three prerequisites for HDFN
  - Mother lacks antigen (exposed through pregnancy or transfusion)
  - Fetus possesses antigen, inherited from father
  - Mother has made an IgG antibody
    - Sensitization depends on
      - Recognition of foreign antigen
      - Responder
      - Antigen is immunologic
      - Amount of fetal-maternal bleed
      - ABO compatibility
- Complications of HDFN include rising levels of unconjugated bilirubin, which is the biggest risk
  - Decision to perform exchange transfusion driven by bilirubin levels
- Central nervous system damage caused by
  - Prematurity
  - Acidosis
  - Hypoxia
  - Hypoalbuminemia

- Rh HDFN
  - Anti-D alone or in combination with Anti-C or anti-E
- "Other" HDFN
  - Other antigens in Rh system
  - Antigens in other systems
- ABO HDFN
  - Can occur in any pregnancy
  - Group A or B infants born to group O mothers
    - Humans can make IgG anti-A,B
    - ABO IgG antibodies occur without history of prior exposure (Table 7-11)
- Serologic studies
- Early pregnancy
  - Performance of ABO/Rh, weak D if D negative
  - Antibody screen, identify if antibodies detected
- 28 weeks
  - Rh-negative women with initial negative antibody screen
    - Repeat antibody screen
    - Administer RhIG
  - Positive antibody screen
    - Identify antibody
    - Presence of antibody does not mean HDFN will occur
    - Not all antibodies are risk to fetus
      - Anti-Le^a, anti-I
        - Baby may lack corresponding antigen
        - Fetal involvement may be predicted by typing father's RBC antigens
    - Maternal antibody titer
      - Titration studies can aid in treatment decisions
      - Establish baseline in first trimester
      - Repeat at intervals determined by clinician
      - Usually not repeated until 16 to 18 weeks
      - Use is controversial
      - No established critical titers for antibodies other than anti-D
      - Represents a noninvasive means to monitor pregnancy

TABLE 7-11	ABO Versus Rh Hemolytic Disease of the Fetus and Newborn	
ABO HDFN	**Rh HDFN**
Most common	Not caused by Rh immunoglobulin
Cannot be diagnosed	Followed with titers
Can affect first child	Immune exposure (second child)
Weak-to-negative DAT	Very strong DAT
Occurs in group type O mothers	Can affect any Rh-negative mother
Slight rise in bilirubin (treat with phototherapy)	High rise in bilirubin (may need to perform exchange transfusion)

DAT, Direct antiglobulin test; *HDFN,* hemolytic disease of the fetus and newborn.

CERTIFICATION PREPARATION QUESTIONS

For answers and rationales, please see Appendix A.

1. Which immunodominant sugar confers A antigen specificity?
   a. D-Galactose
   b. L-Fucose
   c. N-Acetylgalactosamine
   d. Both A and C

2. If a patient has an A_2 ABO type, which of the following statements is true?
   a. The patient's red cells will react with anti-A_1 lectin
   b. The patient's serum will react with A_2 cells
   c. The patient's red cells will react with anti-A_2 lectin
   d. The patient's serum will react with A_1 cells if anti-A_1 is present

3. Which genotype confers the Bombay blood type?
   a. *Hh*
   b. *hh*
   c. *Sese*
   d. *Lele*

4. Which genes encode for Rh antigens?
   a. *RHDCE*
   b. *RHD*
   c. *RHCE*
   d. Both b and c

5. Testing for the D antigen was conducted at the IAT phase. A control was included in the testing. Both the patient's red cells and the control tube reacted at 4+. How would you interpret this test?
   a. The test is invalid because the control tube was positive
   b. The patient is D positive
   c. The patient is D negative
   d. The test should be repeated and the control tube omitted

6. Of the red cells listed, which has the most D antigen present?
   a. Rh null
   b. D positive
   c. dce/dce
   d. D − −

7. Which is true of the Duffy blood group system?
   a. Antigens are resistant to enzyme treatment
   b. Antibodies never show dosage
   c. Fy^a and Fy^b are codominant alleles
   d. The majority of whites are Fy(a − b −)

8. Which antibody is typically considered to be an autoantibody if found in the serum of an adult?
   a. Anti-K
   b. Anti-I
   c. Anti-D
   d. Anti-Fy^a

9. Which reagent destroys all of the Kell blood group system antigens?
   a. DTT
   b. Chloroquine diphosphate
   c. AHG
   d. LISS

10. Which is true of antibodies to Kidd blood group system antigens?
    a. They are enhanced by enzymes
    b. Titers can quickly drop in patients
    c. Both A and B
    d. None of the above

11. Which of the following is true of the Lewis system?
    a. Lewis antigens are found on type II precursor cells
    b. Lewis antigens are well developed at birth
    c. Antibodies to Lewis antigens always cause HTRs
    d. Antibodies to Lewis antigens rarely cross the placenta

12. Which of the following is true of antibodies to MNS blood group system antigens?
    a. Anti-U is directed at a high-incidence antigen
    b. Anti-N is commonly found
    c. Anti-M is always clinically significant
    d. Anti-S is reactive with enzyme-treated cells

13. Which of the following antibodies is classified as "biphasic" and an autoantibody?
    a. Anti-B
    b. Anti-P
    c. Anti-H
    d. Anti-Le^a

14. You have performed an antibody screen using the tube method. All three screening cells tested negative. The Coombs check cells in all three tubes are also nonreactive. What should you do?
    a. Respin the tubes and reread them
    b. Report the antibody screen as negative
    c. Repeat the antibody screen
    d. Perform an antibody identification panel

15. An antibody panel has six 2+ reactive cells at AHG phase. Panel testing using enzyme-treated cells showed no reactivity. Which is the most likely antibody that is present?
    a. Anti-Fy^a
    b. Anti-e
    c. Anti-k
    d. Anti-Lu^a

16. A patient has a currently nonreactive antibody screen but has a history of anti-Jk^a in the patient file. Which type of crossmatch must be performed on this patient?
    a. Immediate spin crossmatch
    b. IAT crossmatch
    c. Electronic crossmatch
    d. Both a and c

17. A recently transfused patient has a 3+ reactive DAT with anti-IgG. Which procedure should be used to identify the specificity of the IgG antibody attached to the red cells?
    a. Adsorption
    b. Neutralization
    c. Titration
    d. Elution

18. An O-negative mother gave birth to an O-positive baby. Her rosette test was positive. Which of the following is true?
    a. The test is invalid because of the mother's ABO type
    b. A Kleihauer-Betke test should be performed to quantify the fetal maternal hemorrhage
    c. The mother should be given a 300-μg dose of RhIG
    d. A weak D test should be performed on the baby

19. In which of the following settings are platelet transfusions *not* indicated?
    a. Thrombotic thrombocytopenic purpura
    b. Immune thrombocytopenic purpura with severe intracranial hemorrhage
    c. Massive transfusion
    d. Vascular catheter placement, platelet count 24,000/μL
    e. Brain biopsy, platelet count 62,000/μL

20. An obstetric patient presents to the hospital with marked vaginal bleeding and severe lower abdominal pain. During placement of an intravenous catheter, she was noted to have marked oozing. She is diagnosed with disseminated intravascular coagulation as a complication of her primary problem. She is given cryoprecipitate and fresh frozen plasma before going to the operating room. What element of cryoprecipitate is important in treating this patient?
    a. Factor I
    b. Factor II
    c. Factor VIII:c
    d. Factor VIII:vWF
    e. Factor XIII

21. A patient's ABO blood type is determined by which of the following?
    a. Genetic inheritance and environmental factors
    b. Genetic inheritance
    c. Environmental factors
    d. Immune function
    e. Maternal blood type

22. A trauma patient with type AB is seen at a rural hospital. The hospital only has 3 units of type AB RBCs. What blood type of RBCs can the patient receive as an alternative?
    a. Type O
    b. Type B
    c. Type A
    d. None of the above
    e. All of the above

23. A genetic state in which no detectable trait exists is called:
    a. Recessive
    b. Dominant
    c. Incomplete dominance
    d. Amorph

24. Most blood group antigens are expressed as a result of which of the following?

    a. Autosomal recessive inheritance
    b. X-linked dominant inheritance
    c. Y-linked recessive inheritance
    d. Autosomal codominant inheritance

25. What blood type is *not* possible for the offspring of AO and BO parents?
    a. AB
    b. A or B
    c. O
    d. All are possible

26. How many molecules of IgM are needed to fix complement?
    a. 1
    b. 2
    c. 3
    d. 4

27. For lysis of red blood cells to occur after antigen–antibody reaction, which compound is required?
    a. Albumin
    b. Glucose-6-phosphate dehydrogenase (G6PD)
    c. Complement
    d. Antihuman globulin (AHG)

28. An end-point of tube testing other than agglutination that must also be considered a positive reaction is called:
    a. Clumping
    b. Mixed field
    c. Hemolysis
    d. Microscopic

29. Mixed-field (mf) agglutination can be observed in the:
    a. DAT on a person undergoing delayed hemolytic transfusion reaction
    b. IAT result of a patient who has anti-Le^a
    c. DAT on a patient on high doses of penicillin
    d. Typing result with anti-A of a patient who is A$_2$ subgroup

30. In which situation(s) may the ABO serum grouping *not* be valid?
    a. The patient has hypogammaglobulinemia
    b. IgM antibodies are present
    c. Cold autoantibodies are present
    d. All of the above

31. If you knew the DAT is positive, what would you expect the Rh control to be when doing a weak D test through AHG?
    a. Negative
    b. Positive
    c. Mixed field
    d. Hemolysis at 37° C would be seen

32. How can IgG antibodies be removed from red cells?
    a. Elution
    b. Adsorption
    c. Prewarming
    d. Neutralization

33. Testing needs to be done with an antiserum that is rarely used. The appropriate steps to take in using

this antiserum include following the manufacturer's procedure and:

  a. Performing a cell panel to be sure that the antiserum is performing correctly

  b. Performing the testing on screen cells

  c. Testing in duplicate to ensure the repeatability of the results

  d. Testing a cell that is negative for the antigen and one that is heterozygous for the antigen

34. Based on the following antigram, which cell is heterozygous for M?

D	C	E	c	e	M	N	S	s	P₁	Leᵃ	Leᵇ	K	k	Fyᵃ	Fyᵇ	Jkᵃ	Jkᵇ
1 0	+	0	+	+	+	+	+	0	0	+	0	0	+	0	+	0	+
2 +	+	0	0	+	0	+	0	+	+	0	+	0	+	+	+	+	0
3 0	0	+	+	+	+	0	+	+	+	0	0	+	+	+	0	+	+

  a. Cell 1

  b. Cell 2

  c. Cell 3

  d. None of the above

35. Which antibody can be neutralized with a specific reagent?

  a. Anti-D

  b. Anti-Jkᵃ

  c. Anti-M

  d. Anti-Leᵃ

36. Group O red blood cells are used as a source of commercial screening cells because:

  a. Anti-A is detected using group O cells

  b. Anti-D reacts with most group O cells

  c. Weak subgroups of A react with group O cells

  d. ABO antibodies do not react with group O cells

37. The use of EDTA samples for the direct antiglobulin test prevents activation of the classical complement pathway by:

  a. Causing rapid decay of complement proteins

  b. Chelating Mg^{2+} ions, preventing assembly of C6

  c. Chelating Ca^{2+} ions, preventing assembly of C1

  d. Preventing chemotaxis

38. Check (Coombs control) cells are:

  a. Added to every negative antiglobulin test

  b. Added to negative direct antiglobulin tests only

  c. Used to confirm a positive Coombs' reaction

  d. Coated with both IgM and C3d

39. What type(s) of red cells is(are) acceptable to transfuse to an AB-negative patient?

  a. A negative, B negative, AB negative, O negative

  b. O negative only

  c. AB negative only

  d. AB negative, A negative, B negative only

40. A nonbleeding adult of average height and weight with chronic anemia is transfused with 2 units of red blood cells. The pretransfusion Hgb is 7.0 g/dL. What is the expected posttransfusion Hgb?

  a. 8 g/dL

  b. 9 g/dL

  c. 10 g/dL

  d. 11 g/dL

41. An IgA-deficient patient with clinically significant anti-IgA requires which of the following?

  a. Leukocyte-reduced fresh frozen plasma

  b. CMV-seronegative RBCs

  c. Irradiated RBCs and platelets

  d. Washed RBCs

42. Anti-H will react weakest with blood from a person with _____.

  a. Group O

  b. Group A₁

  c. Group A₂

  d. Group A₂B

43. Which of the following antibodies *do not* match the others in terms of optimal reactive temperature?

  a. Anti-Fyᵃ

  b. Anti-M

  c. Anti-K

  d. Anti-S

44. What antibody can an R₁r patient make if transfused with R₂R₂ blood?

  a. Anti-D

  b. Anti-C

  c. Anti-E

  d. Anti-c

  e. Anti-e

45. What is the probability of finding blood negative for the Jkᵃ and Fyᵃ antigens (23% of population is Jk [a −] and 34% of population is Fy[a −])?

  a. 5.1%

  b. 51%

  c. 7.8%

  d. 78%

46. If the following patient's RBCs were tested against anti-H lectin and did not react, this person would be identified as a(an):

Cell typing		Serum typing				Antibody Screening results		
Anti-A	Anti-B	A1 cells	B cells			SCI	SCII	Autocontrol
0	0	4+	4+	IS		4+	4+	0
				37C LISS		4+	4+	0
				AHG		4+	4+	0
				Check cell				2+

  a. Acquired B

  b. Secretor

  c. Oₕ phenotype

  d. Subgroup of A

47. If a person has the genetic makeup *Hh, AO, LeLe, sese*, what substance will be found in the secretions?

  a. A substance

  b. H Substance

  c. Leᵃ substance

  d. Leᵇ substance

48. Before A and B antigens can be expressed, the precursor substance must have the terminal sugar _____.
    a. d-Galactose
    b. N-Acetylgalactosamine
    c. Glucose
    d. L-Fucose

49. A white female's RBCs gave the following reactions: D+, C+, E-, c+, e+. The most probable Rh genotype is:
    a. *DCe/Dce*
    b. *DCe/dce*
    c. *DCe/DcE*
    d. *Dce/dCe*

50. If a D-positive person makes anti-D, this person is most likely:
    a. Partial D
    b. D negative
    c. Weak D as position effect
    d. Weak D because of transmissible genes

51. A serum containing anti-k is not frequently encountered because of which of the following?
    a. People who lack the k antigen are rare
    b. People who possess the k antigen are rare
    c. The k antigen is not a good immunogen
    d. Kell-null people are rare

52. A characteristic of the Xg^a antigen is that the Xg^a antigen:
    a. Has a higher frequency in women than in men
    b. Has a higher frequency in men than in women
    c. Is enhanced by enzymes
    d. Is usually a saline reacting antibody

53. Which of the following is a characteristic of the Kidd system antibodies?
    a. The antibodies are usually IgM
    b. The corresponding antigens are destroyed by enzymes
    c. The antibodies are usually strong and stable during storage
    d. The antibodies are often implicated in delayed hemolytic transfusion reactions

54. Anti-E will react with which of the following cells?
    a. R_oR_o
    b. R_1R_1
    c. R_2R_2
    d. rr

55. Which statement is *not* true concerning anti-Fy^a and anti-Fy^b?
    a. Are clinically significant
    b. React well with enzyme-treated panel cells
    c. Cause hemolytic transfusion reactions
    d. Cause a generally mild hemolytic disease of the newborn

56. Which of the following antibodies can be neutralized with pooled human plasma?
    a. Anti-Hy and anti-Ge:1
    b. Anti-Ch^a and anti-Rg^a
    c. Anti-Co^a and anti-Co^b
    d. Anti-Do^a and anti-Js^b

57. Donors who have received RBC transfusion within the last 12 months are deferred because:
    a. Blood could transmit hepatitis or HIV
    b. Donor red cell hemoglobin level may be too low
    c. Donor health would prohibit the donation process
    d. There will be two cell populations in this donor

58. Autologous presurgical donations are not allowed for which of the following patients?
    a. Weigh less than 100 lb
    b. Under the age of 14
    c. With hemoglobin of 13 g/dL
    d. With bacteremia

59. Which of the following viruses resides exclusively in leukocytes?
    a. HCV
    b. HBV
    c. CMV
    d. HIV

60. Which product is *least* likely to transmit hepatitis?
    a. Cryoprecipitate
    b. Plasma protein fraction
    c. RBC
    d. Platelets

61. In preparing platelets from a unit of whole blood, the correct order of centrifugation is:
    a. Hard spin followed by a hard spin
    b. Light spin followed by a light spin
    c. Light spin followed by a hard spin
    d. Hard spin followed by a light spin

62. Which antibody could cause hemolytic disease of the fetus and newborn?
    a. Anti-I
    b. Anti-K
    c. Anti-Le^a
    d. Anti-N

63. A group A, D-negative obstetric patient with anti-D (titer 256) is carrying a fetus who needs an intrauterine transfusion. The blood needed should be:
    a. Group A, D-negative RBC
    b. Group A, D-negative whole blood
    c. Group O, D-negative RBC
    d. Group O, D-negative whole blood

64. Which of the following mothers should receive RhIG?
    a. A-negative mother; O-negative baby; no prenatal care, anti-D in mother
    b. AB-negative mother; B-positive baby; anti-D in mother
    c. O-negative mother; A-positive baby; no anti-D in mother
    d. A-positive mother; A-positive baby; no anti-D in mother

65. How many doses of RhIG are indicated for a Kleihauer-Betke reading of 0.6%?
 a. 1
 b. 2
 c. 3
 d. 4

66. What should be done *first* if a mother types as O and the baby types as AB?
 a. Report the results with no further testing
 b. Try to get a sample from the father
 c. Recheck all labels, get new samples, if necessary, and retest
 d. Retype using all new reagents

67. A newborn has a positive DAT. What is the best procedure to determine the antibody causing a positive DAT in this newborn?
 a. An antibody titer on the mother's serum
 b. An antibody panel on the mother's serum
 c. An antibody panel performed on the eluate of the mother's cells
 d. An antibody panel performed on the eluate of the baby's cells

68. Which of the following is(are) an example(s) of a record-keeping error?
 a. Use of correction fluid or tape
 b. Using pencil
 c. Documentation after the fact
 d. All of the above

69. Which of the antigens below is considered low incidence?
 a. Fy^a
 b. S
 c. C
 d. Kp^a

70. Which of the antigens below is considered high incidence?
 a. Fy^b
 b. Vel
 c. E
 d. S

71. In performing tube testing, you see many medium-sized agglutinates in a clear background. How would you grade this reaction?
 a. 2+
 b. 1+
 c. 4+
 d. 3+

72. Of the following, which genotypes would result in the B phenotype?
 a. *BB*
 b. *AB*
 c. *BO*
 d. a and b
 e. a and c

73. How would you interpret the following reactions?

Forward Type		Reverse Type	
Anti-A	Anti-B	A_1 Cells	B Cells
0	0	4+	4+

 a. Blood type A
 b. Blood type O
 c. Blood type B
 d. Blood type AB

74. Noting these reactions, if they patient needed blood now, what type of blood should be transfused?

Forward Type		Reverse Type	
Anti-A	Anti-B	A_1 Cells	B Cells
4+	0	1+	4+

 a. Blood type A
 b. Blood type O
 c. Blood type A_2
 d. Blood type A

75. Blood group antibodies made by type A and type B people are predominantly which class?
 a. IgE
 b. IgA
 c. IgG
 d. IgM

76. Based on these reactions, what should be the next step?

Forward Type		Reverse Type	
Anti-A	Anti-B	A_1 Cells	B Cells
4+	0	1+	4+

 a. Test the serum with A_2 cells
 b. Report the patient as type A
 c. Test the cells with anti-A_1 lectin
 d. Both a and c
 e. Request a new specimen

77. A "directed donor" unit of blood is defined as a unit of blood from a person who gives blood for:
 a. Relief of polycythemia or other blood disorder
 b. His or her specific use only
 c. First-degree blood relative
 d. Another person he or she has specified

78. Before the patient can receive a directed donation unit, the patient requires which of the following tests to be completed?
 a. Type and screen only
 b. Type and screen and compatibility testing
 c. Retype of patient and donor unit
 d. No additional testing is required

79. An 18-year-old female with a hematocrit of 38%, temperature of 37° C, and blood pressure of 175/90 mm Hg presents for whole blood donation. Based on this information, would you accept, permanently defer (PD), or temporarily defer (TD) the donor?

a. Accept
b. TD, blood pressure is too high for a person of her age
c. TD, temperature is too high
d. PD, for all values listed

80. A 63-year-old man with a hemoglobin value of 130 g/dL and pulse of 80 beats/min, who received human pituitary growth hormone (PGH) when he was 10 years old, presents for whole blood donation. Based on this information, would you accept, permanently defer (PD,) or temporarily defer (TD) the donor?
a. Accept the donor
b. TD, because of the human PGH
c. PD, because of the human PGH
d. PD, because of the high hemoglobin value

81. A 38-year-old female weighing 153 lb, who received the rubella vaccine 2 months previously, presents to donate whole blood. She also received 2 units of packed cells after the delivery of her eighth child 8 weeks ago. Based on this information, would you accept, permanently defer (PD), or temporarily defer (TD) the donor?
a. Accept the donor
b. TD because of the packed cells 8 weeks ago
c. PD because of receiving blood products
d. TD because of the rubella vaccine

82. A 22-year-old female with a cousin with AIDS who had taken aspirin the day before and with needle marks on both arms presents to donate whole blood. Based on this information, would you accept, permanently defer (PD), or temporarily defer (TD) the donor?
a. PD, needle marks on both arms
b. TD, needle marks on both arms
c. PD, cousin with AIDS
d. TD, because of the aspirin

83. Each unit of blood must be tested for all of the following except:
a. Anti-HIV 1/2
b. HBsAg
c. Anti-HCV
d. Antigen to HCV

84. The principle of the HBsAg test is to detect which of the following?
a. Antigen in patient's plasma
b. Antigen on the patient's RBCs
c. Antibody in patient's serum
d. Antigen and antibody in patient's serum

85. Cryoprecipitate is prepared by first thawing:
a. Fresh frozen plasma at 1° to 6° C, and then doing a cold centrifugation to pack the cryoprecipitate to the bottom so the plasma may be removed
b. Fresh frozen plasma at room temperature, then placing in the freezer for 2 hours, then centrifuging and removing the cryoprecipitate

c. Cryoprecipitate at 1° to 6° C, then pooling the thawed cryoprecipitate in batches of 10 units, then quickly refreezing
d. Cryoprecipitate at room temperature, then centrifugation in the cold to concentrate the cryoprecipitate to the bottom before adding more plasma to reconstitute

86. Platelets must be kept in constant motion for which of the following reasons?
a. Maintain the pH so the platelets will be alive before transfusion
b. Keep the platelets in suspension and prevent clumping of the platelets
c. Mimic what is going on in the blood vessels
d. Preserve the coagulation factors and platelet viability

87. After thawing and pooling cryoprecipitate for transfusion to a patient, the product should be stored at:
a. Room temperature
b. 1° to 6° C
c. 37° C
d. 0° C

88. Fresh frozen plasma must be thawed at which temperature?
a. 1° to 6° C
b. Room temperature
c. 37° C
d. 40° C or higher

89. Frozen red blood cells are prepared for transfusion by thawing at:
a. Room temperature and then washing with saline
b. 37° C in a water bath and then washing with different concentrations of saline
c. 37° C control incubator and then mixing well before transfusion
d. 1° to 6° C for 2 days and then washing with different concentrations of dextrose

90. Which is the most likely reason frozen deglycerolized red blood cells would be used?
a. A patient with antibodies to a high-frequency antigen
b. Pregnant women requiring intrauterine transfusions
c. Emergency transfusion situations
d. Group AB Rh-negative patients

91. One indication for transfusion of thawed/pooled cryoprecipitate would be replacement of which of the following?
a. Factor X in hemophiliacs
b. Factor VIII in massively transfused patients
c. Fibrinogen
d. Volume

92. A contraindication for transfusing red blood cells to a patient is if the patient:

a. Is massively bleeding
b. Has well-compensated anemia
c. Has bone marrow failure
d. Has decreased red blood cell survival

93. Concerning the component and the required quality control results, which of the following is a true statement?
    a. FFP must have 80 international units of fibrinogen in 7 units tested
    b. Cryoprecipitate must have 80 international units of factor VIII
    c. Leukocyte-reduced red blood cells must have fewer than 3.3×10^{11} WBCs in each unit
    d. Platelets must have no red blood cells

94. Fresh frozen plasma must be stored at:
    a. Colder than $-18°$ C for no longer than 1 year from donation
    b. Colder than $-38°$ C for no longer than 1 year from donation
    c. Exactly $-18°$ C for no longer than 1 year from donation
    d. $-18°$ C to $-38°$ C for up to 10 years from donation

95. The storage temperature for packed red blood cells is _____.
    a. $1°$ to $10°$ C
    b. $1°$ to $4°$ C
    c. $1°$ to $6°$ C
    d. $20°$ to $25°$ F

96. Platelets made from a single whole blood donation should contain which of the following?
    a. 3×10^{11} platelets in 90% of samples
    b. 3.3×10^{9} platelets in 75% of samples
    c. 5.5×10^{10} platelets in 90% of samples
    d. 10×10^{10} platelets in 75% of samples

97. Frozen red blood cells must be stored at _____.
    a. $180°$ C or less
    b. $18°$ C or less
    c. $32°$ C or less
    d. $65°$ C or less

98. The temperature for incubation of the indirect antiglobulin test (IAT) should be _____.
    a. $24°$ C
    b. $6°$ C
    c. $37°$ C
    d. $37° \pm 10°$ C

99. The temperature of a blood refrigerator without a continuous recording device should be recorded:
    a. Daily
    b. Every 4 hours
    c. Once every 24 hours
    d. Every 30 minutes

100. When should quality control be performed on routine blood typing reagents?
    a. At the beginning of each shift
    b. Once daily
    c. Weekly
    d. Only when opening a new vial

SELF-ASSESSMENT

Content Area: _____

Score on Practice Questions: _____

List the specific topics covered in the missed questions:

List the specific topics covered in the correct questions:

NOTES

Clinical Chemistry

Janelle M. Chiasera

LIPIDS AND LIPOPROTEINS

Lipids

- Essential components, required for many body functions
- Functions: Hormone precursors, hormones, cell membrane structure and function, fuel, energy storage, aid in nerve conduction, aid in digestion
- Analysis commonly used to assess risk for cardiovascular disease
- Major lipids analyzed in the clinical laboratory include total cholesterol and triglycerides
- Total cholesterol and triglycerides most commonly measured using enzymatic assays (Table 8-1)

Lipoproteins

- Spherical lipid and protein complex (Figure 8-1), lipid core (triglycerides and cholesterol esters) and an outer shell of phospholipids, protein, and free cholesterol
- The smaller the diameter of the molecule, the more dense the molecule
- Each lipoprotein molecule has a different physical and chemical makeup; lipoproteins may be separated and measured based on one or more of these characteristics (Table 8-2)
- High-density lipoprotein (HDL) and low-density lipoprotein (LDL) are the only lipoproteins currently routinely measured in the clinical laboratory (see Table 8-3 for a list of methods used to measure HDL and LDL)
- Functions: Transport lipids through circulatory system, facilitate lipid metabolism
- Five major lipoproteins: Chylomicrons, very-low-density lipoprotein (VLDL), LDL, and HDL
- Additional lipoproteins identified include chylomicron remnant, intermediate density lipoprotein (IDL), and Lp(a)
  - Chylomicron remnant*: A lipolytic product of chylomicron catabolism, rapidly taken into the liver cell by specific receptors

- Intermediate density lipoprotein†: A lipolytic product of VLDL catabolism; taken up into the liver cell or converted to LDL
- Lp(a): An LDL-like molecule with one Apo(a) linked to the Apo B-100, high level of homology with plasminogen, increased concentrations associated with increased risk for coronary heart disease (CHD)

Apoproteins

- Functional and structural protein components of the lipoprotein molecule
- Each lipoprotein molecule contains one or more apoproteins
- Three main functions
  - Activate enzymes to aid in lipid metabolism
  - Maintain structural integrity of the lipoprotein molecule
- Enhance cellular uptake of lipoproteins (apoproteins are recognized by cell surface receptors) (see Table 8-4 for specific apoprotein function by class)

Specimen Considerations

- Serum or plasma after 12- to 16-hour fast (fast required for triglyceride analysis)
- Ethylenediaminetetraacetic acid (EDTA) (1 mg/1 mL blood) plasma preferred for analysis of lipoproteins (EDTA preserves lipoproteins); separate plasma within 2 hours
- National Cholesterol Education Program recommends multiplying plasma concentrations by 1.03 to convert to serum values
- No alcohol 72 hours before blood collection (alcohol transiently increases triglycerides)
- Patient should be seated during collection
- Avoid citrate, fluoride, oxalate anticoagulants (can cause dilution of plasma components) (Box 8-1)

Pathology

- Abnormalities in lipids and lipoproteins are referred to as hyperlipidemias and hyperlipoproteinemias, respectively
- Elevated levels of lipids and lipoproteins are associated with risk for coronary heart disease, specifically, increased total cholesterol, increased LDL, decreased HDL

---

*Remnant lipoproteins have been shown to be predictive of coronary heart disease risk.

TABLE 8-1	Methods to Measure Total Cholesterol and Triglyceride		
Analyte	**Method**	**Principle**	**Comments**
Total cholesterol	Enzymatic, end-point	*Reaction Steps* 1. Cholesterol—Esters $\xrightarrow{\text{Cholesterol esterase}}$ Cholesterol + Fatty acids 2. Cholesterol + O_2 cholesterol oxidase → cholest-4-en-3-one + H_2O_2 *Detection:* A. H_2O_2 + 4-aminophenazone(or other dye) $\xrightarrow{\text{peroxidase}}$ oxidized dye(A_{max}, 500 nm) + H_2O_2 B. Monitor O_2 consumption with an O_2 electrode	Most common method
	CDC-modified Abell reaction	Cholesterol extracted with zeolite, esters chemically hydrolyzed (saponification), and total cholesterol measured by Liebermann-Burchard (L-B) reaction	Reference method
Triglycerides*	Enzymatic	*Common Steps to All Enzymatic Assays Below:* 1. Triglycerides $\xrightarrow{\text{Lipase, Protease}}$ Glycerol + 3 Fatty acids 2. Glycerol + ATP $\xrightarrow{\text{Glycerol Kinase}}$ Glycerol-3 phosphate + ADP *Pyruvate Kinase (NADH Consumption):* 3. ADP + Phosphoenolpyruvate $\xrightarrow{\text{Pyruvate Kinase}}$ ATP + Pyruvate 4. Pyruvate + NADH + H^+ $\xrightarrow{\text{Lactate Dehydrogenase}}$ Lactate + NAD$^+$ *Glycerol Phosphate Dehydrogenase (Formazan Colorimetric):* 3. Glycerol-3-phosphate + NAD$^+$ $\xrightarrow{\text{Glycerol Phosphate Dehydrogenase}}$ Dihydroxyacetone phosphate + NADH + H^+ 4. NADH + Oxidized tetrazolium $\xrightarrow{\text{Diaphorase}}$ Reduced tetrazolium *Glycerol Dehydrogenase:* 3. Glycerol + NAD$^+$ $\xrightarrow{\text{Glycerol Dehydrogenase}}$ Dihydroxyacetone + NADH + H^+ 4. NADH + H^+ + Resazurin $\xrightarrow{\text{Diaphorase}}$ Resorufin + NAD$^+$	Most common methods

CDC, Centers for Disease Control and Prevention.
*National Cholesterol Education Program recommends all laboratories offer glycerol blanking.

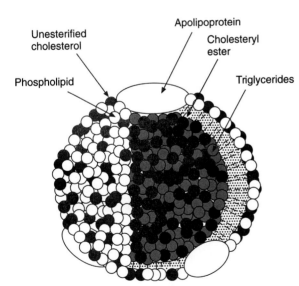

FIGURE 8-1 Lipoprotein particle.

- Tangier disease: Autosomal dominant lipoprotein disorder resulting from catabolism of HDL. Characterized by extremely reduced HDL concentrations and accumulation of cholesterol esters in body tissues, causing orange tonsils, splenomegaly, and peripheral neuropathy

Carbohydrates

- Aldoses or ketoses, nomenclature based on configuration (D or L); D sugars represent majority found in the body
- Three main classes of carbohydrates
  - Monosaccharides
    - Simple sugars
    - Glucose
    - Fructose
  - Disaccharides
    - Two monosaccharides linked by a glycosidic bond
      - Maltose (glucose and glucose)
      - Lactose (glucose and galactose)
      - Sucrose (glucose and fructose)
  - Polysaccharides
    - Two monosaccharides linked by glycosidic bond
    - Starch and glycogen

- Pathologic processes are classified based on lipid levels, lipoprotein pattern, and clinical and biochemical phenotype, with most very rare in occurrence (Table 8-5)

TABLE 8-2	Lipoprotein Characteristics			
Lipoprotein (Diameter (nm)	Density (g/mL)	Major Lipids (%)	Electrophoretic Mobility	Protein Content (%)
Chylomicrons (>70)	<0.95	90 TGex	Origin	1-2
VLDL (26-70)	0.95-1.006	65 TG (end), 15 chol	Pre-β	8-10
LDL (19-23)	1.019-1.063	50 chol	β	20
HDL (4-10)	1.063-1.21	20 chol, 25 phos	α	50-55

Chol, Cholesterol esters; *HDL*, high-density lipoproteins; *LDL*, low-density lipoproteins; *phos*, phospholipids; *TGend*, endogenous triglycerides; *TGex*, exogenous triglycerides; *VLDL*, very-low-density lipoproteins.

TABLE 8-3	Methods to Measure High-Density and Low-Density Lipoproteins		
Analyte	Method	Description	Comments
HDL	Ultracentrifugation*	Sample adjusted to a density of 1.063 (potassium bromide) and centrifuged at high speed for 24 hr. Sample separates based on density (see Table 8-2)	Specialized laboratories only
	Precipitation*	1. Precipitation of Apo B containing lipoproteins using polyanion-divalent cation solutions. HDL quantitated in the supernatant after precipitation and centrifugation	Commonly used method
		2. Precipitation of Apo B containing lipoproteins using dextran sulfate and iron; no centrifugation needed	
	Electrophoresis	Separation based on size and charge; mobility equal to α_1-globulins; agarose gel	Frequently used
	Homogeneous (direct)	Immunologic assay involving blockage of non-HDL lipoproteins; HDL free to react with reagent enzymes	Commonly used method
LDL	Friedewald formula	LDL-C = cholesterol − (VLDL-C + HDL-C) TG/5 approximates VLDL-C	Commonly used; not reliable estimation when TG >400 mg/dL
	β Quantification	Uses ultracentrifugation (to separate VLDL and chylo) and precipitation (to remove HDL), LDL calculated as density >1.006 − HDL	Research only
	Homogeneous (direct)	Uses detergents or other chemicals to block or solubilize lipoprotein classes to allow for quantitation of LDL	Commonly used method

HDL, high-density lipoprotein; *LDL*, low-density lipoprotein; *TG*, triglycerides; *VLDL*, very-low-density lipoprotein.
*Centers for Disease Control and Prevention reference method involves ultracentrifugation (to remove VLDL), heparin manganese precipitation from 1.006 infranatant (to remove LDL), and analysis of supernatant by Abell-Kendall method.

TABLE 8-4	Apoprotein Classes *Function and Carriers*		
Apoprotein Class		Lipoprotein Carrier	Function
A	AI	HDL, chylomicrons	Cofactor for LCAT
	AII	HDL	Unknown
	AIV	HDL, chylomicrons	Activates LCAT
B	48	Chylomicrons	Secretion of TG from intestines
	100	VLDL, LDL	LDL receptor binding
C	I	Chylomicrons, VLDL, HDL	Activates LCAT
	II	Chylomicrons, VLDL, HDL	Activates LpL
	III	Chylomicrons, VLDL, HDL	Inhibits activation of LpL by C-II
E		Chylomicrons, VLDL, HDL	Facilitate uptake of remnant particles (chylomicrons and IDL)

HDL, High-density lipoproteins; *LCAT*, lecithin cholesterol acyltranferase; *LDL*, low-density lipoproteins; *LpL*, lipoprotein lipase; *TG*, triglycerides; *VLDL*, very-low-density lipoproteins.

BOX 8-1   Recommended Ranges
National Cholesterol Education Program: Adult Treatment Panel Recommended Ranges (Based on Serum Samples)

Total cholesterol: <200 mg/dL
Triglycerides: <150 mg/dL
HDL: >40 mg/dL; >60 mg/dL protective (subtract a risk factor)
LDL: <100 mg/dL optimal or:
   <100 mg/dL with CHD or CHD risk equivalent
   <130 mg/dL with two or more risk factors
   <160 mg/dL with 0 to 1 risk factor
Risk factors: Cigarette smoking, hypertension (blood pressure >140/90 mm Hg or on hypertensive medication), HDL <40 mg/dL, family history of premature CHD, age (men ≥45 years, women ≥55 years).

CHD, Coronary heart disease; *HDL,* high-density lipoprotein; *LDL,* low-density lipoprotein.

- Serve as major source of energy for the body; glucose is the only monosaccharide used by the body for energy; all sugars must be digested to this monosaccharide for use
- Glucose regulation involves primarily insulin (decreased glucose) and glucagon (increased glucose), both produced from the pancreas, acting in conjunction. To a lesser extent, epinephrine, cortisol, and growth hormone (all increase glucose) contribute to glucose regulation; insulin is the only hormone that acts to decrease glucose concentrations
- Carbohydrate metabolism terminology
  - Glycolysis: Process that converts glucose to pyruvate for energy purposes
  - Gluconeogenesis: Formation of glucose from non-carbohydrate sources (amino acids, lactate, glycerol [lipids])
  - Glycogenolysis: Breakdown of glycogen to form glucose
  - Glycogenesis: Conversion of glucose to glycogen for storage purposes

- Measurement done to diagnose hyperglycemia (diabetes mellitus) or hypoglycemia
- Hemoglobin A1c is used as a measure of long-term glycemic control (2- to 3-month period). A1c is used to diagnose and monitor treatment of diabetes. The American Diabetes Association (ADA) recommends that A1c measurements be performed at least twice per year in those with stable glycemic control and quarterly in those with unstable glycemic control. The ADA recommends an A1c goal of approximately 7% in those with diabetes to reduce the complications associated with diabetes (microvascular, macrovascular, and neuropathic)
- Hemoglobin A1c is made through the three-step glycation process
  - Glucose reversibly binds to the amino terminal end of hemoglobin to form a labile aldimine
  - The aldimine undergoes irreversible rearrangement (Amadori arrangement) to form a stable ketoamine
  - Glucose undergoes a conformational change to a cyclic structure

Measurement
- Three enzymatic methods are available: Hexokinase, glucose oxidase, and glucose dehydrogenase (Table 8-6)

Specimen Considerations
- Glucose may be analyzed on a variety of samples, including
  - Serum
  - Plasma (5% lower than serum)
  - Whole blood (~15% lower than plasma)
  - Capillary (2 to 5 mg/dL higher than venous collected samples)
  - Urine
  - Other fluids (cerebrospinal fluid [CSF], ascetic, pleural, peritoneal, and drainage fluids) collect in tubes containing fluoride/oxalate preservative; analyze immediately after collection, centrifuge if not clear

TABLE 8-5	Primary Hyperlipoproteinemias			
Name	Fredrickson Phenotype	Increased fraction(s)	Plasma Appearance	Defect
Hyperchylomicronemia	I	TG, chylomicrons	Cream layer over clear plasma	LPL or Apo-CII deficiency
Hyperbetalipoproteinemia	IIA	IIA: LDL, TC	IIA: Clear	LDL receptor mutation
	IIB	IIB: LDL, TG, VLDL	IIB: Turbid	Decreased LDL clearance
Dysbetalipoproteinemia	III	TC, TG, LDL (IDL)	Turbid	Defective ApoE
Hyperprebetalipoproteinemia	IV	VLDL, TG	Turbid	
Mixed hyperlipoproteinemia	V	Chylomicrons, VLDL, TC, TG	Cream layer over turbid plasma	

HDL, High-density lipoproteins; *LCAT,* lecithin cholesterol acyltransferase; *LDL,* low density lipoproteins; *LpL,* lipoprotein lipase; *TG,* triglycerides; *VLDL,* very low density lipoproteins.

TABLE 8-6	Enzymatic Methods to Measure Glucose
Method	**Principle**
Hexokinase	Glucose + ATP $\xrightarrow{\text{Hexokinase}}$ Glucose-6-phosphate + ADP
	Glucose-6-phosphate + NAD$^+$ $\xrightarrow{\text{G6PD}}$ 6-Phosphogluconate + NADH + H$^+$
Glucose oxidase	Glucose + O$_2$ $\xrightarrow{\text{GlucoseOxidase}}$ Gluconic acid + H$_2$O$_2$
	o-Dianisidine + H$_2$O$_2$ $\xrightarrow{\text{Peroxidase}}$ Oxidized o-dianisidine + H$_2$O
Glucose dehydrogenase	Glucose + NAD + $\xrightarrow{\text{Glucose Dehydrogenase}}$ D-Glucono-δ-lactone + NADH + H$^+$

BOX 8-2	**Recommended Ranges** *American Diabetes Association* *Recommended Range for Glucose*
Glucose <100 mg/dL	

- Separate immediately after collection to avoid glycolysis; glucose in whole blood at room temperature undergoes glycolysis at a rate of 5% to 7% per hour. Collect in sodium fluoride if cannot be separated immediately (Box 8-2)
- ADA criteria for the diagnosis of diabetes mellitus are found in Table 8-9
- American Diabetes Association Criteria for the Diagnosis of Gestational Diabetes.
  - Perform in those with high-risk characteristics: Marked obesity, history of gestational diabetes mellitus (GDM), glycosuria, or a strong family history. Initial screening at first prenatal visit; retest at 24 to 28 weeks of gestation if negative
  - Fasting plasma glucose (FPG) greater than 126 mg/dL or random plasma glucose (RPG) greater than 200 mg/dL meets the diagnosis of GDM; if not diagnostic (in women with high-risk characteristics), perform either of the following
    - One-step approach
      - Perform a diagnostic oral glucose tolerance test (OGTT) without prior screening (Table 8-8)
    - Two-step approach

TABLE 8-7	**Oral Glucose Tolerance Test in Diagnosis of Gestational Diabetes** *Samples Drawn After 100-g* Glucose Drink*
Time of Sample Collection	**Target Level**
Fasting (before glucose load)	95 mg/dL
1 Hr after glucose load	180 mg/dL
2 Hr after glucose load	155 mg/dL
3 Hr after glucose load†	140 mg/dL

Interpretation: If two or more values meet or exceed the target level, gestational diabetes mellitus is diagnosed.
*A 75-g glucose load may be used, although this method is not as well validated as the 100-g oral glucose tolerance test.
†The 3-hr sample is not drawn if 75 g is used.

TABLE 8-8	**Screening Oral Glucose Tolerance Test for the Diagnosis of Gestational Diabetes Mellitus**
Gestational Diabetes Screening: Glucose Challenge Test	
Sample drawn 1 hr after a 50-g glucose drink	
Glucose Level	**Interpretation**
<140* mg/dL	Normal screen
140*-199 mg/dL	Abnormal screen; perform diagnostic oral glucose tolerance test

*Some use a cutoff of >130 mg/dL because that identifies 90% of women with gestational diabetes mellitus in contrast to 80% identified using the threshold of >140 mg/dL.

TABLE 8-9	**American Diabetes Association Diagnostic Criteria for Diabetes Mellitus**	
	Criteria	**Comments**
1.	Hemoglobin A1c ≥6.5% or	Using a method traceable to the National Glycohemoglobin Standardization Program
2.	Fasting plasma glucose ≥126 mg/dL or	
3.	Random plasma glucose ≥200 mg/dL or	With symptoms of hyperglycemia
4.	2-Hr plasma glucose ≥200 mg/dL	During an oral glucose tolerance test as described by the World Health Organization with a 75-g glucose load

NOTE: In the absence of symptoms of hyperglycemia, 1-3 should be confirmed by repeat testing.

  - Perform a screening OGTT, if the screening OGTT is abnormal (Table 8-9)
    - Perform the diagnostic OGTT (see Table 8-8)

Pathologic Processes
Hypoglycemia
- Defined as glucose value of 45 mg/dL or less, life-threatening condition
- Diagnosed based on Whipple triad: (1) glucose 45 mg/dL or less, (2) symptoms of hypoglycemia, (3) resolution of symptoms after glucose administration

- Two types
  - Reactive "fictitious" hypoglycemia: Caused by insulin injections
  - Spontaneous: Caused by excessive insulin secretion (insulin-producing tumor)
- C-peptide and insulin levels are helpful in differentiating the types
  - Fictitious: See increased insulin, low or undetectable C-peptide
  - Spontaneous: See increased insulin, increased C-peptide
- Unexplained hypoglycemia in children (<5 years of age) may indicate galactosemia (inborn error of glucose metabolism), Clinitest can aid in the diagnosis
  - Galactosemia suggested when urine glucose (dipstick) is negative and Clinitest positive
- Hypoglycemia in children with liver enlargement is suggestive of one of 14 glycogen storage diseases, von Gierke's disease. This is an inherited disease resulting from a deficiency in glucose-6-phosphatase (enzyme responsible for breaking down glycogen).
- Clinically significant glycogen storage diseases
  - Glycogen storage disease IA (von Gierke's disease): Deficiency in glucose-6-phosphatase
  - Glycogen storage disease II (Pompe's disease): Deficiency in acid maltase
  - Glycogen storage disease III (Cori's disease): Deficiency in debranching enzyme
  - Glycogen storage disease V (McArdle's disease): Deficiency in myophosphorylase
  - Glycogen storage disease VII (Tarui's disease): Deficiency in phosphofructokinase

Hyperglycemia: Diabetes Mellitus

- Defined as a group of metabolic diseases represented by hyperglycemia and caused by
  - Defect in insulin secretion
  - Defect in insulin action
  - Defect in both insulin secretion and action
- Symptoms of hyperglycemia include polyuria, polydipsia, weight loss with polyphagia, blurred vision
- Long-term complications include retinopathy, neuropathy, nephropathy, and atherosclerotic cardiovascular disease
- Diagnostic criteria (see Table 8-9)
- Intermediate group
  - The ADA also defined an intermediate group located between the normal and diagnostic range, referred to as increased risk for diabetes
  - Defined as follows
    - FPG 100 to 125 mg/dL: Impaired fasting glucose
    - 2-hour PG in the 75-g OGTT 140 to 199 mg/dL: Impaired glucose tolerance
    - A1c 5.7 to 6.4%: At risk for developing diabetes mellitus (DM)
    - NOTE: This intermediate group is not a clinical entity, but rather serves as a risk factor for the development of DM and cardiovascular disease

- Types of DM
  - Type 1 DM (T1DM) (5%-10% of all DM cases)
    - Cause: Absolute deficiency of insulin secretion
  - Type 2 DM (T2DM) (90%-95% of all DM cases)
    - Cause: Combination of insulin resistance and inadequate compensatory secretion of insulin
  - Gestational DM (GDM)
    - Any degree of glucose intolerance with onset or first recognition during pregnancy
  - Other specific types
    - Caused by genetic abnormalities, diseases, endocrinopathies, infections, drugs, etc.

Markers of Glucose Control: Analytes Used to Assess Glucose Control

- Glucose: Glucose level at the time of draw
- Hemoglobin A1c (HbA1c) also known as glycated hemoglobin. Measure of glucose control over the previous of 2 to 3 months (life span of a red cell), represents glucose attached to the N-terminal valine of the hemoglobin molecule
  - A very strong association between HbA1c and estimated average glucose
  - The ADA and the American Society for Clinical Chemistry recommend estimated average glucose (eAG) be reported along with every HbA1c result
- eAG: Calculated average glucose that corresponds to a measured HbA1c result.

$$eAG\ mg/dL = 28.7 \times A1c - 46.7$$

- Fructosamine: Refers to glycated albumin. A measure of glycemic control over a 2- to 3-week period

Blood Gases

- Includes pH, pCO_2, pO_2, HCO_3-, base excess, O_2 saturation
- pH, pCO_2, pO_2 are measured, all others are calculated parameters
- Normal acid-base status refers to a pH of 7.40 and a ratio of bicarbonate to carbonic acid of 20:1
- pH
  - Index of acidity or alkalinity of blood
  - $pH = -\log [H^+]$; inverse, nonlinear relationship to $[H^+]$; unitless; increase (H) = decrease pH
    - Decrease in 1 pH unit results in a 10-fold increase in $[H^+]$ activity
  - Decreased pH (<7.35) indicates acidemia, increased pH (>7.45) indicates alkalemia
  - pH is regulated within a very narrow limit, optimal $pH = 7.40$, which corresponds to an $[H^+]$ of 40 nmol/L
- pCO_2 is the respiratory component
  - pCO_2 refers to the pressure of carbon dioxide dissolved in the blood
  - A normal pCO_2 refers to the ability of the body to remove CO_2 at a rate equal to the cellular production of CO_2

- The body rids itself of CO_2 via two mechanisms: The lungs and conversion of CO_2 to carbonic acid that dissociates to HCO_3^- and H^+ (in the presence of carbonic anhydrase)
- Increased pCO_2 indicates respiratory acidosis (see Table 8-11 for causes of acid-base disturbances)
- Decreased pCO_2 indicates respiratory alkalosis (see Table 8-11 for causes of acid-base disturbances)
- Bicarbonate is the metabolic component
  - Calculated parameter, calculated from pH and pCO_2 using the Henderson-Hasselbalch (HH) equation
    - HH equation

$$pH = pK' + \log HCO_3^- / H_2CO_3$$
$$H_2CO_3 = \alpha \times pCO_2 (\alpha = 0.0306)$$
$$\text{Optimal } HCO_3^- / H_2CO_3 = 20:1$$

- An indication of the buffering capacity of the blood
- Increased bicarbonate indicates metabolic alkalosis (see Table 8-11 for causes of acid-base disturbances)
- Decreased bicarbonate indicates metabolic acidosis (see Table 8-11 for causes of acid-base disturbances)
- pO_2
  - Is a measure of the pressure of dissolved O_2 in the blood
  - Value is related to the ability of the lungs to oxygenate blood
  - Decreased pO_2 may be related to decreased pulmonary ventilation, impaired gas exchange, altered blood flow within the heart or lungs

Physiologic Buffers

- Body's first line of defense in all body fluids against changes in pH
- All buffer systems are intercellular
- The body contains four buffer systems
  - Bicarbonate: Carbonic acid buffer system
    - Most physiologically important buffer system, works in conjunction with the hemoglobin buffer system to maintain normal blood gas status
    - Is of primary importance in acid-base regulation because CO_2 (a volatile acidic gas) is produced from energy metabolism
    - Combats the production of large amounts of acid (H_2CO_3) according to the following equation

$$H_2CO_3^- \xrightarrow{\text{Carbonic Anhydrase}} H_2O + CO_2$$

  - Hemoglobin buffer system
    - Reduced hemoglobin has an increased affinity for H^+ rather than oxygenated hemoglobin
    - Buffers by transporting acid from the tissues to the lungs for removal
  - Plasma protein buffer system and phosphate buffer system
    - Of minor importance

Sample Considerations

- Sample is highly susceptible to improper collection and handling

- Arterial, venous, and capillary samples acceptable
- Samples are stable for 15 minutes at room temperature, 45 minutes if stored on crushed ice
- Avoid pneumatic tube transport unless a pressure-sealed container is used
- Anaerobic conditions are essential during collection; room air has a pCO_2 of 0 and a pO_2 of approximately 150 mm Hg, which may affect sample values if they are uncapped or contain air bubbles
  - Samples exposed to room air (uncapped or air bubbles) may result in false elevations in pO_2 and false decrease in pCO_2 as a result of equilibration with room air
- Collect in syringe with dry heparin anticoagulant; glass syringe preferred stored on ice; if collected in plastic syringe, store at room temperature and assay within 15 minutes

Measurement

- pH, pCO_2, and pO_2 are measured using an electrochemical cell (galvanic cell) that contains two half cells (reference and indictor) connected by a salt bridge
  - Reference electrodes include standard hydrogen (SHE), saturated calomel (SCE), and silver/silver chloride (Ag/AgCL) electrodes. Most commonly used reference electrode is the silver/silver chloride electrode
    - Saturated with KCL (SCE and Ag/AgCL) or HCL (SHE) so the electrode has a constant, fixed potential
  - Indicator electrodes include glass, liquid, solid-state, gas sensing, and enzyme
    - Potential of this electrode varies depending on the analyte in the patient sample
- pH and pCO_2 are measured using potentiometry (current is maintained at zero and voltage is measured) and pO_2 is measured using amperometry (voltage is constant and current is measured)
  - pH is measured using a pH-sensitive glass indicator electrode with an Ag/AgCl reference electrode
  - pCO_2 is measured using a modified pH electrode covered by a silicone rubber membrane permeable to gas. The pH electrode is modified by the addition of an aqueous layer of bicarbonate solution on the inside surface of the membrane; the bicarbonate buffer reacts with the CO_2 in the patient sample, producing an H^+ ion that is detected by the internal pH meter
  - pO_2 is measured using a cell containing a platinum cathode, an Ag/AgCL reference electrode, a phosphatase buffer (in contact with both electrodes), and a polypropylene membrane. Voltage is applied to the cathode (-0.6 V) and pO_2 crosses the membrane and reduces, causing four electrons of current to flow for every O_2 molecule
  - Recommended ranges for blood gases are found in Table 8-10
  - Acid-base disorders are presented in Table 8-11

Total Body Water, Electrolytes, and Minerals

Anion Gap

- Accounts for approximately 65% and 55% of total body mass in males and females, respectively
- Divided into two main categories: Intracellular water (ICW) and extracellular water (ECW) (Table 8-12)
- The composition of interstitial fluid is similar to that of plasma, except that plasma contains large protein molecules
- Regulation of fluid volume depends on plasma osmolality and blood volume
- The plasma component of ECW is the only compartment directly measurable
- Electrolytes include bicarbonate, sodium, potassium, chloride, osmolality, and anion gap
  - Sodium: Major cation of extracellular fluid, maintained by Na^+/K^+ ATPase pump (exchanges three sodium ions out of cell for two potassium ions moving into the cell), largely determines osmolality of extracellular fluid
  - Potassium: Major cation of intracellular fluid, maintained by Na^+/K^+ ATPase pump (exchanges three sodium ions out of cell for two potassium ions moving into the cell), involved with neuromuscular excitability and contraction of the heart
  - Chloride: Major extracellular anion, exact function not well understood
  - Bicarbonate: Second most abundant ion in extracellular fluid, major component of the blood buffering system
- Movement of fluid between compartments is a result of osmotic pressure and hydrostatic and oncotic pressure differences
  - Osmotic pressure is the most important factor moving water (from lower concentrations to higher concentrations) between the intracellular space and plasma; caused by the difference in concentrations of solutions on either side of a membrane
  - Hydrostatic pressure drives fluid out of the vessels into the surrounding tissue

Osmotic Pressure, Osmolality, and Volume Regulation

- Osmotic pressure determines water distribution among body water compartments; force that moves water from dilute to concentrated solutions
- Osmolality is a measure of solute concentration of a solution; a measure dependent on the number (not size and charge) of particles in solution

TABLE 8-10	Recommended Ranges for Blood Gases Analytes	
Analyte	**Range**	**Units**
pH	7.35-7.45	No units
pCO_2	35-45	mm Hg
pO_2	80-100	mm Hg
HCO_3	22-28	mmol/L
Base excess	−2-+2	mmol/L
O_2 saturation	≥95	%

TABLE 8-11	Acid-Base Disorders, Cause, and Laboratory Values			
Disorder	**Associated Data**	**Uncompensated**	**Compensated***	**Cause**
Respiratory acidosis	Decreased pH Increased pCO_2	N HCO_3	Increased HCO_3 (1 mmol/L for every 10–mm Hg increase in pCO_2)†	Obstructive lung disease, acute airway obstruction, circulatory failure, impaired respiratory system
Metabolic acidosis	Decreased pH Decreased HCO_3	N pCO_2	Decreased pCO_2 (1-1.3 mm Hg for every 1-mmol/L decrease in HCO_3)	Ketoacidosis, hypoxic acidosis, renal failure
Respiratory alkalosis	Increased pH Decreased pCO_2	N HCO_3	Decreased HCO_3 (1-2 mmol/L for every 10–mm Hg decrease in pCO_2)†	Hypoxia-induced hyperventilation, pulmonary embolism, pulmonary edema, anxiety, overventilation, drugs, CNS disorders
Metabolic alkalosis	Increased pH Increased HCO_3	N pCO_2	Increased pCO_2 (0.6-0.7 mm Hg for every 1-mmol/L increase in HCO_3)	Hypokalemia, excess administration of HCO_3, vomiting, GI suction, corticosteroid excess

↑, Increased; ↓, decreased; *CNS*, central nervous system; *GI*, gastrointestinal; *N*, normal.
*The terms *uncompensated* and *compensated* refer to whether the body has made changes to restore the pH to normal (20:1 ratio). *Uncompensated* means the body has not yet attempted to restore the pH to normal; *compensated* refers to the fact that the body has made changes to restore the pH to normal.
†Refers to compensation for acute situations only. Chronic situations will increase or decrease HCO_3 by 3-5 mmol/L for every 10–mm Hg change in pCO_2

TABLE 8-12	Total Body Water Compartments and Electrolytes			
Compartment	**Components**	**Percent of Total Body Water (%)**	**Major Cations**	**Major Anions**
Intracellular		~60	K, Mg	PO$_4$
Extracellular	Plasma	~10	Na, K, Ca	Cl, HCO$_3$
	Interstitial fluid	~30	Na, K, Ca	Cl, HCO$_3$

TABLE 8-13	Major Cations and Anions in Extracellular and Intracellular Fluid Compartments
Primary Cations	**Primary Anions**
Sodium (Na$^+$)	Chloride (Cl$^-$)
Potassium (K$^+$)	Bicarbonate (HCO$_3^-$)
Calcium (Ca$^+$)	Phosphate (HPO$_4$)
Magnesium (Mg$^+$)	Sulfate (SO$_4^{2-}$)

TABLE 8-14	Recommended Ranges for Electrolytes	
Analyte	**Range**	**Units**
Sodium	135-145	mmol/L
Potassium	3.5-5.0	mmol/L
Chloride	98-107	mmol/L
Total carbon dioxide	21-28	mmol/L
Osmolality (plasma)	275-295	mOsm/kg
Anion gap	8-16 (without potassium) 12-20 (with potassium)	mmol/L

- Osmolality formula

$$\text{Osmolality}_{calculated}(mOsm/kg) = 2(Na) + (\text{Blood urea nitrogen[mg/dL] 2.8}) + (\text{Glucose[mg/dL]}/18)$$

- The measured osmolality and calculated osmolality may be used to calculate the osmolal gap. A difference between the calculated and measured osmolality may be due to the following
  - Presence of other osmotically active substances (other than sodium, glucose, urea)
  - Metabolic acidosis caused by nonelectrolytes (lactic acid, ketoacids, alcohol, ethylene glycol, organic acids)
  - Osmolal gap formula

$$\text{Osmolal gap} = \text{Measured osmolality} - \text{Calculated osmolality}$$

- Regulation of osmolality and volume depends mainly on thirst and to a lesser extent antidiuretic hormone (ADH), renin-angiotensin-aldosterone (RAA) system, natriuretic peptides
  - Thirst, stimulated by increased osmolality and decreased volume, acts to increase water intake and decrease osmolality
  - ADH, stimulated by increased osmolality and decreased volume, results in the reabsorption of water by the kidneys and decreased osmolality
  - RAA system, stimulated by decreased volume and decreased sodium, increases blood pressure, serum sodium, urine potassium, and urine hydrogen and decreases serum potassium and hydrogen
  - Natriuretic peptides, stimulated by increased cardiac volume, increase urine sodium and decrease blood volume and aldosterone

Electrolytes

- The term *electrolytes* refer to the majority of osmotically active ions (cations and anions) in the body
- Primary cations and anions are listed in Table 8-13

- Electrolytes are molecules capable of carrying a charge and are characterized as anions or cations
  - Anions carry a negative charge
  - Cations carry a positive charge
- Electrolytes are essential components in numerous processes
  - Volume and osmotic regulation: Sodium, chloride, and potassium
  - Heart contractility: Potassium and magnesium
  - Enzyme activation: Magnesium
  - Acid-base balance: Bicarbonate, potassium, and chloride
  - Blood coagulation: Calcium and magnesium
- Sodium is the major cation in extracellular fluid, and potassium is the major cation in intercellular fluid
- The Na$^+$/-K$^+$ ATPase pump maintains the distribution of sodium inside the cell and potassium outside the cell by exchanging three sodium ions moving out of cells for two potassium ions moving into the cell
- The kidneys maintain or excrete sodium based on osmolality and blood volume
- Reference ranges for electrolytes are found in Table 8-14

Pathologic Processes
Sodium
- Hyponatremia
  - Defined as plasma sodium less than 135 mmol/L; weakness and confusion seen at values less than 20 mmol/L; paralysis and severe mental impairment seen at values less than 110 mmol/L
  - Hyponatremia should be confirmed by decreased plasma osmolality; both urine and plasma osmolality are helpful in differentiating between causes of hyponatremia

TABLE 8-15	Causes of Hypernatremia and Hyponatremia	
Pathology	**Volume Status**	**Cause**
Hyponatremia	Hypovolemia	Sodium loss in excess of water Thiazide diuretics GI factors, burns, sweat Potassium depletion
Hyponatremia	Normovolemia	Water balance issues SAIDH Hyperlipidemia (artifactual) Adrenal insufficiency Altered osmolality regulation
Hyponatremia	Hypervolemia	Movement of fluid from intravascular to interstitial fluid CHF Hepatic cirrhosis Advanced renal failure Excess water intake Nephrotic syndrome
Hypernatremia		Renal loss GI loss Sweating Inadequate thirst mechanism Those without access to water Ingestion of excessive salt

CHF, Congestive heart failure; *GI,* gastrointestinal; *SIADH,* syndrome of inappropriate antidiuretic hormone.

- Pathogenesis of hyponatremia is associated with volume status (hypovolemic, normovolemic, and hypervolemic) (Table 8-15)
- Diagnosis of hyponatremia includes decreased plasma sodium, decreased plasma osmolality, and differentiation of cause by urine sodium
  - Urine sodium less than 15 mmol/L: Hypovolemia with fluid replacement (diarrhea, vomiting)
  - Urine sodium greater than 20 mmol/L: Syndrome of inappropriate secretion of antidiuretic hormone, thiazides, aldosterone deficiency, renal failure with excess water
- Hypernatremia
  - Defined as plasma sodium greater than 150 mmol/L
  - Rarely occurs in those with a normal thirst response
  - Results from excess water loss relative to sodium levels, including renal loss, gastrointestinal (GI) loss and sweating, fever, burns, and exposure to heat
  - Measurement of osmolality is used to differentiate the causes of hypernatremia
  - Diagnosis of hypernatremia includes increased plasma sodium and differentiation of cause by urine osmolality
    - Urine osmolality greater than mOsm/kg: GI loss, diminished thirst, excessive intravenous or oral intake of sodium

  - Urine osmolality 300 to 800 mOsm/kg: Impaired ADH release, diuretics, osmotic diuresis
  - Urine osmolality less than 300 mOsm/kg: Diabetes insipidus

Potassium

Hypokalemia
- Defined as potassium less than 3 mmol/L
- Poses a serious concern in all people; characterized by muscle weakness, irritability, paralysis, cardiac abnormalities
- Potassium less than 2.5 mmol/L induces cardiac arrhythmias, including premature atrial and ventricular beats and ventricular tachycardia and fibrillation
- Potassium less than 3.5 mmol/L before surgery is associated with increased incidence of arrhythmias requiring cardiopulmonary resuscitation
- Causes include
  - GI or urinary loss
    - Vomiting, diarrhea, gastric suction
    - Kidney disorders, including tubular acidosis
    - Excess aldosterone
    - Hypomagnesemia
  - Increased cellular uptake
    - Alkalemia increases cellular uptake of potassium
    - Insulin increases uptake of potassium into muscle and liver cells
  - Reduced dietary intake

Hyperkalemia
- Defined as potassium greater than 5 mmol/L
  - Potassium 6 to 7 mmol/L associated with altered electrocardiogram
  - Potassium greater than 8 mmol/L associated with muscle weakness
  - Potassium greater than 10 mmol/L associated with cardiac arrest
- Poses a serious concern in all people; characterized by muscle weakness, cardiac arrhythmias, and cardiac arrest
- Often multiple underlying conditions exist
- Causes
  - Excess intake (oral or intravenous)
    - Likely seen with renal impairment
  - Cellular loss
    - Processes that promote the release of potassium from cells (trauma, severe tissue hypoxia, massive hemolysis, metabolic acidosis, administration of cytotoxic agents, hypothermia)
  - Decreased renal excretion
    - Glomerular filtration impairment
    - Tubular function impairment
    - Conditions that reduce aldosterone production
  - Factitious (artifactual)
    - Prolonged tourniquet use during collection
    - Excessive clenching of fist during venipuncture

○ Storage of blood on ice; whole blood samples for potassium analysis should be collected and stored at room temperature

○ Hemolysis

Chloride

Hyperchloremia (Chloride >107 mmol/L)
- Frequently follows hypernatremia
- Causes: GI loss, renal tubular acidosis, mineralocorticoid deficiency
- Compensated respiratory alkalosis
- Often indicates an acidotic process

Hypochloremia (Chloride <98 mmol/L)
- Causes: Excessive loss (GI loss), mineralocorticoid excess, salt-losing renal disease
- Often indicates an alkalotic process

Bicarbonate

Increased Bicarbonate
- Causes: Severe vomiting, hypokalemia, excessive alkali intake

Decreased Bicarbonate
- Causes: Hypoxia, ketoacidosis, diarrhea

Anion Gap (AG)

- The difference between the sum of routinely measured cations and anions (Table 8-16)
- Anion gap formulas

$$AG = (Na^+ + K^+) - (Cl^- + HCO_3^-); \text{normal range 10 to 20 mmol/L}$$
$$AG = (Na^+) - (Cl^- + HCO_3^-); \text{normal range 8 to 16 mmol/L}$$

○ Potassium is frequently omitted because its contribution is so small and it is found elevated as a result of hemolysis

- Clinical utility: Acid-base disturbances, laboratory error (quality control), assessment of increases in unmeasured cations and anions

Bone and Minerals

Bone
- Two main functions of bone: Support and mineral homeostasis
- Bone contains 99% of calcium, 85% of phosphorus, and 55% of magnesium
- Classification of bone: Long bones (i.e., limbs) or flat bones (i.e., skull)
- Three main cell types in bone
  - Osteoblasts: Synthesize bone, very rich in alkaline phosphatase (ALP), contain receptors for parathyroid hormone (PTH), calcitriol, and estrogen
  - Osteocytes: Synthesize small amount of matrix for bone integrity, capable of bone resorption when mineral concentrations are altered
  - Osteoclasts: Demineralize and digest bone
- Strength of bone determined by bone density (peak bone mass and amount of bone loss) and bone quality (structure, turnover, damage, and mineralization

Bone Remodeling
- Remodeling of bone involves a coupling process of bone resorption and formation
- 10% of bone mass participates in the remodeling process
- The coupled processes differ according to age; as people age, they are predisposed to overall net bone loss (Table 8-17)
- Hormonal regulation of remodeling is controlled by PTH, calcitonin, vitamin D (systemic regulators), and prostaglandin and growth factors (e.g., insulin like growth factor) (local regulators) (see Table 8-18 for role of PTH, calcitonin, and vitamin D on calcium and phosphorus

Minerals
- Include calcium, magnesium, and phosphorus
- Found predominantly in bone; bone contains 99% of calcium, 85% of phosphorus, 55% of magnesium

TABLE 8-16	Causes of Increased and Decreased Anion Gap	
Anion Gap	**Cause**	**Example**
Increased	Decreased unmeasured cations	Uremia
	Increased unmeasured anions	Lactic acidosis, ketoacidosis, ingestion of toxic substances (methanol, ethanol, ethylene glycol)
	Laboratory error	Overestimation of sodium, underestimation of chloride or bicarbonate
Decreased	Increased unmeasured cations	Calcium, magnesium
	Decreased unmeasured anions	Hypoalbuminemia
	Laboratory error	Underestimation of sodium, overestimation of chloride or bicarbonate

TABLE 8-17	Effect of Age on Bone Homeostasis
Age Group	**Net Effect**
Infancy and adolescents	Bone formation > bone resorption
Young adults	Bone formation = bone resorption
Older adults	Bone formation < bone resorption

TABLE 8-18	Effect of Hormones on Mineral Homeostasis	
Hormone	**Effect**	**Net Effect**
Parathyroid hormone	*Bone:* Activates osteoclasts, mobilizes calcium and phosphorus *Kidney:* Calcium reabsorption, phosphorus excretion *Kidney:* Stimulate 1-α-hydroxylase activity (activates vitamin D)	Increased calcium Decreased phosphorus Activation of vitamin D
Calcitonin	Activates osteoblasts, retention of calcium in bone	Decreased calcium Decreased phosphorus
Vitamin D	*Intestines:* Reabsorption of calcium and phosphorus *Kidneys:* Reabsorption of calcium and phosphorus	Increased calcium Increased phosphorus

TABLE 8-19	Recommended Ranges for Minerals	
Analyte	**Range**	**Units**
Calcium	8.5-10.5	mg/dL
Ionized calcium	4.48-4.92	mg/dL
Magnesium	1.5-2.5	mEq/L
Phosphorus	2.8-4.0	mg/dL
PTH	10-65	pg/mL
Vitamin D		

PTH, Parathyroid hormone.

- Metabolism depends on mineral availability and the interaction of bone, kidney, and GI tract with PTH, calcitonin, and vitamin D
- Calcium
  - Three forms present in plasma: 45% ionized calcium (biologically active form), 45% protein bound, and 10% complexed with anions
  - Controlled by action of PTH and vitamin D on bone and kidney and intestines
  - Has widespread functions, including formation of bone, coagulation, neurologic and neuromuscular function, and nonspecific binding
- Phosphorus
  - Functions in energy metabolism, nucleic acid metabolism, bone formation, cell signaling, and acid-base homeostasis
  - Regulated secondary to calcium
  - Recommended ranges for minerals are found in Table 8-19
  - Specimen considerations are found in Table 8-20
  - Calcium, magnesium, and phosphorus status, symptoms, and causes are presented in Table 8-21

TABLE 8-20	Specimen Considerations for Calcium, Magnesium, and Phosphorus	
Analyte	**Specimen**	**Comments**
Calcium	Serum or plasma (heparin only) Separate as quickly as possible to avoid uptake of calcium by cells No hemolysis	pH will alter calcium levels (every 0.1 decrease in pH will increase the ionized calcium (IoCa) by 0.16 mg/dL
Magnesium	Serum or plasma (heparin only) Separate as quickly as possible to avoid elution of magnesium from cells) No hemolysis	
Phosphorus	Serum or plasma (heparin only) Separate as quickly as possible	

- Most commonly used methods to measure calcium, magnesium, and phosphorus are found in Table 8-22

Proteins

- Serve a key role in transport, synthesis, storage, and clearance of substances.
- May be classified by their function (Table 8-23)
- Comprise 50% to 70% of dry weight of cells
- Are classified as positive and negative acute phase reactants (see Table 8-23)
  - Positive acute phase reactants: Serum proteins that increase in response to inflammation
  - Negative acute phase proteins: Serum proteins that decrease in response to inflammation
- Complex macromolecules composed of amino acids linked by peptide bonds in a head to tail fashion
- Measured clinically in blood, urine, CSF, amniotic fluid, saliva, feces, peritoneal fluid, and pleural fluid
- May be separated by electrophoresis into the following regions: Albumin, α_1, α_2, β, and γ (see Table 8-24 for list of globulins in each category and the function)

Proteins and Their Function

- Synthesized in the liver except for the immunoglobulins, which are synthesized by plasma cells
- Metabolism originates in the GI tract by proteolytic enzymes, absorbed through the jejunum, and transported through portal circulation to amino acid pools
- May be classified by their function (see Table 8-23)
- Are amphoteric in nature, therefore contain two ionizable sites (proton-donating and proton-accepting sites)

TABLE 8-21 · Calcium Magnesium and Phosphorus Status, Symptoms, and Causes

Analyte	Status	Symptoms	Causes
Calcium	Hypocalcemia	Hyperreflexia Tetany Muscle pain Cramps Paresthesias Seizures Heart arrhythmias	Hypoparathyroidism Vitamin D deficiency Pseudohypoparathyroidism (PTH resistance) Calcitonin Magnesium deficiency Dietary deficiency Phosphate infusion
Calcium	Hypercalcemia	Fatigue/malaise Weakness Depression Apathy Nephrolithiasis	Hyperparathyroidism Tumors/malignancies Endocrine disturbances (thyrotoxicosis and Addison's disease) Thiazide diuretics
Phosphorus	Hyperphosphatemia		Increased intake Increase GI absorption Cell injury/lysis Decreased renal excretion
Phosphorus	Hypophosphatemia		Decreased intake Vitamin D deficiency Redistribution into the cell (i.e., respiratory alkalosis, insulin administration, epinephrine injection, healing bone) Excessive loss (renal disorders, proximal convoluted tubule injury Increased GFR
Magnesium	Hypermagnesemia		Iatrogenic Increased intake Increased GI absorption Cellular release
Magnesium	Hypomagnesemia		Malabsorption\malnutrition Diuretics Endocrine disorders (hyperaldosteronism, hyperthyroidism)

GFR, Glomerular filtration rate; *GI,* gastrointestinal; *PTH,* parathyroid hormone.

TABLE 8-22 · Most Commonly Used Methods to Measure Calcium, Magnesium, and Phosphorus

Method	Principle	Comments
Calcium	Calcium + OCPC red complex →	Colorimetric using OCPC or arsenazo III
Ionized calcium	Calcium-specific ion selective electrode	Potentiometry
Magnesium	Magnesium + Calmagite → Colored product	Most current methods use metallochromic indicators or dyes that change color as they bind magnesium (calmagite, methylthymol blue, formazan dye, arsenazo)
Phosphorus	Phosphate ions + Ammonium molybdate → Phosphomolybdate *Detection steps:* 1. Read phosphomolybdate at 340 nm 2. Reduce phosphomolybdate to molybdenum blue and read at 600-700 nm	

OCPC, Orthocresolphthalein complexone.

TABLE 8-23 · Classification of Proteins by Function

Function	Description	Example(s)
Immune defense	Immunoglobulins used for the elimination of foreign antigens	IgA, IgG, IgM, IgD, and IgE
Acute phase reactants (APR)	Proteins associated with inflammation	*Negative APR:* Albumin, prealbumin, and transferrin *Positive APR:* $\alpha1$, $\alpha2$, β, δ globulins
Transport	Proteins used to bind and transport substances	Prealbumin, albumin, ceruloplasmin, $\alpha2$-macroglobulin, transferrin
Coagulation	Proteins aid clot formation and work with complement	Complement

TABLE 8-24	Serum Protein Electrophoresis Regions With Associated Proteins and Their Function		
Region	**Relative (%)**	**Proteins**	**Function**
Albumin	60	Albumin	Transport, oncotic pressure, amino acid reserve
α_1	3	1. α_1-Antitrypsin 2. α_1-Acid glycoprotein 3. α_1-Antichymotrypsin	1. Binding, inactivation of trypsin-like enzymes 2. Binds and inactivates progestin and neutral or cationic drugs 3. Inactivation of chymotrypsin-like enzymes
α_2	10	1. Ceruloplasmin 2. α_2-Macroglobulin 3. Haptoglobin	1. Copper oxidase, oxidation of iron and incorporation into transferrin 2. Inhibitor of proteolytic enzymes, transport of cytokines and growth factors 3. Binds and transports free hemoglobin
β	11	1. Transferrin 2. Complement (C3 and C4)	1. Transports iron to tissues 2. Essential factors in complement pathways
γ	16	1. Immunoglobulins 2. C-reactive protein	1. Protection against foreign antigens 2. Nonspecific acute phase protein

- Can use total protein and albumin to calculate an A/G ratio

$$\text{Globulin} = \text{total protein (g/dL)} - \text{Albumin (g/dL)}$$

$$\text{A/G Ratio} = \text{Albumin (g/dL)}/\text{Globulin (g/dL)}$$

- High A/G suggests underproduction of globulins found in some leukemias and genetic deficiencies
- Low A/G suggests overproduction of globulins (multiple myeloma or autoimmune disease) or underproduction of albumin (liver disease or nephrotic syndrome)

$$\text{Normal A/G} = 1.0 \text{ to } 1.8$$

- Prealbumin: Negative acute phase protein, transport protein for thyroxine and triiodothyronine sensitive, marker of poor nutritional status, increased concentrations seen with steroid use and in alcoholics
- Albumin: Negative acute phase protein, nonspecific binder of many substances, major function is to maintain colloid osmotic pressure
- Globulins: Includes α_1, α_2, β, and δ fractions
  - α_1 Region
    - α_1-Antitrypsin: Positive acute phase protein; major component of the α_1 region (90%); functions to inhibit protease neutrophil elastase; deficiency is associated with a mutation in the *SERPINA1* gene causing α_1-antitrypsin deficiency. α_1-Antitrypsin is associated with emphysema and sometimes cirrhosis
    - Others include α_1-fetoprotein, α_1-glycoprotein, and α_1-antichymotrypsin
  - α_2 Region
    - Haptoglobin: Positive acute phase protein; serves to bind free hemoglobin in the blood for clearance; used clinically to detect and evaluate hemolytic anemia. Laboratory data in hemolytic anemia includes decreased haptoglobin, red blood cell (RBC) count, hemoglobin, and hematocrit with an increased reticulocyte count
    - Ceruloplasmin: Positive acute phase protein, functions to bind serum copper (90% bound by ceruloplasmin), used clinically to aid in the diagnosis of Wilson's disease (see decreased total serum copper and ceruloplasmin with increased urine copper)
    - Other includes α_2-macroglobulin
- β Region
  - Transferrin: Negative acute phase protein; functions in iron transport to the tissues; used clinically to investigate causes of anemia, gauge iron metabolism, and determine iron-carrying capacity in the blood
  - Others include hemopexin, β_2-microglobulin, and complement
- γ Region
  - C-reactive protein (CRP): Positive acute phase protein, marker of inflammation, but more recently high sensitivity CRP
    - Used to determine risk for development of cardiovascular disease
  - Immunoglobulins: Includes IgG, IgA, IgM, IgD, and IgE
- Separated by electrophoresis from anode to cathode (Figure 8-2)
- Common abnormal electrophoretic patterns
  - β-γ Bridge: Fusion of the β and γ bands caused by fast moving γ-globulins; most common cause is cirrhosis, but this also may be seen in rheumatoid arthritis and respiratory and skin infections

Anode Prealbumin Albumin α_1 α_2 β δ Cathode

FIGURE 8-2 Electrophoresis from anode to cathode.

TABLE 8-25	Methods to Measure Total Protein and Albumin	
Method	**Principle**	**Comments**
Albumin	Albumin + BCG → Color change	Dye binding methods using BCG or BCP
Total protein	Protein + Cupric divalant ions $\xrightarrow{\text{Alkaline}}$ Violet chelate	Biuret reaction based on the presence of peptide bonds
Serum protein electrophoresis	Electrophoresis at pH 8.6 on cellulose acetate or agarose gel resulting in an electrophoresis pattern as follows: Anode prealbumin albumin α_1, α_2, β, δ cathode	Uses barbital buffer at pH 8.6, conferring a net negative charge on proteins; proteins migrate from cathode to anode

BCG, Bromocresol green; *BCP,* bromocresol purple.

- Acute phase reaction: Increased bands in the α_1, α_2, and β regions with a decreased albumin band; seen with infection, tumor growth, hepatitis, surgery, trauma, burns
- Nephrotic syndrome pattern: Decrease in albumin and γ bands, with an increase in α_2-globulins
- M-spike: Diffuse increase in the γ-globulin band, found in polyclonal gammopathy

Specimen Considerations

- Albumin: Serum or plasma (heparin), marked lipemia, may interfere with the bromocresol green assay
- Protein: Serum or plasma, plasma values will be 2 to 4 g/L higher than serum because of the presence of fibrinogen
- Methods to measure total protein and albumin are found in Table 8-25
- Recommended ranges for proteins are found in Table 8-26

Liver

- Largest internal organ, weighing 1200 to 1600 g
- Extremely vascular organ, receives 1500 mL blood/min from two major vessels—the hepatic artery and the portal vein
- Performs many diverse functions, including metabolism (carbohydrate, amino acid, lipid, and bilirubin), detoxification (serves as a barrier between potentially harmful substances absorbed in the GI tract and systemic circulation), elimination (through the production of bile), and storage (provides a source of energy during fasting states)
- Functional unit of the liver is the lobule
  - Lobules contain two cell types
    - Hepatocytes
      - Responsible for metabolic function of the liver
    - Kupffer cells
      - Line the vascular spaces and are phagocytic macrophages capable of ingesting bacteria and other foreign material
- The liver is the only organ involved in bilirubin metabolism, because bilirubin is formed from the breakdown of old RBCs (Figure 8-3)

TABLE 8-26	Recommended Ranges for Proteins	
Analyte	**Range**	**Units**
Albumin	3.5-5.0	g/dL
α_1	0.1-0.3	g/dL
α_2	0.6-1.0	g/dL
β	0.7-1.1	g/dL
γ	0.8-1.6	g/dL
Total protein	6.5-8.3	g/dL

Jaundice

- Condition characterized by yellow discoloration of skin, sclera, and mucous membranes
- Most commonly caused by increased bilirubin, not clinically seen until bilirubin values exceed 3 to 5 mg/dL
  - Total bilirubin is composed of three fractions
    - Conjugated bilirubin (soluble and excretable)
    - Unconjugated (water-insoluble and nonexcretable)
    - δ Bilirubin (bilirubin covalently bound to albumin)
  - Elevations in unconjugated bilirubin pose great risk for development of kernicterus, especially in infants
- Jaundice may be divided into three categories
  - Prehepatic
    - Occurs when increased amounts of bilirubin are brought to the liver cell, most commonly resulting from increased RBC destruction
      - Causes
        - Hemolytic anemia
        - Exposure to chemicals
        - Some cancers
        - Autoimmune hemolytic anemia
        - Transfusion reaction
        - Hemolytic disease of the newborn
        - Congestive heart failure
  - Hepatic
    - Occurs from direct damage to the liver cell
      - Causes
        - Gilbert's disease
        - Crigler-Najjar syndrome
        - Dubin-Johnson syndrome
        - Rotor's syndrome
        - Cirrhosis

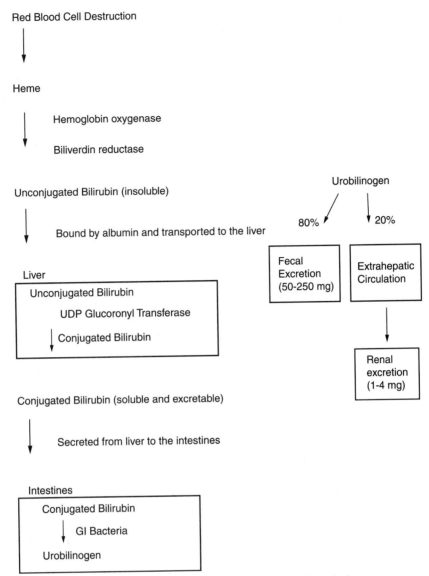

FIGURE 8-3 Bilirubin metabolism. *GI*, Gastrointestinal.

- Viral hepatitis
- Alcoholic liver disease
- Drug-induced liver disease
- Hepatocellular carcinoma
- Neonatal physiologic jaundice
- Posthepatic
  - Occurs from the blockage of the flow of bile from the liver
    - Causes
      - Bile duct stones
      - Gallbladder stones
      - Cancer of the bile ducts
      - Bile duct stenosis
- Typical laboratory findings in prehepatic, hepatic, and posthepatic jaundice
  - Prehepatic
    - Total bilirubin: Normal to increased
    - Conjugated bilirubin: Normal to increased
    - Unconjugated bilirubin: Increased
    - Urine urobilinogen: Increased
  - Hepatic
    - Total bilirubin: Increased
    - Conjugated bilirubin: Increased
    - Unconjugated bilirubin: Normal or increased
    - Urine urobilinogen: Normal or increased
  - Posthepatic
    - Total bilirubin: Increased
    - Conjugated bilirubin: Increased
    - Unconjugated bilirubin: increased
    - Urine urobilinogen: Decreased

Description of Disorders of Bilirubin Metabolism
Gilbert's Disease
- Inherited unconjugated hyperbilirubinemia
- Mild, benign condition, bilirubin only slightly elevated (usually <3 mg/dL)
- Affects 2% to 12% of population (male gender bias)
- Caused by defective transport of bilirubin through the liver cell membrane

- Activity of uridine diphosphate (UDP)–glucuronyl transferase is 20% to 50%
- Requires no treatment

Crigler-Najjar Syndrome

- Rare, inherited condition
- Caused by decreased or absent UDP–glucuronyl transferase
- Classified as type 1 (no UDP–glucuronyl transferase, bad prognosis) and type 2 (decreased UDP–glucuronyl transferase)

Dubin-Johnson Syndrome

- Chronic, benign condition producing obstructive liver disease
- Results in the ineffective removal of conjugated bilirubin from the hepatocyte
- Causes conjugated hyperbilirubinemia
- Requires no treatment

Rotor's Syndrome

- Similar to Dubin-Johnson syndrome
- Benign conjugated hyperbilirubinemia
- Caused by a reduction in the concentration or activity of the intracellular binding protein ligandin

Other Liver Disorders

Reye's Syndrome

- Acute and often fatal childhood condition (5-15 years)
- Hypothesized to be caused by a virus that improves within 2 and 4 days and then is followed by the abrupt onset of vomiting and diarrhea that may progress to coma, respiratory arrest, and often death
- Hallmark signs include encephalopathy and fatty degeneration of the liver
- Aspirin has been found to be associated with Reye's syndrome

Alcoholic Liver Disease

- Relatively common condition resulting from long-term consumption of alcohol
- Disease is caused by the hepatotoxic effects of acetaldehyde in high concentrations
- Acetaldehyde is formed from the catabolism of alcohol in the presence of alcohol dehydrogenase
  - Three associated stages
    - Alcoholic fatty liver: Occurs with moderate alcohol consumption for 6 to 12 months; reversible condition resulting in the infiltration of fat into the liver; condition is reversible, with cessation of alcohol resulting in complete recovery; very few laboratory abnormalities seen
    - Alcoholic hepatitis: Occurs with moderate alcohol consumption over a longer period; presents with a variety of symptoms, including hepatomegaly, vomiting, jaundice, abdominal pain. Laboratory results reflect liver damage and include increased aspartate aminotransferase (AST), alanine aminotransferase (ALT), γ-glutamyl transferase (GGT), ALP, and bilirubin increased acute phase reactants
    - Alcoholic cirrhosis: Occurs with heavy alcohol consumption over an extended period; results in the most severe damage to the liver that is irreversible; symptoms include weight loss, weakness, hepatomegaly, splenomegaly, jaundice, ascites, fever, malnutrition, and edema. Laboratory findings include elevated AST and ALT, decreased albumin, prolonged prothrombin time, and elevations in ALP and bilirubin associated with the cholestatic form

Specimen Collection and Handling

- Bilirubin: Serum or plasma acceptable, protect from light (bilirubin will deteriorate 30% to 50%/hr when exposed to light), no hemolysis, fasting sample preferred
- Methods
  - Most commonly used methods to measure bilirubin are modifications of the diazotized sulfanilic acid method (diazo method) described by Jendrassik and Grof in 1938 (Table 8-27)
- Recommended ranges for bilirubin are found in Table 8-28

General Endocrinology

- Hormone: A chemical substance produced by an organ to result in an effect on a target organ
- Hormones are classified into three groups: Protein, steroid, and aromatic amino acid derivatives

TABLE 8-27	Commonly Used Methods to Measure Bilirubin	
Method	**Principle**	**Comments**
Total bilirubin	Bilirubin + Diazotized sulfanilic acid + Accelerator → Azodipyroles (reddish-purple)	Classic diazo reaction described by Ehrlich; accelerator is caffeine and sodium benzoate; all fractions of bilirubin react with this method
Direct bilirubin	Bilirubin + Diazotized sulfanilic acid → Azodipyroles (reddish-purple)	Classic diazo reaction minus the accelerator; only conjugated and δ bilirubin react in this method
Indirect bilirubin	Indirect bilirubin = Total bilirubin − Direct bilirubin	Calculation

- Protein hormones are produced by the hypothalamus, pituitary gland, and other target glands and circulate in a free form (unbound)
- Steroid hormones are all derived from cholesterol, majority circulate bound to carrier plasma proteins
- Aromatic amino acid derived hormones are synthesized from tyrosine
- Hormone concentrations in the body are tightly controlled by feedback control of the hypothalamic-pituitary-target organ axis (HPT axis) (Figure 8-4)
- Two types of feedback exist
  - Positive
    - Positive feedback begins when the hypothalamus receives input to produce a releasing factor that acts on the pituitary gland. The pituitary responds by releasing tropic hormones that act on a specific target gland to promote hormone synthesis and release
  - Negative
    - Negative feedback: Hormones that are synthesized and released from target glands feed back to the pituitary gland and hypothalamus to stop further production of releasing and tropic hormones

- The hypothalamus (located in the brain) synthesizes and secretes releasing or inhibiting factors to turn on or shut off the HPT axis; the central nervous system and concentration of target gland hormones regulate the release of these hormones
- The pituitary gland (found at the base of the skull) produces hormones (tropic and nontropic) that act directly on a target organ to produce hormones
- Hypothalamus and pituitary hormones are synthesized and released in a minute-to-minute pulsatile fashion; pituitary hormones also exhibit circadian rhythm
- Transport proteins (found in circulation) carry steroids from the organ of synthesis to the target organ or tissue (see Table 8-29 for a list of common transport proteins)
- See Table 8-30 for a list of hypothalamus and pituitary hormones, their associated target glands, and hormones produced
- Disorders occur as a result of hyperfunction or hypofunction of an endocrine gland; classified as primary, secondary, or tertiary depending on the site of the defect
  - Primary disorders refer to a defect in the target gland

TABLE 8-28	Recommended Ranges for Bilirubin	
Analyte	**Range**	**Units**
Total bilirubin	0.2-1.0	mg/dL
Conjugated bilirubin	0.0-0.2	mg/dL

TABLE 8-29	Hormone Transport Proteins and Associated Hormones
Protein	**Hormone(s)**
Cortisol-binding globulin	Cortisol
Sex hormone–binding globulin	Estradiol, testosterone
Thyroid-binding globulin	T_3, T_4
Thyroxine-binding prealbumin	T_4
Albumin	All hormones

T_3, Triiodothyronine; T_4, thyroxine.

TABLE 8-30	Major Hypothalamus and Pituitary Hormones: Their Target Organs and Hormones		
Hypothalamus Hormones	**Pituitary Hormones**	**Target Gland**	**Hormones**
CRH	ACTH	Adrenal gland	Glucocorticoids Mineralocorticoids Catecholamines
TRH	TSH	Thyroid gland	T_3 and T_4
GnRH	LH/FSH	Ovaries/ testes	Sex steroids
GHRH	GH	Bone	Insulin-like growth factor

ACTH, Adrenocorticotropic hormone; *CRH,* corticotropin-releasing hormone; *FSH,* follicle-stimulating hormone; *GH,* growth hormone; *GnRH,* gonadotropin-releasing hormone; *LH,* luteinizing hormone; *TRH,* thyrotropin-releasing hormone; *TSH,* thyroid-stimulating hormone; T_3, triiodothyronine; T_4, tetraiodothyronine or thyroxine.

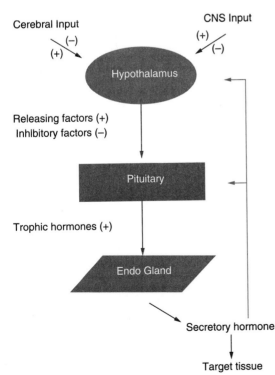

FIGURE 8-4 Hormone feedback control system. *CNS,* Central nervous system; *Endo gland,* endocrine gland.

TABLE 8-31	Thyroid Testing Recommended Ranges	
Analyte	**Range**	**Units**
sTSH	0.4-4.2	μU/mL
fT4	0.8-2.7	ng/dL
fT3	1.4-4.4	pg/mL
THBR	0.72-1.25	

fT3, Free triiodothyronine; *fT4*, free thyronine; *sTSH*, serum thyroid-stimulating hormone; *THBR*, thyroid hormone–binding ratio.

BOX 8-3	**Function of Thyroid Hormones**

Fetal growth and development
Sexual maturation
Central nervous system development
Caloric and metabolic activity
Stimulate protein synthesis
Stimulate carbohydrate and lipid metabolism
Influence calcium and phosphorous metabolism
Increased blood flow, cardiac output, and heart rate

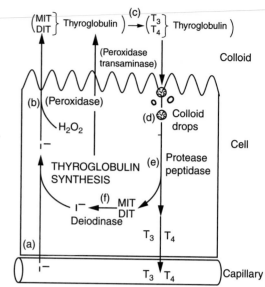

FIGURE 8-5 Thyroid hormone synthesis. *DIT*, diiodotyrosine; *MIT*, moniodotyrosine; T_3, triiodothyronine; T_4, thyroxine.

- Secondary disorders refer to a defect in the pituitary gland
- Tertiary disorders refer to a defect in the hypothalamus
- Recommended ranges for thyroid testing can be found in Table 8-31

Thyroid Function, Hormones, and Disorders

- The thyroid gland is a small bilobed organ located in the lower front of the neck
- The thyroid gland contains two main cell types: Follicular and parafollicular
  - Follicular cells produce thyroid hormones (triiodothyronine [T_3] and thyroxine [T4]), which are stored in the colloid of the follicle cell
  - Parafollicular cells produce calcitonin and are referred to as C-cells
- The production and secretion of thyroid hormones (T_3 and T_4) is regulated by the anterior pituitary hormone, thyroid-stimulating hormone (TSH), also known as thyrotropin
- Production and secretion of TSH are regulated by thyrotropin-releasing hormone (TRH) produced by the hypothalamus
- TRH and TSH secretion is turned on and off depending on thyroid hormone levels by positive and negative control of the HPT axis
- Thyroid hormones are responsible for multiple physiologic processes (Box 8-3)
- Thyroid hormone production involves four steps
  - Iodide trapping by the thyroid gland
  - Incorporation of iodide into tyrosine using peroxidase

- Coupling of iodinated tyrosyl residues to thyroglobulin (Tg)
- Release of iodothyronines through the cleavage of follicular Tg by proteases (Figure 8-5)
- The synthesis of thyroid hormones requires iodine, which is ingested in the form of iodide; the transport of iodide to the follicle is the rate-limiting step in the synthesis of thyroid hormones
- Approximately 80% of secreted hormone is T_4 and 20% is T_3; most of the physiologically available T_3 is produced from the deiodination of T_4; deiodination of the β ring of T_4 produces T_3; deiodination of the α ring of T_4 produces reverse T_3 (rT_3), a biologically inactive compound
- T_3 and rT_3 are produced in approximately equal amounts
- T_3 and T_4 circulate bound to carrier proteins (99% bound)
- Disorders of the thyroid gland are divided into three main groups
  - Hyperthyroidism (overproduction of thyroid hormones)
    - Caused by autoantibodies to TSH receptors (Graves' disease), thyroidal nodules (toxic nodular goiters), thyroidal TSH receptor sensitivity to human chorionic gonadotropin (seen in pregnancy)
    - Most common of all causes is Graves' disease
    - Occurs most commonly in females
    - Manifests with characteristic symptoms, including goiter and exophthalmos
    - Anti–thyroid peroxidase and TSH receptor antibodies are present in up to 95% of cases
    - May manifest as subclinical or overt (see Table 8-32 for laboratory findings in thyroid disorders)

TABLE 8-32	Laboratory Findings in Thyroid Disorders				
Disorder	**TSH**	**fT$_4$**	**T$_3$**	**Antibodies**	**Comment**
Subclinical hypothyroidism	Increased	N	N	+/−	Symptoms generally not present
Overt hypothyroidism	Increased	Decreased	Decreased	Often present	
Subclinical hyperthyroidism	Decreased	N	N	+/−	
Overt hyperthyroidism	Decreased	Increased	Increased	Often present	
Euthyroid sick syndrome	Increased or decreased	N	Decreased	Not present	Increased rT$_3$

N, Normal; *rT$_3$*, reversed triiodothyronine.

- ○ Symptoms include nervousness, tremor palpitations, fatigue, weakness, weight loss, heat intolerance, menstrual change, neck mass, muscle weakness, and exophthalmos (prominence of the eyes)
- Hypothyroidism (underproduction of thyroid hormones)
  - ○ Primary hypothyroidism may be caused by insufficient iodine or autoimmune destruction of the thyroid gland (Hashimoto's thyroiditis)
  - ○ Most common primary cause is Hashimoto's thyroiditis
  - ○ Secondary and tertiary hypothyroidism are caused by pituitary and hypothalamus dysfunction, respectively
  - ○ May present as subclinical or overt (see Table 8-32)
  - ○ Symptoms include cold intolerance, dyspnea, weight gain, cognitive dysfunction, constipation, dry skin, hoarseness, edema, myalgia, depression, menorrhagia
- Euthyroid sick syndrome (abnormal thyroid hormones in the absence of thyroid disease)
  - ○ Refers to abnormalities in thyroid hormone concentrations in the absence of thyroid disease
  - ○ Common in hospitalized patients
  - ○ Characterized by decreased conversion of T$_4$ to T$_3$ with an increase in rT$_3$; TSH may be low and the response to TRH blunted
  - ○ There is no benefit to treating this with thyroid hormone replacement
- Disorders may be further characterized as the following depending on the site of the defect
  - Primary: Disease originates in the thyroid gland
  - Secondary: Disease originates in the pituitary gland
  - Tertiary: Disease originates in the hypothalamus
- American Thyroid Council (ATC) published recommendations for thyroid disease screening; high-risk persons should be screened (high risk includes elderly, neonates, postpartum females, those with a family history of autoimmune disease or thyroid disease)
- Diagnosis of hyperthyroidism and hypothyroidism should include TSH and free thyroxine (fT$_4$)
- The ATC recommends delaying thyroid testing in those who are sick until the illness subsides. If unavoidable, FT$_4$ is the most reliable indicator of thyroid status in sick individuals

- A battery of tests is available to assess thyroid function, including TSH, fT$_4$, total thyroxine (TT$_4$), free triiodothyronine (fT$_3$), total triiodothyronine (TT$_3$), index methods (thyroid hormone–binding ratio [THBR] or free thyroxine factor [T-7]), Tg, thyroid antibodies, and thyroxine binding globulin (TBG) measurements
- Free hormone levels (fT$_4$ and fT$_3$) are better indicators of thyroid status because they are independent of binding protein concentrations
- The ATA recommends using TSH and fT$_4$ for diagnostic purposes; if necessary, test for fT$_3$ also may be ordered
- A log linear relationship exists between TSH and fT$_4$ such that a doubling of thyroid hormones results in a 100-fold inverse change in TSH; therefore, TSH is the most sensitive indicator of thyroid status
- TSH
  - ○ Assays are labeled as "generation" assays, which refers to the sensitivity of the method; first-generation methods refer to assays with analytical sensitivities of 1.0 mIU/L, second-generation assays have a sensitivity of 0.1 mIU/L, third-generation assays have a sensitivity of 0.01 mIU/L, etc.
  - ○ Most current assays for TSH employ a two-site (sandwich) heterogeneous immunoassay that uses a capture antibody directed toward the α subunit and a second antibody (labeled) directed toward the β subunit of the TSH molecule. The second antibody is commonly labeled with peroxidase, ALP, and/or chemiluminescent or fluorescent labels
- fT$_4$
  - ○ Reference method involves dialysis of sample to which a known tracer amount of iodinated T$_4$ has been added
    - Sample is assayed for TT$_4$ and fT$_4$ and calculated using the formula

$$\% \, fT_4 = TT_4 \times \% \, \text{Tracer T4 (dialyzed)}$$

  - ○ Current method includes measurement of fT$_4$ using immunometric assays

- THBR
  - Used to estimate the number of unoccupied thyroid hormone binding sites
  - Represents the percent uptake of patient sample relative to the percent uptake of a euthyroid person; formula

$$THBR = \frac{\% \ Uptake \ (patient \ serum)}{\% \ Uptake \ (reference \ serum)}$$

  - A THBR of 1.0 indicates that the patient uptake and the reference sample uptake are the same
  - More accurately reflects thyroid status in those with abnormal binding protein concentrations
  - THBR is directly proportional to the free hormone fraction

Sample Collection and Handling
- Serum or plasma (some methods require serum only)
- Preferable free from hemolysis and lipemia
- Newborn screening is whole blood collected by heel puncture within 48 to 72 hours after birth
- Sample should be stored at 2° to 8° C if not analyzed within 24 hours

Adrenal Cortex and Medulla

- Adrenal glands are located at the upper pole of each kidney
- Adrenal cortex constitutes 90% of total gland volume, and the medulla constitutes 10% of total gland volume
- Adrenal cortex secretes corticosteroids, including glucocorticoids (cortisol), mineralocorticoids (aldosterone), and sex steroids (androgens and estrogens)
- Adrenal medulla secretes catecholamines (epinephrine, norepinephrine, dopamine)
- All hormones are steroid hormones that are produced from cholesterol

Adrenal Cortex Hormones
- Glucocorticoids: Cortisol
  - Regulated by HPA axis (adrenocorticotropic hormone [ACTH] at the pituitary; corticotropin-releasing hormone [CRH] at the hypothalamus)
- Mineralocorticoids: Aldosterone
  - Regulated by the RAA system and to a lesser extent ACTH (pituitary) and potassium levels
- Androgens: Dehydroepiandrosterone sulfate (DHEA-S), dehydroepiandrosterone (DHEA), and androstenedione

Adrenal Medulla Hormones
- Catecholamines
  - Epinephrine
  - Norepinephrine
  - Dopamine

Adrenal Cortex Disorders
- Diseases of this organ are classified as resulting from hypofunction or hyperfunction of the adrenal cortex
- Adrenal gland hyperfunction may result in three broad categories of disorders: Hypercortisolism (Cushing's syndrome), hyperaldosteronism (Conn's syndrome), and congenital adrenal hyperplasia
- Cushing's syndrome (hypercortisolism)
  - General term used to describe any condition resulting from increased cortisol
  - A condition referred to as pseudo-Cushing's syndrome may exist with chronic alcoholism and/or a high level of cortisol-binding globulin associated with pregnancy or the use of contraception, which can be confused with Cushing's syndrome
  - Causes include iatrogenic and noniatrogenic; noniatrogenic causes include pituitary tumors (60% of all cases), ectopic ACTH (20% of all cases), and adrenal adenoma and adrenal carcinoma (combined 20% of all cases)
  - Cushing's syndrome is divided into two broad categories: ACTH dependent (Cushing's disease) and ACTH independent (Cushing's syndrome)
    - Cushing's disease is caused by an ACTH-producing pituitary tumor; the feedback control system is nonfunctional. Condition is characterized by
      - Increased cortisol and ACTH
      - Increased glucose, sodium, and aldosterone
      - *NOTE:* Cortisol in very high levels can have mineralocorticoid activity
    - Cushing's syndrome is caused by adrenal adenoma that produces excess cortisol; the feedback control system is functional. Condition is characterized by
      - Increased cortisol and decreased ACTH
      - Increased glucose, sodium, and aldosterone
  - Clinical features of Cushing's syndrome are listed in Box 8-4
- Laboratory diagnosis of Cushing's syndrome
  - Includes two phases of testing
    - Screening tests: Used to detect hypercortisolism
      - Overnight dexamethasone test (1 mg dose at 11 PM); at 8 AM plasma cortisol levels are collected
      - Cortisol 5 µg/dL or less: Normal

BOX 8-4   Clinical Feature of Adrenal Hypercortisolism

Truncal obesity
Hypertension
Glucose intolerance
Plethoric facies
Skin atrophy
Muscle weakness
Menstrual and gonadal dysfunction
Acne
Hirsutism
Osteoporosis
Psychiatric problems

- Cortisol 10 µg/dL or greater: Hypercortisolism
  - Urine free cortisol test, involves a 24-hour urine collection
    - Urine cortisol less than 50 µg/24 hours: Normal
  - Cortisol at midnight (when cortisol levels are at their lowest); a plasma sample or more commonly a salivary sample is collected at midnight
    - Cortisol less than 5 µg/dL: Normal
    - Cortisol 5 µg/dL or greater: Hypercortisolism
- Differentiating tests: Used to differentiate the causes of hypercortisolism
  - Plasma ACTH
    - Less than 2 pmol/L: Cushing's syndrome
    - Approximately 11 pmol/L: Cushing's disease
    - 50 pmol/L = Ectopic sources
  - Bilateral petrosal sinus sampling after CRH (100 µg) administration. Three venous catheters are placed: one each in the left and right inferior petrosal sinus sampling (IPSS) that drain the pituitary gland and one in the inferior vena cava (IVC). Baseline samples are collected, CRH is administered, and collections are taken at 2, 5, and 10 minutes. The ratio of IPS to IVC is interpreted as follows
    - IPSS:IVC greater than 2: Cushing's disease
    - IPSS:IVC less than 1.4: Ectopic cause
- Conn's syndrome (hyperaldosteronism)
  - Results from an excess of mineralocorticoids, mainly aldosterone. Aldosterone in excess will cause reabsorption of sodium (water and chloride secondarily) and excretion of potassium and hydrogen
  - Characterized by hypertension, hypokalemia, and alkalosis as a result of the action of aldosterone
  - Caused mainly by two disorders: Aldosterone-producing adrenal adenoma (Conn's syndrome) or idiopathic hyperaldosteronism (IHA); differentiation is critical, because 70% of the cases of Conn's syndrome are medically curable
  - Conn's syndrome is the most common cause of hyperaldosteronism; condition is characterized by
    - Increased aldosterone and decreased renin
  - Idiopathic adrenal hyperplasia characterized by
    - Increased aldosterone and renin
- Diagnosis of primary hyperaldosteronism involves a two-step approach
  - Screening for hyperaldosteronism
  - Confirmation of hyperaldosteronism using one of three aldosterone suppression tests
  - Screening involves a morning (between 8 AM and 10 AM) plasma aldosterone–to–plasma renin ratio. Ratios above 25 in the presence of

increased aldosterone are considered suspect for hyperaldosteronism. The positive screen test must be confirmed using an aldosterone suppression test
  - Confirmation of hyperaldosteronism can be accomplished using one of three tests
    - Oral salt load test
    - Intravenous saline infusion test
    - Fludrocortisone suppression test
- Once the diagnosis is made, differentiation between aldosterone-producing adrenal adenoma and IHA is required to ensure proper treatment
  - Bilateral adrenal venous sampling coupled with simultaneous determination of ACTH-stimulated cortisol from both glands may be used
- Congenital adrenal hyperplasia
  - Describes a group of inborn errors of metabolism caused by enzyme deficiencies in the biosynthesis of cortisol and aldosterone
    - Can cause adrenal insufficiency and excess androgen synthesis
    - Can cause females at birth to appear masculinized
  - At least six defects are known to exist. Most common defect is 21-hydroxylase deficiency (partial), which occurs in 95% of all congenital adrenal hyperplasia cases
  - 21-Hydroxylase deficiency is inherited as an autosomal recessive disorder affecting 1 in 10,000 births. Much higher frequencies may be seen in Ashkenazi Jews (1 in 30)
  - Diagnosis involves demonstration of low cortisol, elevated 17-hydroxyprogesterone, low aldosterone
- Adrenal gland hypofunction results in adrenal insufficiency and is caused by
  - Primary adrenal disease (Addison's disease)
  - Secondary adrenal insufficiency (decreased levels of ACTH or CRH)
  - Long-term suppression of the HPT axis by exogenous administration of glucocorticoids
- A relatively rare disorder (prevalence of 1 in 50,000)
- Most common cause is autoimmune adrenalitis and is commonly associated with other autoimmune disorders
- This disorder develops slowly with the gradual loss of cortisol and increased ACTH. The melanocyte-stimulating property of ACTH is what results in the clinical feature of hyperpigmentation
- Symptoms appear after approximately 90% of the adrenal gland is destroyed
- Generally the disorder is considered in people with uncontrollable hypertension and unexplained hypokalemia with increased urinary potassium (>30 mmol/day). Clinical features of Addison's disease are listed in Box 8-5.

BOX 8-5	Clinical Features of Primary Adrenal Insufficiency
Muscle weakness	
Fatigue	
Weight loss	
Pigmentation	
Anorexia	
Fever	
Dehydration	
Nausea	
Hypotension	
Abdominal pain	

BOX 8-6	Clinical Features of Pheochromocytoma
Hypertension	
Headache	
Palpitations	
Pallor	
Dyspnea	
Nausea	
Anxiety attacks	
General weakness	

- Diagnosis of Addison's disease may be made one of two ways
  - Symptoms alone
    - Symptoms alone are enough to diagnose this condition in most cases
    - Symptoms include
      - Hyponatremia
      - Hyperkalemia
      - Acidosis
      - Hypovolemia
      - Hypotension
  - Plasma aldosterone and renin results
    - An elevated plasma renin result and decreased plasma aldosterone result are diagnostic for Addison's disease

Adrenal Medulla Disorders
- Disorders of the adrenal medulla are divided into catecholamine excess and catecholamine deficiency
  - Catecholamine excess results as a consequence of adrenal medullary chromaffin cell tumors; the most important tumor clinically is pheochromocytoma
    - Although rare in occurrence (0.2% occurrence) and mostly benign, accurate and timely diagnosis is essential because pheochromocytoma will cause severe cardiovascular complications and death if not identified and properly treated
    - 10% to 15% may be malignant
    - Pheochromocytoma is divided into two types: Multiple endocrine neoplasia (MEN) 1 and MEN 2
    - Clinical features are presented in Box 8-6
    - Vanillylmandelic acid (VMA), a metabolite of epinephrine and norepinephrine, is used to aid in the detection of excess catecholamine production caused by neuroblastomas, pheochromocytomas, and other neuroendocrine tumors
      - NOTE: VMA is subject to many interferences; therefore an increased VMA is not diagnostic of the previously mentioned disorders

TABLE 8-33	Common Enzymes and Reactions Catalyzed	
Enzyme	**Reaction Catalyzed**	**Comments**
AST	L-Aspartate + α-Ketoglutarate ↔ Oxaloacetate + L-Glutamate	P-5'-P required for full catalytic activity
ALT	L-Alanine + α-Ketoglutarate ↔ L-Glutamate + Pyruvate	P-5'-P required for full catalytic activity
ALP	p-Nitrophenyl phosphate ↔ p-Nitrophenol + HPO_4	Magnesium required for full catalytic activity
LD	L-Lactate + NAD ↔ Pyruvate + NADH + H^+	pH 8.3-8.9 favors forward reaction pH 7.1-7.4 favors reverse reaction
CK	Creatine + ATP ↔ Creatine phosphate + ADP	Magnesium required for full catalytic activity

ALP, Alkaline phosphatase; ALT, alanine aminotransferase; CK, creatine kinase; LD, lactate dehydrogenase.

Enzymology
- Enzymes play an integral role in many cellular processes
- Thousands have been identified; the clinical laboratory routinely measures fewer than 15 for diagnostic purposes
- Enzymes are proteins with catalytic activity; they accelerate the rate at which a chemical reaction takes place without themselves being consumed in the process (see Table 8-33); different forms of enzymes exist that are referred to as isoenzymes
  - Lactate dehydrogenase is a tetramer containing two subunits, heart and muscle, that form five isoenzymes: LD-1 (HHHH), LD-2 (HHHM), LD-3 (HHMM), LD-4 (HMMM), and LD-5 (MMMM); historically the LD-1, LD-2 flipped ratio was used in the diagnosis of acute myocardial infarction

TABLE 8-34	Rise and Fall Pattern of Creatine Kinase–Myocardial Bound and Troponins After Acute Myocardial Infarction		
Analyte	Rise (hr After AMI)	Peak (hr After AMI)	Back to Normal
CK-MB	4-6	12-24	72 hr after AMI
Troponin I	4-6	12-24	3-7 days
Troponin T	4-6	12-24	7-10 days

AMI, Acute myocardial infarction; *CK-MB,* creatine kinase–myocardial bound.

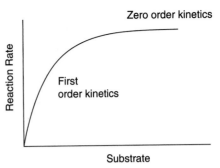

FIGURE 8-6 Zero order kinetics.

- Creatine kinase is a dimer containing two subunits, muscle and brain, that form three isoenzymes: CK-BB (brain type), CK-MB (myocardial bound), and CK-MM (muscle type); CK-MB is used in the diagnosis of acute myocardial infarction (AMI) (CK-MB >6% of total CK is diagnostic for AMI); additionally, CK-MB has a typical rise and fall pattern after an AMI that is used in conjunction with troponin levels to diagnose AMI (Table 8-34)
  - According to the Joint European Society for Cardiology/American Heart Association (AHA) Science Advisory and the Coordinating Committee/AHA/World Heart Federation Task Force for the redefinition of myocardial infarction, the diagnosis of acute myocardial infarction, is based on meeting two of the following three criteria
    - Clinical symptoms of ischemia
    - Electrocardiographic changes
    - Rise and fall of highly sensitive biochemical markers (preferably troponins)
  - Additionally, the European Society of Cardiology and the American College of Cardiology consensus report recommended that samples for the determination of AMI be collected as follows
    - Admission
    - 6 to 9 hours after admission
    - 12 to 14 hours after admission (if the earlier samples were negative)
- Enzymes combine with substrate to form enzyme/substrate complexes that dissociate, releasing enzyme and product according to the following Michaelis-Menten theory

$$E + S \leftrightarrow ES \leftrightarrow E + P$$

- Rates of the forward and reverse reaction = k_1 and k_2
- Enzyme assays in chemistry are designed for zero order kinetics in which the rate of reaction is proportional to enzyme present (Figure 8-6)

Test Procedures

- Enzymes are measured using activity or mass assays
  - Activity assays measure the catalytic effect of an enzyme on a substrate; activity is measured at optimal temperature and pH for enzymes of interest; substrate is added in excess so reaction rate depends only on the amount of enzyme in the reaction (zero order kinetics)
  - Activity assays are also referred to as kinetic assays; kinetic assays measure enzyme activity over a specified period
  - Activity assays report activity as an international unit (IU)
    - The IU is defined as the amount of enzyme needed to convert 1 µmol of substrate per minute using standardized conditions
    - Enzyme concentrations (international units per liter) are calculated using the formula

      $$IU/L = \Delta A/E \times L \times 10^6 \times 1/T \times TV/SV$$

      where ΔA = Average change in absorbance per minute
      E = Molar absorptivity
      T = Time
      TV = Total volume
      SV = Sample volume
      10^6 = Conversion factor from moles to micromoles
      L = Light path
  - Mass assays that measure either protein mass or enzyme concentrations have been developed and are in use clinically for determining isoenzymes such as CK-MB, LD-1, and the bone fraction of ALP
- Diagnostic utility is related to their tissue distribution (Table 8-35)
- Recommended ranges for commonly measured enzymes can be found in Table 8-36

Sample Collection and Handling

- Serum or plasma (heparin)
- Calcium and magnesium chelating anticoagulants must be avoided because calcium and/or magnesium are required for full catalytic activity of certain enzymes

TABLE 8-35	Enzyme Distribution and Clinical Significance	
Enzyme	**Tissue Distribution**	**Clinical Significance**
Alkaline phosphatase	Placenta, intestinal mucosa, kidney, bone, liver	Hepatobiliary damage
Alanine aminotransferase	Liver, kidney	Hepatocellular damage
Aspartate aminotransferase	Heart, liver, skeletal muscle, kidney, pancreas	Hepatocellular damage
γ-Glutamyltransferase	Kidney, biliary tract of liver	Hepatobiliary damage
Lactate dehydrogenase	Brain, heart, erythrocytes, kidney, lung, skeletal muscle, liver, pancreas, stomach	Nonspecific
Creatine kinase	Skeletal muscle, myocardium, brain, colon, stomach, urinary bladder	Myocardial damage and skeletal muscle injury
Amylase	Pancreas, salivary glands, fallopian tube	Pancreatitis
Lipase	Pancreas	Pancreatitis

TABLE 8-36	Recommended Ranges for Commonly Measured Enzymes	
Enzyme	**Recommended Range**	**Units**
Alkaline phosphatase	30-90	Units/L
Alanine aminotransferase	6-37	Units/L
Aspartate aminotransferase	5-30	Units/L
γ-Glutamyltransferase	6-45	Units/L
Lactate dehydrogenase	(L ↔ P) 100-225 (P ↔ L) 80-280	Units/L
Creatine kinase	15-160	Units/L
Amylase	60-180	Units/L
Lipase	10-200	Units/L

CERTIFICATION PREPARATION QUESTIONS

For answers and rationales, please see Appendix A.

1. Which of the following is considered a lipid?
   a. Chylomicrons
   b. LDL
   c. Cholesterol
   d. HDL

2. In the laboratory procedure for the quantification of HDL, the purpose of the dextran sulfate is to:
   a. Precipitate all Apo A1 containing lipoproteins
   b. Covert cholesterol esters to cholesterol for detection
   c. Precipitate all Apo B and Apo A containing lipoproteins
   d. Precipitate all Apo B containing proteins

3. Which of the following lipoproteins is the smallest of all the lipoproteins and is composed of 50% protein?
   a. HDL
   b. Chylomicrons
   c. LDL
   d. Triglycerides

4. Which of the following would be most adversely affected by a nonfasting sample?
   a. HDL
   b. LDL
   c. Cholesterol
   d. Triglycerides

5. Which of the following apoproteins is responsible for receptor binding for IDL and the chylomicron remnant produced in fat transport?
   a. Apo A1
   b. Apo C
   c. Apo E
   d. Apo B

6. Which of the following enzymes is found bound to HDL and LDL in blood plasma and acts to convert free cholesterol into cholesteryl esters?
   a. Cholesterol esterase
   b. Cholesterol oxidase
   c. Lecithin-cholesterol acyltransferase
   d. Lipase

7. Which of the following blood samples would serve best to assay lipoproteins because this anticoagulant acts to preserve lipoproteins?
   a. EDTA plasma sample
   b. Heparin plasma sample
   c. Citrate plasma sample
   d. Fluoride plasma sample

8. Exogenous triglycerides are transported in the plasma in which of the following forms?
   a. VLDL
   b. Chylomicrons
   c. LDL
   d. Cholesteryl esters

9. A patient presents to his physician for a lipid profile. The following results are received:
   HDL = 50 mg/dL
   Total cholesterol = 300 mg/dL
   Triglycerides = 200 mg/dL
   The calculated LDL cholesterol is:
   a. 200
   b. 210
   c. 290
   d. 350

10. According to the National Cholesterol Education Program, which lipid or lipoprotein class is more important for therapeutic decision making (diet and medication decisions)?

a. Chylomicrons
b. LDL
c. HDL
d. Cholesterol

11. Which of the following mechanisms accounts for the elevated plasma level of β-lipoproteins seen in hyperbetalipoproteinemia (Fredrickson's type II lipoproteinemia)?
    a. Elevated insulin found in these patients
    b. Apo B-100 receptor defect
    c. Apo C-II–activated lipase deficiency
    d. LCAT deficiency

12. Which enzyme is common to all enzymatic methods for triglyceride measurement?
    a. Glycerol phosphate oxidase
    b. Glycerol phosphate dehydrogenase
    c. Pyruvate kinase
    d. Glycerol kinase

13. A patient sample is assayed for fasting triglycerides and a triglyceride value of 1036 mg/dL. This value is of immediate concern because of its association with which of the following conditions?
    a. Coronary heart disease
    b. Diabetes
    c. Pancreatitis
    d. Gout

14. Which of the following apoproteins is inversely related to risk for coronary heart disease and is a surrogate marker for HDL?
    a. Apo A-I
    b. Apo B
    c. Apo B100
    d. APO E

15. What is the most appropriate fasting procedure when a lipid study of triglycerides, total cholesterol, HDL, and LDL tests are ordered?
    a. 8 hours, nothing but water allowed
    b. 10 hours, water, smoking, coffee, tea (no sugar or cream) allowed
    c. 12 hours, nothing but water allowed
    d. 16 hours, water, smoking, coffee, tea (no sugar or cream) allowed

16. John Smithers (21 years of age) is in to see his physician for a pre-college physical and checkup. John has always been extremely healthy. The following laboratory results are received:

    $A_{Standard} = 0.679$ $A_{Control} = 0.650$
    $A_{Smithers} = 0.729$ $C_{Standard} = 200$ mg/dL
    Control range 190-195 mg/dL

    John's cholesterol concentration is approximately:
    a. 186 mg/dL
    b. 199 mg/dL
    c. 209 mg/dL
    d. 215 mg/dL

17. Sucrose is considered a disaccharide that on hydrolysis yields which of the following sugars?

a. Glucose
b. Galactose and glucose
c. Maltose and glucose
d. Fructose and glucose

18. Laboratory tests are performed for a postmenopausal, 57-year-old woman as part of an annual physical examination. The patient's random serum glucose is 220 mg/dL, and the glycated hemoglobin (HbA1c) is 11%. Based on this information, this patient would mostly likely be classified as:
    a. Normal
    b. Impaired
    c. Having type 1 diabetes
    d. Having type 2 diabetes

19. Which of the biochemical processes below is promoted by insulin?
    a. Glycogenolysis
    b. Gluconeogenesis
    c. Esterification of cholesterol
    d. Uptake of glucose by the cells

20. Laboratory results for a patient with type 2 diabetes are as follows:

Analyte	Result
Glucose	128 mg/dL
Total cholesterol	195 mg/dL
HDL	45 mg/dL
LDL	105 mg/dL
BUN	38 mg/dL
Creatinine	2.1 mg/dL
Microalbuminuria	54 μg/Ml
AST	28 U/L
ALT	38 U/L

Which of the following statements is correct regarding this patient?
    a. Patient is at increased risk for cardiovascular disease
    b. Patient is at increased risk for diabetic nephropathy
    c. Patient is at increased risk for liver failure
    d. Patient is at risk for hypoglycemia

21. At what serum glucose concentration would glucose begin to appear in the urine?
    a. 50 mg/dL
    b. 75 mg/dL
    c. 100 mg/dL
    d. 170 mg/dL

22. Which of the following laboratory tests is the best marker to detect patients with diabetes who are at risk for developing diabetic nephropathy?
    a. Creatinine
    b. BUN
    c. Microalbuminuria test
    d. Glucose

23. A 68-year-old obese woman visits her doctor reporting increased urination (especially at night), increased thirst, and increased appetite. Her glucose on examination was 210 mg/dL (fasting). Which of the following statements best fits with the given information above?

a. The patient most likely has type 1 diabetes mellitus
b. The patient would show a positive glucose in her urine
c. The patient would have a decreased glycated hemoglobin
d. Additional testing of this patient should include assessment of hypoglycemia

24. Which of the following hemoglobin A1c results represents an impaired state according to the American Diabetes Association?
a. 4.5%
b. 5.5%
c. 6.0%
d. 6.5%

25. A plasma glucose result is 100 mg/dL. The corresponding glucose in whole blood would approximate:
a. 58 mg/dL
b. 87 mg/dL
c. 98 mg/dL
d. 114 mg/dL

26. Which of the following methods is virtually specific for glucose and employs G6PD as a second coupling step requiring magnesium?
a. Hexokinase
b. Glucose oxidase
c. Glucose dehydrogenase
d. Pyruvate kinase

27. A 62-year-old patient presents to the physician with report of increased thirst and increased urination, particularly at night. The physician requests a series of tests over the next few days. The following data are received:

Analyte	Result
Random glucose	186 mg/dL
Fasting glucose	114 mg/dL
2-Hour OGTT	153 mg/dL
HbA1c	5.9%

Which of the following conclusions may be made regarding these data?
a. Data represents normal glucose status
b. Data represents an impaired glucose status
c. Data represents the presence of an insulinoma
d. Data represents the diagnosis of diabetes

28. Which of the following renal conditions is associated with a recent group A β-hemolytic streptococcus infection?
a. Kidney obstruction
b. Acute renal failure
c. Uremic syndrome
d. Acute glomerulonephritis

29. The red complex developed in the Jaffe method to determine creatinine measurements is a result of the complexing of creatinine with which of the following?
a. Alkaline picrate
b. Diacetyl monoxide
c. Sulfuric acid
d. Sodium hydroxide

30. The kidney is responsible for acid-base balance through the removal of H ions via four major mechanisms. Which of the following describes one of those mechanisms?
a. Reabsorption of H ions in the proximal convoluted tubule
b. Reaction of H ions with Na in the descending loop of Henle
c. Reaction of H ions with filtered bicarbonate ions
d. Reaction of H ions with ADH in the collecting ducts

31. Given the data below, the calculated creatinine clearance corrected for body surface area approximates _____.

Analyte	Result
Serum creatinine	1.2 mg/dL
Urine creatinine	120 mg/dL
Urine volume	1.75 L/day
Surface area	1.80 m²

a. 16 mL/min
b. 115 mL/min
c. 126 mL/min
d. 210 mL/min

32. Which formula is most accurate in predicting plasma osmolality?
a. $Na + 2(Cl) + BUN + Glucose$
b. $2(Na) + 2(Cl) + Glucose + BUN$
c. $2(Na) + Glucose/18 + BUN/2.8$
d. $2(BUN) + Glucose/18 + Cl/2.8$

33. Which of the following statements regarding serum urea is true?
a. Levels are independent of diet
b. High BUN levels can result from necrotic liver disease
c. BUN is elevated in prerenal as well as renal failure
d. BUN rises earlier and quicker than creatinine in renal damage

34. Osmolality can be defined as a measure of the concentration of a solution based on:
a. The number of particles present
b. The number and size of particles present
c. The density of particles present
d. The isoelectric point of a particle

35. An increased osmole gap is most commonly seen in which of the following?
a. Type 2 diabetes
b. Pancreatitis
c. Presence of toxins such as ethanol and ethylene glycol
d. Liver failure

36. A patient with type 2 diabetes is in for a routine examination with the physician. A series of laboratory tests are performed, including calculation of an eGFR. The patient's calculated eGFR is 64 mL/min. This result is most indicative of:

a. A normal state
b. Abnormal glucose control
c. Mild kidney damage
d. Kidney failure

37. A healthy 28-year-old female sees her physician for a routine examination and receives a "relatively" clean bill of health except for the results below.
Total bilirubin 2.8 mg/dL
Direct bilirubin 0.1 mg/dL
Indirect bilirubin 2.7 mg/dL
These results most likely indicate which of the following?
a. Normal bilirubin metabolism
b. Extrahepatic obstruction
c. Dubin-Johnson syndrome
d. Gilbert's disease

38. Which of the following is measured using glutamate dehydrogenase and is a measure of advanced stages, poor prognosis, and coma in liver disease?
a. Total bilirubin
b. Ammonia
c. Unconjugated bilirubin
d. Urea

39. In which of the following disease states would you see an elevation in total bilirubin and conjugated bilirubin only?
a. Biliary obstruction
b. Hemolysis
c. Neonatal jaundice
d. Hepatitis

40. In which of the following conditions does no activity of glucuronyl transferase result in increased unconjugated bilirubin and kernicterus in neonates and eventual death within 18 months?
a. Gilbert's disease
b. Dubin-Johnson syndrome
c. Crigler-Najjar syndrome
d. Intravascular hemolysis

41. As a reduction product of bilirubin catabolism, this compound is partially reabsorbed from the intestines through the portal circulation for reexcretion by the liver. What is this compound?
a. Urobilinogen
b. Azobilirubin
c. Biliverdin
d. Urobilin

42. In the liver, bilirubin is conjugated in the presence of which of the following?
a. β-Glucuronidase
b. Bilirubin oxidase
c. Uridine diphosphate (UDP)–glucuronyl transferase
d. Peroxidase

43. Hepatocellular damage may be best assessed by which of the following parameters?
a. Serum AST and ALT levels
b. GGT and ALP
c. Bilirubin, GGT, and ALP
d. Ammonia and urea

44. Which of the following conditions is caused by deficient secretion of bilirubin into the bile canaliculi?
a. Gilbert's disease
b. Physiologic jaundice of the newborn
c. Dubin-Johnson syndrome
d. Hemolytic jaundice

45. Which of the following enzymes is responsible for the conjugation of bilirubin?
a. Biliverdin reductase
b. Peroxidase
c. UDP–glucuronyl transferase
d. β-Glucuronidase

46. Which of the following analytes is the best indicator of hepatobiliary damage?
a. AST
b. ALT
c. ALP
d. Bilirubin

47. Which of the following fractions of bilirubin in high concentrations is associated with kernicterus in newborns?
a. Delta bilirubin
b. Unconjugated bilirubin
c. Conjugated bilirubin
d. Unconjugated and delta bilirubin

48. The characteristic laboratory finding in alcoholic cirrhosis includes:
a. Moderate elevations in AST and ALT, normal GGT, and normal ALP
b. Slight elevations in AST and ALT, marked elevations in ALP, normal GGT
c. Slight elevations in AST, ALT, and GGT and marked elevations in 5' nucleotidase
d. Slight elevations in AST and ALT (AST>ALT), marked elevations in GGT, slight elevations in ALP

49. Which of the following liver conditions shows an increase in both conjugated bilirubin and ALP, manifests with antimitochondrial antibodies, and shows a characteristic lipoprotein X on electrophoresis?
a. Hemochromatosis
b. Primary biliary cirrhosis
c. Alcoholic fatty liver
d. Hepatic tumors

50. Which set of results is consistent with uncompensated metabolic acidosis?
a. pH 7.25, HCO_3 15 mmol/L, Pco_2 37 mm Hg
b. pH 7.30, HCO_3 16 mmol/L, Pco_2 28 mm Hg
c. pH 7.45, HCO_3 22 mmol/L, Pco_2 40 mm Hg
d. pH 7.40, HCO_3 25 mmol/L, Pco_2 40 mm Hg

51. A patient with emphysema who has fluid accumulation in the alveolar sacs (causing decreased ventilation) is likely to be in which of the following acid-base clinical states?
a. Respiratory alkalosis
b. Respiratory acidosis
c. Metabolic acidosis
d. Metabolic alkalosis

52. Which of the following buffer systems is the most important physiologic buffer system in the body?
a. Hemoglobin
b. Protein
c. Phosphate
d. Bicarbonate/carbonic acid

53. To maintain electrical neutrality in the red blood cell, bicarbonate leaves the red blood cell and enters the plasma through an exchange mechanism with which of the following?
a. TCO_2
b. Sodium
c. Chloride
d. Phosphate

54. Increased PCO_2 in a patient most commonly results in which of the following primary acid-base abnormalities?
a. Respiratory acidosis
b. Metabolic acidosis
c. Respiratory alkalosis
d. Metabolic alkalosis

55. Which of the following changes will occur with a blood gas sample exposed to room air?
a. pH increased
b. $pCOO_2$ increased
c. pO_2 decreased
d. Ionized calcium increased

56. Which of the following is the correct collection and handling for the analysis of blood gases?
a. Plastic syringe, dry heparin, store on ice, assay within 1 hour
b. Glass syringe, liquid heparin, store on ice, assay within 15 minutes
c. Glass syringe, no additive, store on ice, assay within 15 minutes
d. Plastic syringe, dry heparin, store at room temperature, assay within 15 minutes

57. What is the blood pH when the partial pressure of carbon dioxide (pCO_2) is 45 mm Hg and the bicarbonate is 28 mmol/L?
a. 7.00
b. 7.11
c. 7.33
d. 7.41

58. What is the normal ratio of bicarbonate to dissolved carbon dioxide in arterial blood?
a. 1:10
b. 10:1
c. 20:1
d. 1:20

59. Which of the following sets of blood gas data is considered normal?
a. pH 7.33, HCO_3 18 mmol/L, pCO_2 32 mm Hg
b. pH 7.30, HCO_3 16 mmol/L, pCO_2 28 mm Hg
c. pH 7.45, HCO_3 22 mmol/L, pCO_2 40 mm Hg
d. pH 7.40, HCO_3 25 mmol/L, pCO_2 40 mm Hg

60. Which of the following values would be seen in uncompensated metabolic acidosis?
a. pH 7.38
b. pCO_2 52 mm Hg
c. HCO_3 15 mmol/L
d. pH 7.53

61. Which of the following blood gas disorders is most commonly associated with an abnormal anion gap?
a. Metabolic acidosis
b. Metabolic alkalosis
c. Respiratory acidosis
d. Respiratory alkalosis

62. Which of the following statements best describes the predominant feedback system associated with endocrinology?
a. Decreased levels of circulating hormones directly result in the production of hormone from the target organ
b. Increased circulating levels of hormones directly result in the production of releasing factor from the hypothalamus
c. Increased circulating levels of hormones directly result in the production of inhibiting factor from the hypothalamus
d. Normal levels of circulating hormones directly result in the production of hormone from the target organ

63. The following laboratory results are from a 54-year-old woman complaining of weight gain, intolerance to heat, fatigue, and not being able to stay awake.

Analyte	Result
Na	140 mmol/L
K	4.0 mmol/L
Glucose	75 mg/dL
Aldosterone	8 ng/dL
Ionized Ca	4.8 mg/dL
Mg	2.0 mEq/L
Phos	3.0 mg/dL
TSH	7.2 μU/mL
FT_4	1.0 ng/dL
Cortisol	10 μg/dL

Which of the following conditions best fits with the history and data?
a. Hyperthyroidism
b. Cushing's syndrome
c. Hyperaldosteronism
d. Hypothyroidism

64. A 42-year-old woman presents to her physician with truncal obesity, bruising, hypertension, hyperglycemia, and increased facial hair. The physician suspects an endocrine disturbance. Significant test results are as follows:

Analyte	Result
TSH	3.0 μU/mL
FT_4	1.0 ng/dL
Glucose	90 mg/dL
Serum cortisol (8 AM)	45 μg/dL

Plasma ACTH (8 AM)   152 pg/mL
Urine free cortisol   Increased
Dexamethasone suppression tests
   Overnight   300 nmol/L
   High dose   >50% suppression

What is the most probable condition?
a. Pituitary tumor
b. Addison's disease
c. Adrenal adenoma
d. Ectopic ACTH production

65. Hypothyroidism is best characterized by which of the following sets of test results?
a. TSH 0.2 μU/mL, FT_3 8.9 pg/mL, FT_4 4.5 ng/dL
b. TSH 8.5 μU/mL, FT_3 1.0 pg/mL, FT_4 0.5 ng/dL
c. TSH 0.1 μU/mL, FT_3 1.1 pg/mL, FT_4 0.8 ng/dL
d. TSH 3.9 μU/mL, FT_3 3.0 pg/mL, FT_4 1.0 ng/dL

66. The release of thyroid-releasing hormone (TRH) would result in which of the following actions from the HPT axis?
a. Decreased release of thyroid-stimulating hormone from the pituitary gland
b. Increased release of thyroid-stimulating hormone from the thyroid gland
c. Increased release of thyroid hormones from the thyroid glands
d. Increased release of thyroid hormones from the pituitary gland

67. A serum thyroid panel reveals an increase in total T_4, normal TSH, and a normal fT_4. What is the most likely cause of these results?
a. Increased thyroxine-binding protein
b. Secondary hyperthyroidism
c. Subclinical hypothyroidism
d. Subclinical hyperthyroidism

68. Thyroid hormones are derived from which of the following?
a. Histidine
b. Cholesterol
c. Tyrosine
d. Phenylalanine

69. In patients with developing subclinical hyperthyroidism, TSH levels will likely be _____, and fT_4 will likely be _____.
a. Decreased, increased
b. Increased, decreased
c. Decreased, normal
d. Increased, normal

70. A 30-year-old woman is admitted to the hospital. She has truncal obesity, buffalo humpback, moon face, purple striae, hypertension, hyperglycemia, increased facial hair and amenorrhea. The physician orders endocrine testing. The results are as follows:

Analyte	Result
Urine free cortisol	Increased
Serum cortisol (8 AM)	Increased

Plasma ACTH   Decreased
Dexamethasone   Overnight: No
   suppression test   suppression
             High dose: No
                suppression

What is the most probable condition?
a. Addison's disease
b. Cushing's disease
c. Conn's syndrome
d. Cushing's syndrome

71. Trophic hormones are produced by the _____, and releasing factors are produced by the _____.
a. Hypothalamus; pituitary
b. Pituitary; hypothalamus
c. Specific endocrine glands; hypothalamus
d. Pituitary; target gland

72. When free thyroxine cannot be measured directly, the free thyroxine index (FT_4I) may be calculated by using which measured laboratory data?
a. TSH and T_3 resin uptake
b. T_4 and T_3 resin uptake
c. TSH and T_4
d. T_3 and T_3 resin uptake

73. The most commonly used challenge test to assist in evaluating a potential growth hormone deficiency is the:
a. Insulin challenge test
b. Dexamethasone suppression test
c. Oral glucose tolerance test
d. Captopril suppression test

74. Symptoms of primary adrenal insufficiency (Addison's disease) include which of the following?
a. Hypercortisolism
b. Hypokalemia
c. Hypertension
d. Acidosis

75. A TRH stimulation test is performed, and a flat response is received from this test procedure. This most likely indicates:
a. Secondary hypothyroidism
b. Tertiary hypothyroidism
c. Primary hypothyroidism
d. Secondary hyperthyroidism

76. The first step in the synthesis of thyroid hormones is:
a. Iodide trapping
b. Binding of thyroglobulin
c. Oxidation of iodine
d. Oxidation of TG molecule

77. Which of the following conditions is a result of catecholamine excess, includes two classifications (MEN 1 and MEN 2), and may result in death from severe cardiovascular complications?
a. Cushing's syndrome
b. Conn's syndrome
c. Addison's disease
d. Pheochromocytoma

78. The main estrogen produced by the ovaries and used to evaluate ovarian function is:
a. Estriol
b. Estradiol
c. Epiestriol
d. Estrogen

79. The Michaelis-Menten theory states which of the following?
a. $E+S+I \rightarrow ES+EI+ESI \rightarrow E+P$
b. $E+S \leftrightarrow ES \rightarrow E+P$
c. $E+S+I \rightarrow ES+EI \rightarrow E+P$
d. $E \leftrightarrow ES \rightarrow E+P$

80. Which of the following enzymes is the best indicator of pancreatic function?
a. AST
b. ALT
c. GGT
d. Lipase

81. Which of the following enzymes catalyzes the conversion of *p*-nitrophenyl phosphate to a colored *p*-nitrophenol product?
a. AST
b. ALT
c. ALP
d. GGT

82. One international unit of enzyme activity is the amount of enzyme that under specified reaction conditions of substrate concentration, pH, and temperature, causes usage of substrate at the rate of:
a. 1 millimole/min
b. 1 micromole/min
c. 1 nanomole/min
d. 1 picomole/min

83. A physician calls to request a CK test on a sample already in the laboratory for coagulation studies. The sample is 1 hour old and has been stored at 4° c. The plasma shows very slight hemolysis. What is the best course of action and the reason for it?
a. Perform the CK assay because no interferent is present
b. Reject the sample because it is slightly hemolyzed
c. Reject the sample because it has been stored too long
d. Reject the sample because the citrate will interfere

84. Which of the following statements regarding CK is true?
a. Levels are unaffected by strenuous exercise
b. Levels are unaffected by repeated intramuscular injections
c. Highest levels are seen in Duchenne's muscular dystrophy
d. The enzyme is highly specific for heart injury

85. Which of the following conditions can "physiologically" elevate serum alkaline phosphatase?
a. Hyperparathyroidism
b. Diabetes
c. Third-trimester pregnancy
d. Nephrotic syndrome

86. Kinetic enzymatic assays are best performed during which phase of an enzymatic reaction?
a. Linear phase
b. Lag phase
c. Plateau phase
d. Any phase as long as temperature and pH are constant

87. A nurse calls the laboratory technologist on duty asking about blood collection for the analysis of enzymes (AST, ALP, ALT, GGT, CK). Which of the following tubes would you suggest the technologist collect?
a. Red top
b. EDTA
c. Oxalate
d. Fluoride

88. Which of the following enzymes catalyzes the conversion of starch to glucose and maltose?
a. Lipase
b. Amylase
c. ALT
d. GGT

89. Hyperparathyroidism is most consistently associated with which of the following?
a. Hypocalcemia
b. Hypercalciuria
c. Hypophosphatemia
d. Metabolic alkalosis

90. What percentage of serum calcium is in the ionized form?
a. 30%
b. 50%
c. 60%
d. 80%

91. Which of the following best describes the action of parathyroid hormone?
a. PTH increases calcium and phosphorus reabsorption in the kidney
b. PTH decreases calcium and phosphorus release from bone
c. PTH decreases calcium and increases phosphorus reabsorption in the liver
d. PTH increases calcium reabsorption and decreases phosphorus reabsorption in the kidney

92. Which of the following is most likely to produce an elevated plasma potassium result?
a. Hypoparathyroidism
b. Cushing's syndrome
c. Diarrhea
d. Hemolysis

93. Which of the following hormones involved in calcium regulation acts by decreasing both calcium and phosphorous?
a. PTH
b. Calcitonin
c. Vitamin D
d. Cortisol

94. Which of the following electrolytes is the chief plasma cation whose main function is maintaining osmotic pressure?
    a. Chloride
    b. Potassium
    c. Sodium
    d. Bicarbonate

95. Which of the following conditions is associated with hypernatremia?
    a. Diabetes insipidus
    b. Hypoaldosteronism
    c. Diarrhea
    d. Acidemia

96. Which of the following conditions will elevate ionized calcium?
    a. Diabetes mellitus
    b. Hyperlipidemia
    c. Acidosis
    d. Alkalosis

97. The anion gap is useful (among other things) as an inexpensive measure of quality control for which of the following analytes?
    a. Blood gas analyses
    b. Sodium, potassium, chloride, and total carbon dioxide
    c. Calcium, phosphorus, and magnesium
    d. AST, ALT, GGT, and ALP

98. Psuedohyperkalemia is most commonly a result of which of the following?
    a. Metabolic acidosis
    b. Hemolysis
    c. Hyperaldosteronism
    d. Hyperparathyroidism

99. The following results were seen on a blood sample:

Analyte	Result
$Na^+ = 140$ mEq/L	$K^+ = 15.0$ mEq/L
$Cl^- = 105$ mEq/L	$HCO_3 = 22$ mmol/L

    The technologist should do which of the following?
    a. Report the results
    b. Repeat and check the chloride result
    c. Repeat and check the Na^+ result
    d. Check the sample for hemolysis

100. The major intracellular cation is which of the following?
    a. Potassium
    b. Sodium
    c. Chloride
    d. Bicarbonate

SELF-ASSESSMENT

Content Area: _____

Score on Practice Questions: _____

List the specific topics covered in the missed questions:

List the specific topics covered in the correct questions:

NOTES

Molecular Diagnostics

Gideon H. Labiner

MOLECULAR BIOLOGY BASICS

Chromosomes

- Genetic material is contained on chromosomes
  - Maternal and paternal inheritance of genetic material
    - Haploid: A single copy is 23 chromosomes
    - Diploid: Two copies of each chromosome, 46 chromosomes
  - Parts of a chromosome
    - Telomeres: Area at the end of a chromosome
    - Centromere: Area in the middle of the chromosome where the chromatids ("arms") meet
      - Metacentric
      - Submetacentric
      - Acrocentric
    - Heterochromatin: Tightly packed DNA
    - Euchromatin: Looser packaging of DNA, which could indicate that a gene is actively being transcribed
  - Chromosome structure
    - Primary structure: Sequence of nucleic acids
    - Secondary structure: Folding of sequence based on hydrogen bonding
    - Tertiary structure: Three-dimensional shape displaying the turns of the helix and major and minor groove
      - B-DNA: Right-handed helix and most common form
      - A-DNA: Right-handed and similar to B form
      - Z-DNA: Left-handed DNA
  - Organization of DNA (Figure 9-1)
    - Chromatin: Nuclear DNA strand and its associated structural proteins
      - Arranged and organized in a hierarchical fashion in which the degree of its condensation increases with higher levels of structural organization
    - Solenoid: Supercoiled chromatin fibers
    - Nucleosome: Eight histone proteins with a strand of DNA (~170 base pairs long) wrapped around them, giving a "beads-on-a-string" appearance
    - Histone: Protein involved in the organization of nuclear DNA
    - Double helix: Sugar-phosphate backbone with base pairs oriented in the core

Nucleic Acid Structure

- Molecular composition of DNA and RNA (Figure 9-2)
  - Base
    - Purines: Double carbon–nitrogen rings
      - Adenine
      - Guanine
    - Pyrimidines: Single carbon–nitrogen ring
      - Cytosine
      - Thymine
      - Uracil: Replaces thymine as base in RNA
  - Sugar: Pentose or five-carbon ring
    - Deoxyribose in DNA
    - Ribose in RNA
  - Phosphate bonds: Monophosphate, diphosphate, triphosphate
  - Nucleotide: Base + Sugar + Phosphate
    - Phosphodiester bond links the $5'$ carbon of one nucleotide to the $3'$ carbon of another
    - Nucleotides always join in a $5'$ to $3'$ orientation
      - This bonding makes the alternating sugar and phosphate backbone of DNA
      - Nucleoside: Base + Sugar
  - Base pairing: Joining of a purine with a pyrimidine by hydrogen bonding
    - Adenine binds with thymine: Two hydrogen bonds
    - Guanine binds with cytosine: Three hydrogen bonds
  - Orientation of molecules
    - Forms right-handed double helix
      - 10 bases per turn
      - One helical turn = 3.4 nm
    - Polymers of sugar and phosphates run in opposite direction
      - Antiparallel
      - Complementary strands join together to form double-stranded DNA (dsDNA)
    - RNA has a hydroxyl group at the $2'$ carbon
    - RNA is usually found in the single-stranded form

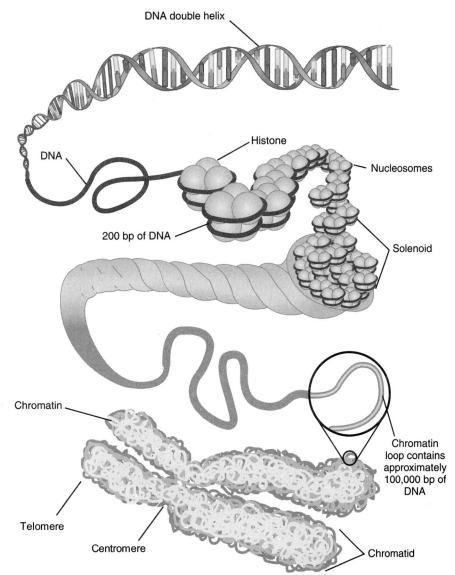

FIGURE 9-1 Structural organization of human chromosomal DNA. *bp*, Base pairs. *(From Jorde B, Carey J, Bamshad M: Medical genetics, ed 4, Philadelphia, 2009, Mosby.)*

Nucleic Acid Physiology and Function

- Central dogma
  - DNA replicates itself to produce DNA
  - DNA is transcribed to make RNA
  - RNA is translated to produce protein
- Replication: Generating or producing new DNA from parent DNA
  - Both strands of parent DNA act as the template for synthesizing daughter stands
    - Process is semiconservative
    - New dsDNA will be made up of one parent and one daughter strand
  - Replication forks are produced through the unwinding enzymes (helicase and topoisomerase)
    - Primase: Enzyme that synthesizes a short RNA to prime DNA synthesis

- DNA polymerases: Enzymes that synthesize DNA with proofreading and exonuclease capabilities
- Okazaki fragments
  - Leading strand: Continuous synthesis of daughter strand
  - Lagging strand: Discontinues synthesis of daughter strand
- DNA ligase: Digests primer and joins Okazaki fragments
- Transcription
  - Genes are located within DNA
    - Allele: A form of a gene that is variable
      - Two alleles make up a genotype
- Locus: Location on the chromosome where the gene/ alleles are located, plural is loci

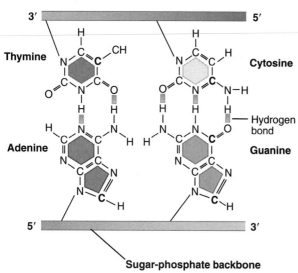

FIGURE 9-2 Chemical structure of the four bases, showing hydrogen bonds between base pairs. Three hydrogen bonds are formed between cytosine–guanine pairs, and two bonds are formed between adenine–thymine pairs *(From Jorde B, Carey J, Bamshad M: Medical genetics, ed 4, Philadelphia, 2009, Mosby.)*

- Genes contain information needed for the production of RNA and proteins
  - Also needed for cellular maintenance
  - Transcription is similar to replication
    - DNA is the source and produces single-stranded RNA (ssRNA) from dsDNA
    - The process uses the enzyme RNA polymerase
- Only specific genes are transcribed at any given time
- Genes contain both coding and noncoding sections

- Exons: Coding regions
- Introns: Noncoding regions, sometimes referred to as junk DNA
- Promoter: Regulatory region that influences the initiation and rate of transcription
- Messenger RNA (mRNA) is the ultimate product of transcription
  - Chain termination: When RNA polymerase reaches a termination sequence
    - pre-mRNA and heterogeneous nuclear (hnRNA) are the sequences before processing
    - Introns are removed by splicing
      - Spliceosomes are formed from small nuclear ribonucleic particles (snRNPs)
      - Exons are placed next to one another
    - Capping: Guanine added at 5′ end
    - Polyadenylation: Poly A tail added to the 3′ end
  - The mature mRNA can now leave the nucleus and enter the cytoplasm
- Translation
  - Transfer RNA (tRNA) and ribosomal RNA (rRNA) form the site for protein synthesis
  - Genes are composed of nucleic acids arranged into codons
  - Codons are 3 nucleic acids that together code for 1 amino acid
    - 64 possible codons for 20 amino acids
      - Redundancy protects against possible mutations
  - Amino acids are the building blocks for protein
  - 20 amino acids are involved in protein synthesis (Table 9-1)

TABLE 9-1	The Genetic Code: Translation of Messenger RNA to Amino Acids During Protein Synthesis			
		Nucleotide Position in the Codon			
First	**Second**	**Third**			
		U	**C**	**A**	**G**
U	U	Phenylalanine	Phenylalanine	Leucine	Leucine
	C	Serine	Serine	Serine	Serine
	A	Tyrosine	Tyrosine	Stop	Stop
	G	Cysteine	Cysteine	Selenocysteine*	Tryptophan
C	U	Leucine	Leucine	Leucine	Leucine
	C	Proline	Proline	Proline	Proline
	A	Histidine	Histidine	Glutamine	Glutamine
	G	Arginine	Arginine	Arginine	Arginine
A	U	Isoleucine	Isoleucine	Isoleucine	Methionine
	C	Threonine	Threonine	Threonine	Threonine
	A	Asparagine	Asparagine	Lysine	Lysine
	G	Serine	Serine	Arginine	Arginine
G	U	Valine	Valine	Valine	Valine
	C	Alanine	Alanine	Alanine	Alanine
	A	Aspartic acid	Aspartic acid	Glutamic acid	Glutamic acid
	G	Glycine	Glycine	Glycine	Glycine

*The codon UGA can code for either selenocysteine or stop.
From Bruns D, Ashwood E, Burtis, C: *Fundamentals of molecular diagnostics*, St. Louis, Saunders, 2007.

- One start codon: Acts as initiation point for reading
  - AUG
- Three stop codons: Terminates the elongation of the polypeptide chain
  - UAA
  - UAG
  - UGA
- tRNA and anticodon
  - tRNA carries amino acids specified by the codon in the mRNA
- Wobble principle: Allows for loose-fitting match between the tRNA anticodons and the mRNA codons
- Epigenetics
  - Alteration of gene function without changing DNA sequence
    - DNA methylation
    - Genomic imprinting
    - Histone modification
- Mitochondrial DNA
  - Circular DNA that is 16,569 base pairs
  - Maternal inheritance pattern
  - Number of mitochondria per cell is variable, some cells have thousands

GENOMES AND NUCLEIC ACID ALTERATIONS

- Human genome
  - 3.2 billion base pairs
  - 23 chromosome pairs (46 chromosomes)
  - Approximately 30,000 genes
    - Sequence variation
      - 99.9% of the genome between random individuals is identical
      - Intron sequences are often simple repeat sequences
  - Microsatellites also called short tandem repeats (STRs)
    - Repeat units are two to six base pairs in length
  - Minisatellites also called variable number of tandem repeats (VNTRs)
    - Repeat units are 40 to 500 base pairs in length
- A polymorphism is a sequence variation occurring in more than 1% of a population
  - Single nucleotide polymorphism (SNP)
- Nucleic acid enzymes
  - Used in molecular laboratory procedures to manipulate nucleic acids
    - Polymerase: Catalyzes the extension of nucleotides in the presence of a template strand
    - Ligase: Catalyzes the linkage between two nucleotides by a phosphodiester bond
    - Nuclease: Cleaves nucleic acids
      - Endonuclease: Acts on internal bonds
      - Exonuclease: Acts on external bonds

- Reverse transcriptase
  - Synthesizes a DNA strand from either DNA or RNA
  - Found in retroviruses
- Kinase: Transfers phosphate groups
- Phosphatase: Removes phosphate groups
- Methylase: Adds methyl groups to nitrogen bases
- Deaminase: Remove amino groups from nitrogen bases

NUCLEIC ACID ISOLATION

- DNA and RNA isolation
  - The process of separating nucleic acid material from its surroundings
    - Surrounding can include tissues, debris, cells, proteins, lipids, or carbohydrates
  - Cell lysis, extraction, and purification are part of the isolation process
  - DNA is fairly stable over a wide range of temperatures; hydrolysis poses a major threat to nucleic acids remaining intact
  - RNA is easily degraded by environmental RNase enzymes
  - Considerations for choosing an isolation method
    - Specimen type (Table 9-2)
    - Amount of sample and desired yield
    - Purity and size of isolate
    - Ease of operation and throughput
    - Costs and hazards
- Extraction methods
  - Liquid phase
    - Used for large sample volumes
    - Phenol-chloroform is a biphasic organic extraction method
      - Hydrophobic portion: Lipids and debris on the bottom
      - Hydrophilic portion: Aqueous phase contains the DNA on top
    - Inorganic method substitutes the harsh chemicals of organic extraction with high salt conditions at a low pH
      - The DNA is collected from the upper phase and then precipitated with isopropyl alcohol
  - Solids phase
    - More commonly used because of ease of use, fewer safety concerns, ability for high throughput, and automation
      - Column filter
      - Magnetic beads
  - General steps of extraction
    - Cell lysis step to disrupt membranes
    - Salt preparation to remove proteins
    - DNA precipitated by alcohol
- Assessment of nucleic acid yield and quality
  - Ultraviolet (UV) light is absorbed by DNA and RNA at a wavelength of 260 nm

TABLE 9-2	Specimen Collection and Storage		
Specimen	**Collection and Transport**	**Storage Temperature (° C) (Short/Long)**	**Considerations**
Whole blood or bone marrow	Lavender or yellow-top tube for whole blood	4/-70	Avoid heparin tube, remove red blood cells before storage to avoid hemolysis
Tissue	Freeze solid tissues or on ice	4/-70	May be paraffin-embedded
Buccal swabs	Rinse or swab oral cavity, collect in buffer or transport medium	4/-20	Less invasive collection procedure
Microorganism	Special collection systems for various target organisms	4/-70	Viral RNA should be stored at 24° C, avoid contamination that may result in false-positive findings
Forensic: Blood, hair, nails, secretions, etc.	Evidence labeled, air dry blood-stained clothes, separate paper bags for each item	4/-70 24° C for blood stored on special filter paper	Chain of custody for evidence, avoid heat and contamination, aliquot to avoid repeated heating and thawing

- Yield can be measured with a spectrophotometer
  - 50 mg/L of dsDNA has an absorbance of 1.0 at 260 nm
  - RNA at an absorbance of 1.0 at 260 nm equals 40 mg/L
- Quality and purity can be measured by looking at the absorbance ratio A260/A280
  - 280 nm is the absorbance of proteins
  - If the ratio is less than 1.6, contamination with protein is present
  - If the ratio is 1.6 to 1.9, minimal contamination may be present in the extract and the DNA is not pure
  - Extracts from 1.8 to 2.0 are typically acceptable for clinical specimens
  - A ratio of 2.0 indicates a pure DNA extract

NUCLEIC ACID TECHNIQUES

Electrophoresis

- Both DNA and RNA carry a negative charge and will migrate toward the positive-charge electrode (anode)
- Gels act like a sieve for nucleic acid molecules
  - Slab gel (vertical or horizontal) or using gel polymer inside a capillary
  - Agarose gel: Larger fragments (20 bp - 10 Mb)
  - Polyacrylamide gel: Smaller sequences (1 bp - 2 kb)
    - Neurotoxin
    - Used for sequencing
- Based on molecular weight of the fragment
- Smaller molecules move faster
- Molecules may form secondary structures or heteroplexes
- Restriction fragment length polymorphism (RFLP)
  - Using restriction enzymes to cut dsDNA at specific cleavage sites
    - Restriction enzymes are derived from bacteria and read nucleic acid sequences and cut the

phosphate backbone of the dsDNA making fragments with
  - Blunt ends
  - Stagger or sticky ends (5′ or 3′)
- Changes in DNA may result in loss or gain of a cleavage site
- Result will be a change in fragment size that can be detected by electrophoresis
  - Fragments are compared to a known DNA ladder
  - Tracking dye and a density agent, such as glycerol, are added to the DNA sample
- Southern blotting (Figure 9-3)
  - After digestion of DNA by a restriction enzyme and separation by electrophoresis, Southern blotting is the act of transferring the resulting fragments to a solid support medium
    - Nylon or nitrocellulose membrane/filter is medium of choice
    - DNA can be fragmented using an acid treatment during transfer as part of depurination
    - Alkaline denaturation is used to form ssDNA
    - Neutralization
  - Transfer (blotting) methods
    - Capillary action
    - Vacuum transfer
  - Immobilization on nitrocellulose membrane through UV cross-linkage
    - Single-stranded probes are incubated with the membranes and hybridize to complementary target regions
      - Probes contain a label for detection
      - Wash excess probe under appropriate stringency conditions to discourage nonspecific binding to nontarget nucleic acid
        - Formamide concentration
        - Temperature
    - Fragments are visualized by
      - Autoradiography film exposed to membrane

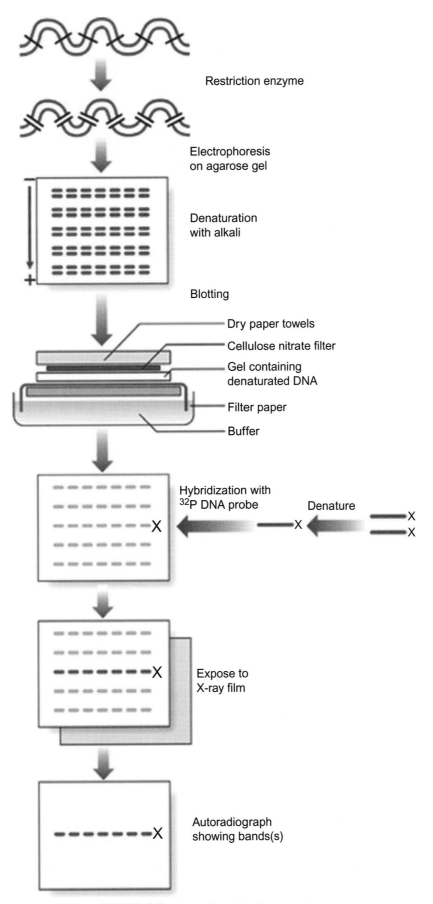

FIGURE 9-3 The Southern blotting procedure.

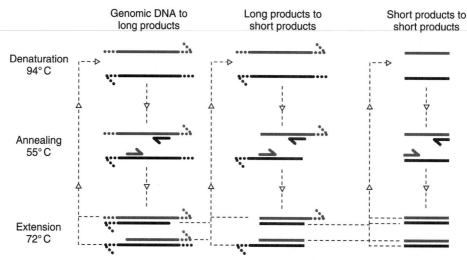

FIGURE 9-4 Schematic diagram of polymerase chain reaction. *(From Bruns D, Ashwood E, Burtis C:* Fundamentals of molecular diagnostics, *St. Louis, Saunders, 2007.)*

- Ethidium bromide (EtBr): Intercalates into DNA and fluoresces under UV light
  - Chemiluminescence signal
- Pulsed-field gel electrophoresis (PFGE)
  - Used for very large pieces of DNA
  - Current applied in alternating orientations
  - Used for epidemiologic studies for infectious diseases
- Northern blotting
  - Technique similar to Southern blotting, but the target is RNA
  - Electrophoresis under denaturing conditions
  - Used for looking at mRNA transcripts
- Western blotting
  - Technique similar to Southern blotting, but the target is proteins
  - Probes are antibodies

Amplification Techniques

Polymerase Chain Reaction. See Figure 9-4.
- Target amplification: Known nucleic acid sequence of interest targeted for enzymatic replication in an amplified manner
- Polymerase chain reaction (PCR) uses a master mix of all components needed for the reaction (Tables 9-3)
  - Template DNA containing target sequence
    - Purified dsDNA
  - Forward and reverse primers
    - Oligodeoxynucleotides (20-30 base pairs)
    - Complementary to the opposing strands flanking the sequences of interest
    - Melting temperature (Tm)

  - When half of the primers are bound (double stranded) and half are unbound (single stranded)
  - Relates to the optimal temperature needed for annealing step
- Magnesium chloride: Cofactor in reaction
- Nucleotide bases
  - Deoxynucleotide triphosphates: dNTP
  - dATP, dCTP, dGTP, and dTTP
- Buffer for optimal pH
- Polymerase adds dNTPs
  - The PCR reaction uses a thermocycler, which allows for the rapid change in temperature needed for each step
- Thermostable *Taq* polymerase withstands the extreme temperature fluctuations necessary to complete the three steps of a PCR cycle
  - Derived from *Thermus aquaticus*, which lives in hot springs
- Steps in PCR (Table 9-4)
  - Denaturation: dsDNA is heated and separated in ssDNA
  - Annealing: Cooler temperature allows for primers to bind to target sequence
  - Extension: Temperature optimal for polymerase activity
- Traditional PCR also is referred to as end-point PCR

Polymerase Chain Reaction Kinetics
- Allows for exponential expansion of products
- Typical PCR run has 25 to 30 cycles, making millions of copies of the target sequence
  - Amplified product is known as an amplicon
    - Clones or replicas of target sequence

TABLE 9-3	Polymerase Chain Reaction Components
Components	**Function**
Template DNA	Includes target sequence
Primers	20-30 base pairs long, flank target sequence at 5′ ends
Magnesium chloride	Enzyme cofactor
dNTP	Nucleotides being added (A, G, T, C)
Buffer	Maintains pH of reaction
Polymerase	Allows for addition of dNTPs at 5′ end during extension

TABLE 9-4	Polymerase Chain Reaction Cycles
Steps	**Temperature (° C)**
Denaturation	~94 (30-60 sec)
Annealing	~55 (30-90 sec)
Extension	~72 (30-90 sec)

- ○ At some point in the PCR run, the production of amplicons plateaus
- Amount of product is related to the efficiency of the cycles

Variations on Polymerase Chain Reaction
Reverse-Transcriptase Polymerase Chain Reaction
- Technique used if the template of interest is RNA
- Uses RNA viral polymerase reverse transcriptase
  - Makes RNA/DNA complex
  - Then replaces the RNA with DNA
    - ○ The resulting strand is referred to as cDNA or complementary DNA
    - ○ Used to measure or detect various types of RNA
    - ○ Does not include the intron sequences of a gene

Multiplex Polymerase Chain Reaction
- The use of multiple primer pairs in one reaction tube
- Allows for detection of multiple targets
  - Internal amplification controls
  - Multiple pathogens
  - Multiple polymorphism in identity testing
- Multiplex ligation-dependent probe amplification
  - Method that uses multiple probes for areas of interest and then amplifies with a single primer

Real-Time Polymerase Chain Reaction
- Also referred to as quantitative PCR (qPCR) because data, by way of florescence signaling, are collected during nucleic acid amplification
- Amplification and fluorescence monitoring takes place in same reaction tube, minimizing risk for contamination
- Real-time PCR dyes
  - EtBr

- SYBR green I: Specific dye for dsDNA
  - ○ Lets off signal when DNA is denatured
  - ○ Safer to use than EtBr
- Probes-specific detection
  - Hybridization probes
    - ○ Fluorescence resonance energy transfer (FRET)
      - Uses two probes: Acceptor probe and donor probe
      - Energy is transferred from donor to acceptor, and a fluorescent signal is released
  - Hydrolysis probes
    - ○ Reporter and quenchers
    - ○ TaqMan is an example that uses the 5′ exonuclease activity of *Taq* polymerase for signal generation
  - Molecular beacons and Scorpion probes
- Melting curve analysis
  - Separation of strands based on temperature
    - ○ For short strands this can be estimated by

$$2(AT) + 4(GC) = T_m$$

  - ○ More complicated for longer strands, must account for
    - Salt concentration
    - GC versus AT binding (GC has more H bonds)
    - Total length of fragment
  - Allows for genotyping
  - SNP selection

Polymerase Chain Reaction Controls and Contamination Issues
- Controls in PCR must monitor for
  - False positive findings resulting from carryover or other contamination
  - False negative findings resulting from presence of inhibitors and/or error in master-mix components
- Purpose for controls
  - Positive control: Contains sequence of interest
  - Negative control: Does not contain sequence of interest
  - Reagent blank control: All reactants except DNA
  - Amplification control
    - ○ Amplification of a different target region
    - ○ Tests for inhibition of PCR
      - If amplification control is negative, corrective action is to repurify DNA extract
    - ○ Differentiates true negative from false negative
      - Sensitivity control: Defines the lower limits of testing
- Primer-dimers
  - Result of unintended binding of primers to one another
  - Distinguished from true target by molecular weight or T_m
- Cleaning and decontamination
  - Uracil-N-glycosylase: Degrades carryover amplicons
  - UV light
  - 10% bleach

- Laboratory design
  - Separate preamplification and postamplification steps
  - Dedicated equipment: Pipettes
  - Prealiquoted reagents
  - Negative airflow and unidirectional processing

Alternative Amplification Techniques

Ligase Chain Reaction
- Uses four primer/probes and DNA ligase
- When the oligonucleotide primer/probes bind to target region separated by a few base pairs, the ligase will join the probes together

Transcription-Based Amplification
- Target is dsDNA or ssRNA and is used to synthesize cDNA
- Isothermal reaction conditions, do not need thermocycler
- Uses reverse transcriptase, RNase H, RNA polymerase, and primers
- End result is ssRNA amplification
  - Examples of transcription-based amplification
    - Transcription-mediated amplification (TMA)
    - Nucleic acid sequence–based assay (NASBA)

Strand Displacement Amplification
- Isothermal application reaction that takes place in two stages
  - Stage one: Target generation
  - Stage two: Probe amplification
- Uses a modified deoxynucleotide
- During the extension step the modified deoxynucleotide is nicked by a restriction enzyme
- The act of nicking and extension allows for amplification of the probes

Signal Amplification

Branched-Chain DNA (bDNA)
- Capture probes on a microtiter well plate used to hybridize target
  - Extenders
  - Preamplifiers
  - Amplifier probes

Hybrid Capture
- RNA probes
- Make DNA-RNA hybrids
- Sandwich assay

Cleavage-Based Amplification
- Invader system: Cuts overlapping regions of nucleotides
  - Use the enzyme cleavase
  - FRET probe
  - Reporter molecule

Additional Molecular Technologies

Microarrays: DNA Hybridization Arrays
- Also known as a DNA chip
- Solid support: Silicon, plastic, or glass
- Oligonucleotide probes are added by photolithography or printing to specific locations to form the array
- Thousands of probes are contained on the support chip
- Applications
  - Bacterial identification
  - SNP and mutation detection
  - Gene expression
  - DNA sequencing
  - Comparative genome hybridization

Mass Spectrometry
- Matrix-assisted laser-desorption ionization time-of-flight (MALDI-TOF)
- No labeling needed
- Genotype derived from differing mass of alleles received by a detector

Nucleic Acid Sequencing

Maxam-Gilbert Chemical Sequencing
- Strong reducing agents used to break nucleotide fragments in predictable places
  - Dimethyl sulfate
  - Formic acid
  - Hydrazine and salt
- Electrophoresis run on polyacrylamide gel
- Method is not amenable to automation and uses hazardous chemicals

Sanger Sequencing
- Uses four dideoxynucleotide (ddNTP) base analogs
  - Results in chain termination as ddNTPs are incorporated randomly among the other dNTPs
  - Dideoxynucleotide lacks 3′ hydroxyl group (OH)
- Separated by polyacrylamide gel electrophoresis or capillary electrophoresis
- Automated methods use fluorescent labeling
  - Dye primer
  - Dye terminator

Pyrosequencing
- Uses four enzymes: DNA polymerase, adenosine triphosphate (ATP) sulfurylase, luciferase, and apyrase
- Uses two substrates: Adenosine 5′ phosphosulfate and luciferin
- Pyrophosphate (PPi) is released, light is produced that corresponds to the dNTP added

Next-Generation Sequencing
- Instruments with the capacity to sequence large volumes of samples
- Whole-genome sequencing for affordable cost (<$1000)
- Used for personalized medicine

Detection Techniques

- Labeled probes
  - Radioactive
    - Phosphorus atoms (^{32}P)
  - Nonradioactive
    - Digoxygenin
    - Biotin
    - Streptavidin and alkaline phosphatase
    - Fluorescent labels

INHERITED DISEASES

Diseases With Mendelian Inheritance

- Inheritance pedigree that follows a dominant and recessive pattern
  - Punnett square (Figure 9-5)
    - Recurrence risk
  - Genes carrying the mutation are on autosomes (chromosomes 1-22)
  - Typically equal frequency for being affected
  - Heterozygous: One normal gene (wild-type) and one abnormal gene (mutation)
  - Homozygous: Inherited two genes with the same mutation

Autosomal Recessive Diseases
Cystic Fibrosis
- Gene on chromosome 7
  - Codes for the cystic fibrosis (CF) transmembrane conductance regulator protein (CFTR)
  - Over 1300 mutations have been identified
  - Most common mutation is delta-F508, which is a three–base pair deletion
  - Phenotypic expression will vary based on mutation
  - Sweat chloride test performed as part of diagnosis

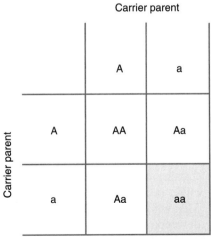

Carrier parent

Carrier parent

	A	a
A	AA	Aa
a	Aa	aa

FIGURE 9-5 Punnett square illustrating the mating of two heterozygous carriers of an autosomal recessive gene. The genotype of the affected offspring is shaded. *(From Jorde B, Carey J, Bamshad M: Medical genetics, ed 4, Philadelphia, 2009, Mosby.)*

- Mutations detected by many platforms, including
  - PCR-RFLP
  - Single-strand confirmation polymorphism (SSCP)
  - Invader (cleavage-based assay)
  - Microarray

Hereditary Hemochromatosis
- Excess iron absorption
- Treatment is via therapeutic phlebotomy
- Several common base substitutions in *HFE* gene have been found
  - G to A at amino acid 282 (C282Y)
  - C to G in exon 63 (H63D)
  - A to T in codon 65 (S65C)
- Individuals with mutations may be asymptomatic because of incomplete penetrance

Autosomal Dominant Diseases
- Presence of one mutated gene is enough to cause disease

Factor V Leiden
- Hereditary hypercoagulability
- Factor V gene is on chromosome 1 (1q23)
  - Leiden mutation is 1691 A→G (R506Q)
- Oral contraceptives increase risk for thrombosis
- Mutations detected by many platforms, including
  - Invader
  - PCR followed by electrophoresis
  - Real-time PCR using melting curve analysis

Huntington's Disease
- Late-onset neurodegenerative disorder
- Gene for Huntington's disease is *huntingtin* and is on chromosome 4
- Trinucleotide repeat
  - Expansion of CAG
  - Normal repeat range from 10 to 27 copies
  - Repeats of 28 to 35 "mutable"
  - Repeats of 36 to 39 reduced penetrance
  - Repeats of 40 or greater are associated with disease
- Anticipation: Higher number of repeats in offspring with earlier onset
- Ethical issues surround testing for Huntington disease
- PCR with fluorescent primers to determine the exact repeat number

X-Linked Diseases
- X-linked recessive females are carriers and usually not affected
- Males will receive the mutated gene only from their mother and will be affected
  - Hemizygous
- Many cases are due to new mutations

Hemophilia A
- Deficiency of coagulation factor VIII (FVIII)
- X-linked recessive
  - Mostly male cases, but female cases have been reported

- Female cases related to skewed X-inactivation of mutated *FVIII* gene
  - Female cases could be due to two mutated *FVIII* genes
- PCR assay for detection of inversion mutation
- Sequence the *FVIII* gene for mutation if inversion assay is negative

Duchenne's Muscular Dystrophy

- X-linked recessive
  - Mostly male cases, but female cases have been reported
- Largest gene in the human genome with a length of 2.2 megabases
  - Dystrophin is the protein product
- Most common neuromuscular disorder
  - Progressive myopathic weakness
  - Elevated serum creatine kinase
  - Diagnosis can be made through immunohistochemical studies
- Multiplex PCR for prenatal testing

Fragile X Syndrome

- X-linked dominant disorder with reduced penetrance
  - Penetrance increases in subsequent generations
- Common inherited form of learning disability
- Name derived from cytogenetic abnormality of a breakpoint or fragile spot within the telomere of a metaphase X chromosome
- Trinucleotide repeat expansion of CGG
  - *FMR-1* gene
  - Normal range alleles contain 5 to 45 repeats
  - Premutation 55 to 200 repeats
  - Mutation with more than 200 repeats
- Southern blotting for genotype analysis
- PCR with capillary electrophoresis for repeat number

Diseases With Non-Mendelian Inheritance

Mitochondrial DNA Diseases

- Mitochondria generate energy by producing ATP through oxidative phosphorylation
- Mitochondria contain their own circular DNA molecule, mtDNA
  - 16,569 base pairs containing 37 genes
  - Heteroplasmy: Normal and mutated mtDNA copies can coexist in a cell
  - Two types of mtDNA mutations
    - Those that affect mitochondria protein synthesis
      - tRNA genes
      - rRNA genes
    - Mutations with the protein coding changes
  - Acquired mtDNA deletions are part of the aging process
- Sequencing of mtDNA is ideal
- PCR and Southern blotting

Imprinting

- Histone or DNA modification
  - Results in transcriptional silencing

- Deletion of allele during egg and sperm production (gametogenesis)
- Different phenotypic presentation depending on maternal or paternal deletion inheritance
  - Imprinting on chromosome, 15 del(q11q13)
    - Prader-Willi syndrome: Paternal inheritance
      - Learning disability
      - Short stature
      - Behavioral issues
    - Angelman's syndrome: Maternal inheritance
      - Learning disability
      - Attacks of laughter
      - Absences of speech
    - Loss of gene expression caused by several mechanisms
- Mutations detected by many platforms, including
  - Cytogenetic detection
    - Karyotyping: For chromosome rearrangement
    - Fluorescence in situ hybridization (FISH): For deletion detection
  - Methylation-specific PCR (mPCR)
  - PCR for STRs for uniparental disomy
  - Sequencing

Complex Diseases

- Mulitfactoral inheritance patterns
  - One or more genes with one or more environmental factors
  - Difficult-to-study combined effects of environmental and genetic factors
    - Twin studies are often used
      - Greater concordance of disease among monozygotic twins who share all genes than dizygotic twins who share half their genes
      - Less than 100% concordance in monozygotic twins indicates environmental contributors

Inherited Breast Cancer

- Familial breast cancer accounts for only 5% to 10% of all breast carcinomas
- Mutations in two major breast cancer genes predispose individuals to breast and ovarian cancer
  - *BRCA1* gene also associated with increased risk for prostate and colon cancer
  - *BRCA2* gene also associated with increased risk for pancreatic cancer
    - Mutations in *BRCA1* and *BRCA2* are inherited in an autosomal dominant manner
      - Inheriting gene does not mean that an individual will develop cancer
      - Cannot tell what type of cancer might develop
      - Cannot tell at what age onset of cancer might occur
      - Men who carry the genes have greater risk for developing cancer
    - *BRCA1* and *BRCA2* are tumor-suppressor genes
- DNA sequencing for mutations on *BRCA1* and *BRCA2*
- Genetic counseling for individuals before testing

Reporting of Test Results

- Result should be written so easily understood and interpreted in an accurate manner
- Along with typical information found on a laboratory report (name, birth date, laboratory name), a DNA test for an inherited disease should include
  - Clinical history and reason for referral
  - Explanation of the methodology used
  - Description of patient's results
  - Diagnostic accuracy
  - Clinical significance of results
  - Statement from or meeting with genetic counselors
    - Implications of results
    - Potential risk for disease for family members
  - Statement regarding whether the test is approved by the U.S. Food and Drug Administration

IDENTITY ASSESSMENT

Forensic DNA Typing

- Genetic variation useful in identity testing
  - Genetic locus variations in a population are called alleles
  - A locus is polymorphic if the least common allele is present in greater than 1% of the population
  - Typically introns (noncoding regions) are used for identity testing
    - VNTR or minisatellite
    - STR or microsatellite
  - Ideal for identity testing because
    - Thousands are scattered throughout the genome
    - Automated fluorescence analysis
    - A specific allele can be identified against a known ladder of alleles
    - STRs are typically transmitted in mendelian fashion
    - The greater the number of alleles present in a locus, the more informative the identification of a specific allelic combination will be
    - Extensive information is available about allele frequency in many populations

Forensic Applications

- Exclusion results are often found during DNA identity testing
- One or more alleles different from known sample needed for exclusion
  - Suspect did not commit the crime
  - Alleged man did not father the child
- Likelihood of inclusion of tested individuals
  - Discriminatory power: Ability to distinguish an individual from the rest of a population
    - Based on allelic frequency over several loci
  - ABO system has a poorer discriminatory factor than DNA identity testing using RFLP or STRs

- Amelogenin gene: Codes for tooth enamel and is used to identify the presence of X chromosomes or an X and a Y chromosome
- The Y chromosome has polymorphic loci that are used forensically to differentiate the male fraction (sperm) from the female fraction (epithelial cells) from rape kit evidence
- Y-chromosome DNA can be used for ancestry studies
  - Fathers and sons will have the same Y chromosome STRs
- mtDNA can be used forensically
  - When nuclear DNA is not available
  - When nuclear DNA is highly degraded
  - When only distant relatives are available for reference sample
- SNP: Locus for which a single base pair varies in a population
  - Microarray
  - Large number must be obtained for significant discriminatory value

Statistical Interpretation

- Loci used in DNA typing exhibit Hardy-Weinberg equilibrium
  - $p^2 + 2pq + q^2 = 1.0$
  - In a population containing the genotypes *AA*, *Aa*, and *aa*
    - p is the frequency of A
    - q is the frequency of a
    - frequency of *AA* is p^2
    - frequency of *Aa* is 2pq

Combined DNA Index System

- DNA evidence from crime scene is added to Combined DNA Index System (CODIS) database
  - Convicted offender database
  - Missing person database
  - 13 core STR loci
    - A "hit" is a match between offender and DNA left at crime scene
    - Ethical issues surround how these databases can be searched

Human Leukocyte Antigen Typing

- Genetic features of human leukocyte antigen (HLA) typing genes
  - Alleles determine the tissue compatibility of transplanted grafts from another donor (allograft)
  - HLA genes code for highly polymorphic surface molecules which serve as strong alloantigens
  - HLA genes are located in the major histocompatibility complex (MHC)
    - Chromosome 6

- o HLA class I
  - ▪ A, B, and C
- o HLA class II
  - ▪ DR, DQ, and DP
- o HLA genes are codominantly expressed
  - ▪ Variability exists among both racial and ethnic groups
- Applications of HLA typing
  - Transplantation
    - o Matching donor and recipient HLA alleles improve long-term organ graft survival
    - o Hematopoietic cell transplantation (HCT) also has the risk for developing acute or chronic graft-versus-host disease (GVHD)
  - DNA-based HLA allele identification
    - o DNA sequencing
    - o Allele-specific PCR
    - o Nomenclature for HLA alleles is frequently updated because of new discoveries
- Hematopoietic cell engraftment (HCT) analysis
  - May display chimerism, which is a mosaicism consisting of the coexistence of cells derived from the recipient and the donor
  - Methods for performing engraftment analysis
    - o Obtain sample from recipient before transplant for native genotype
    - o Posttransplantation STR loci are informative (nonidentical genotype) and a calculation is performed from this data

MOLECULAR METHODS IN INFECTIOUS DISEASES

Indications for Molecular Testing

- Molecular methods are faster than microbial culture methods or are slow growing
- Can detect pathogens that might not culture by traditional methods
- Provides genetic information that can be used for antimicrobial drugs
- Used to monitor therapy or provide prognosis
- Trace outbreak of infection
- Provides greater sensitivity and specificity
- Capable of high throughput

Molecular Bacteriology

- Bacterial genomes
  - Less complex than human genomes
  - Usually circular DNA
  - Approximately 4.5 million base pairs
  - Plasmids: Additional genetic material carried by bacteria
    - o dsDNA and circular
    - o Codes for antibiotic resistance and pathogenicity
    - o Used for identification purposes

Specific Pathogens

- *Chlamydia trachomatis* and *Neisseria gonorrhoeae*
  - Usually run together on multiplex assays
  - Many platforms for detection, including
    - o Hybrid Capture
    - o PCR
    - o Strand displacement amplification (SDA)
    - o Transcription-mediated amplification (TMA)
- Group B streptococcal disease
  - Important in perinatal testing to decrease infection of neonate
  - Real-time PCR
- *Mycobacterium tuberculosis*
  - Standard growth methods take 6 to 8 weeks
  - Molecular testing is rapid and allows for prompt treatment
    - o TMA of ribosomal RNA
    - o PCR for 16S ribosomal RNA gene
  - Detection of antimicrobial resistance is possible
  - Drawback to nucleic acid detection of *M. tuberculosis* nonviable organisms
    - o Should not test individuals who have received antituberculosis medication for infection
- Methicillin-resistant *Staphylococcus aureus* (MRSA)
  - *mecA* gene is responsible for resistance
    - o Gene allows for drug resistance
  - Tests using PCR and real-time PCR
- Vancomycin-resistant enterococcus (VRE)
  - *vanA*, *vanB*, and *vanC* genes are responsible for resistance
  - Tests using PCR and real-time PCR

Molecular Virology

- Viral genomes
  - Less complex then bacterial and human
  - Range from 5000 to 250,000 base pairs
  - Variable in structure
    - o DNA or RNA
    - o ssDNA or dsDNA
    - o Linear or circular
  - Sequence variations are common
    - o Single base changes
    - o Insertions
    - o Deletions
- Viral-load testing
  - Test to quantify amount of viral nucleic acid in host
    - o Used to predict time and course of disease
    - o When to initiate antiviral therapy
    - o Monitor response to therapy
  - Test platforms include
    - o RT-PCR
    - o Branch DNA testing
    - o Nucleic acid sequence–based amplification (NASBA)

- Human immune deficiency virus (HIV) type 1
  - RNA retrovirus
    - Uses reverse transcriptase to enter into host DNA
    - *gag* and *pol* genes are targets for identification
  - CD4 count and viral load are factors in therapy and progression to acquired immunodeficiency syndrome
    - Goal of therapy is to obtain viral loads below 50 copies/mL
  - Enzyme-linked immunosorbent assay for screening test followed by Western blot for confirmation
  - Resistance testing
    - Sequencing for nucleotide changes, which might decrease effectiveness of antiviral therapy
    - Reverse transcriptase has no proofreading capabilities, so errors are common
    - Phenotypic resistance measures viral replication when combined with an antiviral drug
- Hepatitis C virus
  - RNA virus
  - Test platforms include
    - RT-PCR
    - TMA
    - bDNA
    - Real-time PCR
- Cytomegalovirus (CMV)
  - dsDNA virus in the herpesvirus family
  - Test platforms include
    - Hybrid Capture
    - NASBA
- Human papillomavirus (HPV)
  - dsDNA
  - Test platforms include
    - Hybrid Capture
    - Real-time PCR
- Herpes simplex virus
  - dsDNA virus in the herpesvirus family
  - Test platforms include
    - PCR
    - Real-time PCR
- Enteroviruses
  - Group of RNA viruses
  - Test platforms include
    - RT-PCR
    - NASBA

Bioterrorism Agents

- The key elements of a biologic weapon are difficulty of detection, ease of dissemination, and ability to cause severe illness or death
- Molecular testing is well suited for the rapid detection of bioterrorism organisms
  - *Bacillus anthracis*
  - *Yersinia pestis*
  - *Francisella tularensis*
  - *Brucella abortus*
  - Variola virus (smallpox)

MOLECULAR GENETICS IN HUMAN CANCERS

Oncogenes and Tumor Suppressor Genes

- Oncogenes
  - Proto-oncogene is a normal gene that codes for proteins that regulate cell growth and differentiation
  - When the proto-oncogene has been altered by mutations that affect gene function it becomes an oncogene
  - Oncogene proteins also function on the stages of cell division
    - Growth factor signaling pathways
    - Promote the transformation of cells into cancer cells
- Tumor suppressor genes
  - Genes that suppress oncogenesis by suppressing malignant phenotypes
  - Cancers can develop when there is loss of function of the gene
  - Involved in the regulation of progression through the cell cycle or the regulation of DNA repair

Molecular Diagnosis of Hematopoietic Neoplasms

Leukemias Versus Lymphomas

- Lineage and stage of differentiation
- Acute and chronic forms

Clonality of Lymphomas

- Important step in detecting malignant from benign proliferation of lymphocytes
  - B lymphocytes: Are able to rearrange segments of the DNA that code for immunoglobulins
  - T lymphocytes: Are able to rearrange segments of the gene that codes for T-cell receptors (TCRs)
  - Some malignant lymphomas and leukemias demonstrate both immunoglobulin and TCR rearrangements
- Assays to determine clonality
  - Southern blotting of antigen-receptor gene rearrangements
    - Positive for clonality when one or two distinct non-germline bands appear
    - SNPs could lead to false identification of monoclonality
  - PCR analysis of antigen-receptor gene rearrangements
    - Amplification of DNA across the V(D)J junctions
    - Evaluation of products by electrophoresis
    - Monoclonal populations yield one or two bands or peaks
    - For polyclonal mixture each cell carries a unique gene rearrangement and would appear as a smear on a gel

Hematopoietic Malignancies
Follicular Lymphoma
- t(14:18) translocation brings the gene for *BCL-2* from chromosome 18 and the gene for the immunoglobulin heavy chain (IgH) from chromosome 14
- FISH analysis can detect via DNA probes
  - Fluorescent red dye probes for the IgH locus
  - Fluorescent green probes for the *BCL-2* gene
  - When the translocation is present, the signal appears as yellow fluorescence

Chronic Myeloid Leukemia
- Translocation of chromosomes 9 and 22
  - Philadelphia chromosome
  - Diagnostic hallmark for chronic myeloid leukemia (CML)
  - *BCR-ABL* gene fusion encodes for a chimeric protein with constitutively activated tyrosine kinase activity
  - 210-kDa protein (p210$^{BCR/ABL}$)
  - t(9:22) may be seen in acute lymphocytic leukemia (ALL) with poor prognosis
- Detection can be done using
  - Conventional cytogenetics
    - Minimal residual disease detection
  - FISH
  - RT-PCR
  - Real-time PCR to quantify *BCR-ABL* transcripts
    - Tyrosine kinase inhibitor imatinib mesylate (Gleevec) is used very successfully for treatment of CML

Myeloproliferative Disorders (non–BCR-ABL)
- *Jak2* mutation: Janus kinase 2, a protein tyrosine kinase
  - Polycythemia vera
  - Essential thrombocythemia
  - Idiopathic myelofibrosis
- Specific change is *V617F* can be detected by:
  - Real-time PCR with melting curve analysis
  - PCR
  - DNA sequencing

Molecular Genetics of Solid Tumors
- *HER2/neu* (human epidermal growth factor 2)
  - Transmembrane protein with tyrosine kinase activity
  - *HER2/neu* is overexpressed in some forms of breast cancer
    - Its presence is an indication for the use of trastuzumab (Herceptin), an anti-*HER2/neu* antibody drug
    - Overexpressed products resulting from the *HER2/neu* gene can be detected by immunohistochemistry
    - FISH can detect increase in DNA copy number
- Epidermal growth factor receptor (*EGFR*)
  - Receptor on cell membrane that when activated initiates proliferation
  - Drugs designed to inhibit binding to the *EGFR* when overexpressed
    - Some mutations to *EGFR* respond to drugs better
    - Sequencing the EGFR gene for these mutations can support optimal treatment
- *K-ras* (Kirsten rat sarcoma viral oncogene)
  - This protooncogene family is the most commonly found mutation in human cancers
  - In G-protein family
    - Act as components for energy production
    - Part of pathway to communicate growth signals from cell membrane to nucleus
    - When mutation is present, remains in an active state
  - Detection can be through DNA sequencing, pyrosequencing, or PCR

MUTATIONS AND CYTOGENETIC ANALYSIS
- Cytogenetics analysis
  - Karyotyping
    - Metaphase chromosomes
    - Arrest mitosis at metaphase with colcemid
  - FISH
  - Microarray
    - Comparative genome hybridization (CGH)
- Mutation classifications
  - A polymorphism is a genotypic change found in more than 1% of the population
  - A mutation or variant is a genotypic change found in less than 1% of the population
    - Types of point mutations
      - Silent
      - Conservative
      - Missense
      - Nonsense
      - Frameshift
    - Several platforms can be used to identify point mutations
      - SSCP
      - Allele-specific oligomer hybridization
      - Real-time PCR with melting curves
      - Sequence-specific primer–PCR
      - MALDI-TOF
- Aneuploidy: Loss or gain of a chromosome
- Chromosome abnormalities
  - Translocation
  - Deletion
  - Inversion
  - Insertion

PHARMACOGENETICS
- Study of genetic variations in drug response using data from many assayed across a genome

- Approach to personalized medicine
- Clinical application of pharmacogenetic testing
  o Polymorphism that can inhibit or induce drug metabolism
  o Cytochrome P450 polymorphisms
  o Drug metabolism enzymes
  o Test can predict response or effectiveness of certain drugs
  o Test platforms
    - PCR
    - Microarray
    - Mass spectrometry

CERTIFICATION PREPARATION QUESTIONS

For answers and rationales, please see Appendix A.

1. During replication the "parent" strand of DNA serves which purpose?
   a. It is completely excised by exonuclease enzymes when replication of the strand is complete
   b. It has a sequence that is complementary to the daughter strand that is being replicated
   c. It is also referred to as the lagging strand
   d. It will be copied by a DNA polymerase to form two new daughter DNA strands

2. Which of the following are forms of nucleic acids?
   a. Nucleosides
   b. DNA or RNA
   c. Base pairs
   d. Trinucleotide sequences

3. The central dogma speaks to the function of the molecular components of DNA and states that:
   a. The main function of genes is to store and transmit genetic information
   b. There are specific nucleotide triplets that code for specific amino acids
   c. Genes are perpetuated as sequences of nucleic acid, but function by being expressed in the form of protein
   d. All sequences of DNA in the human genome will result in the production of RNAs

4. An exon is defined as:
   a. A region of DNA present in a mature strand of mRNA and can be translated into protein
   b. A region of DNA that is recognized by RNA polymerase to start transcription
   c. A region of DNA that is transcribed then removed from mRNA by excision and is not translated into protein
   d. A region of DNA comprising three base pairs that signal for termination of replication

5. During the replication process the addition of bases occurs:
   a. At the telomeric end of a DNA strand
   b. In the 3' to 5' direction
   c. In the 5' to 3' direction
   d. In both the 5' to 3' and 3' to 5' directions

6. Transfer RNA (tRNA):
   a. Is a gene silencing RNA used in cancer research
   b. Is a macromolecular complex delivered from the nucleus by ribosomal RNA
   c. Contains the codon sequence that synthesizes an amino acid
   d. Contains the anticodon region that binds to mRNA codon in the ribosome

7. Which one of the following statements concerning mitochondrial DNA (mtDNA) is incorrect?
   a. Pseudogenes are small pieces of nuclear DNA that share significant homology with mtDNA
   b. mtDNA is circular and contains approximately 16,500 base pairs
   c. mtDNA is inherited from the mother because only ova contain mitochondria
   d. Follows mendelian inheritance patterns

8. The enzyme ligase joins the Okazaki fragments of the
   _____.
   a. Template strand
   b. Lagging strand
   c. Leading strand
   d. Primer fragments

9. How does ribonucleic acid (RNA) differ from deoxyribonucleic acid (DNA)?
   a. RNA has a uracil and DNA has a thymine
   b. RNA does not contain nucleotides and DNA does
   c. DNA resides in the cytoplasm of the cell and RNA is in the nucleus
   d. DNA has a messenger form and RNA does not

10. The chromosomes in a eukaryotic cell:
    a. Are in their most compact state and appear as chromatin arms joined at the center during the cell division stage called metaphase
    b. Contain genomic regions that are rich in genes, less compactly organized, and termed heterochromatin
    c. Contain two specialized regions of euchromatin, telomeres, and centromeres
    d. Are highly ordered structures of a single RNA molecule, compacted many times with the aid of structural RNA-binding proteins

11. Which of the following is a description of restriction endonucleases?
    a. A family of bacteria from which endonuclease that cuts DNA into fragments is produced
    b. Only able to digest specific genes on specific chromosomes with their endonuclease action
    c. Enzymes that specifically degrade DNA in nucleic acid mixtures when plasmids are present
    d. Enzymes produced by bacteria to prevent invasion and replication of foreign DNA in their bacterial genome

12. Which enzyme catalyzes DNA replication?
    a. Endonuclease
    b. Ligase

    c. Polymerase

    d. Reverse transcriptase

13. Which of the following is a block of specific sequence variants that are inherited together?
    a. Allele
    b. Haplotype
    c. Locus
    d. Polymorphism

14. Messenger RNA (mRNA) is produced in the _____.
    a. Golgi
    b. Mitochondria
    c. Nucleus
    d. Ribosomes

15. In the organic liquid phase (phenol-chloroform) DNA extraction procedure, proteins are precipitated out of solution:
    a. In the aqueous phase
    b. As a pellet on the filter
    c. In the organic phase
    d. On the silica-based gel

16. The purity of an extract of nucleic acid can be determined by which of the following?
    a. Measuring absorbances at 260 nm and 280 nm and dividing A260 by A280
    b. Measuring the bands on an agarose gel
    c. Measuring absorbances at 260 nm and 280 nm and subtracting A280 from A260 and then multiplying the result by a dilution factor
    d. Multiplying the concentration of the nucleic acid by the dilution factor

17. Solid-phase DNA extraction procedures are more commonly used in a clinical laboratory because:
    a. They can be coupled with a gas chromatograph linked to a mass spectrometer
    b. They perform best when a large volume of sample is submitted for DNA extraction
    c. They are adaptable to automation
    d. They involve organic solvents that are easily found in a laboratory

18. The rate of DNA migration in a gel electrophoresis depends primarily on the _____.
    a. Buffer temperature
    b. Pore size of the gel
    c. Shape of the DNA molecule
    d. Size of the genomic DNA

19. Signal amplification differs from target amplification when designing protocols for identification of nucleic acids. Which of the following is an example of a signal amplification technique?
    a. Branched-chain DNA detection
    b. Ligase chain reaction
    c. Polymerase chain reaction
    d. Reverse-transcriptase PCR

20. Identify the correct sequence of events for a polymerase chain reaction (PCR) cycle.
    a. Anneal, extend, and denature
    b. Denature, anneal, and extend
    c. Extend, anneal, and denature
    d. Extend, denature, and anneal

21. When RNA is to be used in a PCR amplification procedure, what is the first step that must be performed?
    a. RNA cannot be used in a PCR reaction because it will disintegrate during the denaturation step
    b. RNA must be denatured to form single strands to allow for the annealing of primers
    c. A reverse-transcription procedure must be performed to form cDNA
    d. RNA must first be treated with RNases to remove interfering substances from the target

22. In the PCR, a _____ initiates extension of the sequence of interest by allowing *Taq* polymerase to begin adding nucleotides to single-stranded DNA.
    a. Probe
    b. Ligase
    c. Promoter
    d. Primer

23. When performing a PCR procedure, which is the most important control to run to check for the presence of amplicons?
    a. Blank control
    b. dTTP control
    c. Control
    d. Oligo dT control

24. The process of transferring the digested DNA out of a gel after electrophoresis and onto a nylon membrane is referred to as:
    a. Hybridization blotting
    b. Northern blotting
    c. Southern blotting
    d. Western blotting

25. In a real-time PCR assay, which probe type is used in conjunction with fluorescence resonance energy transfer (FRET) on the formation of a duplex?
    a. Hybridization
    b. Hydrolysis
    c. Hexamere
    d. Primer

26. The increase in quantifiable signal observed early in a real-time PCR run depends on which of the following?
    a. The wavelength of the fluorescent dye in the reaction
    b. The number of cycles in the run
    c. The amount of fluorescent quencher
    d. The initial amount of target DNA

27. Which of the following practices should be employed to prevent contamination of patient samples and reagents with amplicons?
    a. Use bleach solution for cleaning work area
    b. Use UV lights in hooded work area
    c. Maintain closed analytical systems
    d. All of the above

28. Which of the following statements is true regarding agarose gel electrophoresis?
    a. Nucleic acids are separated in an electrical field because of their net positive charge
    b. Larger nucleic acid molecules are able to migrate through the agarose gel faster than smaller molecules
    c. Nucleic acids are separated in agarose by shape, charge, and size
    d. Agarose is a dye that binds in double-stranded DNA

29. PCR requires all of the following components except:
    a. Deoxynucleotide triphosphates
    b. DNA endonuclease
    c. DNA polymerase
    d. Oligonucleotides (primers)

30. What is the purpose of the primer extension?
    a. To cut the native DNA into small pieces with a restriction enzyme
    b. To hybridize the oligonucleotide primers to the single-stranded DNA pieces
    c. To produce PCR amplicons
    d. To activate the DNA polymerase to form hybrids with the oligonucleotide primers

31. The most common nucleic acid stain used after separation by agarose gel electrophoresis is:
    a. Bromothymol blue
    b. Bromocresol green
    c. Ethidium bromide
    d. Phenolphthalein

32. This method is based on the microscopic grouping of probe DNA molecules attached to a solid support mechanism such as glass, silicon, or plastic chips.
    a. DNA microarray
    b. Multilocus enzymes electrophoresis
    c. Restriction fragment length polymorphism (RFLP)
    d. Polymerase chain reaction (PCR)

33. The field of proteomics studies which of the following?
    a. Proteins on a cellular level
    b. Serum proteins
    c. Proteins in genes
    d. The human genome

34. Which of the following is *not* a factor that influences hybridization reactions?
    a. Degree of complementarity between the probe and target nucleic acid
    b. pH
    c. Size of the target's genome
    d. Temperature

35. Which of the following is false about primers?
    a. Primers should be at least 100 nucleotides long
    b. Primers are typically 15 to 30 nucleotides long
    c. Primers should have a GC percentage of 40% to 60%
    d. Primers should anneal to a specific target

36. In a chain-termination DNA sequencing reaction, which one of the following components are tagged with a fluorescent dye?
    a. Dideoxynuclotide triphosphates (ddNTP)
    b. Deoxynucleotide triphosphates (dNTP)
    c. Pyrophosphates (PPi)
    d. Capillary probe (CaP)

37. Pyrosequencing sequence analysis and quantification depends on the release of _____ in a quantity equal to that of an incorporated dNTP.
    a. Apyrase
    b. Luciferase
    c. Nucleotides
    d. Pyrophosphate

38. In which of the following inheritance patterns are homozygous alleles necessary to express the disease phenotype?
    a. Autosomal dominant
    b. X-linked dominant
    c. Autosomal recessive
    d. Trinucleotide repeats

39. The differential activation of genes depending on the parent from which they are inherited is referred to as:
    a. Allelic heterogeneity
    b. Imprinting
    c. Mosaicism
    d. Pleiotropy

40. What is the preferred specimen type for molecular studies for the diagnosis of inherited mutations?
    a. RNA extracted from peripheral mature red cells
    b. RNA extracted from fresh serum
    c. DNA extracted from peripheral blood white cells
    d. DNA extracted from peripheral blood mature red cells

41. A type of polymorphism that consists of a series of trinucleotide repeats that can be two to seven base pairs in length and is known as a microsatellite sequence is also referred to as a:
    a. Restriction fragment length polymorphism (RFLP)
    b. Variable number tandem repeat (VNTR)
    c. Restriction endonuclease
    d. Short tandem repeat (STR)

42. The site of a particular nucleotide sequence on a chromosome is referred to as a(n):
    a. Allele
    b. Locus
    c. Polymorphism
    d. Genotype

43. The HLA A, B, and C molecules are encoded for by which class gene(s)s within the major histocompatibility complex (MHC)?
    a. Class I
    b. Class II
    c. Class III
    d. All groups in MHC class

44. The detection of the DNA from cytomegalovirus (CMV) and human papillomavirus (HPV) is typically performed using the Hybrid Capture assay. What type of assay is Hybrid Capture?
a. Target amplification assay
b. Signal amplification assay
c. Reverse transcriptase assay
d. Viral load assay

45. The major advantage for using nucleic acid techniques for the identification of infectious disease is:
a. The lower cost involved with molecular analysis
b. The high specificity for identification of an organism
c. The lack of false negatives
d. The ability to distinguish normal flora from disease-causing organisms

46. Which of the following genes is not found in retroviruses?
a. *Gag*
b. *Pol*
c. *Env*
d. *Onc*

47. In chronic myeloid leukemia (CML) the fusion of chromosomes 9 and 22 produces a hybrid gene, *BCR-ABL*. This chromosome is referred to as the:
a. Cincinnati chromosome
b. Legionnaires chromosome
c. Myeloprolifererative chromosome
d. Philadelphia chromosome

48. The technique that uses fluorescent DNA probes to detect chromosomal abnormalities within cells in cytogenetic studies is referred to as:
a. Fluorescence in situ hybridization (FISH)
b. Karyotype in situ hybridization (KISH)
c. Fluorescence in situ PCR
d. Microarray

49. A tumor-suppressor gene performs which of the following task(s)?
a. Codes for normal growth-promoting proteins
b. Codes for proteins that control cell division
c. Repairs nucleotide mismatches in the DNA strand
d. All of the above

50. Which term describes a normally occurring gene that when altered is often associated with cancers?
a. Oncogene
b. Proto-oncogene
c. Meta-oncogene
d. Post-oncogene

BIBLIOGRAPHY

Bruns D, Ashwood E, Burtis C: Fundamentals of molecular diagnostics, St. Louis, 2007, Saunders.

Buckingham L: Molecular diagnostics: fundamentals, methods, and clinical applications, ed 2, Philadelphia, 2011, F. A. Davis.

Mahon C, Lehman D, Manuselis G: Textbook of diagnostic microbiology, ed 4, St. Louis, 2011, Saunders.

Rodak B, Fritsma G, Keohane E: Hematology: clinical principles and applications, ed 4, St. Louis, 2012, Elsevier.

Turnpenny PE, Ellard S: Emery's elements of medical genetics, ed 14, Philadelphia, 2012, Churchill Livingston.

SELF-ASSESSMENT

Content Area: _____

Score on Practice Questions: _____

List the specific topics covered in the missed questions:

List the specific topics covered in the correct questions:

NOTES

Laboratory Operations

Paul R. Labbe and Linda J. Graeter

ORGANIZATIONAL MANAGEMENT STRUCTURE FOR THE CLINICAL LABORATORY

- Many types of management organizational charts, depending on whether it is in an academic medical center, a large hospital network system, an independent laboratory, research laboratory, or a physician office laboratory organization. General laboratory management structures include
  - Laboratory director: Strategic oversight of laboratory services
  - Laboratory manager: Daily workflow of the laboratory team
  - Technical managers: Specialists in ensuring total service quality and accurate testing
  - Logistical supervisors: Specialists in preanalytical and postanalytical collection to reporting and billing of laboratory testing
  - Medical laboratory scientists and technicians: Daily testing production and evaluation of results
  - Laboratory assistants: Support services to the laboratory workflow (pretesting, testing, and posttesting)

LEADERSHIP

Management and Motivation

Leadership Styles (Kurt Lewin, 1939)
- Authoritative/autocratic: Leader informs employees what is to be done and how it is to be performed—closed system
- Participative/democratic: Includes one or more employees in the decision-making process, with the leader maintaining the final decision-making authority—open system
- Delegative: Leader confers the decision-making ability to the employees, with the leader still responsible for the decisions made by the employees—free reign or laissez faire system
- Combination: All three styles are used, depending on the issues involved—generally an indication of a good leader

Management Styles
- Management by objective (MBO): Targets organizational and employee performance by aligning goals and objectives throughout the organization, including timelines, tracking, and feedback in the process
- Continuous quality improvement (CQI): Analytical decision-making tool that determines when a process is working predictably and when it is not, and identifying the variation to lessen or eliminate it, using process control charts (Figure 10-1)
- Total quality management (TQM): Management approach to long-term success through customer satisfaction, incorporating all members of an organization participating in improving process, products, services, and the culture in which they work

Motivational Theories and Styles
- Maslow's Hierarchy of Needs: Psychology theory proposed by Abraham Maslow in 1943 in which all individuals focus on the fundamental needs and once those are fulfilled will progress to higher needs (Figure 10-2)
- Frederick Herzberg's Motivator-Hygiene Theory: Theory of motivation in which employees base their satisfaction or dissatisfaction with work on hygiene factors (company policies, wages, job security) and motivator factors (status, advancement opportunity, recognition, personal achievement)
- McGregor's Theory X and Y: Theoretical assumptions proposed by Douglas McGregor in 1960 based on behavior of individuals at work
  - Theory X is that humans have an inherent dislike of work and will avoid it if they can—therefore they need to be "controlled" (boss-centered leadership)
  - Theory Y is that the expenditure of physical and mental effort in work is as natural as in play or rest—therefore, if the job is satisfying, the employee will be self-motivated (employee-centered leadership)
- Tannenbaum Schmidt Theory: Continuum of leadership proposed in 1958 by Robert Tannenbaum and Warren Schmidt and later updated in 1973 suggests a manager uses a broad range of leadership styles based on the prevailing circumstances in the current environment

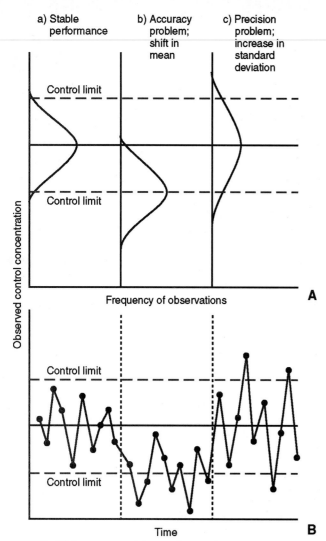

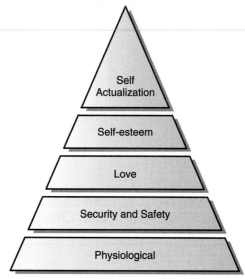

FIGURE 10-2 Maslow's hierarchy of human needs. *(From Fuller J: Surgical technology: principles and practice, ed 6, St. Louis, 2012, Saunders.)*

FIGURE 10-1 Conceptual basis of control charts. **A,** Frequency distributions of control observations for different error conditions. **B,** Display of control values representing those distributions when concentration is plotted versus time on a control chart. *(From Burtis C, Ashwood E, Bruns D: Tietz fundamentals of clinical chemistry, ed 6, St. Louis, 2008, Saunders.)*

- Blake Mouton: Robert Blake and Jane Mouton in 1964 plotted leadership behavior on a grid based on concern for people versus concern for production, with a scale of 1 to 9 based on the level of concern. Snapshots of five styles of leadership include impoverished, country club, politician, authoritarian, and team
- Hershey Blanchard: Ken Blanchard and Paul Hershey conceived a leadership theory in the mid-1970s based on situational models; there is no single "best" style of leadership, but is more dependent on the task, knowledge, and group dynamics for each situation
- Fiedler Theory: Developed by Fred Fiedler, this leadership theory is based on two factors of situational contingency: leadership style and situation control. An index designated the least-preferred coworker (LPC) scale is a rating used by leaders, with a high score

suggesting a human relations orientation in contrast to a low LPC score indicating a task orientation
- Myers-Briggs Type Indicator (MBTI): Uses a theory of psychological types to make insights of type theory applicable to individuals and groups. A grid displays the 16 personality types based on your indicators: Extraversion(E)/Introversion(I), Sensing (S)/Intuition(N), Thinking(T)/Feeling(F), and Judging(J)/Perceiving(P) and is determined using the MBTI instrument

PROFESSIONALISM

- Profession: Principle, vocation, employment, or calling that requires specialized knowledge and intensive academic preparation
- Professional: Member of a vocation who has obtained a degree in a highly specialized field, commonly engaged in creative and intellectually challenging work
- Professionalism: Practice of an activity using the conduct, aims, and qualities based on a code of ethics for that profession
- Code of ethics: American Society for Clinical Laboratory Science sets forth the principles and standards by which clinical laboratory professionals practice their profession, based on
  - Duty to patient
  - Duty to colleagues and the profession
  - Duty to society

COMMUNICATION

- Effective laboratory operation depends on individual specialists working as an effective team within the health care system of professionals

- Communication is a key to an effective laboratory
  - Verbal communication: Using sounds, words, speech, and language to interact between individuals and to groups
  - Nonverbal communication: Using touch, body language, timeliness, and personal space to convey interaction and listening attentiveness with others
  - Paraverbal communication: Messages transmitted through the tone, pitch, and pacing of the voice
  - Informative communication: Using data, instructions, and knowledge to convey information to others
- Communication styles can be affective (emotional), imaginative (perceived image), persuasive (inducing or commonly accepted), and ritualistic (cultural or routinely established)
- Active listening requires the listener to be attentive to the communicator and is a structured way of responding to others. Suspending one's own frame of reference, using good judgment, and avoiding other activities will focus the listener on evaluation of what the communicator is conveying. Roadblocks to active listening are performing other tasks and multitasking during the communication process

REGULATORY

- U.S. clinical laboratories are governed by the laws and regulatory guidelines of the following federal and state agencies and programs
  - Department of Health and Human Services (DHHS): Oversight federal government agency that regulates clinical laboratories based on the federal laws passed by the U.S. Congress
  - Centers for Medicare & Medicaid Services (CMS): Within the DHHS, regulates all laboratory testing (except research) performed on humans in the United States through the Clinical Laboratory Improvement Amendments (CLIA)
  - CLIA Program: Program administered through the federal and state agencies to ensure high-quality laboratory testing
  - CLIA 88: Law established by the U.S. Congress to create uniform federal standards for regulating clinical laboratories; also extended government oversight to all testing facilities, including physician office laboratories. The government agencies responsible for overseeing the laboratory standards are CMS, Centers for Disease Control and Prevention, and Food and Drug Administration
  - CLIA Certificates: CLIA 88 requires clinical laboratories to obtain one of four certificates to perform laboratory testing: Certificate of Waiver, Certificate of Provider Performed Microscopy, Certificate of Compliance, or Certificate of Accreditation. CMS issues the first three certificates, and the Certificate of Accreditation is obtained through

CLIA-approved accrediting organizations. Currently more than 200,000 laboratories are registered under CLIA, approximately 50% of which are physician office laboratories
- CLIA-approved providers: 2013 current listing of approved accreditation organizations for issuing a CLIA accreditation certificate: American Association of Blood Banks, American Osteopathic Association, American Society for Histocompatibility and Immunogenetics, College of American Pathologists, COLA, Joint Commission http://www.cms.gov/MLNProducts/downloads/CLIABrochure.pdf
- *Family Medical Leave Act* (FMLA): Supplies any employee who has been on the job for over 1 year up to 12 weeks of unpaid, job-protected leave each year
- *Fair Labor Standards Act* (FLSA): In 1938 it set guidelines on pay practices in government, businesses, and health care and defined overtime pay practices. The *Equal Pay Act* of 1963 is a section of the FLSA that affirms equal pay for equal work
- Food and Drug Administration (FDA): Government agency that regulates clinical laboratories through approval of laboratory test kits and medical devices and provides clarification on how workload should be calculated when using current FDA-approved semiautomated gynecologic cytology screening devices
- Centers for Disease Control and Prevention (CDC): Government laboratory working on the Battelle Project to identify best practices in laboratory medicine
- Department of Transportation (DOT): Provides the regulations for shipment of biological and hazardous materials, including clinical laboratory specimens
- Environmental Protection Agency (EPA): Regulates and oversees the disposal of contaminated wastes from the clinical laboratory
- *Health Insurance Portability and Accountability Act* (HIPAA): In 1996 identified rules to protect individuals' identifiable health information, the rights granted to that individual, enforcement activities, and methods to monitor and file a complaint
- *Health Information Technology for Economic and Clinical Health Act* (HITECH): In 2009 defined regulations requiring all health providers to notify individuals when their health information has been breached; is monitored by the Office for Civil Rights
- National Labor Relations Board (NLRB): Federal agency to safeguard employee rights and determine whether they have the right to form a union; the laboratory is recognized as a bargaining unit by the NLRB
- National Institute for Occupational Safety and Health (NIOSH): Division of the CDC responsible

for conducting research and making recommendations for the prevention of work-related illnesses and injuries

- Occupational Safety and Health Administration (OSHA): Main federal agency charged with enforcement of safety and health legislation
- Office of Inspector General (OIG): Monitors the business aspects of the clinical laboratory and establishes guidelines to prevent fraud and abuse from unethical and improper reimbursement for laboratory services under government programs such as Medicare and Medicaid

ACCREDITATION

- All U.S. clinical laboratories that apply for a Certificate of Accreditation must be certified by one of the seven deemed status accreditation organizations designated on the CMS website
  - American Association of Blood Banks (AABB): Accreditation is granted for collection, processing, testing, distribution, and administration of blood and blood components; hematopoietic progenitor cell activities; cord blood activities; perioperative activities; relationship testing activities; immunohematology reference laboratories; and Specialist in Blood Bank schools
  - American Association for Laboratory Accreditation: provides acceditation services and training
  - American Osteopathic Association (AOA): The AOA Healthcare Facilities Accreditation Program (HFAP) is authorized by the CMS to survey hospitals, clinical laboratories, and other health care facilities for compliance with CMS standards
  - American Society for Histocompatibility and Immunogenetics (ASHI): Accreditation program to evaluate laboratory personnel, procedures, and facilities to determine if they are in compliance with published standards of ASHI and standards of organizations by which ASHI is deemed: HCS/BM Transplantation—Related and Unrelated Donor; Solid Organ Transplantation—Deceased and Live Donor; Parentage Testing; Histocompatibility Testing; and Transfusion Support
  - College of American Pathologists (CAP): Laboratory Accreditation Program meets the needs of a variety of laboratory settings from complex university medical centers to physician office laboratories. The program also covers a complete array of disciplines and testing procedures. Because of its comprehensive nature, CAP accreditation can help achieve a consistently high level of service throughout an institution or health care system
  - COLA: First organization to be renewed since increased government scrutiny of survey organizations and was given permission to accredit

laboratories for the next 6 years to help laboratories meet CLIA requirements. The increase in oversight by CMS was driven by a government investigation in 2006 into how some highly publicized laboratory errors had occurred and could have been prevented

- The Joint Commission (TJC) accredits more organizations than any other agency in health care. It accredits more than 18,000 health care organizations, including approximately 3000 clinical laboratories
- Individual state health departments issue the other three CLIA certificates as a governmental arm of CMS
- Other certification and accreditation agencies for specific health or specialty laboratories
  - Det Norske Veritas (DNV): Recently instituted accreditation organization within the United States for accreditation of hospitals using the International Standards Organization (ISO) 9001 certification. If a hospital uses DNV for accreditation, it then partners with one of the other deemed organizations for accreditation of the hospital laboratory
  - Substance Abuse and Mental Health Services Administration (SAMHSA): Offers a certification required by all laboratories that are performing federal workplace drug testing programs
  - National Accrediting Agency for Clinical Laboratory Sciences (NAACLS): International agency for accreditation and approval of educational programs in the clinical laboratory sciences and related health professions

HUMAN RESOURCES

- Job position: Determination of a job position is done through an evaluation instrument or job position analysis checklist
  - The job analysis is a review of the job to be done and the work to be performed. Once this is completed a job description, performance analysis, training assessment, and promotional criteria may be set
- Job advertisement: Once a vacancy in a job position occurs, a job advertisement is placed to attract applicants and list the role of the job, experience required, purpose, location, general schedule, and responsibilities. The advertisement should be short and to the point, using terminology that will attract the professional laboratory personnel desired for the position
- Job description: Written statements that describe the duties, responsibilities, outcomes expected, qualifications needed, and reporting responsibilities to co-workers and supervisor
- Full time equivalent (FTE): Defined by the Government Accountability Office (GAO) as the number of hours worked divided by the compensable hours in a work year as defined by law
  - 2080 hours/year equates to 1 FTE
  - 1040 hours/year equates to 0.5 FTE

- Interview and selection process: An interview is conducted to determine the best candidate for the position
  - A standard set of questions should be used with all candidates that are job-related and review objective criteria based on the job description. Not all candidates need to be interviewed for the job they apply to, but standard cutoff criteria should be applied to all candidates to avoid bias and discrimination
- Employee orientation and training: A checklist should be used to ensure all pertinent issues are reviewed with the new employee to ensure complete understanding of the responsibilities of the position
  - This review should cover administrative policies, the general layout of the work environment, organizational policies, department and job duties, and an identified mentor to assist in the new employee training
  - Many organizations have a probationary period for the new training to take place to determine if the employee is a good fit for the job and the job is a good fit for the employee
- Employee evaluation/annual review: Assessment and review of a worker's job performance
  - Employees are evaluated on a regular basis (often once per year)
  - Reminds workers what is expected of them in the workplace and provides employers with information to use when making employment decisions, such as promotions, pay raises, and layoffs
- Employee corrective action and discipline: Used to redirect the poor or inappropriate performance of a laboratory employee through specific goals and retraining
  - Step-wise action plan documented through a set of targeted objectives and a timeline for completion
- Team building: Uses a skill set to bring members of different backgrounds and skill sets together for a common purpose
  - Within the laboratory, among phlebotomists, aides, technicians, technologists, specialists, and pathologists
  - Outside the laboratory, incorporating the health care team of physicians, nurses, and ancillary health care team members
- Conflict management: Uses strategies to improve the positive aspects of conflict and decrease the negative aspects of conflict, for improving the group outcome and improving learning and performance of the group
  - Conflict is an expected process within a group and when managed properly may increase the performance outcome of the group
  - Five approaches to conflict management: Avoiding, accommodating, compromising, forcing, and collaborating
- Customer service applies to internal and external customers
  - The three Rs of customer service: Results, Relationship, and Resource

- Good customer service is the best public relations and positive advertising strategy
- Successfully handling a dissatisfied customer will 95% of the time ensure that this customer will use your services again, because you have attempted to "right the wrong"
- Legal considerations guide the policies and procedures of the laboratory in relation to human resources and the appropriate practices of laboratory testing
  - Refer to the accreditation and certification section of this chapter, along with the definitions of the various governmental institutions and regulations, such as the National Labor Relations Board, *Fair Labor Standards Act, Equal Pay Act,* and *Family Medical Leave Act*

FINANCIAL ASPECTS OF LABORATORY

- Budget preparation: A template for forecasting revenue and expenses for an organization
  - A budget involves four processes: Development of goals, forecasting of revenue using budget assumptions, forecasting of expenses, and ongoing monitoring of both revenue and expenses
- Capital versus operational expense: Capital expense is money used for physical assets such as acquiring or upgrading facilities or equipment and is often depreciated over a 5-plus year period. Operating expense is money used for day-to-day operations, such as employee wages, taxes, and the general costs of doing business
- Justification for both capital and operating costs often use return on investment process thinking
  - Determine if the expenditure is essential, necessary, or desired; will reduce day-to-day costs over a period; or will add additional revenue
- Classification of expenses: Fixed versus variable and direct versus indirect
  - A fixed cost is a routine charge that does not change with test production (rent of facility space, taxes, etc.)
  - A variable cost changes based on fluctuations in test volume (reagent usage) and hours worked (regular and overtime costs)
  - A direct expense is related to all components associated with performing the test (laboratory equipment, reagents, service contract, quality control)
  - Indirect expense is related to all components considered overhead or administrative, such as marketing/sales, insurance, etc.
  - A laboratory could have fixed indirect and fixed direct costs and the same with variable classifications
- Cost allocations: Cost/billable is calculated using the total direct costs of performing a test as the numerator and the revenue generated sample as the denominator
  - Cost/billable is used in many reagent rental agreements in which the instrument is placed in the laboratory and an agreed-on cost per billable test

(does not count quality control, standards, or patient repeat samples tested) is calculated for the laboratory to pay the instrument vendor on an ongoing basis via their operating budget instead of a capital expense for buying the instrument outright

- A cost/test may be different from a cost/billable because this ratio includes all tests performed on the instrument, including quality control and standards

- Reimbursement: Fee for service—before the 1980s all laboratory testing was reimbursed at the fee charged for the service
  - Diagnostic related groups (DRGs): Established in 1982 to determine the level of payment for the service provided—laboratory services were combined with other ancillary services for the inpatient population of hospitals
  - Resource-Based Relative Value Scale: AMA coding system to reimburse physicians for outpatient work or Part B of Medicare reimbursement—based on relative value units of (1) work, (2) practice expense, (3) malpractice expense
  - Ambulatory Payment Categories (APCs): Are assigned to outpatient and emergency room procedures and tests and determine the outpatient prospective payment system
  - Current Procedural Terminology (CPT): A registered product of the AMA to standardize the language of various medical procedures
  - International Classification of Diseases 9 (ICD-9). Procedure-based classifications assigned to all tests within the laboratory
  - Healthcare Common Procedure Coding System (HCPCS): Standardized identification system to ensure claims are processed in a consistent manner for reimbursement (originally HCFA for the earlier name of the CMS Health Care Financing Administration)
  - Since 1984 and the enactment of the *Deficit Reduction Act,* laboratories must bill Medicare directly based on a universal laboratory fee schedule that is capped, and the Act eliminated any copay by the patients under Medicare versus other insurances

WORKLOAD AND PRODUCTIVITY

- CAP workload is a measurement that is over 25 years old; it is a productivity measurement based on the time to perform a test, the specimen processing involved, and the reporting time aspects of completing a report
  - Hospitals often use an adjusted patient day–to–FTE ratio to determine productivity for the laboratory. However, the inpatient-to-outpatient testing ratio along with revenue received rather than number of tests performed could skew the data
  - Billable tests/FTE could be used but does not take into account the variance in the test menu complexity

- Laboratory Management Index Program (LMIP): CAP service that accounts for workload recording for labor per billable test plus the expenses for non-billable tests (quality control)
- Test/FTE is often used today to benchmark with other laboratories using a standardized test terminology and the FTE, which equals 40 hours/week or 2080 hours/year
- Scheduling to maximize efficiency, productivity, and customer service is based on the workload units, budget, test menu and volume, education and experience level of employee, and complexity of the work
  - By assigning a standard unit (estimate of time) to each billable test allows you to calculate the number of FTEs needed for scheduling and the approximate costs to budget
    - Standard unit measured as 0.25 (time to perform one test)

$0.25 \times 12,000$ tests over a 4-week period $= 3000$ hours needed
3000 hours/160 hours(4 weeks) $= 18.75$ FTEs

- Staff mix is determined by the work complexity, the hours of operation (days only or 24 hours), and the resources available for checks/balances and supervision
  - Experience, training, and maturity within the profession will aid in determining aide/technician/technologist mix per shift in the laboratory setting
- Pool/as-needed (PRN)/contract staff are often used to fill temporary vacancies in the laboratory workforce
  - Pool staff may be employees who work only as needed and when called by the laboratory
  - PRN: Acronym for Latin term *pro re nata,* or "as needed"
  - Staff also may be acquired through temporary staffing agencies and are contracted for a period to fulfill specific job duties but are not employees of the organization

SAFETY

- OSHA mandates personal protective equipment and ergonomic work stations be supplied to all employees within the laboratory
  - A safety manual, training, and safety officer are critical to ensure a safe work environment within the laboratory, with appropriate documentation and counseling for employees who improperly skip safety protocols when performing their job
- Safety "right to know" addresses hazards and provides guidelines for employees to understand the general laboratory information on safety, including occupational exposure to blood-borne pathogens and hazardous chemicals and the protection devices and communications necessary to ensure a safe work environment
  - The mandate of right to know lists the hazardous substances with which the employees work, what protection is available, training and education,

and the ability of employees to make a written request for further information on safety for their job

- Blood-borne pathogens and chemical hygiene plan are specific and targeted plans that describe the hazards, the education and training on those hazards, annual documentation of this training, protective equipment, and medical surveillance for exposures
  - Hepatitis B vaccine must be offered to all employees at no cost, because of the significant risk for infection of employees through needle sticks, cuts, or splashes to mucous membranes
- Safety program must be present in all laboratories to deal with the multiple regulatory agencies' guidelines (OSHA, EPA, DOT, NIOSH, etc.) and to ensure a safe work environment
  - A safety officer develops and maintains safety procedures, with ongoing updates through communication and training and comprehensive documentation of these processes
  - All laboratory employees and students must play a proactive role in their own safety and the safety of their co-workers

PROCEDURES

- Laboratory procedures are the standard written processes that all laboratory employees follow to function effectively in their roles
  - CAP requires procedures based on the guidelines presented in the CLSI Laboratory Documents Development and Control
  - This guideline follows the common elements that should be in all procedures: Title, purpose/principle, procedure instructions, references, author, approval signatures, safety information, reagents, supplies and equipment needed, limitations of the method, calculations, and expected values

QUALITY

- Daily quality control: Process used to ensure that the daily laboratory reports are generated from appropriate patient specimens following standard procedures and using metrics and monitors throughout the preanalytical, analytical, and postanalytical processes to ensure accurate and precise results
- Quality assurance: Systematic process that ensures a quality laboratory service and result every time, all of the time. A quality assurance leader or team reviews the processes in place for a consistent standard accurate laboratory result and evaluates these processes to be proactive in process improvement techniques
- Westgard's quality management framework: James Westgard developed multiple-rule quality control for the laboratory known as the "Westgard Rules," a series of statistical calculations to determine whether variations in quality control are random or systemic, giving guidance on acceptability and reportablity of accurate laboratory test values
- Troubleshooting: Erroneous laboratory results are investigated through evaluation of the preanalytical, analytical, and postanalytical steps
- Process improvement: Six Sigma, Lean, and TQM are proactive process improvement techniques and systems
  - Six Sigma improves laboratory processes by removing the causes of errors and minimizes variations (improving precision). Six Sigma is a statistical term defined as 3.4 errors/million opportunities or 99.99966% free from defects
  - Lean, or Kaizen, is a method to remove non–value added steps in any process within the laboratory, with the result of improving turnaround time or space usage efficiency
  - Total Quality Management promotes a philosophy that everyone involved in the laboratory workflow has a responsibility for a quality product; this encompasses suppliers/vendors, the health care team, management, and patients
- Continuing education: Professional development and professionalism depend on ongoing education throughout a 40-year career
  - CLIA 88 recommends and some state agencies and employers require, continuing education on an annual basis
  - Professional Acknowledgment for Continuing Education (P.A.C.E.) credits are offered through ASCLS and are approved for laboratory-focused programs

EDUCATION

Medical Laboratory Education

- Encompasses training new employees, current employees, students, other health care professionals, and the community; includes continuing education programs
- Overseen by the National Accrediting Agency for Clinical Laboratory Sciences (NAACLS). NAACLS accredits educational programs in Cytogenetic Technology, Medical Laboratory Scientist, Medical Laboratory Technician, Diagnostic Molecular Scientist, Histotechnician, Histotechnologist, and Pathologists' Assistant
  - NAACLS publishes and administers the Guide to Accreditation and Accreditation Standards for each program type
  - The goals and responsibilities of laboratory educational training programs are guided by NAACLS and the profession itself through its various professional societies
    - Scope of practice: Defines the roles of and the services provided by laboratory professionals

○ Body of knowledge: Within the scope of practice, describes the knowledge, skills, and attitudes that are required of laboratory professionals. Educational programs are obligated to provide the content of its discipline's body of knowledge to students

○ Curriculum: Defined course of studies; the total content encompasses the various components of the body of knowledge

Learning Domains

- Learning is categorized into three domains: Cognitive, Psychomotor, and Affective. Each domain is further divided into levels of learning called taxonomy levels. Taxonomy levels within each domain begin at the respective fundamental level and progress to the more complex level. This provides a performance continuum for the learner
- Cognitive: Knowledge based on the following
  - Recall: Remembering facts
  - Comprehension: Understanding of the material
  - Application: Relating learned material to new situations
  - Analysis: Breaking down a situation into interrelated components
  - Synthesis: Tying interrelated components together in a useful way
  - Evaluation: Judging the value of information, "critical thinking"
- Psychomotor: Performance based, includes coordination, thoroughness, and efficiency
  - Observing
  - Preparing
  - Performing
- Affective: Behavior and attitude based
  - Listening and learning
  - Applying appropriate behavioral patterns
  - Commitment to and a respect for life-long professionalism

Bloom's Taxonomy

- Developed by Dr. Benjamin Bloom, Bloom's Taxonomy is a set of principles that outline the learning levels within the cognitive domain. Bloom's Taxonomy has become an underlying guideline for the education community, regardless of the discipline

Learning Objectives

- Learning objectives (LOs) are statements that explicitly describe what the learner should know or be able to do after a period of instruction
- LOs are also categorized as Cognitive, Psychomotor, or Affective
- LOs are further categorized into levels I, II, and III from simple to complex
- LOs must be measurable with respect to student performance

- Cognitive LOs: Cognitive LOs are based on knowledge; the student must possess the knowledge needed to meet the objective
  - Level I: Recall of learned information; verbs include define, describe, list
  - Level II: Applying the learned information; verbs include calculate, discuss, explain
  - Level III: Analyzing information, making decisions; verbs include analyze, compare, distinguish
  - Cognitive LO examples
    ○ Define the term *nosocomial*
    ○ Discuss the advantages of using automatic pipettors
    ○ Give a patient's medical history and laboratory results accurately
- Psychomotor LOs: Psychomotor LOs are based on skill; the student must be able to successfully utilize learned motor skills to meet the objective.
  - Level I: Awareness of ability to perform a motor skill; verbs include prepare, label, set up
  - Level II: Proficiency in performing the skill; verbs include operate, measure, perform
  - Level III: Ability to alter the procedure; verbs include revise, design, develop
  - Psychomotor LO examples
    ○ Motor skills to meet the objective
      ▪ Label the tubes for a serial dilution procedure
      ▪ Perform a manual platelet count within 20% of the automated analyzer result
      ▪ Design the procedure using the new automated instrument
- Affective LOs: Affective LOs are behavior based; the student must exhibit appropriate and professional behaviors and attitudes
  - Level I: Awareness of activity; verbs include comply, attend, obey
  - Level II: Associating a value to an activity; verbs include cooperate with, assist, share
  - Level III: Commitment to a set of values; verbs include defend, exhibit, influence
  - Affective LO examples
    ○ Complies with the class attendance policy
    ○ Assists classmates with maintaining an organized laboratory space
    ○ Exhibits a respectful demeanor at all times

LEARNING ASSESSMENTS

- Learning assessments are measures of student performance within the three learning domains. Assessments can include examinations (tests) and quizzes, practical examinations, writing a paper, doing a presentation, and being observed by an instructor in class or in the laboratory
- Examination questions are categorized into three taxonomy levels: I, II, and III

- Level I: Simple recall questions—examples
  - What color is a positive spot indole test?
  - What is the normal value for serum chloride?
- Level II: Using learned material to interpret and answer the question—examples
  - A Gram stain of a pleural fluid specimen shows gram-negative coccobacilli. Which of the following is the organism most likely seen in the Gram stain?
  - An anion gap was found to be 28 mmol/L. Which of the following is a possible cause of this result?
- Level III: Using learned materials to solve a problem—examples
  - A patient was found to have circulating blasts. The marrow blast count was 43%. No Auer rods were identified, and the peroxidase and nonspecific esterase were negative. Flow cytometry immunophenotyping revealed the presence of CD 13, CD 33, and CD 34 in the abnormal cells. CD 41, CD 19, and TdT were negative. Which of the following is the most likely cause of these findings?
  - The image shown is an auramine-rhodamine stain of an organism recovered from an infected finger wound that was slowly progressive in spite of topical antibiotic treatment. The infection developed after the patient cut his finger while cleaning his home aquarium. The organism grew optimally at 30° C on Middlebrook 7H11 medium and formed deep yellow pigment when exposed to light. The organism was negative for nitrates and heat-stable catalase, but hydrolyzed Tween and produced urease and pryazinamidase. Which of the following is the most probable identification of this organism?

Learner Types
- The three fundamental types of learners are visual, auditory, and kinesthetic
  - Visual learners learn primarily from written materials and by sight
  - Auditory learners learn primarily by listening and talking
  - Kinesthetic learners learn primarily by doing
- Instructional materials and methods should be designed with consideration for all three learning types

Teaching Methods
- Lecture: Instructor presents material to a group of students
- Laboratory demonstration: Method, technique, or instrument is demonstrated
- Discussion: Topics are interactively discussed in class by the instructor and students
- Role playing: Students assume roles in a given scenario; helpful in demonstrating affective behaviors
- Case study based: Students are provided with patient case studies, typically used to facilitate critical thinking in patient diagnoses
- Problem-based learning: Students work in groups to solve a problem
- Cooperative learning: Students work in groups, discussing and learning material
- Distance education: Students participate and learn from a distance using online materials

Clinical (Bench) Teaching
- For laboratory professionals, the first type of teaching often encountered is training students or new employees "at the bench." Teaching clinical skills requires a basic understanding of the educational process, including planning. The steps involved in clinical training are
  - Students are provided with the didactic knowledge and psychomotor skills necessary to accurately understand and perform the procedure
  - Students observe the procedure step by step, demonstrated by the instructor. This step includes obtaining specific information about the procedure from the Standard Operating Procedure manual (SOP)
  - Students practice the procedure as the instructor observes until the expected competency is attained. The instructor assesses performance and provides feedback to the students
  - Students perform the procedure under the supervision of an instructor

CERTIFICATION PREPARATION QUESTIONS

For answers and rationales, please see Appendix A.

1. During the morning rush, your laboratory manager comes into the laboratory and starts explaining a new policy regarding vacation requests. Word spreads of the change throughout the day, and the message has changed somewhat. Several in the laboratory are upset and complain to the laboratory manager. Which of the following actions is the *most* appropriate way to handle such a situation?
   a. Nothing should be changed, it was handled appropriately
   b. The manager should have posted the change on the bulletin board in the break room
   c. The manager should have announced the policy on each shift
   d. The manager should have discussed and distributed the policy at a laboratory meeting, or several laboratory meetings, so that all employees heard the policy from the manager

2. What is the most important role of the manager in charge?
   a. Independent decision making
   b. Communication
   c. Informal discussions
   d. None of the above

3. Your laboratory was just inspected by CAP. Your inspector noted a phase I (lower level) citation that

the hematology laboratory space is quite small. What action should the laboratory take?

  a. Submit a written plan to CAP outlining that the laboratory will reorganize the space to meet the needs of the department

  b. Immediately begin remodeling the laboratory, because this type of citation must be corrected within 30 days

  c. Ignore the phase I citation, because it is only a recommendation

  d. Reply to the CAP that space issue is not their concern

4. The role of NAACLS is to:

  a. Accredit laboratories

  b. Offer certification examinations

  c. Offer continuing education

  d. Accredit educational programs

5. COLA is similar to which of the following agencies?

  a. CAP

  b. TJC

  c. AABB

  d. ASCLS

6. Your laboratory is going to begin offering drug testing to local employers. While setting up the laboratory, you will likely work with which of the following agencies for accreditation of the laboratory?

  a. COLA

  b. SAMHSA

  c. AABB

  d. CLSI

Match the following three agencies with the correct application they oversee.

7. __ CMS

8. __ FDA

9. __ DOT

  a. Regulates shipments of human specimens

  b. Approves new testing procedures and methods

  c. Regulate laboratory testing via CLIA

10. Job descriptions can be viewed as a summary of the findings obtained from a job analysis.

  a. True

  b. False

11. Which of the following items should not be contained within a job advertisement?

  a. Name of organization

  b. Starting salary

  c. Position title

  d. Certification/licensure requirements

12. Which of the following qualifications is(are) necessary to be an effective evaluator?

  a. Knowledge of job and work being done

  b. Proximity to the person being judged

  c. Time to conduct the review

  d. All of the above

13. There is no relationship between an evaluation instrument and the job description.

  a. True

  b. False

14. Rewards such as a reserved parking spot or the ability to attend conferences may be used to recognize employee accomplishments.

  a. True

  b. False

15. Which of the following is a benefit of teams in the workplace?

  a. Sense of accomplishment

  b. Increased communication

  c. Relief for employees

  d. All of the above

16. Which of the following is a category for justification of capital expenditures?

  a. Replacement

  b. Cost reduction

  c. New equipment

  d. All of the above

17. Which of the following government regulations apply standards for employers to apply for medical leave of absence:

  a. CAP

  b. FMLA

  c. CLMA

  d. CLSI

18. You are the lead chemistry MLS. Your laboratory manager has asked you to evaluate two new methods for cholesterol analysis. In your evaluation, you found that method A was very accurate and precise and that method B was not very accurate and precise. However, the laboratory will make more money by investing in method B. Which of the following decisions would exhibit professionalism?

  a. Recommend method A to your laboratory manager. It is important that the laboratory produce the most accurate and precise results

  b. Recommend method B to your laboratory manager. It is important that the laboratory make as much money as possible

  c. State that you are unable to make a recommendation, because no difference in the methods was noted

  d. Recommend that you need more time to evaluate both methods

19. The three Rs of customer service include results, relationships, and reliability.

  a. True

  b. False

20. Legal personnel issues in the clinical laboratory include all of the following except:

  a. Medical leaves

  b. Reimbursement

  c. Termination procedures

  d. Interview questions

21. Which of the following regulates overtime pay?

  a. NLRB

  b. FLSA

  c. EPA

  d. FMLA

22. A hospital is reimbursed under the Medicare DRG program according to which of the following?
    a. Amount of service provided
    b. Costs incurred in providing care
    c. Nature of the illness
    d. Profit margin of the laboratory

23. Which statement describes the appropriate scheduling process?
    a. Matching the people presently working in the laboratory with current workload requirements
    b. The setting of long-term goals and objectives for the number and types of personnel needed to meet the labor requirements of the laboratory
    c. Allow a democratic approach and have the staff schedule when they want to work
    d. Placing all of the experienced personnel on one shift

24. Which of the following is a goal of an interview?
    a. Establish social contacts
    b. Evaluate applicant's skills and personality
    c. Discuss the religious background of the applicant
    d. Discuss prior arrests of the applicant

25. Annual budget assumptions are based on _____.
    a. Estimated direct costs
    b. Estimated indirect costs
    c. Projected reimbursement and revenue
    d. All of the above

26. Ambulatory Payment Category (APC) codes are used for reimbursement purposes for which of the following?
    a. Inpatients
    b. Medicare inpatients
    c. Outpatient and emergency room patients
    d. None of the above

27. According to most managed care plans, the type of reimbursement similar to federal systems is:
    a. Capitation
    b. Per diem
    c. Per case
    d. Carve out

28. Budgets should be reviewed _____ to identify budget variances.
    a. Weekly
    b. Monthly
    c. Quarterly
    d. Annually

29. When calculating the costs per billable tests, the total test volume in the laboratory is not needed.
    a. True
    b. False

30. Which of the following agency(ies) developed the Medical Compliance Plan (MCP)?
    a. CAP
    b. TJC
    c. HHS OIG
    d. NAACLS

31. The *Clinical Laboratory Improvement Act* of 1988 applies to which of the following?
    a. All clinical laboratories
    b. Hospital laboratories only
    c. Laboratories engaged in interstate commerce only
    d. Physician office laboratories only

32. What is the purpose of a compliance plan?
    a. Reduce fraud and abuse billing practices
    b. Monitor employee compliance to safety practices
    c. Train employees on customer satisfaction
    d. Ensure fairness in scheduling

33. Which organization publishes guidelines for writing technical procedures that are usually acceptable to agencies that govern laboratory operations, such as CAP and COLA?
    a. AABB
    b. CLSI
    c. OSHA
    d. ASM

34. Which of the following arrangements offers the most instrument service coverage and "piece of mind" for laboratory managers?
    a. Pay as needed for time and materials
    b. Establishing a service contract for key instruments
    c. Fingers crossed that nothing breaks down
    d. Order new instruments when the warranty runs out on the old one

35. Given the following information, calculate the needed FTEs.
    Standard unit: 0.5
    Number of billable tests in 14 days: 10,000
    a. 62.5
    b. 125
    c. 250
    d. None of the above

36. Productivity can be calculated by which of the following?
    a. Dividing actual hours worked by earned hours and multiply by 100
    b. Dividing earned hours by actual hours and multiply by 100
    c. Calculating the number of people on your staff and dividing by the number of shifts
    d. Comparing the number of radiology technicians in comparison to laboratory technicians

37. Legal institutional issues in the clinical laboratory include all of the following except:
    a. Confidentiality
    b. Job announcements
    c. Procedures
    d. Chain of custody

38. PRN employees are useful in the scheduling process because they help to decrease overtime and increase flexibility.
    a. True
    b. False

39. When using the 8 and 80 payroll regulation and guidelines, are employees paid overtime when they work more than 8 hours in one day?
    a. Yes, the employees would be paid overtime
    b. No, the employees would not be paid overtime because they must have worked more than 80 hours also
    c. It depends on how the employees desire to be paid
    d. The employees are not paid overtime regardless of how many hours are worked

40. You are in charge of planning the schedule for the day shift. Your laboratory manager asks that you identify three ways to reduce the labor costs for that shift. Of the following, which is not a way to reduce the costs?
    a. Use PRN employees to reduce overtime costs
    b. Switch to a 40-hour work week
    c. Schedule your most educated and trained employees during first shift
    d. Use a mix of highly educated employees and relatively new employees

41. As part of the Blood-borne Pathogens Plan, employers must offer the hepatitis B vaccine to all employees at the expense of the clinical laboratory (or organization).
    a. True
    b. False

42. Which of the following components should not be included in a written procedure?
    a. Test method
    b. Cost per billable test
    c. Quality control procedures
    d. Reagents and media needs

43. Which of the following agencies has the inspection authority for laboratory accreditation?
    a. CAP
    b. TJC
    c. State health departments
    d. All of the above

44. Which of the following questions can be legally asked during an interview?
    a. What is your date of birth?
    b. Where have you previously worked?
    c. Do you have any dependents?
    d. Do you have any long-term health problems?

45. Which of the following methods would be most helpful during the interview to assess an applicant's abilities to resolve problems in a mature manner?
    a. Read a scenario and ask the applicant how he or she would react if in the situation
    b. Directly ask the applicant if he or she is mature
    c. Observe the applicant during the interview
    d. There is no way to assess these abilities during the interview process

46. An educational learning objective must:
    a. Be written in broad terms
    b. Not be measurable
    c. Be provided after the educational unit ends
    d. Explain exactly what the student should be able to do

47. The cognitive learning domain includes which of the following?
    a. Evaluation
    b. Demonstration
    c. Attitudes
    d. Motor skills

48. Being described as a team player falls primarily within which learning domain?
    a. Cognitive
    b. Psychomotor
    c. Affective
    d. Level III

49. Which of the following learning objectives is appropriately written?
    a. The student will understand how to perform urine microscopy
    b. The student will be able to accurately list the steps in performing a venipuncture
    c. The student will be aware of professional behavior
    d. The student will not make mistakes

50. An examination question that includes a comprehensive list of laboratory tests from a given patient and requests the examinee to make a diagnosis is an example of a question that belongs to which taxonomic level?
    a. Level I
    b. Level II
    c. Level III
    d. Level IV

BIBLIOGRAPHY

American Association for Clinical Chemistry: Communicating the laboratory's value to health care: an interview with Rodney Forsman, Clin Lab News: 12–13, 2004.

Cohen C, Cohen SL: Lab dynamics: management skills for scientist, ed 1, New York, 2005, Cold Spring Harbor Laboratory Press.

Drucker P: The practice of management, ed 1, New York, 1993, Harper Business.

Garcia L: Clinical laboratory management, ed 1, Washington, DC, 2004, ASM Press.

Harmening DM: Laboratory management: principles and processes, ed 2, St. Petersburg, Fla, 2007, D.H. Publishing Consulting.

Hudson J: Principles of clinical laboratory management: a study guide and workbook, ed 1, Upper Saddle River, NJ, 2003, Prentice Hall.

Jones S: Clinical laboratory pearls, ed 1, Philadelphia, Pa, 2000, Lippincott Williams & Wilkins.

Lewin K, Lippitt R: An experimental approach to the study of autocracy and democracy: a preliminary note, Sociometry 1:292–300, 2003.

de Kieviet W, Frank E, Stekel H: Essentials of clinical laboratory management in developing regions, 2008, Committee on Clinical Laboratory Management, Education and Management Division, International Federation of Clinical Chemistry.

Hofstede G: "Cultures and Organizations: Software of the Mind," Admin Sci Quart (Johnson Graduate School of Management, Cornell University) 38(1):132–134, March 1993, JSTOR 2393257.

CLINICAL LABORATORY MANAGEMENT WEBSITES

CMS: http://www.cms.hhs.gov/

CLIA application: http://www.cms.gov/Medicare/CMS-Forms/CMS-Forms/Downloads/CMS116.pdf

Credentialing Agencies

CAP: http://www.cap.org/apps/cap.portal

ASCP: http://www.ascp.org/

TJC: http://www.jointcommission.org/

COLA: http://www.cola.org/

NAACLS: http://naacls.org/

ASHI: http://www.ashi-hla.org/

AO: http://www.osteopathic.org/Pages/default.aspx

DNV: http://dnvaccreditation.com/pr/dnv/default.aspx

Laboratory Resource Sites

CLSI http://clsi.org/

A2LA: http://A2la.org

POCT: http://www.pointofcare.net/

NIT: http://www.nih.gov/

LOINC: /https://loinc.org/

SNOMED: http://www.ihtsdo.org/

Lab Tests Online: http://labtestsonline.org/

Labs Are Vital: http://www.labsarevital.com/

Results for Life: http://www.labresultsforlife.org/

Professional Organizations and Associations

CLMA: http://clma.org/

AACC: http://aacc.org/AACC/

ASM: http://www.asm.org

ASCLS: http://www.ascls.org/

NILA: http://www.aab.org

AAB http://www.aab.org/

AMT: http://www.amt1.com/

Continuing Education

MTS: http://www.medtraining.org/

Body of Knowledge: http://www.clma.org/?page=BOK_Logo

CE organizer: http://ceorganizer.ascls.org/

Government and Legislative

Library of Congress: http://thomas.loc.gov/

House of Representatives: https://writerep.house.gov/writerep/welcome.shtml

Senate: http://www.senate.gov/general/contact_information/senators_cfm.cfm

SaveOurLabs: http://www.saveourlabs.com/

Quality Control Reference

Westgard Rules: http://www.westgard.com/

Human Resources Reference

Performance reviews: http://performancesolutions.com/

SELF-ASSESSMENT

Content Area: _____

Score on Practice Questions: _____

List the specific topics covered in the missed questions:

List the specific topics covered in the correct questions:

NOTES

Laboratory Calculations

Melanie J. Giusti and Mark W. Ireton

SIGNIFICANT FIGURES AND ROUNDING

- Measured numbers include a certain amount of certainty and uncertainty
  - The uncertainty is in the digit furthest to the right, and it reflects the precision of the measuring instrument and the skill of the person using it
- The significant figures in a measured number include every digit *except* nonmeasured zeroes that only hold the decimal place
- Table 11-1 shows examples of numbers and the number of significant figures in each one
- When making calculations, the final answer is rounded off to reflect the value with the least certainty (the fewest significant figures)
- For multiplication and division, the answer must have the same number of significant figures as the starting value with the least number of significant figures
  - For example, multiplying 2.5 g/L by 0.5250 L results in a product of 1.3125 g. However, this must be rounded to 1.3 g because 2.5 g/L has only two significant figures
- For addition and subtraction, the answer must have the same number of decimal places as the starting value with the fewest number of decimal places
  - For example, the sum of 15.5 mL of solution plus 25.92 mL of solution (measured with a more precise instrument) equals 41.42 mL. This number must be rounded to 41.4 mL because 15.5 mL has only one decimal place
- When rounding numbers
  - If the left-most digit removed is greater than 5, round up the final retained digit by one
  - If the left-most digit removed is less than 5, the final retained digit remains the same
  - If the left-most digit to be removed is 5, the final retained digit is increased if it is odd, or it stays the same if it is even
- Only measured numbers determine significant figures
  - Exact, counted, or ideal numbers do not determine significant figures. For example, 1000 mg in 1 g is an exact amount
  - Counted numbers, such as 5 nucleated RBCs on a blood smear, or the valence of a molecule, also do not affect significant figures
  - When a practice problem asks to make a 1-L solution, that volume does not affect significant figures because it is a theoretical amount, with no indication of how it would be measured
  - Numbers are rounded only after all calculations are complete. Rounding before calculations are complete introduces inaccuracies that can become exaggerated in further calculations

EXPONENTIAL NOTATION

- Very large and very small numbers are written in exponential notation—usually one to three digits to the left of the decimal place and a multiplier based on 10^x
  - When this exponential x is a positive integer, the number is multiplied by 10 x-number of times
  - When the exponential x is a negative integer, the number is divided by 10 x-number of times
  - In other words, if the exponential form is written out in standard notation, the decimal point is moved x number of digits to the right when x is positive and x number of digits to the left when x is negative
  - Example
    - $2.5 \times 10^2 = 2.5 \times 10 \times 10$: Move the decimal point two digits to the right = 250
    - $2.5 \times 10^{-2} = 2.5 \div 10 \div 10$: Move the decimal point two digits to the left = 0.025
- In mathematical operations involving exponential notation, the significant digits and the exponential powers are handled separately

TABLE 11-1	Example Numbers and Their Significant Figures	
Measurement		**Significant Figures**
10		1
10.		2
10.0		3
35		2
0.35		2
0.0035		2
0.00350		3

- In multiplication, the exponents are added
- In division, the exponents are subtracted
- Example

$$(3 \times 10^4)(5 \times 10^5)$$

  - Answer: The product of the significant digits is 15. The sum of the exponents is 9. Therefore the answer is 15×10^9 or 1.5×10^{10}
- Example

$$\frac{4 \times 10^3}{2 \times 10^5}$$

  - Answer: The quotient of the significant digits is 2. The exponent in the denominator is subtracted from the exponent in the numerator. Therefore the answer is 2×10^{-2}
- If it is necessary to add or subtract numbers in exponential notation, convert the exponential number to standard notation before making calculations, then convert back to exponential notation when finished

UNITS OF MEASURE

Metric System

- The metric system is used for measuring size, volume, and weight
- Very large and small amounts are modified by prefixes based on factors of 10
  - For example, "kilo" is equal to 1000 units or 1×10^3, so there are 1000 meters per kilometer, or 10^{-3} kilometers per meter (Table 11-2)
- Knowing these values, it is possible to convert between units using the factor-label method
  - Example
    - How many grams are in 2 kg?
      - Answer: Knowing that a kilogram is equivalent to 10^3 g, multiply 2 kg by 10^3 g/kg and cancel the kilogram units

$$2 \text{ kg} \times \frac{10^3 \text{g}}{\text{kg}} = 2 \times 10^3 \text{g or } 2000 \text{g}$$

TABLE 11-2	Metric System
Prefix	**Factor**
mega- (M)	1,000,000 or 1×10^6
kilo- (k)	1,000 or 1×10^3
deci- (d)	0.1 or 1×10^{-1}
centi- (c)	0.01 or 1×10^{-2}
milli- (m)	0.001 or 1×10^{-3}
micro- (μ)	0.000001 or 1×10^{-6}
nano- (n)	0.000000001 or 1×10^{-9}
pico- (p)	0.000000000001 or 1×10^{-12}
femto- (f)	0.000000000000001 or 1×10^{-15}

- Example
  - What is 20 mg converted to micrograms?
    - Answer: Knowing that a gram is equivalent to 10^3 mg, and that a gram is also equivalent to 10^6 μg, use the factor-label method to solve for micrograms

$$20 \text{ mg} \times \frac{\text{g}}{10^3 \text{ mg}} \times \frac{10^6 \text{ μg}}{\text{g}} = 20 \times 10^3 \text{ μg}$$

TEMPERATURE CONVERSIONS

- Temperatures are measured in degrees Celsius (°C), degrees Fahrenheit (°F), or Kelvins (K)
- In the medical laboratory, the Celsius scale is most often used
- Formulas used to convert between these scales
  - °F = 9/5 °C + 32
  - °C = 5/9 (°F − 32)
  - K = °C + 273
- To use any of these equations, insert the known values to solve for the unknown values
  - Example
    - 99.2° F equals how many degrees Celsius?
      - Answer: Insert the known Fahrenheit value into the equation for Celsius, and solve

$$°C = 5/9 (99.2 - 32)$$
$$°C = 5/9 (67.2)$$
$$°C = 37.3$$

      - Hint
        - If in doubt about correctly remembering the Celsius/Fahrenheit conversion formulas during an examination, it is possible to double-check the correctness of the equation by using the known freezing and boiling points of water: 0° C or 32° F and 100° C or 212° F, respectively
        - Insert either the Celsius or Fahrenheit boiling point or freezing point of water into a formula, and if the answer is correct then so is the formula

FACTORS AND DILUTIONS

Dilutions and Ratios

- A dilution can be expressed as a fraction of specimen volume divided by the sum of specimen volume and diluent. The resulting fraction is the dilution (or dilution factor)

$$\text{Dilution} = \frac{\text{Specimen volume}}{\text{Specimen volume} + \text{diluent volume}} = \frac{\text{Specimen volume}}{\text{Total volume}}$$

- Example
  - 10 mL of saline is added to 10 mL of blood. What is the dilution?
    - Answer: Divide the volume of blood (10 mL) by the total volume contained
    - This is a ½ dilution

$$\text{Dilution} = \frac{10\ \text{mL}}{10\ \text{mL} + 10\ \text{mL}} = \frac{10\ \text{mL}}{20\ \text{mL}} = \frac{1}{2}$$

- Example
  - What is the dilution if 10 μL is diluted to 100 μL?
  - Answer: Divide the sample volume by the total volume

$$\text{Dilution} = \frac{10\ \mu L}{100\ \mu L} = \frac{1}{10}$$

- Example
  - How do you prepare a solution of 20 mL of serum that is diluted to 100 mL, and what is the dilution?
    - Determine the volume of diluent by subtracting the specimen volume from the total volume

$$100\ \text{mL} - 20\ \text{mL} = 80\ \text{mL}$$

- Next divide the amount of sample (20 mL) by the total volume (100 mL), which equals 1/5
- Answer: Add 80 mL of diluent to the 20-mL sample, which makes a 1/5 dilution
- The concentration of a diluted solution is the product of its original concentration times the dilution factor
  - Example
    - 20 mL of a 20-mg/dL reagent is diluted 1/5
    - What is the final concentration?
      - Answer: Multiply the initial concentration by the dilution factor

$$\frac{20\ \text{mg}}{\text{dL}} \times \frac{1}{5} = \frac{4\ \text{mg}}{\text{dL}}$$

- Dilutions written as fractions are always considered to be volume of sample per total volume
- Ratios can be used to express part-per-part or part-per-whole, and are written with a colon between figures
- In a solution containing 1 mL of serum and 4 mL of saline (total volume 5 mL), the following dilution and ratio relationships exist
  - Dilution is 1/5
  - Ratio of serum to total volume is 1:5
  - Ratio of serum to saline is 1:4
  - Ratio of saline to total volume is 4:5
  - Ratio of total volume to serum is 5:1
  - Ratio of saline to serum is 4:1

Dilution Series

- When a diluted solution is diluted again, the final dilution is the product of its dilution factors (Figure 11-1)
  - Tube A is an undiluted patient sample
  - Tubes B to D contain 9 mL diluent

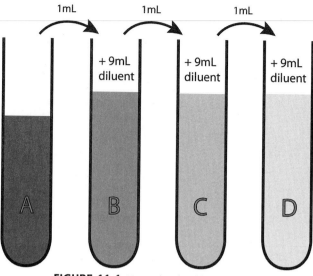

FIGURE 11-1 Example of a dilution series.

- If a 1-mL aliquot is taken from tube A and added to tube B, this represents a 1/10 dilution in tube B
- If 1 mL of the dilution in tube B is added to tube C, and 1 mL of the tube C dilution is added to tube D, each of these represents a 1/10 dilution
- The dilution factors in each tube are
  - Tube A = Undiluted (neat)
  - Tube B = 1/10
  - Tube C = (1/10) (1/10) = 1/100
  - Tube D = (1/10) (1/10) (1/10) = 1/1000
- The concentration of the solution in any selected tube is the product of the concentration of tube A times the dilution factor of the selected tube

CONVERSION AND CORRECTION FACTORS

- Factor: A fraction that can be used to:
  - Correct a variance in procedure
  - Express a quantity in different terms
  - Combine calculations
- The most basic factor is a unit-conversion, which is the basis for the factor-label method
  - Example
    - To convert a volume measured in milliliters to liters, multiply the original figure by a fraction with equivalent numerator and denominator and cancel out the corresponding units

$$450\ \text{mL} \times \frac{1\text{L}}{1000\ \text{mL}} = 0.45\ \text{L}$$

- To use a factor to correct for a variance in procedure, the equation is:

$$\text{Measured value} \times \frac{\text{Volume that should be used}}{\text{Available sample volume}} = \text{Corrected value}$$

- In the case of a dilution, the numerator in the previous fraction example would be volume of the diluted specimen
- Example
  - A urine specimen is delivered to the laboratory for a sodium measurement. The procedure calls for 5.0 mL but the specimen is only 4.0 mL, and acquiring a new specimen is not possible. The medical laboratory scientist at the bench dilutes the specimen with 1.0 mL of water to 5.0 mL. The analyzer measures a sodium concentration of 44 mEq/L. What is the corrected (actual) concentration of the patient sample?
    - Answer: To correct for the dilution, multiply the result by the diluted volume (how much should have been used) and divide by the available specimen volume

$$44 \text{ mEq/L} \times \frac{5.0 \text{ mL}}{4.0 \text{ mL}} = 55 \text{ mEq/L}$$

- When the dilution factor is known, the corrected value can also be found by multiplying the measured result by the inverse of the dilution factor. In the previous example, the dilution factor was 4/5, so the measured value can be multiplied by 5/4 for the corrected value

UNITS OF CONCENTRATION AND PREPARATION OF SOLUTIONS

Concentration as Parts per Parts and as Percent

- Solution concentration can be expressed proportionally as:
  - Weight per volume (w/v)
    - Weight per volume concentrations are often expressed as grams per deciliter or milligrams per deciliter
    - Example
      - 3.2 g glucose dissolved in 2 dL of water has a concentration or 3.2 g/2 dL or 1.6 g/dL
    - In a weight per volume solution, addition of solute does not affect volume (assuming the solution is not saturated)
  - Volume per volume (v/v)
  - Weight per weight (w/w)
    - The addition of solute adds to the mass of the solute and to the total solution but not to the mass of solvent
    - Example
      - 1 g sodium chloride in 100 g H_2O describes a solution that is 1 g/100 g or 0.01 g/g NaCl
  - Number per volume (n/v)
  - Percent solution

- Amount per 100
- In the clinical laboratory, percent solutions are expressed as grams per 100 mL
- Example
  - 0.9% saline solution contains 0.9 g NaCl per 100 mL water

Molarity

- Molarity (M) is the number of moles (mol) of solute per liter of solution

$$M = \frac{\text{mol}}{L}$$

- Example
  - What is the molarity of a solution containing 3 mol of glucose in 500 mL of water?
    - Answer: Use the equation previous and the factor-label method to solve for moles per single liter

$$M = \frac{3 \text{ mol}}{500 \text{ mL}} \times \frac{1000 \text{ mL}}{L} = \frac{6 \text{ mol}}{L} = 6M$$

- Example
  - How many moles of glucose are in 400 mL of a 5-M glucose solution?
    - Answer: Multiply molarity (which is converted from Moles to moles per liter) by volume to solve for moles

$$400 \text{ mL} \times 5 \text{ M} = 400 \text{ mL} \times \frac{5 \text{ mol}}{L} \times \frac{L}{1000 \text{ mL}} = 2 \text{ mol}$$

- Molarity and weight/volume are interchangeable using molecular weight (MW), also called molar mass, which is based on atomic mass and is equal to grams per mole

$$MW = \frac{g}{\text{mol}}$$
$$MW \times M = \frac{g}{\text{mol}} \times \frac{\text{mol}}{L} = \frac{g}{L}$$

- Example
  - How many moles are in 23.4 g of potassium chloride? (MW of KCl = 74.5 g/mol)
    - Answer: Use the factor-label method to multiply mass by the inverse of MW to eliminate grams and solve for moles

$$23.4 g \times \frac{\text{mol}}{74.5 \text{ g}} = 0.314 \text{ mol}$$

    - NOTE: Grams per mole can be inverted to moles per gram when solving for moles because proportionally 1 mol of KCl represents the same amount as 74.5 g of KCl

- Example
  - How much water is needed to make a 0.5-M solution from 150 g of NaCl? (MW of NaCl = 58.5 g/mol)
    - Answer: Knowing that 0.5 M equals 0.5 mol/L, solve for volume by multiplying the weight of the sample by the inverse of the molarity by the inverse of molecular weight (to isolate liters in the numerator)

$$150 \text{ g} \times \frac{L}{0.5 \text{ mol}} \times \frac{\text{mol}}{58.5 \text{ g}} = 5.1L$$

Molality

- Molality (m) is the number of moles of solute per kilogram of solvent

$$m = \frac{\text{mol}}{\text{kg}}$$

- Remember that the denominator is the mass of solvent, *not* of the entire solution
  - Example:
    - What is the molality of a solution containing 5.0 mol glucose and 4.0 kg water?
      - Answer: Insert the measurements into the molality formula and divide to determine moles per 1 kg

$$m = \frac{5.0 \text{ mol}}{4.0 \text{ kg}} = \frac{1.2 \text{ mol}}{\text{kg}}$$

Normality

- Normality (N) is a term of concentration based on the ability of some substances to release hydrogen (H^+) or hydroxide (OH^-) ions in solution
- In biological systems, the number of H^+ or OH^- ions that are released per molecule in solution is equivalent to valence, which is the bonding ability of a molecule
- The simplest definition of normality is based on molarity and valence

$$N = M \times \text{Valence}$$

- Example, $Ca(OH)_2$ dissociates in solution to release two OH^- ions per molecule, so the valence is 2. Therefore the normality of a 1-M solution of Ca$(OH)_2$ is 2 N

$$N = M \times \text{Valence} = 1 \times 2 = 2$$

- For substances with a valence of 1, normality equals molarity
- Normality is also defined as equivalents per liter and can be determined given the weight of solute and the volume of solution using the following steps:
  - Determine valence to calculate the gram equivalent weight of the solute, which is the weight of 1 mole

of the substance (also known as formula weight) divided by its valence
- Calculate the number of equivalents in solution, which is the weight of the solute in the sample divided by the gram equivalent weight
- Solve for normality with the equation, N = Eq/L
- Equation review

$$\text{Gram equivalent weight} = \frac{MW \times 1 \text{ mol}}{\text{Valence}}$$

$$\text{Equivalents (Eq)} = \frac{\text{Grams in sample}}{\text{Gram equivalent weight}}$$

$$N = \frac{Eq}{L}$$

- Example
  - What is the normality of a 1-L solution containing 46.3 g $Ca(OH)_2$? (MW of $Ca(OH)_2 = 74.1$ g/mol)
    - Answer
      - Determine the valence to calculate gram equivalent weight. $Ca(OH)_2$ dissociates into two OH^- ions per molecule, so the valence is 2. Gram equivalent weight is

$$\text{Gram equivalent weight} = \frac{MW \times 1 \text{ mol}}{\text{Valence}} = \frac{74.1 \text{ g}}{2} = 37.0g$$

- Determine the number of equivalents in the sample

$$Eq = \frac{\text{Grams in sample}}{\text{Gram equivalent weight}} = \frac{46.3 \text{ g}}{37.05 \text{ g}} = 1.25$$

- Finally, solve for the normality of this solution

$$N = \frac{Eq}{L} = \frac{1.25 \text{ Eq}}{1L}$$

- The normality of this solution can be written as 1.25 N or 1.25 Eq/L

Osmolality

- One osmole is equivalent to a mole of substance multiplied by the number of osmotically active particles per mole the substance dissociates into in solution
- For example, glucose molecules do not dissociate into smaller particles in water, so 1 osmole of glucose equals 1 mole of glucose
- NaCl dissociates into one Na^+ and one Cl^- (two total particles) per mole, so 1 mole of NaCl equals 2 osmoles NaCl
  - Osmoles = Number of moles × number of osmotically active particles per mole
- Osmolality measures concentration in terms of osmoles per kilogram of solvent
  - Osmolality = Osmoles per kilogram

- Osmolality is the preferred unit in the clinical laboratory for osmometry measurements of electrolytes, freezing point depression, and vapor pressure depression. Note that in the abbreviation for milliosmoles, the "O" is capitalized—mOsmol
  - Example
    - What is the osmolality of 32.7 g NaCl dissolved in 2.0 kg water? (MW of NaCl = 58.5 g/mol)
    - Answer: Multiply the weight of NaCl by the inverse of its molecular weight to determine how many moles are present

$$32.7g \times \frac{mol}{58.5g} = 0.55897 \; mol$$

  - NaCl dissociates into two osmotically active particles per molecule in solution
  - Determine number of osmoles

$$Osmoles = Moles \times Active \; particles = 0.55897 \times 2 = 1.1179$$

  - Solve for osmolality

$$Osmolality = \frac{osmol}{kg} = \frac{1.1179 \; osmol}{2.0 \; kg} = 0.56 \; osmol/kg$$

Proportionally Equivalent Solutions

- Calculations with two solutions whose concentrations do not change are known as ratio and proportion calculations
- The general formula for ratio and proportion is

$$\frac{w_1}{v_1} = \frac{w_2}{v_2}$$

- Weight per volume (w/v) is most common, but weight per weight (w/w), volume per volume (v/v), number per volume (n/v), and other combinations are also used
  - Example
    - If a 5.0-dL solution contains 4.5 mg of bilirubin, how much bilirubin would there be in a 2.0-dL aliquot of the solution?
      - Answer: Assign values to set up the equation
        - $w_1 = 4.5$ mg
        - $v_1 = 5.0$ dL
        - $w_2 = $ Unknown
        - $v_2 = 2.0$ dL
    - Insert these values into the equation and cross-multiply to solve for the unknown mass (w_2) in the 2.0-dL aliquot

$$\frac{4.5 \; mg}{5.0 \; dL} = \frac{w_2}{2.0 \; dL}$$

$$\frac{4.5 \; mg \times 2.0 \; dL}{5.0 \; dL} = w_2$$

$$1.8 \; mg = w_2$$

  - Example
    - The total carbon dioxide concentration of a serum sample is 25 mEq/L

- How many milliequivalents of CO_2 are contained in the 10-mL collection tube?
  - Answer: Assign values to set up the equation
    - $n_1 = 25$ mEq
    - $v_1 = 1$ L = 1000 mL
    - $n_2 = $ Unknown
    - $v_2 = 10$ mL
  - Insert these values into the equation and cross-multiply to solve for the unknown number of milliequivalents (n_2) in the 10-mL tube:

$$\frac{25 \; mEq}{1000 \; mL} = \frac{n_1}{10 \; mL}$$

$$\frac{25 \; mEq \times 10 \; mL}{1000 \; mL} = n_1$$

$$0.25 \; mEq = n_1$$

Dilution Equations (Changing Concentrations)

- When making a dilution, the volume of the original solution is less than the volume of the diluted solution
- The amount of solute remains the same
- Because volume (V) times concentration (C) equals amount of solute, and the amount of solute remains the same, the resulting equation can be used to solve for any one missing factor in this type of dilution problem

$$V_1 \times C_1 = V_2 \times C_2$$

- Example
  - What volume of a 0.5-M glucose solution can be made from 100 mL of a 3-M glucose stock solution?
    - Answer: Assign values for the equation
      - $V_1 = 100$ mL
      - $C_1 = 3$ M
      - $C_2 = 0.5$ M
      - $V_2 = $ Unknown
  - Divide both sides of the equation $V_1 \times C_1 = V_2 \times C_2$ by C_2 to isolate V_2, then insert the known quantities and solve for V_2

$$V_2 = \frac{V_1 \times C_1}{C_2} = \frac{100 \; mL \times 3 \; M}{0.5 \; M} = 600 \; mL$$

  - Note that in this problem there is no need to convert M to moles per liter because these units cancel each other
- Example
  - A 3.5-L solution was diluted with 1.5 L of water to create a 0.5-M solution with a total volume of 5.0 L
  - What was the concentration of the original solution?
    - Answer: Assign values for the equation
      - $V_1 = 3.5$ L
      - $C_1 = $ Unknown

- $V_2 = 5.0 \text{ L}$
- $C_2 = 0.5 \text{ M}$
  - o Divide both sides of the formula $V_1 \times C_1 = V_2 \times C_2$ by V_1 to solve for C_1, which represents the concentration of the original solution

$$C_1 = \frac{V_2 \times C_2}{V_1} = \frac{5.0 \text{ L} \times 0.5 \text{ M}}{3.5 \text{ L}} = 0.7 \text{ M}$$

STATISTICS AND QUALITY ASSESSMENT

Measures of Center

- Mean
  - The mean ($\bar{x}$) is the average of the individual values (x or x_i) in the sample set
  - Calculated by dividing the sum (Σ) of all the individual values by the number (n) of values in the set

$$\bar{x} = \frac{\sum x}{n}$$

- Example
  - o What is the mean of the following data set: 2.5, 3.1, 4.3, 4.0, 5.2, 4.7, 4.8?
    - Answer: Divide the sum of the values by the total number of values

$$\bar{x} = \frac{28.6}{7} = 4.1$$

- Median
  - The number in the middle of an ordered data set
    - o Place the data set in numerical order
    - o If an odd number of values, select the number in the middle
    - o If an even number of values, the median is the average of the two middle numbers
  - Example
    - o What is the median of the following data set: 1, 2, 3, 9, 10, 12, 14
      - Answer: The median is 9
  - Example
    - o What is the median of the following data set: −2, 0, 2, 4, 5, 8
      - Answer: The median is $(2+4)/2 = 3$
- Mode
  - The most frequently found number(s) in a data set
  - Example
    - o In the data set {2, **5, 5, 5**, 7}, the mode is 5
    - o In the data set {1, **4, 4, 4**, 8, **9, 9, 9**, 15, 20}, the modes are 4 and 9
- Midrange (M)
  - The average of the lowest (L) and highest (H) values in a data set
  - Example
    - o In the data set {2, 3, 5, 6, 8}, what is the midrange?
      - Answer

$$M = \frac{L + H}{2} = \frac{2 + 8}{2} = 5$$

Measures of Variability

- Range (R)
  - The difference between the highest value and the lowest value in a sample set

$$R = H - L$$

  - Not often used, but an easy calculation for quick assessment of the comparative precision of test runs
    - o A larger range indicates decreased precision
- Variance (SD^2 or s^2) and standard deviation (SD or s)
  - First, determine the mean of the sample set
  - Next, a data table is created
    - o Each x value is placed in the first column
    - o The mean subtracted from each x value is in the second column ($x - \bar{x}$)
    - o The square of the difference between each x and the mean is listed in the third column $[(x - \bar{x})^2]$
    - o The sum of the values in the third column is inserted into the equation for variance

$$\text{Variance} = SD^2 = \frac{\sum (x - \bar{x})^2}{n - 1}$$

- Example
  - o For the data set {2.4, 2.6, 2.8, 3.3, 3.6, 3.9}, the number of values (n) is 6. The mean is

$$\bar{x} = \frac{\sum x}{n} = \frac{18.6}{6} = 3.1$$

  - o Create the data table as described previously using each x value and the mean

x	$(x - \bar{x})$	$(x - \bar{x})^2$
2.4	−0.7	0.49
2.6	−0.5	0.25
2.8	−0.3	0.09
3.3	0.2	0.04
3.6	0.5	0.25
3.9	0.8	0.64
		$\sum (x - \bar{x})^2 = 1.76$

  - o Solve for variance

$$SD^2 = \frac{\sum (x - \bar{x})^2}{n - 1} = \frac{1.76}{5} = 0.352$$

  - o Standard variation is, by definition, the square root of variance

$$\text{Standard deviation} = SD = \sqrt{SD^2} = \sqrt{\frac{\sum (x - \bar{x})^2}{n - 1}} = \sqrt{0.352}$$
$$= 0.593$$

Coefficient of Variation

- To use standard deviation to compare the precision of one assay to the precision of another assay, the relative differences in the size of values between the different assays must be normalized
- The standard deviation of an assay is divided by the mean of its results
- The resulting quotient is the coefficient of variability (CV), which is expressed as a percent

$$CV = \frac{SD}{\bar{x}} \times 100\%$$

- The assay with the lower CV value is the more precise assay
  - Example
    - Using the figures from the earlier section on standard deviation, the CV for that assay would be

$$CV = \frac{0.593}{3.1} \times 100\% = 19.1\%$$

    - If another assay has a standard deviation of 0.235 and a mean of 2.12, its CV would be

$$CV = \frac{0.235}{2.12} \times 100\% = 11.1\%$$

    - The second assay is more precise because its CV is lower

Accuracy and Precision

- Accuracy
  - Closeness of an individual result to the true value
  - In terms of the multiple results in a test procedure, accuracy can be judged in terms of measures of center
    - Example: An assay whose mean and/or median are close to the actual result would be considered accurate
- Precision
  - The reproducibility of a test procedure
  - Can be evaluated in terms of the measures of variability
    - Example: An assay with a low standard deviation or coefficient of variability can be considered a precise assay

Sensitivity, Specificity, and Predictive Values

- Four terms that correlate a patient's disease state to the test results
  - True positive (TP)
    - Patient has the disease and correctly tests positive
  - True negative (TN)
    - Patient does not have the disease and correctly tests negative
  - False positive (FP)
    - Patient does not have the disease, but the test results are positive
  - False negative (FN)
    - Patient has the disease, but the test results are negative
- Clinical sensitivity
  - Total number of patients with the disease can be defined as the sum of the true positives and false negatives
  - Proportion of true positive test results to the total patients with the disease

$$\text{Sensitivity} = \frac{\text{True positives}}{\text{Total diseased patients}} = \frac{TP}{TP + FN} \times 100\%$$

  - The sensitivity describes the ability to detect the target analyte even in low concentrations
  - A highly sensitive test can detect disease even when the disease marker is present in small amounts, thus preventing false negatives
  - A test with poor sensitivity has many false negatives because the test often misses the marker for the disease in specimens
- Clinical specificity
  - The total number of patients who do not have the disease is the sum of the true negatives and false positives
  - Proportion of the true negative test results to the total number of patients who do not have the disease

$$\text{Specificity} = \frac{\text{True negatives}}{\text{Total patients without disease}} = \frac{TN}{TN + FP} \times 100\%$$

  - Describes the ability to correctly detect only the intended marker of disease, not similar analytes that may be present
  - A highly specific test will have few false positives because only the specific analyte of disease is detected
  - A test with poor specificity will have many false positives because it will incorrectly interpret benign analytes as markers of disease
- Positive predictive value (PPV or PV$^+$)
  - Indicates the degree of certainty that positive or negative test results are correct
  - Proportion of the patients with positive results who actually have disease
  - Calculated by dividing the true positives by all positive test results

$$PPV = \frac{\text{True positives}}{\text{Total positives}} = \frac{TP}{TP + FP} \times 100\%$$

  - Indicates the certainty that a positive test result is correct
- Negative predictive value (NPV or PV$^-$) of a test is the proportion of the patients with negative results who are actually disease free
  - Calculated by dividing the true negatives by all negative test results

$$NPV = \frac{\text{True negatives}}{\text{Total negatives}} = \frac{TN}{TN + FN} \times 100\%$$

- Example
  - Determine the sensitivity, specificity, and predictive values in a new assay to detect influenza infection was developed and tested on 500 people; 200 people tested positive for the flu. Of these 200 positives, 185 were confirmed as being infected using the reference method. Of the remaining 300 people who tested negative, 6 were later shown to be infected with influenza
    - Answer
      - First, define basic information
        - Of the 200 total positive test results, 185 were shown to be true positive results, with the remaining 15 patients with positive results actually having false positive results
        - Of the 300 negative test results, 294 were confirmed as true negatives and the remaining 6 were shown to be false negatives
        - The total number of patients with disease is the sum of the true positives and false negatives: 191
        - The total number of patients who were disease free is the sum of the true negative and false positive results: 309
        - True positive (TP) = 185
        - False positive (FP) = 15
        - True negative (TN) = 294
        - False negative (FN) = 6
      - Next, use the previous equations to solve for sensitivity, specificity, PPV, and NPV

$$\text{sensitivity} = \frac{TP}{TP + FN} \times 100\% = \frac{185}{191} \times 100\% = 96.8\%$$

$$\text{specificity} = \frac{TN}{TN + FP} \times 100\% = \frac{294}{309} \times 100\% = 95.1\%$$

$$PPV = \frac{TP}{TP + FP} \times 100\% = \frac{185}{200} \times 100\% = 92.5\%$$

$$NPV = \frac{TN}{TN + FN} \times 100\% = \frac{294}{300} \times 100\% = 98.0\%$$

QUALITY CONTROL

Normal Distribution

- In any large sample of random data, if the data points on the x-axis are plotted against frequency on the y-axis, a bell-shaped curve will form, with its peak coinciding on the x-axis with the mean of the sample
- Normal (Gaussian) distribution
  - Curve is symmetrical around the vertical line that passes through the mean on the x-axis, and the curve approaches but never touches the x-axis—is considered a normal, or Gaussian, distribution

- The area under the curve represents the sum of all the frequencies of the numbers in the sample, and the total sum is 1
- The normal curve is useful in the clinical laboratory when the units on the x-axis are SD on either side of the mean
- In a normal curve
  - 68% of all numbers will fall between −1 SD and +1 SD of the mean
  - 95% will fall between −2 SD and +2 SD
  - 99% will fall between −3 SD and +3 SD
  - The values that fall within ±2 SD of the mean are considered normal and within the 95% *confidence interval*
  - The values outside ±2 SD but within ±3 SD of the mean are questionable
- The Levey-Jennings chart
  - Horizontal graph of quality control data
  - X-axis of the normal curve is converted to the vertical axis
    - Median flanked by 3 positive standard deviation increments above and 3 negative standard deviation increments below
    - Data points for each day plotted horizontally
    - Once the mean and standard deviations for an assay are determined, the Levey-Jennings chart provides an easy-to-read visual representation of quality control data generated over time
- Westgard Multirule set
  - Monitor quality control performance is based on control rules
  - Refer to Figure 11-2 for examples listed parenthetically in the following list
    - 1_{2s}: One control exceeds ±2 SD of the mean (day 1, level 1)
    - 1_{3s}: One control exceeds ±3 SD of the mean; indicative of random error (day 2, level 1)
    - 2_{2s}: Two consecutive controls are either +2 SD or −2 SD of the mean; indicative of systematic error (day 4, levels 1 and 2; or day 4 and 5, level 1)
    - R_{4s}: Combination of one control +2 SD of the mean and another −2 SD of the mean; indicative of random error (day 6, levels 1 and 2)
    - 4_{1s}: Four consecutive controls exceed either +1 SD or −1 SD of the mean; indicative of systematic error (days 7-10, level 1; or days 8-9, levels 1 and 2)
    - 10_x: 10 consecutive controls falling on one side or the other of the mean; indicative of systematic error (no example illustrated)
  - Whether violation of these rules constitutes a warning or a rejection depends on individual laboratory policies
- Some patterns in quality control results are defined more qualitatively
  - Shift

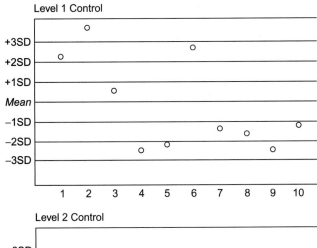

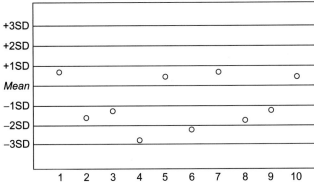

FIGURE 11-2 Examples of Levey-Jennings chart used for evaluation of quality control data.

- o Six or more control values fall on the same side of the mean
  - o The distance from the mean does not matter
  - o The problem does not necessarily grow steadily worse
  - o A shift represents that a new mean has been established
- Trend
  - o Six or more consecutive control values get continuously larger or smaller (i.e., a linear direction of values)
  - o Can move away from, toward, or across the mean
  - o Represents a progressively worsening problem
- Dispersion
  - o Uneven distribution of control values outside ±1 SD but within ±3 SD of the mean
  - o Increased dispersion represents loss of precision without loss of accuracy

CERTIFICATION PREPARATION QUESTIONS

For answers and rationales, please see Appendix A.

1. How many liters are in 4 dL?
   a. 400
   b. 40
   c. 0.4
   d. 0.04

2. How many liters are in 3 μL?
   a. 0.003
   b. 0.000003
   c. 0.0000003
   d. 0.000000003

3. How many micrograms are in 10 mg?
   a. 100
   b. 1000
   c. 10000
   d. 100000

4. How many grams are in 0.85 kg?
   a. 8.5
   b. 85
   c. 850
   d. 8500

5. 25° C is equivalent to how many degrees Fahrenheit?
   a. 31.7
   b. 45.9
   c. 77
   d. 102.6

6. 80° F is equivalent to how many Kelvin?
   a. 285.4
   b. 299.7
   c. 353.0
   d. 359.4

7. How would you prepare a 1/5 dilution of a urine sample?
   a. 1 part urine + 3 parts diluent
   b. 1 part urine + 4 parts diluent
   c. 1 part urine + 5 parts diluent
   d. 1 part urine + 6 parts diluent

8. A 50-g/L solution was diluted 1:5. This diluted sample was then diluted 1:10. What is the concentration of the final solution?
   a. 0.8 g/L
   b. 1 g/L
   c. 2.9 g/L
   d. 3.3 g/L

9. How much diluent is needed to prepare 300 mL of a 0.2-M working solution from a 0.8-M stock solution?
   a. 75 mL
   b. 225 mL
   c. 900 mL
   d. 1200 mL

10. What is the molarity of a solution containing 2 mol of sodium in 400 mL of water?
   a. 0.005 M
   b. 0.5 M
   c. 5 M
   d. 50 M

11. How many moles of glucose are in 300 mL of a 2-M glucose solution?
   a. 0.6
   b. 6
   c. 60
   d. 600

12. How many grams of NaCl are required to make 0.50 L of a 1.5-M NaCl solution? (MW of NaCl=58.5 g/mol)
    a. 4
    b. 19.5
    c. 44
    d. 175.5

13. What volume of diluent is in a 4-M solution containing 125.6 g of KCl (MW=74.5 g/mol)?
    a. 0.42 L
    b. 2.37 L
    c. 6.74 L
    d. 421 L

14. What is the normality of a 2-L solution of 54.2 g H_2SO_4 (MW=98.0 g)?
    a. 0.28 N
    b. 0.56 N
    c. 0.91 N
    d. 1.11 N

15. How many grams of NaCl (MW=58.5 g/mol) are in a 0.67-osmol/kg solution that was made from 3.0 kg of water?
    a. 39.4
    b. 59.1
    c. 102.2
    d. 236.4

16. In the calculation of the mean, what does "n" represent?
    a. The sum of the values
    b. The number of values in the set
    c. The average of the values
    d. The middle number of the set

17. What is the mode a reflection of in a data set?
    a. The average of the individual values in the data set
    b. The most frequent number in the data set
    c. The average of the lowest and highest numbers in the data set
    d. The number in the middle of the date set

18. Which of the following statistics is equivalent to the square root of the variance?
    a. Coefficient of variation
    b. Standard deviation
    c. Sensitivity
    d. Specificity

Use the data in Box *11-1* to answer questions 19 to 21.

BOX 11-1	Cholesterol Results for 10 Patients	
180	150	150
200	165	168
150	205	145
170		

19. Using the data in Box 11-1, what is the mean of the cholesterol results?
    a. 150
    b. 168
    c. 187
    d. 189

20. Using the data in Box 11-1, what is the mode of cholesterol results?
    a. 150
    b. 165
    c. 168
    d. 187

21. Using the data in Box 11-1, what is the standard deviation of the cholesterol results?
    a. 13.8
    b. 15.1
    c. 21.2
    d. 26.1

22. What is the midrange of the following data set: 10, 4, 6, 7, 12, 9, 14?
    a. 7
    b. 8.8
    c. 9
    d. 9.5

23. Which of the following is correct when rounding 2.25 to one decimal place?
    a. 2.2
    b. 2.3

24. What is the sum of the following figures: 0.125+3.45+32.981?
    a. 36.556
    b. 36.55
    c. 36.56
    d. 36.6

25. Which of the following represents the product of $(4 \times 10^3)(6 \times 10^2)$?
    a. 10×10^5
    b. 10×10^6
    c. 24×10^5
    d. 24×10^6

26. The closeness of a test value to the actual value describes which of the following?
    a. Accuracy
    b. Precision
    c. Reproducibility
    d. Reliability

27. Which of the Westgard rules is violated in the control data below? (Figure 11-3)
    a. 2_{2s}
    b. R_{4s}
    c. 4_{1S}
    d. 10_x

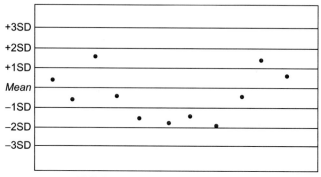

FIGURE 11-3 Quality control data.

28. Which of the following Westgard rules is indicative of random error?
    a. 1_{3S}
    b. 2_{2s}
    c. 4_{1s}
    d. 10_x

29. Which of the following pairs of concepts are correctly matched?
    a. Sensitivity: prevent false negatives :: specificity: prevent false positives
    b. Sensitivity: prevent false positives :: specificity: prevent false negatives
    c. Sensitivity: precision :: specificity: accuracy
    d. Sensitivity: coefficient of variation :: specificity: standard deviation

30. Which of the following equations represents the clinical sensitivity of a test?
    a. $\frac{TP}{TP + FN} \times 100\%$
    b. $\frac{TN}{TN + FP} \times 100\%$
    c. $\frac{TP}{TP + FP} \times 100\%$
    d. $\frac{TP}{TP + FP} \times 100\%$

BIBLIOGRAPHY

Bettelheim FA, March J: Introduction to organic & biochemistry, ed 3, Fort Worth, Tex, 1998, Harcourt Brace College.

Burtis CA, Ashwood ER, Bruns DE: Tietz fundamentals of clinical chemistry, ed 6, St. Louis, 2008, Saunders.

Campbell JB, Campbell JM: Laboratory mathematics: medical and biological applications, ed 5, St. Louis, 1997, Mosby.

Davidsohn I, Henry JB, editors: Todd-Sanford clinical diagnosis by laboratory methods, ed 14, Philadelphia, 1969, W.B. Saunders.

Pauling L, Pauling P: Chemistry, San Francisco, 1975, W.H. Freeman.

SELF-ASSESSMENT

Content Area: _____

Score on Practice Questions: _____

List the specific topics covered in the missed questions:

List the specific topics covered in the correct questions:

NOTES

A

Answers and Rationales to Certification Preparation Questions

---

CHAPTER 1

1. a. Some bacteria form thick-walled structures termed spores. These structures are formed during a process that makes a copy of a chromosome and encloses it with a thick protein coat. This spore is resistant to heat, cold, drying, most chemicals, and boiling. Spores can remain viable for many years in soil or dust.

2. c. Genus and species are italicized or underlined. Genus is capitalized; species is lowercase.

3. b. Bacterial cells generate stored energy in the form of ATP by one of two basic mechanisms: respiration or fermentation. Fermentation is metabolism in the absence of oxygen, an anaerobic process. In fermentation, glucose is converted into pyruvate by either the Embdem-Meyerhof pathway or glycolysis. Pyruvate can then enter several other cycles, and the end-products vary depending on cycle entered. In aerobic respiration, glucose usage under aerobic conditions and pyruvate enters the Kreb's cycle (TCA cycle). The end-products of respiration are carbon dioxide and water. The unique metabolic pathways and end-products produced by bacteria can be used to aid in the identification of particular genera or species.

4. d. Bacteria can acquire or exchange genetic material with other bacteria through several basic mechanisms: conjugation, transformation, or transduction. Conjugation involves cell-to-cell contact, a series of complex chemical signals between cells, and usually the formation of a bridge or sex pilus. Transformation is the uptake of free DNA by a recipient cell. Transduction is the acquisition of DNA through the action of a bacteria phage.

5. d. Transduction refers to moving genetic information from one prokaryote to another via a bacteriophage or virus.

6. c. The Gram stain procedure involves four steps: applying crystal violet—the initial purple dye that enters the cell; applying Gram's iodine—the mordent or chemical that binds to the crystal violet forming a complex; decolorizing—alcohol or acetone/alcohol is used to remove the crystal violet/iodine complex from gram-negative cells; and safranin counter stain—the red dye is used as a second stain. Gram-positive bacteria retained the initial crystal violet, the red counter stain blends with the violet, and gram-negative bacteria are only stained with the safranin and appear red.

7. d. Although many different bacteria can be isolated from skin and soft tissue infections, the two most common organisms are *Staphylococcus aureus* and *Streptococcus pyogenes*. We should be aware of these likely organisms as we read and report gram-stained smear results. *S. pneumoniae and N. gonorrhoeae* are important pathogens but rarely associated with skin infections. Although *Pseudomonas* can be associated with some unique infections of the skin, they are uncommon.

8. d. The two major uses for gram-stained smears are to evaluate the quality of a specimen (inflammation versus normal flora contamination) and describe the types of bacteria—gram-positive versus gram-negative. For sputum specimens, expectorated lower respiratory tract specimens, the following criteria are often applied: (1) more than 25 epithelial cells/low-power field = saliva, significant number of normal flora bacteria. (2) Few epithelial cells, many white blood cells = specimen more likely to yield a pathogen. In adult patients, specimens with significant numbers of epithelial cells often are not cultured and new samples are collected.

9. b. The atmosphere in which specimens are incubated can have a significant effect on the growth of potential pathogens. Many bacteria isolates will grow easily in routine air or with a slight increase in carbon dioxide, 3% to 5% CO_2 (aerobes). Other pathogens require special atmospheres for optimal growth, including increased CO_2, nitrogen, or decreased or complete absence of oxygen:
Microaerophilic: 5% O_2, 10% CO_2, 85% N
Anaerobic: 85% N_2, 10% H_2, 5% CO_2

10. d. Hektoen enteric (HE) contains meat peptones and yeast extract, bile salts (inhibit gram-positive organisms), lactose, sucrose, salacin (carbohydrate sources), pH indicators (bromophenol blue and acid fuchsin), and ferric ammonium citrate for the detection of H_2S production. This medium is very selective for enteric pathogens and is differential for *Salmonella* and *Shigella*. Yellow-orange colonies = lactose fermenter *(E. coli)*, colorless/green colonies with unchanged medium = non–lactose fermenter *(Shigella, Providencia)*, and black colonies = H_2S production *(Salmonella)*.

11. c. The genus *Staphylococcus* represents one of the most important groups of potentially pathogenic bacteria and most common normal flora organisms. This genus has the general characteristics of gram-positive cocci in clusters and is catalase-positive, facultative anaerobic, ferments glucose, and nonmotile.

12. a. A unique pathogenic factor of *Staphylococcus aureus* is the production of coagulase. This protein is responsible for the formation of fibrin clots in the host. Coagulase is found in two basic forms: bound to the surface of the cell, also known as clumping factor, and free in the medium. The bound form can be detected with several tests that demonstrate clumping of the bacterial cell or sensitized red blood cells, and the free form is most often detected by clot formation with rabbit plasma.

13. d. The initial testing of an isolate of a gram-positive cocci is catalase to differentiate the staphylococci (catalase-positive) from enterococci and streptococci (catalase-negative). If an isolate is catalase-positive and fits the general characteristics of a *Staphylococcus* spp., the coagulase test is used to differentiate S. *aureus* from the other species of the genus.

14. a. *Staphylococcus saprophyticus* is normal flora of the mucous membranes of the urogenital tract.

It causes urinary tract infection in some populations, especially young, sexually active women. In this population, it is considered significant in urine cultures even if it is found in small numbers.

15. d. *Staphylococcus aureus* is capable of producing a large number of molecules, which may contribute to its ability to cause disease. Toxic shock syndrome is a disease associated with the production of a specific toxin, toxic shock syndrome toxin–1 (TSST-1), which belongs to the group of toxins known as enterotoxins.

16. a. Several media can be used for selection of *Staphylococcus aureus* from mixed cultures. PEA or CNA would select for gram-positive organisms but are not specific for S. *aureus*. Mannitol salt agar was developed specifically to select for *Staphylococcus* spp. and to differentiate between S. *aureus* and other *Staphylococcus* spp., because S. *aureus* ferments mannitol and other species generally do not. More recently, chromogenic agars have been developed that are more specific for S. *aureus* and some have been designed to specifically detect methicillin-resistant S. *aureus*

17. a. Although some bacterial pathogens can cause vomiting and diarrhea, the hallmark of the staphylococcal enterotoxins is that because the toxins are preformed in the contaminated food, the organism does not need to grow in the host and therefore the action is very rapid. Most other enteric pathogens need to proliferate before the host experiences disease.

18. b. Of the organisms listed, only *Streptococcus pneumoniae* exhibits these characteristics. The two laboratory tests are bile solubility, which is the characteristic of S. *pneumoniae* isolates lysing when a solution of bile is dropped on the colony, and resistance to optochin. The optochin test is performed by streaking a lawn of organism onto a blood agar plate and then placing a standardized disk containing the chemical optochin onto the plate. After incubation, S. *pneumoniae* will not grow up to the disk—that is, growth is inhibited, demonstrating that the organism is susceptible to the chemical agent. Viridans group streptococci, S. *pyogenes,* and enterococci, do not autolyze in the presence of bile and are resistant to optochin.

19. b. Of the organisms listed, only *Streptococcus pyogenes* exhibits these characteristics. Clinically, S. *pyogenes* is the most important bacterial cause of pharyngitis. All isolates are susceptible to penicillin at this time. In the laboratory, β-hemolytic streptococci that are susceptible to bacitracin,

also known as the A disk, are presumptively identified as *S. pyogenes*, or group A β-hemolytic *Streptococcus*. The PYR test also can be used, because this pathogen is PYR-positive.

20. c. Of the organisms listed, only *Streptococcus agalactiae* exhibits these characteristics. Clinically, this organism, also known as group B *Streptococcus*, is an important cause of neonatal meningitis and sepsis. Of the β-hemolytic streptococci, it is unique in being hippurate hydrolysis–positive and CAMP test–positive. Latex or other grouping tests are usually used in clinical laboratories rather than hippurate or CAMP testing.

21. a. Rapid antigen detection tests are often used to aid in the diagnosis of group A pharyngitis. The present generation of tests are rapid, approximately 15 minutes, and reasonably sensitive—65% to 85% in general. Therefore (1) they can be useful in quickly identifying most cases of streptococcal pharyngitis. (2) Because of limits to the sensitivity, a negative test does not mean that the patient does not have the bacteria present and additional testing is often needed, so this statement is not true. (3) As stated, the major limitation in this test method is the limits to detecting small numbers of organisms—sensitivity. (4) The rapid antigen tests for group A streptococci is only for those bacteria and is not useful for the detection of viruses. Rapid antigens for viruses may detect some, but not all, causes of pharyngitis and are in general designed for bronchitis, bronchiolitis, and pneumonia.

22. c. The ability of streptococcal species to produce compounds that can alter the appearance or integrity of the red blood cells in 5% sheep blood agar can be used to help presumptively identify potential pathogens. α-Hemolysis is the appearance of a "green" band of red blood cells around a colony. This greening is due to the conversion of hemoglobin to methemoglobin. β-Hemolysis is the actual lysis of the red blood cells resulting in a clear area around the colony, γ-hemolysis is a term that historically was applied to colonies that did not alter the red blood cells, hence no zone around the colony. κ-Hemolysis is a nonsensical term. This image shows greening and thus α-hemolysis.

23. a. Two easily performed laboratory tests allow the differentiation of clinically important isolates of the genera *Enterococcus* from *Streptococcus*: growth in presence of 6.5% salt and growth on bile/esculin medium. Streptococci and enterococci are catalase-negative, do not produce coagulate, and will grow on PEA medium.

24. d. Of the organisms listed, only *Streptococcus* sp., not groups A, B or D meets these criteria. *Streptococcus pyogenes* is PYR positive and bacitracin susceptible. *S. agalactiae* is CAMP and hippurate positive. *Enterococcus faecalis* is bile esculin and salt positive.

25. b. Some bacteria that are environmental have a broad range of permissive growth temperatures. Among potentially pathogenic, gram-positive bacilli, the ability of *Listeria monocytogenes* to grow well at refrigerator temperatures can be used to select for this organism.

26. a. Among the gram-positive bacilli, several basic characteristics can be used to help differentiate the groups, including catalase, acid-fast, and modified acid-fast stains; bacterial cells that branch; and spore formation. Of the organisms listed, only *Corynebacterium* is a catalase-positive, gram-positive bacillus that is not acid-fast, does not branch, and does not form spores; the genus *Bacillus* forms spores, *Mycobacterium* is acid-fast, and *Nocardia* cells branch.

27. c. This clinical description is of diphtheria. *Corynebacterium diphtheriae* grows on tellurite medium, grows as black colonies with brown halos in Tinsdale medium, and shows gram-positive bacilli in irregular clublike shapes on gram-stained smears.

28. d. The genus *Corynebacterium* is a catalase-positive, gram-positive bacillus that is not acid-fast, does not branch, and does not form spores. It shows gram-positive bacilli in irregular clublike shapes on gram-stained smears. Group B *Streptococcus* would be seen as cocci in chains on gram-stained smear and would be catalase-negative, *Erysipelothrix* is H$_2$S-positive, and *Listeria* is motile.

29. c. The clinical description is classic for *Erysipelothrix* infection. This organism is positive for the production of H$_2$S on triple sugar iron (TSI) slants. The genus *Corynebacterium* is catalase-positive, gram-positive bacillus. Group B *Streptococcus* would be seen as cocci in chains on gram-stained smear and would be catalase-negative and β-hemolytic. *Listeria* would be motile and show hemolysis on blood agar.

30. c. Although the clinical disease has little overlap, in the laboratory *Erysipelothrix* and *Listeria monocytogenes* can appear similar. The most common tests for differentiating these organisms include: CAMP test (*Listeria*, positive; *Erysipelothrix*, negative), hydrogen sulfide production (*Listeria*, negative; *Erysipelothrix*, positive), and esculin hydrolysis (*Listeria*, negative; *Erysipelothrix*, positive).

31. b. Although *Streptococcus agalactiae* and *Listeria monocytogenes* may cause somewhat similar diseases and appear similar on 5% sheep blood agar, they can be differentiated with gram-stained smear (*S. agalactiae*, gram-positive cocci in chains from *L. monocytogenes*, gram-positive bacilli), catalase (*S. agalactiae*, negative from *L. monocytogenes*, positive), and motility (*S. agalactiae*, negative from *L. monocytogenes*, positive).

32. b. Endospores are unique to *Bacillus* sp. among aerobic gram-positive bacilli. All *Bacillus* spp. are catalase-positive. Once the genus is established, confirmation of *B. anthracis* requires additional testing such as demonstration of a capsule and lysis of the strain by specific bacteriophages.

33. d. *Bacillus anthracis* and *Bacillus cereus* can be differentiated in the laboratory by a variety of different test results. Of the combinations listed, motility (*B. anthracis* nonmotile and *B. cereus* motile) and β-hemolysis on 5% sheep blood agar (*B. anthracis* nonhemolytic and *B. cereus* hemolytic) best differentiate these two potential pathogens.

34. d. In a food-borne outbreak, *Bacillus cereus* can be found in the food. It does not cause a systemic infection but rather a toxin-mediated disease.

35. c. The single biggest challenge for the laboratory isolation of *Mycobacterium tuberculosis* from respiratory samples is the presence of normal organisms that grow more rapidly. Therefore the decontamination of these sputum samples with processes such as decontaminating the specimen with N-acetyl-L-cysteine (NALC)–sodium hydroxide mixture is critical for the successful isolation of *M. tuberculosis*.

36. c. The clinical description, the presence of acid-fast bacilli (AFB) in the sample, and the lack of growth in the laboratory, would raise suspicion that this sample contained an unusual and potentially non-cultivatable AFB, such as *Mycoplasma leprae*. The other organisms listed should grow within 8 weeks on standard medium.

37. d. The *Mycoplasma tuberculosis* complex is made up of several closely related organisms that primarily cause disease in humans. This group includes: *M. tuberculosis*, *M. bovis* (historically found in cattle), *M. bovis* BCG (vaccine strain for the BCG vaccine), and *M. africanum* (found in Western Africa and clinically similar to *M. tuberculosis*).

38. c. Nontuberculous mycobacteria (atypicals, mycobacteria other than tuberculosis [MOTT]), can be classified by a system first described by Ernest Runyon in 1959. This system classified organisms into four Runyon groups, based on:
Presence or absence of pigmentation?
Pigment production light dependent or not?
Growth rate slow or fast?
Runyon I: Photochromogens—slow growing, and produce a yellow-orange pigment when exposed to light.
Runyon II: Scotochromogens—slow growing, and produce a yellow-orange pigment in light or in the dark.
Runyon III: Nonchromogenic—slow growing, and do not produce pigment. Note that some may produce very pale yellow, buff, or tan pigment but do not intensify upon light exposure
Runyon IV: Rapid growers.

39. b. In identification of mycobacterial isolates, the Tween 80 test involves testing for lipase using polysorbate 80 (Tween 80). Certain mycobacterial species possess a lipase that splits polysorbate 80 into oleic acid and polyoxyethylated sorbitol. The test contains phenol red, which is stabilized, when the polysorbate 80 is hydrolyzed, the pH shifts and the phenol red indicator changes from yellow to pink.

40. b. For the organisms listed, the Enterobacteriaceae are, in general, oxidase-negative (this entire listed group). Traditionally, various biochemical characteristics are used to differentiate members of the large group of organisms. *Salmonella enteritidis* is oxidase-negative, nitrate-positive, indole-negative, citrate-positive, methyl red–positive, urease-negative, H_2S-positive; *Klebsiella pneumoniae* is indole-negative, citrate-positive, usually methyl red–negative (variable), urease-positive, H_2S-negative; *Escherichia coli* is indole-positive, citrate-negative, methyl red–positive, urease-negative, H_2S-negative; *Shigella sonnei* is indole-negative, citrate-negative, methyl red–positive, urease-negative, H_2S-negative.

41. c. For the organisms listed, the Enterobacteriaceae are, in general, oxidase negative (this entire listed group). Traditionally, various biochemical characteristics are used to differentiate members of the large group of organisms. *Proteus aerogenes* is not a valid name. *Escherichia coli* is indole-positive, H_2S-negative, and, although usually motile, not described as swarming. *Proteus mirabilis* and *Proteus vulgaris* can be differentiated using indole; *P. mirabilis* is negative and *P. vulgaris* is positive.

42. a. A significant cause of worldwide clinical disease is diarrhea. Cholera is an important cause of diarrhea and results in massive fluid loss, "rice water stools" (white blood cells and blood absent), and often death within 24 hours. Shiga toxin is a cytotoxin that causes inflammation and ulcerative lesions, destroys epithelial cells, and results in bloody, mucous-laden stools.

43. a. Thiosulfate-citrate-bile salts-sucrose agar (TCBS agar) is selective medium designed to aid in the isolation of *Vibrio* spp. TCBS agar contains sodium thiosulfate and sodium citrate to inhibit members of the Enterobacteriaceae. Gram-positive bacteria are inhibited by bile salts. Ferric citrate is used to detect hydrogen sulfide production. Sucrose is included as a fermentable carbohydrate to help differentiate *V. cholera* from other species. Bromothymol blue is included as an indicator of pH changes.

44. b. *C. jejuni* is the most common human pathogen of this genus. It is associated with food-borne gastroenteritis because of its presence in poultry, raw milk, and water. It is one of the most common causes of human bacterial gastroenteritis in numerous parts of the United States.

45. a. The urea slant can be used to aid in identification of enteric gram-negative bacilli. The test detects the ability of bacteria to hydrolyze urea to ammonia and CO_2; ammonia release causes pH change. A positive test yields a bright pink slant.

46. b. *Salmonella enteritidis* grows well on XLD agar and is a nonfermenting organism that produces H_2S, resulting in the black pigment. *Shigella sonnei* would appear as clear colonies, *Serratia* and *Klebsiella* are both lactose fermenting and would appear as yellow colonies.

47. c. Growth on CIN agar with this characteristic colonial morphology is indicative of *Yersinia enterocolitica*.

48. d. Decarboxylation of the amino acids lysine, ornithine, and arginine results in the formation of the following amine end-products: Ornithine decarboxylase (ODC), ornithine → putrescine; lysine decarboxylase (LDC), lysine → cadaverine; arginine dihydrolase (ADH), arginine → citrulline.

49. b. Triple sugar iron (TSI) slants have traditionally been used to help identify and differentiate stool pathogens. These reactions are characteristic of *Shigella* spp.

50. c. *Bordetella pertussis* infects the upper airway. The best specimen for identification of this pathogen has been shown to be collected from the nasopharynx.

51. c. When stained using the Gram stain, members of the genus *Brucella* usually appear as gram-negative coccobacilli.

52. a. *Legionella pneumophila* requires specialized medium, 35° C, carbon dioxide, and extended incubation; hold for 2 weeks.

53. c. Of the media listed, only chocolate agar provides the X and V factors required for the growth of *Haemophilus* spp.

54. a. Most members of the genus *Haemophilus* require X and V factors, and these factors are a key characteristic in the identification of this genus. The factor requirement test involves inoculation of unsupplemented media with a light suspension of the organism and placement of X and V factor disks on the agar surface. Growth around only the X/V combination supports the identification of *Haemophilus* spp.

55. a. *Eikenella corrodens* is an asaccharolytic, oxidase-positive bacillus that does not grow on MacConkey agar and that produces a bleachlike odor. *Eikenella* has been referred to as part of the HACEK group of organisms along with *Hemophilus*, *Actinobacillus*, *Cardiobacterium*, and *Kingella*. It is most often associated with wounds of the mouth or teeth or other wounds originating with contact with the mouth or teeth, but has been known to cause subacute bacterial endocarditis.

56. c. Reporting of a sexually transmitted infection (STI) from a child younger than 12 years of age usually has significant social and legal ramifications. Because other *Neisseria* spp. can be incorrectly identified as *Neisseria gonorrhoeae*, particular care and additional confirmatory testing are often the most appropriate course of action.

57. a. Of the species of *Neisseria* found in humans, *N. meningitidis* is a glucose-positive, maltose-positive, sucrose-negative, lactose-negative major cause of bacterial meningitis.

58. b. Of the species of *Neisseria* found in humans, *N. gonorrhoeae* is an oxidase-positive, glucose-positive, maltose-negative, sucrose-negative, lactose-negative major cause of venereal disease.

59. b. When seen in a gram-stained smear, *Nesseria spp.* are gram negative diplococci.

60. a. The Hugh-Leifson oxidative-fermentative (OF) test shows a pH shift in the open glucose tube and no pH in the closed tube. This indicates that this organism is an oxidizer.

61. b. The oxidase test detects the presence of cytochrome oxidase. This enzyme is part of the energy transfer cascade of intermediate metabolism.

62. d. In the laboratory, *Stenotrophomonas maltophilia* has unique characteristics, including growth on blood agar and chocolate agar with a green-lavender or yellow pigment. Colonies are non–lactose fermenting on MacConkey agar, oxidase-negative, catalase-positive, and esculin-positive. This gram-negative bacillus strongly oxidizes maltose but only weakly oxidizes glucose.

63. b. Melioidosis is caused by *Burkholderia pseudomallei*.

64. a. *Stenotrophomonas maltophilia* is oxidase-negative, and *Burkholderia cepacia* is oxidase-positive.

65. b. *Acinetobacter* and *Stenotrophomonas* are oxidase-negative. The soluble green pigment differentiates *Pseudomonas aeruginosa* from *Burkholderia*.

66. a. Key tests can be used to differentiate *Acinetobacter* from *Pseudomonas*. Two easy tests are oxidase (*Pseudomonas* is positive and *Acinetobacter* is negative) and motility (*Pseudomonas* is positive and *Acinetobacter* is negative).

67. a. Cystic tryptic agar (CTA) sugar reactions are used to differentiate *Neisseria* species. If *Moraxella catarrhalis* is tested in this system, the isolate will be glucose-negative, maltose-negative, lactose-negative, and sucrose-negative.

68. b. Of the organisms listed, only *Pseudomonas aeruginosa* produces the pigment pyocyanin.

69. b. Of the tests listed, the oxidase test is the only test that exhibits a dark purple color.

70. c. An important characteristic of *Mycoplasma* and *Ureaplasma* is that both genera have only a cell membrane with no cell wall.

71. c. Nongonococcal urethritis (NGU) is an infectious clinical condition that is most often associated with *Ureaplasma urealyticum*.

72. c. Traditional methods for the detection of *Chlamydia trachomatis* infections included cytology, culture, antigen detection, and serology. These methods are all much less sensitive than nucleic acid amplification methods, which have become the standard detection methods for this infection in most situations.

73. c. Because of the clinical signs and symptoms, including the rash, the most likely of those listed is Rocky Mountain spotted fever. Additional testing may be required. Rocky Mountain spotted fever is the most common rickettsial disease in the United States. The disease is characterized by abrupt onset of fever, chills, headache, and myalgia. A rash is common and usually begins on the hands and feet and spreads toward the trunk. Diagnosis is often based on the clinical disease but fluorescent antibody (FA) or polymerase chain reaction (PCR) for antigen in skin biopsies can be performed.

74. a. Primary syphilis is characterized by a chancre that typically heals within 6 weeks.

75. c. Of the tests listed, only the VDRL is a valid nontreponemal test.

76. b. This patient's signs and symptoms are classic for Lyme disease. Laboratory testing is often performed to support the diagnosis.

77. c. The characteristic lesion, lack of demonstrable organism in the lesion by gram-stained smear, and the reactive rapid plasma reagin (RPR) test all support the diagnosis of syphilis (*Treponema pallidum*).

78. c. Based on the gram-stained smear and basic biochemical reactions, the best identification of this organism is *Bacteroides fragilis*.

79. a. Pseudomembranous colitis caused by *Clostridium difficile* is best confirmed by the presence of toxin in the stool. In some unusual circumstances, the organism may need to be isolated from the stool and then tested for its ability to produce toxin.

80. a. Lecithinase production, double-zone hemolysis on sheep blood agar, and gram-stained morphology are key criteria in the identification of *Clostridium perfringens*.

81. c. The most common way to confirm that an anaerobic system has the correct gas mixture is to use the change in color of the methylene blue indicator.

82. b. The presence of sulfur granules in a clinical specimen from the neck, mouth, or respiratory tract of the patient strongly indicates the presence of *Actinomyces* spp.

83. a. Both the E test and agar disk diffusion or Kirby-Bauer test are used for antimicrobial susceptibility testing and are based on the diffusion of an antibiotic into an agar-based medium. In the medium, both systems establish an antibiotic gradient.

84. b. The most important clinical need for minimum inhibitory concentration (MIC) testing is when the organism isolated does not have a predictable pattern or the organism is isolated in an isolated body site such as the central nervous system.

85. b. The best definition of minimum inhibitory concentration (MIC) is the lowest concentration of an antibiotic in a dilution series that inhibits growth of the bacteria.

86. c. When comparing minimum inhibitory concentration (MIC) testing to Kirby-Bauer or disk diffusion testing, the lower the MIC, the larger is the zone of inhibition.

87. a. The antibiotic concentration in a disk used for Kirby-Bauer testing is designed to give a specific zone of inhibition for control stains of bacteria. If the organism is able to grow closer to the disk than expected, the concentration of the antibiotic in the disk is too low.

88. a. Of the definitions listed, only urethritis refers to an infection of the lower urinary tract.

89. c. *Streptococcus pneumoniae* commonly associated with Otitis Media; its identification includes the Optochin test.

90. b. *Streptococcus pyogenes* causes impetigo, of the organisms listed.

91. a. Staphylococci produce hyaluronidase which can break down connective tissue, allowing for the spread of infection.

92. d. Because of the need to isolate potentially fastidious pathogens and anaerobic bacteria, routine cultures of cerebrospinal fluid should include 5% sheep blood agar, chocolate agar, or thioglycolate broth. Other clinical conditions may warrant additional specialized media.

93. c. The clinical symptoms exhibited by the patient are consistent with a potential diagnosis of meningitis.

94. a. In cases of vaginitis, clue cells are a common finding. Clue cells are epithelial cells covered with small gram positive bacilli found in vaginal discharge.

95. b. The term aseptic meningitis describes meningitis that is characterized by negative bacterial and fungal culture.

96. c. Most patient samples for bacteriology cultures only can be semi-quantitated, because of sampling and plating limitations. Urine cultures, however, are routinely quantitated to aid the differentiation of true infection from contamination.

97. b. Quality control practices ensure that the test results are accurate. Therefore Gram staining and reading a glass slide with a mixed smear of *Staphylococcus* and *Escherichia coli* along with each gram-staining run of specimens examined within the microbiology laboratory that day is an example of quality control. Quality assurance is the overall process of ensuring the quality of the results reported by the laboratory and includes quality control, employee training and certification, etc.

98. d. Tracking the rate of skin organism contamination among a laboratory's blood culture results on a monthly basis and introducing specific training to phlebotomists when rates exceed the norm would be an example of quality assurance. Quality assurance is the overall process of ensuring the quality of the results reported by the laboratory and includes quality control, employee training and certification, etc.

99. b. Infectious substances are substances known or reasonably expected to contain pathogens.

100. d. Because of the need to quantitate the sample and the fact that bacteria grow in urine, making storage and transport of sample critical, a 24-hour urine sample for bacteriology culture is inappropriate.

CHAPTER 2

1. c. In contrast to bacteria, yeasts reproduce by a process known as budding. The process in the mother yeast cell begins with a weakening and outpouching of the yeast cell wall and then formation of a cell wall septum between the mother and daughter yeast cells. When the cells separate, there is a "bud scar" left on the surface of the mother cell.

2. d. The loose intertwined network of basic structural units of the molds that grows in a matlike structure is known as the mycelium.

3. c. Molds that form hyphae and reproductive structures with little or no pigment are often referred to as hyaline molds.

4. b. Certain molds form two types of conidia: macroconidia and microconidia. Macroconidia are large, multiseptate and club-shaped or spindle-shaped spores, whereas microconidia are small, nonseptate teardrop-shaped spores.

5. d. The structure indicated in the image is a conidiophore of an isolate of *Aspergillus*.

6. c. Historically, the differentiation of dermatophytes was accomplished using a variety of morphologic characteristics and growth characteristics. The characteristics listed support the identification of *Microsporum audouinii*. The most suggestive of these characteristics is the rare distorted macroconidia and rare microconidia.

7. b. *Blastomyces dermatitidis* is endemic to North America, specifically the Mississippi river valley. When seen in tissue samples it appears as large, spherical, thick-walled yeast cells 8 to 15 μm in diameter, usually with a single bud that is connected to the parent cell by a broad base.

8. c. *Coccidioides immitis* is endemic in hot, semi-arid climates such as the southwestern United States and northern Mexico. It is a saprobe in mold form (desert soil). It is the most virulent of all agents of human mycoses. *Coccidioides* causes mild infection in everyone who inhales it, but is usually asymptomatic and self-limiting. Dissemination in the immunocompromised population is much higher than found for other fungal agents. The part of its life cycle in the mammalian host is highlighted by the endosporulating spherules in tissue.

9. a. These are the characteristic large, spherical, thick-walled yeast cells 8 to 15 μm in diameter showing broad-based budding.

10. b. *Sporothrix schenckii* is found worldwide (soil saprobe). It is a thermal dimorph. Infections with this fungus is an occupational risk and is often referred to as rose gardeners disease. The clinical disease of sporotrichosis usually involves chronic cutaneous and subcutaneous mycosis characterized by ulcers and abscesses along lymphatic channels.

11. c. The most common phenotypic test for the identification of *Candida* spp. is the germ tube test. *C. albicans* is defined as germ tube–positive. *Torulopsis glabrata (Candida glabrata)* is urease negative and unable to assimilate dextrose, maltose, or sucrose. CMT agar morphology shows blastoconidia only.

12. d. *Cryptococcus neoformans* can be differentiated from other *Cryptococcus* species through the use of the Niger seed test; *C. neoformans* is Niger seed–positive (dark colonies).

13. c. The most common phenotypic test for the identification of *Candida* spp. is the germ tube test. *C. albicans* is defined as germ tube–positive. The standard procedure needs to be followed because it is well described that changes in incubation conditions can significantly affect the test. *Candida albicans* and *Candida tropicalis* can be used a positive and negative control, respectively.

14. a. The classification of *Pneumocystis jiroveci* has been contested. It has been considered many different things over the years, including a fungus and a protozoan. It is known to cause opportunistic infections in the immunocompromised patient. Diagnosis requires demonstration of the organism in tissue, lavage, or sputum. It cannot be cultured except in animal models. In the laboratory, Grocott's methenamine silver (GMS) stain is commonly used to identify the organism, which appears as "cups and saucers" or "deflated balls."

15. b. The appearance and biochemical characteristics of this organism support the identification of *Candida albicans*. The germ tube test is a key indicator.

16. b. *Malassezia furfur* is normal skin flora in 90% of humans. Clinically it is responsible for tinea versicolor and catheter-related infections in patients on long-term intravenous lipids. Macroscopically the organism appears as cream/brown wrinkled colonies that grow better in the presence of oil. Microscopically it grows as yeastlike cells, often with distinct collarettes.

17. c. Conidiation of dematiaceous fungi includes three basic types of structures: (1) *Cladosporium* type—resembles a tree, in which conidiophore is the trunk and branched chains of conidia form the branches; (2) *Phialophora* type—short conidiophores plus phialide, vase-shaped conidia extruded from phialide and then clustered; and (3) *Rhinocladiella* type—stalked conidiophores that become knobby as conidia are produced. Conidia are produced sequentially until a *Cladosporium*-type conidiation is reached.

18. b. *Acremonium* sp. is a mold that displays a white cottony macroscopic morphology and, on microscopic evaluation, exhibits hyaline, septate hyphae, and "toothbrush"-like conidiophores.

19. a. *Penicillium* sp. is a mold that displays a velvety, gray-green colony morphology. On microscopic evaluation, flask-shaped conidiophores arranged in a brushlike formation are seen.

20. a. The macroscopic morphology, color, temperature tolerance, and growth rate, combined with the microscopic characteristics, supports *Aspergillus* as the genus and *A. fumigatus* as the species.

21. b. The protein coat that surrounds the nucleic acid is called the capsid.

22. b. Viral envelopes are acquired as the virion buds through the membrane of the mammalian host cell and picks up components of the membrane.

23. b. Prions are unique infectious proteins with no associated nucleic acids.

24. a. Viruses have different structures than bacterial or mammalian cells. The viral nucleocapsid is the protein coat that contains or covers the nucleic acid (genome) of the virus particle.

25. c. Norovirus is an important cause of gastroenteritis in several settings, including closed environments such as cruise ships and long-term care facilities. None of the other viruses listed are associated with gastroenteritis as a major symptom.

26. b. The severe acute respiratory syndrome (SARS) virus arose as a previously unrecognized organism causing serious respiratory tract infections. This virus has been shown to be part of the coronavirus group.

27. c. This is the description of the coronavirus group.

28. d. Rotaviruses are responsible for significant outbreaks of gastroenteritis and are an enteric virus. The specimen of choice for detecting this virus is stool.

29. b. Nucleic amplification assays such as polymerase chain reaction are the most sensitive method for the detection of many/most viruses and patient samples, including cerebrospinal fluid for the diagnosis of meningitis.

30. a. This typical fibroblastic cell line is showing the rapid development of foci of rounding and degenerating cells. This is typical of herpes simplex virus in culture.

31. d. The trophozoite form is the motile, feeding, and multiplying form of amoeba. Trophozoites require a moist or liquid environment; when such an environment is not present, the trophozoite has the ability to convert to the cyst form.

32. b. Polyvinyl alcohol (PVA) is most often used for fixed smear preparation. It is less effective when used in concentration methods than is formalin-ethyl acetate. Formalin fixatives do not preserve the morphology of organisms well enough for use in fixed smear preparation. Merthiolate-iodine-formaldehyde (MIF) is not used for the same reason.

33. a. *Taenia solium*, the pork tapeworm, is known to cause cysticercosis. The oncosphere form can migrate through the bloodstream and invade tissue, forming a cystlike structure.

34. d. *Strongyloides stercoralis* is not often recovered in the ovum stage in feces. The rhabditiform larval stage is the primary diagnostic stage for strongyloidiasis.

35. c. Identifying multiple parasites in fecal specimens is common, so a full examination of each slide is necessary.

36. a. *Necator americanus*, *Ancylostoma duodenale*, and *Strongyloides stercoralis* all pass through the human lung during their life cycles.

37. a. Morphologically, *Acanthamoeba* spp. appear as a wrinkled, double-walled cyst and are known to cause corneal keratitis.

38. d. *Trichuris trichiura* is known as whipworm because of the appearance of the adult larva. Adult larvae are typically 2.5 to 5.0 cm. in length. The posterior end of the larva is large, and the anterior end is slender and long, resembling a whip handle and whip. Additionally, the adult male larva possesses a curved tail.

39. b. *Schistosoma haematobium* ova are typically 110 to 170 microns by 40 to 70 microns and possess a large terminal spine. *S. haematobium* ova are recovered in urine.

40. c. *Echinococcus granulosus* is found in areas where sheep are raised in close proximity to dogs; the dog is the true definitive host. Sheep and humans are accidental intermediate hosts. *E. granulosus* larvae are typically 4.0 to 5.0 mm in length and comprise a scolex and three proglottids.

41. b. *Entamoeba coli* trophozoites are typically 15 to 50 microns in diameter. Morphologic criteria include one nuclei with an eccentric karyosome and irregular peripheral chromatin, vacuolated cytoplasm, and broad pseudopods.

42. c. *Giardia lamblia* cysts measure approximately 8 to 19 microns in length. Morphologic features include an ovoid shape, two to four nuclei, two to four median bodies, and a smooth wall.

43. c. *Entamoeba histolytica* cysts measure approximately 12 to 15 microns in diameter. Morphologic features include a round shape, two to four nuclei, and a rounded chromatoid bar. Clinically, blood may be seen in stool samples of individuals with an *E. histolytica* infection.

44. a. c.; b. d.; c. a.; d. b.

45. d. The diagnostic criteria of *Wuchereria bancrofti* include the presence of a sheath and nuclei that do not extend to the tail tip. The organism also demonstrates nocturnal periodicity.

46. d. *Necator americanus* rhabditiform larvae possess a long buccal cavity and a small genital primordium. Neither the rhabditiform or filariform larval stage has a notched tail. *Strongyloides stercoralis* rhabditiform larvae possess a short buccal cavity and a prominent genital primordium. Filariform larvae possess a notched tail.

47. a. The morphologic appearance of *B. hominis* is distinct. The organism typically measures 5 to 30 microns in diameter. The center of each comprises a large vacuole that generally stains a teal color with the trichrome stain. The central vacuole is surrounded by a thin rim of cytoplasm that contains two to six small nuclei.

48. a. c.; b. d.; c. a.; d. b.

49. a. Medically important known human tapeworms include *Dipylidium caninum*, *Diphyllobothrium latum*, *Hymenolepis diminuta*, *Hymenolepis nana*, *Taenia saginata*, and *Taenia solium*. *D. latum* is the only one with operculated ova.

50. a. *Trypanosoma* spp. are hemoflagellates that can be identified in peripheral blood smears as a trypomastigote form. Trypomastigotes assume a C, S, or U shape in blood. Each one is characterized by a central nucleus, a posterior kinetoplast, and a full-body undulating membrane.

CHAPTER 3

1. c. Serum ferritin concentrations reflect the body's storage of ferritin. Serum iron measures free iron, and serum transferrin provides a measure of how many binding sites are available to bind iron and is used with transferrin saturation, the percentage of sites available to carry iron.

2. a. Iron-deficiency anemia resulting from the decreased mean corpuscular volume (MCV) and mean corpuscular hemoglobin (MCH), indicating hypochromic microcytic cells. Vitamin B_{12} deficiency typically exhibits macrocytosis. Anemia of chronic inflammation tends to exhibit a mild anemia, with a hemoglobin value of approximately 9 to 11 g/dL. Hemochromatosis is not an anemia and, untreated, exhibits a normal to elevated red blood cell count.

3. b. The inclusions suggest the presence of excess storage iron. Sideroblastic anemia is a disorder characterized by elevated iron stores resulting from an inability to incorporate iron into heme. The inclusions suggest the presence of excess storage iron. Ringed sideroblasts may also be found in bone marrow examinations. Iron-deficiency anemia shows a microcytic hypochromic anemia; however, it is characterized by a lack of iron. Pernicious anemia is a megaloblastic anemia. Thalassemia minor shows a microcytic hypochromic anemia; however, it often has an elevated red blood cell count with hypochromic, microcytic cells but would not normally show iron inclusions (although transfusion-dependent thalassemias may exhibit transfusion-associated iron excess).

4. a. Iron-deficiency anemia is most likely, because sideroblastic anemia and hemochromatosis show increased iron and ferritin with a decreased total iron-binding capacity (TIBC) whereas anemia of chronic inflammation has decreased serum iron and percent saturation but normal-to-increased serum ferritin.

5. c. Gastrointestinal disease may lead to malabsorption, which could possibly affect iron absorption. Alcoholism and lead poisoning can lead to a secondary sideroblastic anemia, and primary sideroblastic anemia may be seen in myelodysplastic syndromes, such as refractory anemia with ringed sideroblasts (RARS).

6. b. Intrinsic factor antibodies would be present in patients with a true megaloblastic anemia, because it is characterized by the destruction of parietal cells, which produce the intrinsic factor needed for B_{12} absorption. Homocysteine is elevated in both vitamin B_{12} and folic acid deficiencies. *Diphyllobothrium latum* can cause megaloblastic

anemia because it competes for vitamin B_{12} in the intestines; however, testing for ova and parasites alone will not define the diagnosis. A bone marrow examination could determine that megaloblastic features were present; however, it would not be specific for pernicious anemia.

7. b. Megaloblastic anemias result from deficiencies in vitamin B_{12} and folic acid. Both are needed for normal cell maturation. Iron and hepcidin play a role in anemias with iron problems, whereas decreased free erythrocyte protoporphyrin (FEP) is seen in some porphyrias. Decreased liver function, alcoholism, and severe hypothyroidism can cause macrocytic anemia, but the anemia is not megaloblastic.

8. c. Pernicious anemia is a megaloblastic anemia that results from defective DNA synthesis from lack of vitamin B_{12}, often showing dysplastic changes in the cells and sometimes requiring a bone marrow examination to confirm the deficiency, particularly to differentiate from myelodysplastic syndromes. The others do not have a need for bone marrow examination.

9. b. Vitamin B_{12} and folic acid are the best place to start in further investigating this patient's anemia, because this will determine the specific follow-up most valuable to the physician. Iron studies could be performed, but a deficiency is unlikely given the macrocytic appearance of the red blood cells. Bone marrow examination is not usually performed unless confirmation of other testing or rule out of myelodysplastic syndrome (MDS) is needed. Intrinsic factor antibody assays may be used to further work up the case if vitamin B_{12} levels are decreased, because the reason for the decrease would need to be confirmed or ruled out.

10. a. Approximately 70% of acquired aplastic anemia cases are idiopathic (Rodak, 2012). It can occur as a result of other stimuli, including various drugs, radiation exposure, and viral infections.

11. c. The absolute lymphocyte count is most likely to be normal, because lymphocytes may also reside in lymphoid tissue beyond the bone marrow. The others and their precursors are primarily found in the bone marrow and tend to have a shorter life span in circulation.

12. a. Fanconi's anemia is characterized by mutations in a group of genes that lead to fragile chromosomes, which break easily and may not be able to repair themselves.

13. c. Haptoglobin is a protein that picks up free hemoglobin, and it frequently decreases as it is used up when free hemoglobin (Hgb) is present in excess of haptoglobin's carrying capacity. Bilirubin, both total and unconjugated, is increased with the increased red blood cell destruction. Plasma Hgb and urine hemosiderin are also increased because of the excesses of free Hgb.

14. b. Macrocytic, normochromic cells with increased polychromasia are present in most cases of hemolytic anemia, because reticulocytes are being released prematurely from the bone marrow to replace cells being destroyed. Microcytic and hypochromic cells are usually seen in disorders of iron/heme metabolism.

15. d. Anemia of chronic disease is characterized by a block in iron incorporation and is a mild anemia, not characterized by increased cell destruction. Sickle cell, active glucose-6-dehydrogenase (G6PD) deficiency, and autoimmune hemolytic anemia are types of hemolytic anemia.

16. b. The direct antiglobulin test (DAT) would be the best test to begin determining the cause of anemia, because it can help determine if spherocytes are the result of immune activity or if they are due to abnormal red blood cell skeletal protein interactions. Osmotic fragility will be decreased in the presence of spherocytes. Glucose-6-dehydrogenase (G6PD) activity would be useful only if G6PD deficiency was present. Vitamin B_{12} is used to determine the cause of macrocytic anemia and does not usually result in spherocytes.

17. a. The *PIGA* gene codes for glycophosphatidylinositol (GPI)-anchored proteins. Paroxysmal nocturnal hemoglobinuria shows a mutation in the *PIGA* gene, which results in deficiencies in GPI proteins, indicated by a negative CD55 and CD59.

18. a. Glucose-6-dehydrogenase (G6PD) deficiency shows lack of enzyme activity that is needed for the reduction of glutathione, which in turn works to deal with protecting hemoglobin from oxidant damage. Defective globin chains can be seen in hemolytic hemoglobinopathies or thalassemia. Antibodies to red blood cells are present in immune-mediated hemolytic anemias, and abnormal protein structure is seen in disorders such as hereditary elliptocytosis or hereditary spherocytosis.

19. c. All are microangiopathic hemolytic anemias, with the exception of traumatic cardiac hemolytic anemia, because they feature intravascular hemolysis resulting from red blood cells (RBCs) shearing when they contact microclots in the circulation. Traumatic cardiac hemolytic anemia is macroangiopathic, because the hemolysis occurs when RBCs move through implanted cardiac devices or patients with cardiac valve issues.

20. d. Thrombotic thrombocytopenic purpura (TTP) is the most likely cause of the laboratory results, because it is consistent with the anemia and thrombocytopenia with the presence of schistocytes. The patient is exhibiting normal coagulation results, which would be increased in disseminated intravascular coagulation (DIC). Chronic myelogenous leukemia could show decreased red blood cell and platelet count; however, this is a younger patient with normal white blood cells. Sickle cell disease is unlikely in a previously healthy female, and the decreased platelets and schistocytes point more to a microangiopathic hemolytic anemia (MAHA).

21. b. The majority of warm autoimmune hemolytic anemia cases involve IgG antibodies, although other antibodies, such as IgA or IgM, may be implicated in rare cases.

22. b. Idiopathic onset is an unknown cause of warm autoimmune hemolytic anemia (WAIHA). Secondary WAIHA is usually associated with chronic lymphoid disorders, viral infections, and autoimmune disorders.

23. a. $\beta^{6Glu \rightarrow Val}$ is the mutation seen in sickle cell anemia. $\beta^{6Glu \rightarrow Lys}$ is the mutation seen in hemoglobin (Hgb) C, $\beta^{26Glu \rightarrow Lys}$ is the mutation seen in Hgb E, and $\beta^{63Glu \rightarrow Arg}$ is seen in Hgb Zurich.

24. d. All of these conditions are associated with sickle cell disease; however, vasoocclusion is common and leads to painful crises that often result in hospital visits.

25. a. Patients with sickle cell trait usually have no clinical symptoms or abnormalities on their complete blood count, although they may exhibit occasional target cells. Under extreme stress or hypoxia, patients may have serious complications similar to those seen in actual sickle cell disease.

26. b. Hemoglobin (Hgb) electrophoresis, high-performance liquid chromatography, or isoelectric focusing is the best means for determining the specific Hgbs present in a patient sample. Solubility testing is a good screen to look for abnormal Hgbs, but does not determine specific Hgb presence or approximate quantities. Bone marrow analysis is an invasive technique and does not provide a

definitive listing for the Hgbs present. Peripheral smear review may show the presence of sickle cells; however, it will not determine if Hgb S is present in the case of someone heterozygous for Hgb S.

27. b. The crystals are likely hemoglobin (Hgb) C, because this abnormal Hgb tends to polymerize in short hexagonal crystals. Hgb S will polymerize into sickle cells. Hgb SC polymerizes into forms that are a hybrid of Hgb S and Hgb C that look like fingers or birds. Hgb E does not form specific crystalloid shapes.

28. c. This patient most likely has thalassemia minor, in addition to his sore throat. The patient has an elevated red blood cell (RBC) count with a disproportionately low hemoglobin and hematocrit, which is often seen in thalassemia minor. Warm autoimmune hemolytic anemia would lead to a decrease in the RBC count. Results are not consistent with a cold agglutinin.

29. a. Hemoglobin H is the result of a three-gene deletion on the α gene. A two-gene deletion would result in α-thalassemia minor.

30. b. This is likely a case of β-thalassemia because hemoglobin (Hgb F) ($\alpha_2\gamma_2$) and Hgb A_2 ($\alpha_2\delta_2$) are increased. Thus α chains are able to be produced; however, β chains are lacking so no Hgb A ($\alpha_2\beta_2$) is present. The other disorders listed are all covered in the α-thalassemia group.

31. c. This is consistent with Pelger-Huet anomaly, which is characterized by mature neutrophils, but hyposegmentation in the majority of neutrophils. Alder-Reilly anomaly features abnormal granulation, leukocyte adhesion deficiency shows relatively normal looking but functionally abnormal neutrophils.

32. a. Acute bacterial infection is the most likely cause of these results, with an elevated white blood cell count and shift to the left. Although some similarities may exist in the complete blood count picture for chronic myelogenous leukemia (CML), the patient is relatively young for the diagnosis. Additionally, the patient appears to have normal red blood cell (RBC) and platelet counts, which may decrease with the neoplastic clone in CML. Viral infections usually show elevations in lymphocyte numbers. Refractory anemia is unlikely because the patient has normal RBC counts.

33. a. α-Naphthyl acetate esterase can be used to exhibit positive esterase activity in monocytes, whereas neutrophils and lymphocytes usually stain

negative. Naphthyl AS-D chloroacetate esterase shows positive activity in granulocytic cells with negative or weak reactions in monocytes. Periodic acid–Schiff stains glycogen and mucoproteins, and staining patterns may be used to help in identification of various cell types. Myeloperoxidase activity is strong in neutrophils from the promyelocyte stage through maturity; however, activity in monocytes is negative or weak.

34. c. A positive tartrate-resistant acid phosphatase (TRAP) stain is indicative of hairy cell leukemia, because hairy cell lymphocytes produce large amounts of acid phosphatase isoenzyme 5, which is inhibited in the presence of tartaric acid. Most other cells of various lines are positive for acid phosphatase; however, they are not resistant to the addition of tartaric acid because of normal or decreased levels of isoenzyme 5.

35. b. The *JAK2 V617F* mutation is present in numerous cases of myeloproliferative neoplasms, including polycythemia vera, essential thrombocythemia, and primary myelofibrosis. *BCR/ABL* mutations are seen in CML, and *PDGFR* mutations are seen in neoplasms with eosinophilia. *RUNX* mutations may be seen in some cases of acute leukemias.

36. b. Although leukocyte alkaline phosphatase (LAP) scores tend to be decreased in chronic myelogenous leukemia (CML) and myeloid cells are present, karyotyping for the presence of the Philadelphia chromosome (9;22 translocation) is required for the confirmation of a diagnosis of CML.

37. a. A bone marrow biopsy would help in confirming a diagnosis of primary myelofibrosis, which is a possible diagnosis suggested by the dacryocytes, left shift, and abnormal platelets. If the patient had primary myelofibrosis, the bone marrow would likely show areas of fibrosis, in addition to increases in megakaryocytes and abnormal platelets. Splenomegaly would be explained by extramedullary hematopoiesis, which is suggested by the presence of dacryocytes. Leukocyte alkaline phosphatase (LAP) staining and karyotyping for the Philadelphia chromosome would be more useful in determining a diagnosis of chronic myelogenous leukemia.

38. d. Myelodysplastic syndromes are characterized by anemias refractory to normal treatment and abnormal cellular appearance resulting from dyspoiesis in the cell lines. Vitamin B_{12}, folic acid, and iron levels usually are normal; however, cells do not mature normally.

39. c. All of these disorders are classified as myelodysplastic syndromes with the exception of chronic myelomonocytic leukemia (CML), which was moved into the World Health Organization classification of myelodysplastic syndrome/myeloproliferative neoplasms, along with juvenile myelomonocytic leukemia, and atypical CML.

40. a. Intermediate B-cell acute lymphoblastic anemia (ALL) is the most likely diagnosis because of the B-cell markers (CD19 and CD22), in addition to CD10, which are specifically seen in common ALL (cALL), also known as intermediate B-cell ALL. This is not a T-cell ALL, because no positive T-cell markers are indicated in the results given.

41. a. Prognosis is currently the best in children, as opposed to in infants and adults. Elevated blast counts or hypodiploidy are associated with a poorer prognosis. The presence of the Philadelphia chromosome has an unfavorable prognosis in acute lymphoblastic anemia.

42. b. The clinical presentation of disseminated intravascular coagulation (DIC), along with the peripheral smear findings, are consistent with acute promyelocytic leukemia (AML with t[15:17]; *PML-RARα*). Acute lymphoblastic leukemia (ALL) is unlikely because of the suggestion of a disorder of the myeloid line because of the presence of Auer rods. AML with t(9:11); *MLLT3-MLL* is a disorder involving the monocytic line, although DIC may be associated with this disorder.

43. c. Acute myelomonocytic leukemia is the most likely because of the presence of both myeloid (CD13, CD33) and monocytic cell lines (CD4, CD14, CD11b, CD11c, CD64, CD36).

44. b. This smear and bone marrow picture is typical of chronic lymphocytic leukemia (CLL) with numerous mature small lymphocytes. Acute lymphocytic leukemia (CALL) would show the presence of blasts; hairy cell leukemia shows a hypocellular, fibrotic bone marrow with hairy lymphocytes. Acute myelogenous leukemia (AML) is not indicated, because there is no evidence of myeloid cells and blasts.

45. c. Sézary syndrome is a disorder of T lymphocytes, whereas the others are plasma cell disorders.

46. a. CD2, CD3, CD4, CD5, CD7, and CD8 are associated with T lymphocytes. CD13, CD14, CD15 are associated with granulocytic/monocytic cells. CD19, CD20, CD22 are associated with B cells. CD34 and CD117 are immature cell markers, and CD71 is an erythroid marker.

47. c. Bone marrow core biopsies are the best indicator of bone marrow architecture and cellularity, because they provide a visual representation of the hematologic cells, fat, and vascular structure. Although a general idea may be obtained by examining the aspirate, it is better used for looking at the specific cell morphology. The buffy coat or concentrated smears concentrate any cells present, particularly in cases of hypocellular samples.

48. c. Fibrotic or hypercellular marrow is seen in all of the following except multiple myeloma, in which sheets of plasma cells may be present.

49. b. Megakaryocytes, with diameters up to 50 μm, are the largest cells present in a normal bone marrow sample. Lymphoblasts and pronormoblasts are less than 20 μm in diameter. Osteoblasts, although large cells, are not hematopoietic cells, and are used in the formation and modeling of bone.

50. a. Hemoglobin (Hgb) A is characterized by pairs of α and β chains, $\alpha_2\beta_2$. $\alpha_2\delta_2$ is Hgb A$_2$, $\alpha_2\gamma_2$ is Hgb F, and $\alpha_2\varepsilon_2$ is Hgb Gower 2, an embryonic Hgb.

51. a. The bone marrow is the site of intramedullary hematopoiesis. The liver and spleen are sites of hematopoietic activity in the embryo, and hematopoietic activity may be renewed in cases of bone marrow compromise, such as primary myelofibrosis. The thymus is a site for lymphoid development.

52. b. Erythropoiesis is stimulated by erythropoietin, which is produced in the kidney, and renal failure can decrease the production of erythropoietin.

53. c. The Rapoport-Luebering shunt is involved in the production of 2,3 diphosphoglycerate, which helps regulate oxygen delivery to the tissues. The overall Embden-Meyerhof pathway is used in the production of adenosine triphosphate (ATP); the hexose-monophosphate shunt functions in reducing glutathione; and the methemoglobin reductase pathway is involved in the reduction of methemoglobin.

54. a. This is most likely a normal child, because children usually have higher relative lymphocyte counts than adults. The patient has normal total white blood cell, red blood cell, and platelet counts and normal differential results.

55. a. Basophils have IgE receptors on their surface membranes. Once IgE is bound to the receptor, it allows the release of the cell's granule contents.

Eosinophils, neutrophils, and monocytes all contain granules; however, they are not associated with IgE.

56. b. The patient most likely has a bacterial infection, because the white blood cell (WBC) count is slightly elevated with increased neutrophils, including the presence of 10% bands. Döhle bodies and toxic granulation, although not exclusive to bacterial infections, are toxic neutrophil changes that may present in these cases. Strenuous exercise may lead to a transient elevation in WBCs and the mobilization of neutrophils from the marginating to circulating pools; however, toxic granulation and Döhle bodies are not usually seen. If the patient had a parasitic infection, elevated numbers of neutrophils would be expected.

57. c. Chediak-Higashi syndrome is characterized by giant fused granules in the white blood cell cytoplasm, with neutropenia and thrombocytopenia as the disease progresses, and patients often die in infancy or early childhood because the granules normally released to aid in the killing of bacteria cannot be released to aid in the kill process. A complete blood count with giant platelets and Döhle-like inclusions in the granulocytes is more characteristic of the May-Hegglin anomaly, and large, dark granules are more associated with Alder-Reilly anomaly.

58. a. Patients with infectious mononucleosis often exhibit an increase in lymphocytes, along with the presence of reactive lymphocytes. Neutrophilia with a left shift is typically seen in bacterial infections or other acute infections.

59. b. CD4 and CD8 markers are monitored in patients with acquired immunodeficiency virus infection. CD33 and CD34 would more likely be used for investigating a suspected acute myeloid leukemia (AML) case.

60. c. Atypical chronic myelogenous leukemia is classified as an MDS/MPD, because it has characteristics of both disorders. Acute promyelocytic leukemia is an acute leukemia, and chronic lymphocytic leukemia is a chronic lymphoid disorder that affects a different cell line than seen in MDS/MPD. Essential thrombocythemia is classified as a myeloproliferative disorder.

61. b. Lymphocytes are derived from the common lymphocyte progenitor cell, whereas the other cells are derived from the common myeloid progenitor (or CFU-GEMM).

62. c. Elevated eosinophil counts are often seen in parasitic infections, particularly those caused by helminths. Aplastic anemia shows decreases in all cell counts. Bacterial infections tend to have increased neutrophil numbers, and viral infections tend to have increased lymphocytes.

63. c. Antibodies are produced by lymphocytes, specifically B cells in the form of plasma cells. None of the other cells can produce antibodies.

64. b. The nitroblue tetrazolium test will reduce nitroblue tetrazolium in normal neutrophils. In cases of chronic granulomatous disease (CGD), the phagocytic cells cannot make nicotinamide adenine dinucleotide phosphate (NADPH) oxidase, which is used in the kill mechanism of neutrophils. Leukocyte adhesion deficiency (LAD) involves problems with adhesion to endothelial cells, and both May-Hegglin and Pelger-Huet anomalies have normal neutrophil phagocytic function.

65. c. Myeloperoxidase (MPO) and terminal deoxnucleotidyl transferase (TdT) would be good initial markers to use. MPO is positive in myeloblasts and promyelocytes, and TdT is positive in early lymphoid cells. Leukocyte alkaline peroxidase (LAP) is used for mature neutrophil activity, nonspecific esterase (NSE) is positive in monocytic cells, Sudan black B is used only for myeloid cells, and brilliant cresyl blue is not used to determine blast origin.

66. a. Imatinib mesylate and related drugs are used to target p210 formed as a result of the *BCR/ABL* fusion gene in chronic myelogenous leukemia (CML). All-*trans* retinoic acid therapy is often used in cases of acute myeloid leukemia (AML), and 2-CDA/cladribine is a drug used for hairy cell leukemia.

67. b. This is most likely a case of polycythemia vera, because the patient exhibits more than two of the diagnostic criteria required by the World Health Organization (hemoglobin >16.5 g/dL, platelet count >400 × 10^9/L, and, additionally, white blood cell count >12 × 10^9/L, although it's not apparent from the information given whether an infection is present). Chronic myelogenous leukemia is less likely because of the lower numbers of immature neutrophils and the higher red blood cell count. Although bacterial infection is not ruled out from this information, the combination of the other elevated parameters is usually seen in cases of polycythemia vera.

68. b. Polycythemia vera differs from secondary polycythemia because it exhibits elevated red blood cell counts while the erythropoietin levels are decreased. Secondary polycythemia shows elevated erythropoietin levels, often as a response to tissue hypoxia resulting from the patient's initial condition.

69. c. The mutation seen in chronic myelogenous leukemia (CML) is t(9;22)(q34;11.2), resulting in the Philadelphia chromosome, with the translocation creating a fusion gene, *BCR-ABL*. t (15;17)(q22; q12) is seen in acute promyelocytic leukemia, t (8;21)(q22;q22) is seen in acute myeloid leukemia (AML) with maturation, and t(11;14)(p15;q11) is seen in precursor T-cell acute lymphoblastic leukemia.

70. d. All are myeloproliferative neoplasms with the exception of Waldenström's macroglobulinemia, which is a plasma cell disorder.

71. b. More than 15% ringed sideroblasts must be present in the bone marrow for a diagnosis of refractory anemia with ringed sideroblasts (RARS). Ringed sideroblasts must have at least five iron granules, surrounding at least one third of the nucleus of a nucleated red blood cell.

72. c. Döhle bodies are found in neutrophils. Multinucleate red blood cells (RBCs), nuclear bridging, basophilic stippling, siderotic granules, and macroovalocytes may be seen in dyserythropoietic RBCs.

73. d. Although iron granules may be seen in some myelodysplastic syndromes, siderotic granules are found in red blood cells, not in neutrophils or platelets. Pelgeroid nuclei in neutrophils and abnormal granulation patterns in neutrophils and platelets are features of dyspoiesis of myeloid cells and platelets.

74. c. Megaloblastic anemia, resulting from a deficiency of vitamin B_{12} or folic acid can look similar to myelodysplastic syndrome, because decreased vitamin B_{12} or folic acid can lead to a similar appearance, such as nuclear-to-cytoplasmic asynchrony and a hypercellular dysplastic bone marrow. Iron-deficiency anemia and α-thalassemia minor exhibit microcytic/hypochromic cells with relatively normal white blood cells (WBCs), and warm autoimmune hemolytic anemia is a hemolytic anemia with normal WBCs, although red blood cells usually show macrocytosis, polychromasia, and spherocytes.

75. a. The most common abnormalities of chromosomes in myelodysplastic syndrome (MDS) occur in chromosomes 5, 7, 8, 11, 13, and 20. Although multiple chromosome abnormalities have been implicated in MDS, currently 5q− syndrome is the only abnormality specific to one disorder subtype in the World Health Organization 2008 classification.

76. d. All are recurrent genetic abnormalities in acute myeloid leukemia (AML) except AML with t (1;19)(q23;q13), *(E2A/PBX1)*, which is an abnormality seen in some cases of precursor B-cell ALL.

77. c. Monocytic precursors are associated with 11q23 *(MLL)* abnormalities. Eosinophils are associated with inv(16)(p13;q22) and t(16;16)(p13;q22), whereas neutrophils are associated with a variety of other genetic abnormalities. Erythrocytes are currently not associated with a specific generality.

78. b. T-cell acute lymphoblastic leukemia (ALL) most commonly affects teenaged males who present with a mediastinal mass, although it also may occur in adult patients in some cases. B-cell ALL is typically seen in children.

79. c. Acute promyelocytic leukemia falls under the classification of acute myeloid leukemia (AML) with recurrent cytogenetic abnormalities, because it manifests with t(15;17)(q22;q12), *(PML/RARα)*. The others currently do not have a specific recurrent cytogenetic abnormality and all are included in the "not otherwise classified" category.

80. a. This is a case of acute myeloid leukemia (AML) with minimal differentiation. Early myeloid cell precursors and stem cell markers are present, while the patient is negative for terminal deoxynucleotidyl transferase (TdT), which rules out lymphoid involvement. The patient also is negative for myeloperoxidase and nonspecific esterase, in the presence of the early myeloid CD markers, which is consistent with AML with minimal differentiation. AML without maturation would have a similar flow cytometry profile, but would have a positive myeloperoxidase result.

81. b. The lumbar puncture would be ordered to determine if there was leukemic involvement in the central nervous system (CNS), because the patient's other results are consistent with possible acute myeloid leukemia (ALL). If blasts are seen in the CNS, intrathecal chemotherapy would be indicated in addition to a standard therapy regimen. Orders for a bone marrow examination and flow cytometry are also indicated. Blasts should not be seen in the peripheral blood in meningitis, infectious mononucleosis, or multiple sclerosis. If the physician suspected infectious mononucleosis, serologic examination specific to infectious mononucleosis would be ordered, not a lumbar puncture.

82. b. The patient most likely has Prolymphocytic leukemia (PLL), because prolymphocytes typically look like lymphocytes with a prominent nucleolus. Sézary syndrome has lymphoid cells with a convoluted nucleus, and plasma cells are the cells seen in multiple myeloma.

83. d. Multiple myeloma shows all of the following laboratory features except for decreased immunoglobulin. Immunoglobulin is increased, because the disorder is a monoclonal gammopathy, with increased IgG.

84. b. Reed Sternberg cells, sometimes described as "owl eye" cells, are present in cases of classic Hodgkin lymphoma. Plasma cells are seen in multiple myeloma and other plasma cell neoplasms.

85. c. Sézary cells are lymphoma cells characterized by cerebriform nuclei and irregular nuclear outlines.

86. b. The hexose monophosphate pathway is used to reduce glutathione, which is used to help the cell combat oxidative damage. Adenosine triphosphate (ATP) is produced via the Embden-Meyerhof pathway. 2,3 diphosphoglycerate (2,3 DPG) results from the Rapoport-Luebering pathway.

87. a. A normal reticulocyte count is 0.5% to 1.5%. Values above 1.5% show the patient is responding to an increased need for red blood cells (RBCs) by pushing out increased numbers of immature RBCs to the bone marrow.

88. d. Bone marrow examination is not indicated in the diagnosis of a standard case of iron deficiency, in which diagnosis can be made by using less invasive measures such as peripheral blood indices and serum iron chemistries.

89. d. The myeloid-to-erythroid (M/E) ratio looks at the number of myeloid cells (M) to nucleated erythroid cells (E) in the bone marrow. A ratio of 1:1 would mean the patient was producing approximately the same number of red blood cells (RBCs) and myeloid cells. A ratio of 2:1 is in the normal range. A ratio of 1:2 indicates the patient is showing erythroid hyperplasia, producing larger numbers of nucleated RBCs than white blood cells, which is often seen in ineffective erythropoiesis. Patients with chronic myelogenous leukemia (CML) will have elevated M/E ratios, because they are producing large numbers of myeloid cells with the malignant cell clone.

90. b. Macrocytosis without megaloblastosis can present in patients with liver disease, chronic alcoholism, and hypothyroidism and in other cases in which reticulocyte production is elevated. Hemochromatosis is a disorder that leads to elevated red blood cell production, not anemia.

91. a. Diagnostic criteria for aplastic anemia include a hypocellular bone marrow, absolute neutrophil count less than 1.5×10^9/L, platelet count less than 50×10^9/L, and hemoglobin value less than 10 g/dL, with decreased reticulocyte response (Rodak, 2012).

92. b. Mutations in α-thalassemia occur as a result of deletions of one or more α-globin genes, and mutations in β-thalassemia occur because of reduced or absent expression of one or more β-globin genes. The α-globin gene is found on chromosome 16, and the β-globin gene is found on chromosome 11.

93. d. This is a patient with α-thalassemia minor. An increased red blood cell (RBC) count would be expected with hemoglobin, mean corpuscular volume, and mean corpuscular hemoglobin values lower than expected for the number of red blood cells present.

94. c. Hemoglobin (Hgb) F is present in larger quantities in fetal development and after a baby is born. As the baby makes more β-globin chains than γ-globin chains, usually between 6 and 9 months of age, the Hgb F decreases and the expression of the missing or mutated gene becomes clinically apparent.

95. b. The thymus is associated with lymphocyte development for precursor T cells, whereas the others all develop in the bone marrow.

96. c. The equation used is number of cells counted/(number of squares counted × area of square × depth of square) × reciprocal dilution to get cells/μL. Cells/μL × 10^6/μL /L will convert the answer to cells per liter. For this patient, 105/(8 × 1 mm^2 × 0.1 mm) × 20/1 = 2625 cells/μL, which converts to 2.6×10^9/L.

97. c. Hereditary elliptocytosis results from an autosomal dominant mutation in the spectrin proteins and protein 4.1R, which will lead to instability in the red blood cell membrane. Spectrin mutations may also appear in hereditary spherocytosis, in addition to mutations of several other proteins.

98. d. Acid β-glycerophosphatase, cathespins, defensins, elastase, myeloperoxidase, and proteinase-3 are found in the primary granules of neutrophils. β$_2$-Microglobulin, collagenase, gelatinase lactoferrin, and neutrophil gelatinase-associated lipocalin are found in the secondary (specific granules). Acetyltransferase, collagenase, gelatinase, lysozyme, β$_2$-microglobulin are found in tertiary granules. Alkaline phosphatase, cytochrome b$_{558}$, complement receptor 1, complement 1q receptor, vesicle-associated membrane–2 are found in the secretory granules.

99. c. This sample, based on the intracellular red blood cell inclusions and boomerang-shaped or banana-shaped structures is suspicious for a malarial infection, particularly based on the patient travel history. The sample should be referred to the pathologist or technical supervisor for confirmation and speciation.

100. b. The Donath-Landsteiner test can be used to demonstrate proximal cold hemoglobinuria by identifying glucose-6-phosphate dehydrogenase deficiency. The osmotic fragility test and direct antiglobulin test (DAT) would be less useful for differential diagnosis. G6PD activity is used to identify cases of glucose-6-dehydrogenase (G6PD) deficiency.

CHAPTER 4

1. b. When damage occurs to the endothelium, primary hemostasis occurs first, resulting in the formation of the primary platelet plug. Secondary hemostasis occurs next, which results in the formation of a stable fibrin clot. The last action is fibrinolysis, which results in the breakdown of the clot.

2. c. Under normal circumstances, vessels are nonthrombotic. Factors that contribute to this include a negatively charged surface; the inhibition of platelet activation through prostacyclin, nitric oxide, and ADPase; and the inactivation of thrombin through heparin sulfate and thrombomodulin. Once damaged, tissue factor is one of the substances released that favors the formation of clots. Other prothrombotic substances include the secretion of platelet-activating factor and von Willebrand factor.

3. a. Aspirin inhibits cyclooxygenase, which blocks thromboxane A$_2$ (TXA$_2$) synthesis, thereby making platelets nonfunctional for the life span of the platelets.

4. c. Both fibrinogen and von Willebrand factor (vWF) bind to platelets. Fibrinogen binds to platelets via the GbIIb/IIIa receptor. vWF binds through the GpIb/IX receptor.

5. a. Platelet agonists include collagen, adenosine diphosphate (ADP), thrombin, epinephrine, thromboxane A$_2$ (TXA$_2$), and arachidonic acid.

6. b. Aspirin inhibits cyclooxygenase, which blocks thromboxane A$_2$ (TXA$_2$) synthesis, thereby making platelets nonfunctional for their life span.

7. a. For secondary aggregation to occur, sufficient stimulus must be present. The stimulus occurs after internal adenosine diphosphate and calcium are released, along with the synthesis and release of thromboxane A$_2$ (TXA$_2$). Primary aggregation is reversible.

8. b. Factor II is also called prothrombin.

9. a. A deficiency of factor XII, as well as prekallikrein and high-molecular-weight kininogen, does not usually manifest with clinical bleeding. Deficiencies of factors IX, VIII, and VII all generally present with clinical bleeding depending on the degree of deficiency.

10. d. Vitamin K is required for the γ-carboxylation step of the formation of factors II, VII, IX, and X and proteins C and S. In this step, an additional carboxyl group is added to the γ-carbon of the glutamic acid residues on the factors. Without this step, the factor is formed, but is not functional because binding to a negatively charged phospholipid surface cannot occur.

11. b. The intrinsic pathway of hemostasis can be monitored through the partial thromboplastin time (PTT) assay. The prothrombin time (PT) assay can be used to monitor the extrinsic pathway. The thrombin time test assesses the formation of fibrin. The fibrinogen assay is used to measure fibrinogen levels.

12. a. The prothrombin time (PT) assay can be used to monitor the extrinsic pathway. The intrinsic pathway of hemostasis can be monitored through the partial thromboplastin time (PTT) assay. The thrombin time test assesses the formation of fibrin. The fibrinogen assay is used to measure fibrinogen levels.

13. b. One of thrombin's many actions is to cleave fibrinopeptides A and B from fibrinogen. This step results in the formation of a fibrin monomer, which can then continue to aggregate with other fibrin monomers. Factor VIII participates in the common pathway. Tissue factor is released by the endothelium during the initial stages leading to primary aggregation. Factor XIII is involved in the covalent cross-linking of D domains of fibrin to form a stable fibrin clot.

14. b. Factor VII is involved in the extrinsic pathway of coagulation, along with tissue factor.

15. c. Protein S is a cofactor for protein C.

16. d. Factor XIII covalently cross-links the D domains of fibrin to form a urea-insoluble clot. Factors II, V, and XI are involved in other parts of the hemostasis pathway.

17. c. Von Willebrand factor circulates as the vWF/VIII complex. If circulating alone, factor VIII will be quickly degraded.

18. b. A deficiency of factor IX is called hemophilia B. Hemophilia A is associated with a deficiency of factor VIII. Hemophilia C is associated with a deficiency of factor XI.

19. c. Fibrinolysis is the process of breaking down a fibrin clot. The activation of plasmin by plasminogen activators begins this process.

20. c. Plasmin is a serine protease with broad specificity against proteins that are susceptible to trypsin degradation. In terms of the hemostatic pathway, plasmin has an effect against fibrin, fibrinogen, and factors V and VIII.

21. c. There are physiologic and exogenous plasminogen activators. The exogenous plasminogen activators include streptokinase and staphylokinase. The physiologic plasminogen activators include tissue-type plasminogen activator and urokinase-type plasminogen activator.

22. d. When plasmin cleaves fibrin, the breakdown products that are formed include fragment X, fragment Y, fragment D, and fragment E. Fragment X has a limited binding ability for thrombin. Fragments Y, D, and E all inhibit fibrin polymerization and inhibit platelet aggregation.

23. a. Plasminogen activator inhibitor-1 has a significant role in limiting the activation of plasminogen.

24. c. α_2-Macroglobulin has wide specificity against many proteases. It generally is not used until α_2-antiplasmin is consumed.

25. c. There are both positive and negative feedback mechanisms in the control of hemostasis. Positive feedback mechanisms include the thrombin activation of platelets, release of platelet factor Va, exposure of the negatively charged surface, and activation of factors Va and VIIIa. Negative feedback mechanisms include thrombin's involvement in the protein C pathway, tissue factor pathway inhibitor (TFPI) inactivation of factor Xa, fibrin binding to thrombin, and the interference of fibrin degradation products (FDPs) in fibrin formation and polymerization.

26. c. In the protein C pathway, protein S serves as a cofactor C. Protein S circulates bound to C4BP. In the presence of protein S and calcium, activated protein C inactivates factors Va and VIIIa.

27. a. Acute idiopathic thrombocytopenic purpura (ITP) is typically observed in children (ages 2-4) and follows viral infections. Affected patients may be asymptomatic or have severe mucosal bleeding. Patients will have a decrease in platelets and increase in lymphocytes and eosinophils. Patients with chronic ITP are usually adults.

28. d. Bernard-Soulier syndrome and Glanzmann's thombasthenia are both qualitative platelet disorders. The bleeding time will be prolonged in both conditions. The platelet count may be affected in either disorder. Platelets are not assessed using prothrombin time (PT). The conditions can be differentiated using platelet aggregation tests. In patients affected with Bernard-Soulier, responses to adenosine diphosphate (ADP), collagen, and epinephrine will be normal, whereas the response to ristocetin is abnormal. The Glanzmann's abnormal responses are observed with ADP, collagen, and epinephrine, but normal with ristocetin.

29. c. The pathophysiology of Glanzmann's thrombasthenia is the deficiency of GpIIb/IIIa.

30. d. In Δ-storage pool deficiency, platelets have a decrease in or absence of dense granules. This results in the lack of a secondary wave of aggregation when the agonist adenosine diphosphate (ADP) is used. Aggregation with collagen and epinephrine is also deficient. A normal response to ristocetin is observed.

31. a. The abnormal partial thromboplastin time (PTT) and normal prothrombin time (PT) suggest a deficiency of a factor in the intrinsic pathway. Given the sex, age, and type of bleeding, evaluations of factors VII and IX should be performed to check for hemophilia A or B. A normal PT rules out the possibility of a common pathway deficiency, which rules out a deficiency of X or V. The symptoms and laboratory results are not suggestive of a platelet abnormality. Factor V Leiden is a condition associated with thrombosis.

32. a. In dysfibrinogenemia, the structure of fibrinogen is abnormal. Fibrin still forms, resulting in normal PT and PTT evaluations. As a result of the structural abnormality, the thrombin time that assesses fibrinogen to fibrin formation is affected.

33. a. Because of compensation of other factors in the hemostatic pathway and the sensitivity of the reagents, factor levels must be reduced to 30% or less before prolongation is observed.

34. c. Disseminated intravascular coagulation is a disorder of consumption. Coagulation proteins, including fibrinogen, and platelets are all consumed in thrombi, resulting in a prolongation of the prothrombin time (PT) and partial thromboplastin time (PTT) and decreased fibrinogen and platelet count. The D-dimer is significant and can help rule out other conditions, because it indicates that thrombi are being formed. The D-dimer would be negative in fibrinogenolysis, fibrinogen deficiencies, and vitamin K deficiency. In vitamin K deficiencies, the fibrinogen assay, platelet count, and D-dimer assay would be normal.

35. d. Factor V deficiency results in a bleeding condition because it is part of the common pathway. Both the prothrombin time (PT) and partial thromboplastin time (PTT) would be abnormal. Protein C deficiency, antithrombin deficiency, and the factor V Leiden mutation are all associated with thrombosis.

36. c. Heparin is an anticoagulant that functions by significantly accelerating the activity of antithrombin.

37. d. Fibrinogenolysis is a condition in which plasmin is generated without the generation of thrombin or thrombi. As clots are not formed, D-dimers are not produced. In disseminated intravascular coagulation, thrombi are formed, and after fibrinolysis, D-dimers are measurable in the blood.

38. a. An abnormal prothrombin time (PT) will be observed in deficiencies or in the presence of an inhibitor. When patient plasma is mixed with normal pooled plasma, the deficient factor is added back, resulting in a correction of the PT. If an inhibitor was present, the PT mix with normal pooled plasma would not result in a correction.

39. c. The principle of the platelet aggregation assays is that the formation of platelet aggregates will decrease the optical density of platelet-rich plasma when an agonist is added. If added to platelet-poor plasma, aggregation would not occur, because of the lack of platelets.

40. b. The goal of the platelet aggregation assay is to assess platelet function. If platelets are not functional, as is the case when aspirin is ingested, the results will not be reflective of the patient's platelets. Fasting is not required. Freezing the plasma will cause the platelets to aggregate before evaluation.

41. b. Fibrinogen is an acute phase protein that will cause levels to increase in conditions in which an acute phase reaction is observed. In disseminated intravascular coagulation, fibrinogen is a protein that is consumed. Fibrinogen levels are absent in afibrinogenemia. In liver disease, fibrinogen production is decreased.

42. c. The thrombin time test is performed by adding an excess of thrombin to the patient specimen to assess fibrinogen-to-fibrin formation. Thromboplastin is used in the prothrombin time (PT) assay. The 5 M urea solubility test is used to assess factor XIII levels.

43. c. Factor IX–deficient plasma contains all coagulation factors with the exception of factor IX. If added to asses a patient's factor VIII level, the factor VIII present in the deficient plasma will result in an analytical error.

44. c. Calcium chloride and partial thromboplastin are the needed reagents for the partial thromboplastin time (PTT) assay.

45. a. The international normalized ratio (INR) is reported out in conjunction with the prothrombin time (PT) result. It helps to standardize the PT results for variations in instrumentation, reagents, and personnel.

46. c. von Willebrand's disease is a qualitative platelet disorder. In this condition, the platelet aggregation response to ristocetin is abnormal. The bleeding time is increased as a result of the qualitative defect in the platelets. Although von Willebrand factor

(vWF) is not assessed in the partial thromboplastin time (PTT) assay, vWF also carries around factor VIII in the circulation to protect it from degradation. Therefore a decrease in vWF sometimes results in a prolongation of the PTT assay because of the lower factor VIII levels, which are corrected by the addition of normal pooled plasma.

47. c. International normalized ration (INR) results of 1.75 and 1.74 are essentially the same. The INR is used to standardize the prothrombin time (PT) assays among laboratories and is compared to assess degree of anticoagulation when the testing is performed at different laboratories.

48. c. It is likely that this patient has a deficiency of one of the contact factors (factor XII, prekallikrein, or high-molecular-weight kininogen). Although the deficiency of these factors results in a very prolonged partial thromboplastin time (PTT), bleeding complications are not observed.

49. d. In a patient with a history of miscarriages, one concern is the presence of lupus anticoagulants. To assess this condition, a panel would include the following tests to rule in or rule out the presence of such an anticoagulant: dilute Russell viper venom time (DRVTT, to indicate an anticoagulant against phospholipids), prothrombin time (PT) and partial thromboplastin time (PTT), and PT and PTT with normal pooled plasma (to rule out a factor deficiency and demonstrate the presence of an inhibitor).

50. d. The activated protein C resistance (APCR) test is a screening test that will be abnormal in the presence of a factor V Leiden defect. It is a clot-based test based on the inability of activated factor V to be inactivated that is quick to perform and cheaper than the molecular-based factor V Leiden test. The other tests listed (protein S, antithrombin, and prothrombin 20210) are all associated with deep vein thromboses if abnormal, but will be normal in the presence of the factor V Leiden defect.

CHAPTER 5

1. b. The ultrafiltrate that enters Bowman's capsule from the glomerulus has the same specific gravity as protein-free plasma, roughly 1.010.

2. a. Bacteria will continue to proliferate unless refrigerated, reducing urine nitrates to nitrites.

3. d. Orthostatic or postural proteinuria is characterized by an elevated protein while a person is in the upright (standing) position and normal protein excretion in a sitting or reclined position.

4. c. A timed urine collection, such as a 24-hour collection, involves voiding and discarding the specimen at the beginning of the collection and voiding and collecting the specimen at the end of the timed collection. If all urine collected during that time is not calculated into the total volume, constituents present may be falsely decreased.

5. a. The method of detection includes two indicators, methyl red and bromothymol blue, which produce a color change from blue or blue-green to yellow.

6. c. Testing for protein is based on the research findings by Sorensen and called the protein error of indicators, which is the ability of protein to alter the color of some acid-base indicators without altering the pH.

7. a. Glucose detection is based on the enzymatic oxidase/peroxidase method, in which glucose oxidase catalyzes the formation of gluconic acid and hydrogen peroxide from the oxidation of glucose. The second enzyme, peroxidase, then catalyzes the reaction of hydrogen peroxide with tetramethylbenzidine to form a colored complex.

8. d. Glucosuria is glucose present in the urine. When no hyperglycemia is present in the patient, it can be due to an acquired or inherited defect in the glucose transport or another renal tubular disorder.

9. d. Ketonuria is the presence of ketones in the urine. When carbohydrates are unavailable, fatty acids are used for energy, resulting in the production and excretion of ketones.

10. a. Hemoglobin (Hgb) and myoglobin catalyze the oxidation of the chromogenic indicator by the peroxide in the test pad. This is due to the strong pseudoperoxidase action of Hgb and myoglobin.

11. c. Myoglobin is a protein found in heart and skeletal muscle. When muscle is damaged, myoglobin is released. It may be detected after muscle trauma or strenuous exercise.

12. c. Renal calculi are small crystals or stones present in the kidneys and causing obstruction. Microscopically, red blood cells can be seen.

13. a. Bilirubin accumulates as a result of a block in the bile duct. When bilirubin builds up, it will be present in urine. This is direct, or conjugated, bilirubin and is a result of the obstruction.

14. d. Urobilinogen is a product of bilirubin metabolism. During hemolysis, red cells are broken down and the bilirubin is converted to urobilinogen.

15. b. For specific gravity detection, in the presence of cations, protons are released by a complexing agent to produce a color change.

16. c. Yeast is often associated with patients having diabetes mellitus, where results are consistent with acidic urine and positive glucose on the dipstick.

17. d. The presence of dysmorphic red blood cells (RBCs) in urine suggests glomerulonephritis. Dysmorphic RBCs are misshapen because they have been distorted when passing through the abnormal glomerular structure.

18. c. Renal tubular cells are seldom seen in urine and are found only in the renal tubules. The urinary tract from the pelvis down the ureters to the bladder and the proximal urethra is lined by transitional epithelial cells. Squamous epithelial cells originate from the distal urethra and vagina.

19. a. The proteins involved in cast formation are secreted by the lining cells of the distal tubules and the collecting ducts.

20. c. Ethylene glycol poisoning can result in the presence of calcium oxalate monohydrate crystals in urine.

21. d. Triple phosphate crystals are present in alkaline urine, so the discrepancy lies in the acid pH or the crystal type.

22. c. Goodpasture's syndrome is an autoimmune disease that attacks the kidneys, leading to kidney failure. Anti–glomerular basement antibodies are antibodies to the kidney membranes involved in the disorder.

23. a. Calcium oxalate is the most common renal crystal observed.

24. c. The additional finding of white blood cell casts signifying infections within the tubules is a primary diagnostic indicator for both acute and chronic pyelonephritis.

25. c. Henoch-Schönlein purpura is a disease occurring primarily in children after upper respiratory tract infections and includes symptoms of raised red patches on the skin. Renal involvement may include mild proteinuria with hematuria and red blood cell casts.

26. b. Focal segmental glomerular nephritis affects certain areas of the glomerulus and comprises IgM and C3 deposits. It is associated with heroin abuse, analgesics, and acquired immunodeficiency syndrome.

27. c. Waxy and broad casts are associated with chronic glomerulonephritis. All the other choices are often associated with both acute and chronical glomerulonephritis.

28. d. Renal tubular epithelial cells are present in renal tubular necrosis, not an inflammation of the bladder (cystitis).

29. c. Cerebrospinal fluid is produced in the choroid plexus of the third and fourth ventricle and the lumbar ventricles.

30. b. A traumatic tap can be identified by having the largest concentration of red blood cells in tube 1 and decreasing red cell concentrations present in tube 2 and tube 3.

31. a. IgG index values greater than 0.8 are indicative of IgG production within the central nervous system.

32. a. Low protein values in cerebrospinal fluid indicate the central nervous system is leaking fluid.

33. b. In cerebrospinal fluid, increase in lactate can be associated with bacterial, fungal, and tubercular meningitis at levels greater than 25 mg/dL.

34. c. In protein electrophoresis of cerebrospinal fluid, a transferrin band for τ transferrin is present, which is a protein produced mainly by the central nervous system.

35. c. Protein electrophoresis is performed on cerebrospinal fluid to detect oligoclonal bands migrating in the γ region, unlike the bands detected during serum protein electrophoresis. Detection of the oligoclonal bands aid in diagnosing multiple sclerosis.

36. d. The concentration identifies the amount of sperm per microliter. To identify the total amount of sperm present, multiply the concentration (12,000/μL) with the total volume (3 mL) to yield a total sperm count of 36,000 μL.

37. c. Fructose comprises 99% of normal reducing sugar in semen; with normal levels of semen, fructose is 13 μmols or greater per ejaculate.

38. d. Also called the Ropes test, the extent of polymerization of hyaluronic acid is determined. The stronger the clot, the greater the viscosity of the synovial fluid.

39. b. In the mucin clot test, the presence of a tight rope–like clot indicates the polymerization of hyaluronic acid in the presence of acetic acid.

40. a. Monosodium urate crystals appear needle shaped under polarized light and are yellow when aligned with the slow vibration of compensated polarized light

41. d. An effusion is an accumulation of fluid in a body cavity.

42. d. A transudate is typically clear to pale yellow, with a ratio of fluid to serum lactate dehydrogenase of less than 0.6, fluid-to-serum protein ratio of less than 0.5, and a total cell count of less than 1000 μL

43. b. Increased neutrophils in a pericardial fluid exudate indicate a bacterial infection.

44. c. Thoracentesis is the process of removing fluid from the pleural space, the space between the lungs and the chest wall.

45. a. Peritonitis is an infection of the peritoneum, the abdominal lining, caused by a bacterial infection. Cirrhosis is a chronic degeneration of the hepatocytes along with inflammation in the liver and can be associated with alcoholism or viral hepatitis. The presence of neutrophils would support peritonitis.

46. a. Amniotic fluid for fetal lung maturity testing should be placed on ice on collection and refrigerated up to 72 hours before testing. If testing will not occur within 72 hours, the specimen can be frozen.

47. d. α-Fetoprotein is determined using maternal serum; this value is then converted to multiples of the median (MOM), in which the maternal value is related to the median fetal gestational age at the time of testing. Values greater than 2.5 MOMs are considered positive screen for neural tube defects.

48. c. Steatorrhea, or fatty stool, is characterized by pale color, bulkiness or frothiness, or a greasy appearance.

49. d. The acid steatocrit is a rapid test to estimate fat secretion via stool and is used to monitor therapy or screen for steatorrhea.

50. c. Elastase 1 is an isoenzyme of elastase, a pancreatic enzyme, that can be detected in stool at concentrations 5 times higher than pancreatic secretion. It is measured by enzyme-linked immunosorbent (ELISA) testing.

CHAPTER 6

1. c. Low acidic environment and enzymes in secretions, coughing, and gastrointestinal tract and skin bacteria are natural barriers to invading pathogens and antigens.

2. d. The primary organs are where lymphocytes reside to mature. Once mature, they leave the primary organs and migrate to the secondary organs, where they await activation.

3. a. Toll-like receptors (TLRs) are molecules on phagocytic cells that recognize certain substances or molecules that reside on surfaces of some bacteria. The TLRs recognize and bind to these substances, enhancing the phagocytic process.

4. a. Once bound to a specific antigen, antibodies can act as opsonins. The Fc portion of the immunoglobulin molecule attaches to the receptor molecules on monocytes and neutrophils to enhance phagocytosis.

5. c. CD10 appears early in the B-cell development and is lost after the immature stage, making this an early B-cell marker. CD20 begins to appear during the immature stage of B-cell development; it is found on the later stages and is a marker for the later stages of B-cell development.

6. a. At the double-positive stage of development, this T cell expresses both CD4 and CD8.

7. a. Natural killer (NK) cells are lymphocytes (cells of the adaptive immune system) that have a cytotoxic effect against cellular pathogens without prior known exposure (innate system characteristic). Thus these cells have been considered a bridge between the systems.

8. d. T cells are involved in cell-mediated immunity, whereas B cells that make antibodies are involved in humoral immunity.

9. b. Proteins that are made up of amino acids can be much more structurally and conformationally complex than the sugars of carbohydrates.

10. d. The complement pathways result in cell lysis. Other complement proteins released after complement activation can have chemotactic properties. Complement proteins also act as opsonins to enhance phagocytosis to help clear debris from inactive and dead cells.

11. d. C3 convertase cleaves C3 to C3a and C3b. C3a is released into the plasma and can act as an anaphylatoxin. C3b is released to combine with C42a in the classical pathway or C3bBb in the alternate pathway of complement activation to form C5 convertase. Extra C3b proteins can act as an opsonin by coating pathogens and attachment to the Fc portion of immunoglobulins.

12. d. Certain cytokines produced can enhance the differentiation of lymphocytes to maturity. Cytokines can have many different effects (pleomorphic) on cells outside of the immune system. Also, different cytokines can have the same effect on the same cell, thus making them redundant.

13. b. Variations in the variable regions of the heavy and light chains of an immunoglobulin molecule define the idiotype.

14. c. Mannose-binding lectin (MBL) of the lectin pathway of complement activation is found in circulation complexed with proteinases. It is considered to be similar in structure to C1q of the classical pathway. The MBL-proteinase complex does not require antibody for complement activation.

15. c. Viruses use cellular mechanisms and processes for replication. These antigens synthesized inside a cell are expressed on the cell surface in the form of major histocompatibility complex (MCH) class I molecules, which are then presented to CD8 cytotoxic T lymphocytes for cell lysis.

16. b. Precipitation reactions occur between soluble antigen and soluble antibody that produce a visible end result typically in the form of a visible line of precipitate. Agglutination reactions occur when the antigen is particulate or coated on a particulate such as latex beads.

17. c. In agglutination tests where postzone is occurring, there are so many antigens in the test system, that each antibody reacts singly with the antigen, so no lattice formation occurs and false negative reactions are seen.

18. d. Antibodies that react against different antigenic determinants (epitopes) of the same specific antigen are considered to be polyclonal.

19. b. In radial immunodiffusion, known antibody is added to the gel. Patient serum contains the antigen to be tested.

20. a. The patient serum contains the antigen to be tested. The gel contains known specific antibody. The area of the precipitation ring around the center well is directly proportional to the concentration of the antigen in the sample tested.

21. d. The indirect antiglobulin uses commercial red cells with known antigens to test for unknown antibody in a patient serum sample (e.g., antibody screening test). The direct antiglobulin tests patient red cells coated with antibody that occurred in vivo (e.g., hemolytic disease of the newborn).

22. a. Indirect tests are performed in two steps. The first step is incubating (cytomegalovirus [CMV]) antigen with specific antibody (patient serum). The second step is adding anti-human globulin (antibody to CMV antibody) coupled with the fluorescent dye for visualizing the reaction.

23. d. Nepholometry measures light at angles. The light source used for detection is placed at an angle from the detection device. Turbidometry detection devices are placed directly across from the light source and measures the intensity of the light as it passes through solution.

24. a. A crossed line in the Ouchterlony diffusion indicates the antigens do not share epitopes in common and is therefore considered nonidentity.

25. a. In a twofold serial dilution, a rise in titer results between the initial titer and subsequent titer of more than two tubes or fourfold, the results are considered diagnostic of infection.

26. c. On activation, certain subsets of T lymphocytes produce growth-enhancing cytokines that act on B cells to mature to antibody-secreting plasma cells. B cells would not be able to mature if a deficiency of T cells existed.

27. b. In the serum of a 2-week-old baby, a titer of IgG anticytomegalovirus would be representative of the maternal antibody that crossed the placenta and not the baby's antibody.

28. b. Both rapid plasma reagin (RPR) and Venereal Disease Research Laboratory (VDRL) tests are nontreponemal tests that detect antibody to cardiolipin. The RPR test is a macroscopic agglutination, and the VDRL test is read microscopically.

29. c. The presence of anti-HBs in patient serum is indicative of recovery from a hepatitis B infection. It also may indicate immunity resulting from vaccination.

30. b. Human leukocyte antigen (HLA) genes are inherited as haplotypes; one haplotype from each parent.

31. c. Visible agglutination and precipitation reactions depend on the antigen and antibody concentrations that are in equivalence. It is at this point that precipatation and lattice formation occurs. Too much antigen results in postzone phenomenon, and too much antibody results in prozone.

32. b. Type I hypersensitivity occurs as a result of the release of the granular contents of mast cells when bound to IgE antibodies cross-linked with antigen.

33. c. Anti-dsDNA autoantibodies are present in patients with systemic lupus erythromatosus and, when identified, can be considered diagnostic of the disease.

34. d. The rheumatoid factor is antibody directed against the Fc portion of the IgG molecule.

35. b. Rh disease of the fetus and newborn is not an autoimmune disease but is classified as a type II hypersensitivity reaction.

36. c. Autoantibody to the thyroid-stimulating hormone receptor ultimately causes release of thyroid hormones and a hyperthyroid condition.

37. d. Antithyroglobulin is a common autoantibody in Hashimoto's thyroiditis resulting in elevated levels of thyroid-stimulating hormone and hypothyroidism.

38. d. Type IV hypersensitivity is the delayed-type hypersensitivity. Skin testing for tuberculosis causes a delayed-type hypersensitivity to intradermally injected antigens in individuals previouly exposed to the organism.

39. c. The fluorescent treponemal antibody absorption (FTA-ABS) test is a confirmatory test that detects specific antibodies to *Treponemal pallidum* in patient specimen.

40. c. The most likely answer is acute hepatitis B because of the presence of IgM anti-HBc in combination with the hepatitis surface antigen. Typically the presence of IgM indicates the presence of an acute phase of a disease.

41. a. Lymphomas are generally classified as malignancies of lymphoid tissue. Leukemias are generally classified as malignancies of hematopoietic cells of the bone marrow or peripheral blood. Both can be classified as acute or chronic.

42. b. Bruton's aggammaglobulinemia is typically seen in infancy. These patients present with frequent recurring infections, especially after protective maternal antibody is gone and normal levels of circulating T cells. The syndrome is a genetic B-cell enzyme deficiency in which the B cells fail to differentiate and mature to antibody-producing plasma cells.

43. d. Hereditary angioedema is characterized by recurrent swelling. The condition is genetic or can be acquired and is the result of a deficiency of the complement protein C1 Inhibitor.

44. a. DiGeorge syndrome is the most likely cause. In this syndrome the thymus fails to develop before birth. These patients also show a marked decrease in T cells.

45. d. Severe combined immunodeficiency is a genetic condition diagnosed in infancy. Both B-cell and T-cell development/function are arrested, resulting in no cell-mediated or humoral immunity.

46. b. Chronic granulomatous disease is an inherited disease that impairs the neutrophil's ability to kill certain bacteria. The neutrophils lack the enzyme nicotinamide adenine dinucleotide phosphate oxidase, easily demonstrated by the failure to reduce nitroblue tetrazolium or produce a blue end result. These patients have normal levels of lymphocytes.

47. b. Because common variable immunodeficiency is commonly diagnosed in early adulthood, this is the most likely explanation for this case study. Bruton's, X-linked agammaglobulinemia, and DiGeorge's syndrome are all typically identified in infancy.

48. d. Waldenström's macroglobulinemia is a disease resulting from an overproduction of an IgM producing B-cell population. The monoclonal IgM can be seen as a spike on electrophoresis.

49. c. Inflammation is caused by the increased blood flow and subsequent influx of neutrophils and other cells to an infected site. The increased blood flow and activity of the cells, including cytokine production, results in the redness, pain, and swelling to the area.

50. c. The hyperacute tissue graft reject occurs within minutes to hours of a transplant and is typically associated with transplantation across ABO blood groups and anti-ABO antibodies.

CHAPTER 7

1. c. N-Acetylgalactosamine (GalNAc) confers type A specificity. D-Galactose (Gal) confers type B specificity. L-Fucose (Fuc) confers type O specificity. The type A and type B sugars are built on Fuc.

2. d. The A_2 subgroup is described as having both qualitative and quantitative differences when compared to the A_1 subgroup. This means that there is less A antigen found on the red cells of people with A_2, and their A antigen looks "different" when compared to that of people with type A_1. Therefore the red cells from those with type A_2 will not react with anti-A_1 lectin. Approximately 20% of those with type A have the A_2 phenotype, and between 1% and 8% of those individuals make anti-A_1. There is no anti-A_2 reagent, and people with the A_2 phenotype would not react with A_2 cells, because that would imply an autoantibody is present.

3. b. People with the Bombay phenotype do not express the H antigen. An individual with the *hh* genotype would not express H antigen.

4. d. The *RHD* gene encodes for the D antigen. The *RHCE* gene determines C, c, E, and e specificities. Therefore the correct answer must include both genes.

5. a. In indirect antiglobulin test (IAT) phase, a control tube is included to show that agglutination detected in the patient test tube is appropriate. In weak D testing, the control tube uses saline rather than anti-human globulin (AHG) reagent. Agglutination in the control tube suggests that the patient cells are already sensitized with immunoglobulin, so a positive reaction in the patient test tube should be invalidated and investigated.

6. d. Individuals with the D– – phenotype may possess more D antigen because they have inherited a nonfunctioning *RHCE* gene. Basically, the *RHD* gene of D– – individuals has no competition when building D antigen, so they end up with more. Rh-null individuals do not express any Rh antigens. D-positive individuals possess the D antigen, but without knowing the genotype, the amount of D antigen cannot be estimated. A person with the *dce/dce* genotype would be considered Rh-negative.

7. c. The Duffy blood group system contains two codominant alleles, Fy^a and Fy^b, as well as Fy3, Fy5, and Fy6. The Fy^a, Fy^b, and Fy6 antigens are sensitive to ficin, and antibodies made against the Duffy antigens can show dosage. Approximately 68% of the black population is Fy(a−b−).

8. b. The I antigen is a precursor to the H antigen, so individuals who express the H antigen are presumed to have the I antigen. Therefore, if an individual expresses anti-I, it is typically considered to be an autoantibody. Anti-I typically presents as a cold-reacting, clinically insignificant IgM autoantibody.

9. a. Dithiothreitol (DTT) disrupts the tertiary structure of proteins, and denatures the Kell system antigens on red cells. Chloroquine diphosphate (CDP) can be used to dissociate antibodies from red cells. Anti-human globulin (AHG) reagent is used in the indirect antiglobulin test (IAT). Low ionic strength solution (LISS) is used as a potentiator.

10. c. The Kidd blood group system contains three antigens, Jk^a, Jk^b, and Jk3. Antibodies made against this blood group system are typically IgG, are best detected by indirect antiglobulin test (IAT), are enhanced by treating reagent red cells with enzymes, and can show dosage. Antibody titers have also been found to increase and then quickly decrease in patients.

11. d. The *Le* gene adds fucose to either a type I precursor chain to make the Le^a antigen or adds fucose to the H structure to make Le^b. Type II chains never express Lewis antigen activity. Newborns express the Le(a−b−) phenotype. Antibodies against the Lewis antigens are typically room temperature (RT) reactive, IgM class, and not clinically significant. Because they are typically IgM class, they cannot cross the placenta.

12. a. The U antigen is located near the red membrane on glycophorin B (GYB), so is always present when S or s is inherited. The amino acid structure on GYB is the same as the first 26 amino acid sequence on glycophorin A (GYA), so the only individuals who can make anti-N are those who lack GYB. Anti-M is typically an IgM class antibody, usually considered to be clinically insignificant. The effect of enzymes on the S antigen is variable.

13. b. Allo-anti-P is a rare antibody made by individuals with the P$_2$^{k} phenotype, so most examples of anti-P seen in the blood bank are actually autoanti-P. Autoanti-P is associated with paroxysmal cold hemoglobinuria. This antibody is an IgG antibody, also called the Donath-Landsteiner antibody. It is a biphasic hemolysin that attaches to P-positive red cells at lower temperatures. Complement is attached, and when the red cells are warmed to 37° C, hemolysis occurs. The other antibodies listed are typically RT reactive antibodies.

14. c. Coombs check cells are used to verify that anti-human globulin (AHG) has been added to reagent tubes and that it is active. When the check cells do not agglutinate, either AHG was not added or it was somehow inactivated. This usually occurs because of inadequate washing. If the check cells do not work, the entire test should be repeated.

15. a. Because enzyme treatment removed the reactivity noted in the original panel, we can infer that the unexpected antibody is directed to an antigen that is sensitive to enzymes. Of the antigens given in the list, only the Fy^a antigen is sensitive to enzymes.

16. b. Whenever an unexpected antibody is currently reactive or noted in a patient's history file, an indirect antiglobulin test (IAT) crossmatch must be performed. An immediate spin or electronic crossmatch is performed only on patients with no evidence of clinically significant antibodies, currently and historically.

17. d. A positive direct antiglobulin test (DAT) implies that the patient has an IgG antibody attached to the red cells. An elution procedure would dissociate the antibody from the red cells and collect it so the specificity can be determined. An adsorption removes red cell antibodies from plasma by adsorbing antibody onto red cells. Neutralization is performed to inactivate an antibody present in plasma. A titration is performed to determine how much antibody is present in plasma.

18. b. A positive rosette test is a qualitative indicator that a fetal bleed has occurred. This is important to detect in Rh-negative mothers who have an Rh-positive baby. To provide the correct dosage of Rh immunoglobulin, a quantitative test must be performed to quantify the amount of bleed that occurred. The Kleihauer-Betke test looks for fetal hemoglobin in a sample collected from the mother.

19. a. Thrombotic thrombocytopenic purpura (TTP) is characterized by thrombocytopenia, microangiopathic hemolytic anemia, renal dysfunction, and central nervous system involvement. Basically, giving platelets to a patient with TTP provides fuel that would exacerbate the condition. The other conditions listed are all appropriate indicators for platelet transfusion.

20. a. In disseminated intravascular coagulation, platelets and fibrinogen are inappropriately consumed, and so transfusion therapy should be targeted toward replacing those elements. Cryoprecipitate contains in a concentrated form most of the coagulation factors found in fresh frozen plasma. These include von Willebrand factor, fibrinogen (I), factor VIII, fibronectin, and factor XIII. Cryoprecipitate is primarily used clinically for patients with deficiencies of factor XIII and fibrinogen.

21. b. The best answer to this question is genetic inheritance, which includes but is not limited to the mother's blood type. Inheritance of the ABO antigens are driven by the *ABO, H,* and *Se* genes. Genetic inheritance, environmental factors, and immune function would influence the presence of antibodies against certain ABO antigens.

22. e. The patient can receive all of the blood types listed, but good blood management would dictate the order in which they were transfused. Generally, the best course of action would be to transfuse type A first because it is usually more plentiful than type B. Patients with O type can receive only type O blood, so it is best to conserve type O when possible. If type A is not plentiful, type B can be given. Once either type A *or* type B is given, types should not be mixed, to help avoid potential reactions. If type A or B is exhausted, it is then appropriate to move to type O.

23. d. An amorph, or silent, gene does produce a detectable antigen product. Examples of amorph, or null, phenotypes include Rh_{null}, O, and Lu (a−b−).

24. d. Most blood group systems genes exhibit codominant expression, or equal expression of both traits. In an autosomal recessive inheritance pattern, a trait is observable only when not paired with a dominant allele. X-linked and Y-linked inheritance patterns are complex and not typically seen in most blood group systems.

25. d. This answer is best explained through the use of a Punnett square:

	A	O
B	AB	BO
O	AO	OO

26. a. IgM is classified as having a large pentamer structure. Thus only one IgM is required to initiate the classical pathway in the complement system. In comparison, it takes two IgG molecules to activate complement.

27. c. In vitro, complement is detected through the use of anti-C3b or anti-C3d reagents. When detected, this indicates complement proteins have been attached to the red cell surface as a result of the activation of complement's classical pathway. In vivo, complement activation may proceed to intravascular hemolysis if conditions are right, which would result in the lysis of red blood cells.

28. c. Hemolysis as a reaction end-point indicates the presence of a complement-activating antibody. This reaction is especially important to recognize because it is an indicator of an antigen–antibody reaction. When hemolysis occurs, the red cell button is often smaller than buttons in other tubes and the supernatant may appear to be pinkish or reddish.

29. a. Mixed-field (mf) agglutination indicates the presence of two red cell populations when noted: one that is agglutinating, and one that is not. Of the scenarios presented, a person undergoing a delayed hemolytic transfusion reaction is most likely to have two cell populations in circulation—his/her own red cells and those from the transfusion. In a delayed transfusion reaction, an antibody has been stimulated against the transfused cells. A positive direct antiglobulin test (DAT) in this scenario indicates the antibody has attached to the transfused cells but not to the patient's own cells; therefore mixed-field reactivity is noted.

30. d. Patient's with hypogammaglobulinemia have an overall reduction of γ-globulins and may not be able to reverse grouping antibodies at levels detectable by ABO typing tests. IgM antibodies, other than those normally detected in reverse grouping tests, or cold autoantibodies may interfere with reverse grouping tests, making the results invalid. One example of an IgM antibody that may interfere with reverse grouping is anti-M.

31. b. Cells that are direct antiglobulin test (DAT)-positive or already have IgG attached would give a false-positive reaction when tested by the indirect antiglobulin test (IAT). The IAT is used to detect antibody bound to red cells in vitro. IAT is a two-stage procedure. In the first stage, antibodies are encouraged to combine with their corresponding antigen during an incubation step. If DAT-positive red cells (cells that have antibody already attached) are used in an IAT test, the first step, in effect, has already occurred. The attached IgG molecules will be detected in the second IAT step, the agglutination step, and give a false-positive reaction.

32. a. An elution is a process that dissociates antigen–antibody complexes on red cells. An adsorption is a process that uses red cells to remove red cell antibodies from a solution. Prewarming is a technique in which all reagents and patient samples used in a test procedure are incubated to reach 37° C (or the preferred testing temperature) before the test is conducted. Neutralization combines a soluble antigen with antibody in vitro and is used as an antibody identification technique. Therefore the best answer is elution.

33. d. Before a reagent is used, it should be assessed to determine if it meets preset acceptable performance criteria. For a red cell antiserum, an example of acceptable performance criteria might include reactivity with antigen-positive cells and no reactivity with antigen-negative cells. When testing antigen-positive cells, cells with heterozygous inheritance are generally recommended for use because this would detect the weakest expression of antigen (single-dose).

34. a. M and N are antithetical alleles in the MNS system. A cell with heterozygous expression of the M antigen would therefore need to also express the N antigen. In other words, it would need to be M+N+. Cells that express only M or N antigen (M+N− or M−N+) would be presumed to be homozygous for either the M or N antigen, respectively.

35. d. Neutralization combines a soluble antigen with antibody in vitro and is used as an antibody identification technique. Commercially prepared Lewis substance is available for purchase, so of the list provided, only anti-Le^a could be neutralized.

36. d. O red blood cells possess only the H antigen, and O red cells used for reagent purposes typically also lack D antigen. O-negative reagent red cells do not react with anti-D or any ABO antibodies.

37. c. Ethylenediaminetetraacetic acid (EDTA) chelates calcium ions to form a soluble complex; therefore it prevents the assembly of C1.

38. a. IgG-sensitized red cells (check cells or Coombs control cells) are commercially prepared with IgG antibodies attached. Proper control of anti-human globulin (AHG) tests systems (indirect antiglobulin test [IAT] or direct antiglobulin test [DAT]) require check cells to be added to negative tubes to ensure that AHG reagent was added and is active.

39. a. People with the AB blood type are considered to be universal recipients because they possess all possible ABO antigens; therefore they do not make any antibodies to ABO antigens. People with AB who are also negative for the D antigen may receive any type of blood as long as they have not made an antibody against the D antigen.

40. b. Transfusing 1 unit of red cells usually increases the hemoglobin (Hgb) by approximately 1 g/dL. Therefore transfusing 2 units of red cells to a patient not actively bleeding should increase the pretransfusion Hgb by 2 g/dL.

41. d. A patient with IgA deficiency and clinically significant anti-IgA requires washed red blood cells if a transfusion is necessary, because washing removes plasma proteins. It should be noted that washing is associated with a loss of about 10% to 20% of the original unit.

42. b. Of the types listed, the enzyme that converts H antigen to A_1 antigen is the most active. Therefore group A_1 has very little unconverted H antigen. The order of blood types possessing the most H antigens to the fewest H antigens is $O > A_2 > B > A_2B > A_1 > A_1B$.

43. b. Anti-Fy^a, anti-K, and anti-S all preferentially react at the anti-human globulin (AHG) phase. Although anti-M also can be found to react at the AHG phase, many examples react only at room temperature (RT) phase.

44. c. A patient with R_1r possesses D, C, c, and e antigens. R_2R_2 blood possesses D, c, and E antigens. To determine what antibodies could be made on exposure, determine what is different between the two, or what foreign antigen could be introduced to the patient. In this case, the E antigen would be foreign and could potentially stimulate antibody production.

45. c. To determine the combined phenotype for blood negative for the Jk^a and Fy^a antigens, multiply the percentages of person negative for each antigen.

$$0.23 \times 0.34 = 0.0782 \text{ or } 7.8\%$$

46. c. Persons of the O_h phenotype (Bombay) type as group O, but also possess potent anti-H. This anti-H is usually detected in tests using group O cells (antibody screen or crossmatch), but may be noted in ABO grouping, because the reverse cells could be hemolyzed instead of just agglutinated.

47. c.
- *H* gene: Produces H antigen on type II chains in secretions and H antigen on red cells
- *A* gene: Encodes for a glycosyltransferase that produces A antigen
- *O* gene: Silent gene
- *Le* gene: Encodes for a fucosyltransferase that produces Le^a antigen
- *se* gene: Amorph allele; inheriting two *se* genes means that the person is a nonsecretor

Le and secretor gene interaction: If *Le* is inherited without *Se*, only Le^a will be found on red cells and in saliva. Because this person is a nonsecretor, only Le^a antigen will be present in the secretions.

48. d. N-Acetylgalactosamine (GalNAc) confers type A specificity. D-Galactose (Gal) confers type B specificity. L-Fucose (Fuc) confers type O specificity. The type A and type B sugars are built on Fuc.

49. b. The DCe/dce (R$_1$r) phenotype is found in approximately 35% of whites and 15% of blacks. Although DCe/Dce (R$_1$R$_o$) and DCe/dCe (R$_1$r') are also possibilities, they are statistically less probable than DCe/dce. It is not possible for this person to be DCe/DcE, because she tested negative for the E antigen.

50. a. Individuals who inherit the D antigen with weakened or missing epitopes are described as having partial D antigen and often present with weakened expression of the D antigen. Because the partial D antigen is essentially incomplete, if an individual with partial D antigen is exposed to complete D antigen, the person would theoretically be able to make an alloantibody against the parts of the antigen that were foreign.

51. a. The k antigen is present in 98.8% of white individuals and 100% of black individuals, so it would be very rare to encounter someone who lacked the k antigen.

52. a. Expression of the Xg^a antigen is controlled by an X-linked gene, and prevalence of the antigen is higher in females than in males. Anti-Xg^a is usually IgG and the Xg^a antigen is sensitive to ficin.

53. d. Kidd system antibodies are usually IgG, are enhanced by enzymes, and do not store well. The titer of Kidd system antibodies in individual patients can rise and fall quickly, meaning that they might not be detected in an antibody screen if the titer is below the detection point of the test system.

54. c.
- R$_o$R$_o$ = Dce/Dce
- R$_1$R$_1$ = DCe/DCe
- R$_2$R$_2$ = DcE/DcE
- Rr = dce/dce

Therefore anti-E will react only with R$_2$R$_2$ cells because they are the only ones in this list that possess the corresponding E antigen.

55. b. Antibodies to Duffy system antigens are clinically significant (associated with hemolytic transfusion reactions) and have typically been shown to cause mild hemolytic disease of the fetus and newborn (HDFN). Because the Fy^a and Fy^b antigens are sensitive to enzymes, anti-Fy^a and anti-Fy^b would not react with enzyme-treated panel cells.

56. b. Anti-Ch and anti-Rg are usually IgG and react weakly. Neutralization of these two antibodies with pooled plasma is often used as part of antibody identification when either or both antibodies are present.

57. a. Potential donors who have been transfused in the last 12 months are deferred because of the possibility of exposure to diseases. Although viral marker testing has increased the safety of the blood supply, some diseases have a window in which markers are below the threshold of detection.

58. d. For autologous donors who weigh less than 100 lb, the volume of blood collected and the amount of anticoagulant used should be proportionately less when compared to a donation from a person weighing more than 110 lb. There is no age restriction for autologous donors. Hgb concentration in a potential autologous donor should be no less than 11 g/dL. Therefore the only condition that would preclude donation is current bacteremia. Blood collected while a patient is septic could cause harm if transfused later.

59. c. Cytomegalovirus (CMV) can be transmitted through transfusion via intact white cells contained in cellular blood products. Leukoreduction of blood products reduces the risk for CMV transmission because the CMV virus resides within intact white cells.

60. b. Plasma protein fraction (PPF) is prepared from large pools of human plasma. Although PPF can transmit infectious agents, the risk for doing so is reduced because certain viruses are inactivated or removed during preparation. Of the components listed, PPF is the only component treated in this manner.

61. c. To prepare platelets, whole blood is first centrifuged at a light spin, and platelet-rich plasma is expressed off the red cells into a satellite bag. The platelet-rich plasma is then centrifuged at a hard spin, and plasma is expressed off of the platelets.

62. b. Of the antibodies in this list, anti-K is the one most likely to be IgG and able to cross the placenta. Anti-I, anti-Le^a, and anti-N typically present as IgM class antibodies when encountered in patient specimens.

63. c. Group O red cells are most generally used for intrauterine and neonatal transfusions. Rh-negative blood is used for fetuses and neonates when the blood type is unknown or Rh-negative. In this case, because the mother has anti-D, Rh-negative blood must be used for the intrauterine transfusion.

64. c. Rh immunoglobulin (RhIG) is given to D-negative mothers to prevent the formation of anti-D. If a mother has already formed anti-D, then RhIG will offer no protection.

65. b. To quantify the amount of fetomaternal hemorrhage (FMH), the percentage of fetal red cells counted is multiplied by the mother's blood volume. The mother's blood volume can be calculated based on her height and weight, but often the average of 5000 mL is used for calculation.

$$(0.6/100) \times 5000 \text{ mL} = 30 \text{ mL}$$

66. c. An O mother (genotype *OO*) would contribute an *O* gene to her child, so regardless of the father's type, an O mother could not have an AB child. A clerical error has likely occurred and should be eliminated as a cause of potential error before further serologic studies are conducted.

67. b. Any antibody attached to a baby's red cells would have to come from the mother. Sample from the mother is easily acquired and should be readily available. Although an eluate could be performed on the baby's cells, that is a time-consuming procedure requiring a large sample. The best procedure is to perform an antibody panel on the mother's serum.

68. d. Use of whiteout obliterates the original results, so is not allowed. Use of pencil results in a record that could be changed—that is, the record is not permanent. If it is not recorded, it did not happen, so documentation after the fact is not allowed.

69. d. Kp^a is an antigen in the Kell system that is present in 2% of whites and found only rarely in blacks.

70. b. Vel is an antigen of high prevalence. Vel exhibits variable antigen expression on red cells and is resistant to treatment with enzymes.

71. a. A 1+ reaction has numerous medium and small agglutinates with a turbid background. A 2+ reaction has many medium-sized agglutinates with a clear background. A 3+ reaction has several large agglutinates and a clear background. A 4+ reaction has a solid agglutinate with a clear background.

72. e. *A* and *B* genes in the ABO system have codominant expression, and the *O* gene is a silent allele, producing no detectable gene product. For an individual to have a B phenotype, a *B* gene needs to be inherited either in a homozygous fashion or along with an *O* gene.

73. b. The forward type shows no agglutination, meaning the individual does not possess A or B antigens. The reverse type shows reactivity with both A$_1$ and B cells, meaning the individual possess antibodies to A and B antigens. This is characteristic of the O blood group.

Forward Type (Patient RBCs)		Reverse Type (Patient Serum)		Interpretation
Anti-A	Anti-B	A$_1$ Cells	B Cells	
0	0	+	+	O
+	0	0	+	A
0	+	+	0	B
+	+	0	0	AB

74. b. This patient forward types as group A and reverse types as group O, so an ABO discrepancy is present. In the event that the patient needs blood before the discrepancy can be resolved, group O must be transfused.

75. d. Group A and B individuals predominantly make IgM ABO antibodies, but small quantities of IgG antibody can be seen. Group O individuals tend to make predominantly IgG ABO antibodies. This is important to understand why ABO hemolytic disease of the newborn is more commonly seen in group O mothers.

76. d. This patient forward types as group A and reverse types as group O, so an ABO discrepancy is present. You could not report out results until the discrepancy was explained. The A$_1$ cells are reacting

only at 1 + strength, so this points to possible extra reactivity in the reverse type. Extra reactivity in the reverse type can be caused by rouleaux, cold-reactive antibodies (autoantibody or alloantibody), or passively acquired antibodies. In the case of a group A individual showing weak reactivity with A_1 cells, this is often seen in group A_2 individuals who have made anti-A_1. Testing the cells with anti-A_1 lectin would tell us if the patient possesses A_1 antigen, and testing the serum with A_2 cells would tell us if the extra reactivity noted in the reverse type is likely caused by anti-A_1. If the discrepancy could not be resolved, it would be advisable to request a new specimen.

77. d. A directed unit is donated for a specific person identified by the donor. This is not limited to blood relatives. A therapeutic phlebotomy is performed on individuals with polycythemia or other blood disorders, as ordered by a physician. When an individual donates blood for his or her own use, this is called an autologous donation.

78. b. The only difference between a directed donation and a volunteer donation is that a directed donation is reserved for a specified individual. Testing for transfusion of a directed unit is no different from that conducted on a volunteer unit intended for transfusion.

79. a. Allogeneic donors must meet the following physical examination criteria before donation:

Physical Examination Criteria

Criteria	Acceptable Limit	
	Allogeneic	**Autologous**
Age	Applicable state law or ≥ 16	Determined by medical director
Blood pressure	Systolic ≤ 180 mm Hg Diastolic ≤ 100 mm Hg	Determined by medical director
Pulse	50-100 beats per minute (bpm) without pathologic irregularity, < 50 bpm acceptable if an otherwise healthy athlete	Determined by medical director
Temperature	≤ 37.5° C (99.5° F) if measured orally, or equivalent if measured by another method	Deferral for conditions presenting risk for bacteremia
Hemoglobin/ hematocrit (Hct)	≥ 12.5 g/dL or an Hct value of ≥ 38%	≥ 11 g/dL or an Hct value of ≥ 33%

80. c. Receipt of human pituitary growth hormone (PGH) requires indefinite or permanent deferral because of the theoretical risk for transfusion-transmitted Creutzfeldt-Jakob disease (CJD).

81. b. Receipt of the rubella vaccine results in a temporary deferral of 4 weeks. Because this vaccine was administered 2 months ago in this individual, this would not cause a deferral. Transfusion of blood, components, human tissue, and/or plasma-derived clotting factor concentrates results in a temporary deferral of 12 months, so this individual would be temporarily deferred for 10 months based on the time of transfusion.

82. a. Use of a needle to administer nonprescription drugs is a condition for indefinite or permanent deferral. Casual contact with a person with an infectious disease generally is not a reason for deferral. Potential donors who have ingested aspirin are deferred (48 hours) only if they are donating apheresis platelets.

83. d. Required tests for infectious disease screening include:
- HBsAg
- Anti-HCV
- Anti-HBc
- HCV NAT
- Anti-HIV-1/2
- HIV NAT
- Anti-HTLV-I/II
- Syphilis – RPR or hemagglutination
- West Nile Virus (WNV) NAT
- IgG antibody to *Trypanosoma cruzi* (Chagas disease)

84. a. The HBsAg test detects the surface antigen of the hepatitis B virus in the blood. In an infected person, this antigen can be detected before the antibody to the core antigen (anti-HBc) is produced.

85. a. Cryoprecipitate (CRYO) is defined as the cold-insoluable portion of FFP thawed at 1-6° C and is suspended in 10-15 mL of plasma.

86. a. Platelets must be gently agitated during storage by the use of a rotator to prevent the pH from decreasing below 6.2.

87. a. Thawed cryoprecipitate components are stored at room temperature after thawing.

88. c. FFP is thawed at temperatures of 30° C to 37° C or in an FDA-approved device.

89. b. Frozen red blood cells are prepared for transfusion by first thawing the unit at 37° C. Next, the glycerol cyropreservative must be removed through a stepwise decreasing osmolar solution of saline.

90. a. As frozen units need to be thawed and deglycerolized prior to transfusion, use of frozen units in an emergency transfusion situation is not practical. Group AB Rh-negative patients can receive O, A, B, or AB Rh-negative units, so transfusion needs could likely be handled from available refrigerated units of blood. There are special considerations that must be made for pregnant women who requiring an intrauterine transfusion, but a frozen unit of red cells would likely only be used in the event of an antibody to a high frequency antigen. Therefore the best answer for this question is A. Red cell units are usually frozen for long-term preservation to maintain an inventory of rare units.

91. c. Indications for transfusion of cryoprecipitate include von Willebrand's disease, Hemophilia A, to control bleeding associated with fibrinogen deficiency, and Factor XIII deficiency.

92. b. Indications for transfusion of red blood cells include treatment of anemia in normovolemic patients and physician decision based on the clinical status of the patient. Patients that are massively bleeding, have bone marrow failure, or have decreased red blood cell survival have clinical situations that would warrant transfusion because of the need for hemoglobin replacement. In patients with compensated anemia, the body has adapted to allow for adequate tissue oxygenation. Transfusion should be withheld in this case until the patient shows clinical signs of inadequate tissue oxygenation.

93. b. FFP has no quality control or minimum requirements. Cryo must have ≥ 80 IU of Factor VIII and ≥ 150 mg of fibrinogen. Leukocyte reduced red cells must have $< 5 \times 10^6$ residual leukocytes and 85% of original red cells retained. There are no quality control or minimum requirements for the number of red cells in platelets.

94. a. FFP is stored at $\leq -18°$ C for 12 months, or $\leq -65°$ C for 7 years with FDA approval.

95. c. Per AABB guidelines, packed red cells are stored at 1° C to 6° C.

96. c. Platelets made from a single whole blood donation (random platelets) should contain $\geq 5.5 \times 10^{10}$ platelets in 75% of the units tested.

97. d. RBCs Frozen with 40% glycerol are stored at $\leq -65°$ C for 10 years.

98. c. In the IAT, incubation takes place at 37° C for a specified amount of time to allow antigen-antibody reactions to occur.

99. b. Per AABB Standards, if an automated temperature recording device is not used, then temperatures of the blood component storage environment must be measured manually every 4 hours.

100. b. As suggested by AABB, red cell reagents, antisera, and antiglobulin serum should have quality control performed each day of use.

CHAPTER 8

1. c. Chylomicrons, low-density lipoprotein (LDL), and high-density lipoprotein (HDL) are considered to be lipoproteins that transport lipids throughout the body; cholesterol is classified as a lipid.

2. d. Dextran sulfate precipitates all Apo B–containing lipoproteins (chylomicrons, very-low-density lipoprotein [VLDL], intermediate density lipoprotein [IDL], and low-density lipoprotein [LDL]) leaving high-density lipoprotein (HDL) (Apo A–containing lipoprotein) in the supernatant. HDL is then mixed with the reagent cholesterol esterase and cholesterol oxidase to quantitate HDL concentrations.

3. a. Lipoproteins are characterized by size and density. High-density lipoprotein (HDL) is the smallest, most dense lipoprotein, carrying 50% of its weight as protein.

4. d. Triglycerides are most adversely affected by recent food intake, and therefore a fast is always recommended for triglyceride analysis.

5. c. Apo E is a ligand for the low-density lipoprotein (LDL) receptor, reverses cholesterol transport, and is a regulator of cell growth and immune responses.

6. c. Two enzymes are responsible for esterifying cholesterol, lecithin-cholesterol acyl transferase (extracellular), and acetyl coenzyme A (acyl-CoA) cholesterol acyltransferase (intracellular).

7. a. Although lipoproteins can be assayed using a variety of anticoagulants, the preferred anticoagulant is ethylenediaminetetraacetic acid (EDTA) because it preserves lipoproteins over time.

8. b. Triglycerides are transported throughout the body by means of two lipoproteins: very-low-density lipoprotein (VLDL) and chylomicrons. VLDL carries endogenously derived triglycerides, and chylomicrons carry exogenously derived triglycerides.

9. b. Low-density lipoprotein (LDL) cholesterol is calculated as follows:

$$LDL = TC - (HDL + TG/5)$$
$$LDL = 300 - (50 + 200/5)$$
$$LDL = 300 - 90$$
$$LDL = 210 \text{ mg/dL}$$

10. b. Low-density lipoprotein (LDL) is currently the only lipoprotein or lipid that is recommended for use by physicians for therapeutic lifestyle changes.

11. b. Both forms of hyperbetalipoproteinemia (types IIA and IIB) are due to either a defect in the low-density lipoprotein (LDL) receptor (type IIA) or a defect in Apo B-100 (type IIB).

12. d. All enzymatic methods to measure triglycerides, regardless of the enzyme used, begin with the conversion of triglycerides to glycerol and fatty acids in the presence of the enzyme lipase, followed by the conversion of glycerol to glycerol-3-phosphate in the presence of the enzyme glycerol kinase.

13. c. Marked increases in triglyceride levels, between 1000 and 2000 mg/dL have been associated with increased risk for the development of pancreatitis.

14. a. Apo A-I is the predominant apoprotein associated with the high-density lipoprotein (HDL) molecule, activates (lecithin cholesterol acyltransferase [LCAT]), and is associated with reverse cholesterol transport. As a result, it is protective against coronary artery disease.

15. c. The recommended fasting state for the study of lipids involves nothing but water for 12 hours before the blood sample collection.

16. c. Using Beer's law, the concentration of cholesterol in the patient (Smithers) serum is determined as follows: 0.679

$$Concentration_{cholesterol} = Absorbance_{unknown}/Absorbance_{standard}$$
$$\times Concentration_{standard}$$
$$Concentration_{cholesterol} = 0.729/0.679 \times 200 \text{ mg/dL}$$
$$Concentration_{cholesterol} = 209 \text{ mg/dL}$$

17. d. Sucrose upon hydrolysis yields fructose and glucose.

18. d. According to the American Diabetes Association criteria for the diagnosis of diabetes (below), this patient would most likely be classified as having type 2 diabetes.

Symptoms and a random plasma glucose
≥ 200 *mg/dL or*
Fasting plasma glucose ≥ 126 *mg/dL or*
2-hr OGTT ≥ 200 *mg/dL or*
Hbg A1c $\geq 6.5\%$

19. d. Insulin lowers glucose levels by increasing the uptake of glucose into the cell and through increased glucose metabolism.

20. b. The data presented indicate that the glucose and low-density lipoprotein (LDL) are mildly elevated, and the blood urea nitrogen (BUN), creatinine, and microalbuminuria results are moderately elevated. This information together indicates that the patient is at most risk for the development of diabetic nephropathy.

21. d. The renal threshold for glucose is 160 to 180 mg/dL. Once plasma levels of glucose hit that threshold, it will spill over into the urine.

22. c. Blood urea nitrogen (BUN) and creatinine are markers of kidney function; however, they are not sensitive enough markers to detect early diabetic nephropathy. The best test to use to detect diabetic nephropathy is the microalbuminuria test.

23. b. An obese, elderly patient with report of increased urination at night, increased thirst, and increased appetite is indicative of a diagnosis of diabetes, most likely type 2 diabetes in this case. With the patient being 68 years of age and obese with only mildly elevated levels of glucose, the diagnosis of type 1 is unlikely. Patients with diabetes would have increased glycated hemoglobin. With a fasting glucose of 210 mg/dL, the assessment of hypoglycemia is unwarranted.

24. c. According to the American Diabetes Association, A1c results between 5.7% and 6.4% indicate an impaired state (prediabetes).

25. b. Whole blood glucose levels are 12% to 15% lower than plasma glucose levels. Therefore a plasma glucose level of 100 mg/dL would roughly correspond to a whole blood level of 85 mg/dL.

26. a. Of the three methods to measure glucose, glucose oxidase, hexokinase, and glucose dehydrogenase, the hexokinase method is considered virtually specific for glucose.

27. b. The cutoff points for normal, impaired, and diagnostic states are described below. According to the values below, the data suggest an impaired state.

	Normal	Impaired	Diagnostic
Resting plasma glucose	<200 mg/dL	140-199 mg/dL	≥200 mg/dL
Fasting plasma glucose	<100 mg/dL	100-125 mg/dL	≥126 mg/dL
2-Hr oral glucose tolerance test	<200 mg/dL	140-199 mg/dL	≥200 mg/dL
A1c	<5.7 %	5.7%-6.4%	≥6.5%

28. d. Acute glomerulonephritis is often associated with a recent group A β-hemolytic *Streptococcus* infection. It is hypothesized that immune complex development associated with a group A β-hemolytic *Streptococcus* infection directly injures the glomerular basement membrane of the glomerulus.

29. a. The classic Jaffe reaction involves complexing of creatinine with an alkaline picrate solution to produce a red complex (Janovski complex).

30. c. The kidney is responsible for acid-base balance through the removal of H ions via (1) the reaction of the hydrogen ions with bicarbonate, (2) the reaction of hydrogen ions with filtered buffers such as disodium salt, (3) reaction with ammonia, and (4) excretion of the free hydrogen ions.

31. b.

$$\frac{\text{Urine creatinine (mg/dL)} \times \text{Urine volume (mL/ min)}}{\text{Serum creatinine (mg/dL)}}$$

$$\times \frac{1.73 \text{ m}^2}{\text{Surface area of patient}}$$

Urine volume : 1.75 L/day × 1000 mL/1 L × 1 hr/60 min

$$= 1.22 \text{ mL/ min}$$

$$\frac{120 \text{ mg/dL} \times 1.22 \text{ mL/ min}}{1.2 \text{ mg/dL}} \times \frac{1.73 \text{ m}^2}{1.80 \text{ m}^2} = 117 \text{ mL/ min}$$

32. c. 2× Sodium (mmol/L) + Glucose mg/dL/18 + Blood urea nitrogen (BUN) mg/dL/2.8

33. c. Blood urea nitrogen (BUN) and creatinine are considered markers of kidney function. Renal failure can cause elevations in BUN and other prerenal conditions such as dehydration or a high-protein diet that raise levels of BUN without affecting creatinine levels.

34. a. Osmolality and specific gravity both measure the solute concentration of a solution. Specific gravity measures solute concentration as the solute's density, which is subject to interference from large molecules such as glucose and proteins. Osmolality, on the other hand, measures solute concentration as the number of molecules present by measuring the number of molecules per kilogram of water.

35. c. The osmolal gap (difference between calculated and measured osmolality) when increased is indicative of the presence of osmotically active substances present other than sodium, blood urea nitrogen (BUN), and glucose. Other osmotically active substances may include ethanol, methanol, ethylene glycol, lactate, or β-hydroxybutyrate.

36. c. According to the National Kidney Foundation, a glomerular filtration rate of 60 to 89 indicates mild kidney damage.

37. d. Dubin-Johnson syndrome and extrahepatic obstruction are conditions that cause elevations in total bilirubin, with the major fraction increased being the conjugated fraction (direct). Gilbert's disease is a condition resulting from genetic mutation in the gene that produces the enzyme uridyl diphosphate glucuronyl transferase, the enzyme responsible for the conjugation of bilirubin. Therefore Gilbert's disease will manifest as unconjugated hyperbilirubinemia.

38. b. Severe liver disease is the most common cause of altered ammonia metabolism. Therefore the monitoring of ammonia levels may be used to determine prognosis.

39. a. Hemolysis and neonatal jaundice would manifest with elevations in total bilirubin primarily as a result of the unconjugated fraction. Biliary obstruction manifests as conjugated hyperbilirubinemia.

40. c. Crigler-Najjar syndrome is an inherited disorder of bilirubin metabolism. Neonates with Crigler-Najjar syndrome have no uridyl diphosphate glucuronyl transferase and therefore cannot conjugate bilirubin for excretion. In neonates this increased unconjugated bilirubin will cause kernicterus without aggressive treatment.

41. a. When bilirubin becomes conjugated it can enter the intestines. In the gastrointestinal tract, bacteria convert conjugated bilirubin to urobilinogen. Three things will happen to the urobilinogen: (1) it is excreted in the feces; (2) it enters extrahepatic circulation, where it is absorbed and recirculated to the liver and excreted in the feces;

and (3) it enters systemic circulation and is excreted in the urine.

42. c. The enzyme responsible for bilirubin conjugation is uridyl diphosphate glucuronyl transferase.

43. a. Aspartate aminotransferase (AST) and alanine aminotransferase (ALT) are the most sensitive markers of hepatocellular damage. γ-Glutamyltransferase (GGT) and alkaline phosphatase (ALP) are markers of hepatobiliary damage. Ammonia, although it may be seen in severe cases of liver damage, is not a sensitive marker of hepatocellular damage.

44. c. Dubin-Johnson is an autosomal recessive disorder resulting in a defect in the ability of the liver cell to secrete conjugated bilirubin into the bile.

45. c. UDP-glucuronyl transferase is the enzyme that is responsible for the conjugation of bilirubin.

46. c. Aspartate aminotransferase (AST) and alanine aminotransferase (ALT) are markers of hepatocellular damage, whereas γ-glutamyl transferase (GGT) and alkaline phosphatase (ALP) are markers of hepatobiliary damage.

47. b. Unconjugated bilirubin is insoluble in water and must be transported by albumin to the liver for further metabolism. Albumin binding prevents unconjugated bilirubin from crossing cell membranes and accumulating in cells. Extremely high levels of unconjugated bilirubin can exceed albumin-binding capacity and allow unconjugated bilirubin to cross the immature blood-brain barrier in neonates, causing kernicterus (toxic damage to the cells in the basal ganglia).

48. d. With chronic alcohol abuse, the amount of alanine aminotransferase (ALT) declines, which results in an increased ratio of aspartate aminotransferase (AST) to ALT. γ-Glutamyltransferase (GGT) is a membrane-bound enzyme that is markedly increased with ethanol use, and alkaline phosphatase (ALP) is slightly elevated with alcohol use.

49. b. Primary biliary cirrhosis (PBC) is an autoimmune disorder that targets the bile ducts. PBC is associated with antimitochondrial antibodies and the presence of lipoprotein X (an abnormal lipoprotein produced in individuals with obstructive biliary tract disease).

50. a. Acidosis will manifest with a pH less than 7.35; because it is metabolic, it would be driven by low levels of bicarbonate (HCO_3^- <22 mol/L). Because it is an uncompensated condition, the respiratory parameter would be in the normal range (P_{CO_2} 35-45 mm Hg).

51. b. A decrease in ventilation would cause the accumulation of the acidic gas P_{CO_2}, causing respiratory acidosis.

52. d. The bicarbonate–carbonic acid buffer system is the most important physiologic buffering system in the body, because it is the buffer system that immediately counteracts carbon dioxide normally produced by cell metabolism.

53. c. This process of exchange between bicarbonate and chloride as bicarbonate leaves the red blood cell is termed the chloride shift.

54. a. P_{CO_2} is an acidic gas controlled by the lungs (respiratory system) and when in increased concentrations will cause respiratory-driven acidosis.

55. a. Room air contains a P_{O_2} of 150 mm Hg and a P_{CO_2} of approximately zero. When a blood gas sample is received in the laboratory uncapped or if it contains air bubbles, gas equilibration between the air and the blood will occur, causing a decreased P_{CO_2}, increased P_{O_2}, and increased pH. Blood gas samples from a patient without oxygen supplementation with a P_{O_2} greater than 110 mm Hg should be investigated for air contamination.

56. d. Ideal blood gas collection should include collection in a plastic syringe containing dry heparin; it should be collected, delivered to the laboratory, and assayed within 15 minutes at room temperature. If the process will exceed 15 minutes, samples are stable for 45 minutes stored on crushed ice.

57. d. The pH may be calculated using the Henderson-Hasselbalch equation for the bicarbonate–carbonic acid buffer system as follows (NOTE: In plasma and at body temperature [37° C] the pK_a of the bicarbonate buffering system is 6.1):

$$pH = pK_a + \log(HCO_3^-/(0.03)\,(P_{CO_2})$$
$$pH = 6.1 + \log 28/(0.03)\,(45)$$
$$pH = 6.1 + \log 20.7$$
$$pH = 7.42$$

58. c. In healthy individuals when the kidneys and lungs are functioning at full capacity the ratio of bicarbonate to carbonic acid is 20:1.

59. d. Reference intervals for arterial blood gases are as follows:

pH	7.35-7.45
P_{CO_2}	35-45 mm Hg
P_{O_2}	80-110 mmol/L
HCO_3^-	22-26 mmol/L

60. c. In uncompensated metabolic acidosis the pH would be decreased (<7.35), and this decrease would be driven by the metabolic component (HCO_3^-). HCO_3^- would be decreased (<22 mmol/L). Because it is uncompensated, the respiratory component (P_{CO_2}) would be normal (34-45 mmol/L).

61. a. The anion gap, especially when elevated, is useful in diagnosing the type of metabolic acidosis and in indicating if a mixed disorder exists.

62. c. The predominant feedback system associated with the endocrine system is negative feedback, in which increased levels of hormones feed back negatively to the hypothalamus and pituitary.

63. d. All results are normal except for the result for thyroid-stimulating hormone (TSH), which is increased. Because TSH is produced at the pituitary, increased TSH results indicate a hypothyroid condition.

64. a. The three main noniatrogenic causes of Cushing's syndrome (hypercortisolism) include (1) a pituitary tumor (Cushing's disease), (2) an adrenal adenoma (Cushing's syndrome), and (3) ectopic adrenocorticotropic hormone (ACTH) production. Pituitary-driven Cushing's disease is ACTH dependent and results from a benign pituitary adenoma that produces ACTH. Therefore ACTH values are increased. During bilateral inferior petrosal sinus sampling the gradient between the inferior petrosal sinus and peripheral venous site after corticotropin-releasing hormone administration in Cushing's disease is greater than 3 (often close to 50).

65. b. Hypothyroidism is a condition in which thyroid hormone levels are low; therefore because of positive feedback the thyroid-stimulating hormone will be increased.

66. c. Thyroid-releasing hormone (TRH) is a tripeptide produced from the hypothalamus. TRH acts directly on the pituitary gland to produce TSH, which acts on the thyroid gland to produce T_3 and T_4.

67. a. Thyroid-stimulating hormone (TSH) is the most sensitive indicator of thyroid dysfunction. When TSH levels are normal is it unlikely that a thyroid abnormality exists. The only abnormal result provided is the total T_4 levels, which inherently are subject to false elevations in individuals with abnormal binding proteins. This is why total levels of thyroid hormones (TT_3 and TT_4) are not routinely obtained in clinical practice.

68. c. Two essential components needed for thyroid hormone production include tyrosine and iodine.

69. c. The term *subclinical* refers to a condition that can be detected using sensitive laboratory tests, but has not progressed to the point of producing symptoms or abnormal thyroid hormone levels. In subclinical hypothyroidism, the thyroid-stimulating hormone will be decreased but the thyroid hormone levels will still be normal.

70. d. The three main noniatrogenic causes of Cushing's syndrome (hypercortisolism) include (1) a pituitary tumor (Cushing's disease), (2) an adrenal adenoma (Cushing's syndrome), and (3) ectopic adrenocorticotropic hormone (ACTH) production. Cushing's syndrome driven by an adrenal adenoma is ACTH independent, resulting in an adrenal adenoma producing cortisol. Because the pituitary gland is functional, it is still responsive to negative feedback to the pituitary because of the increased cortisol levels and the ACTH result will be decreased. During a bilateral inferior petrosal sinus sampling the gradient between the inferior petrosal sinus and peripheral venous site after corticotropin-releasing hormone administration in Cushing's syndrome is less than 2.

71. b. Releasing and inhibiting factors are produced from the hypothalamus, and trophic hormones are produced from the pituitary.

72. b. The free thyroxine (FT_4) index is calculated as follows:

$$FT_4I = TT_4 \times \text{Thyroid hormone binding ratio}/100$$

73. a. Assuming that a screening test is abnormal, a definitive stimulation test is often performed. The definitive test involves looking at the growth hormone response after intravenous insulin infusion.

74. b. Pheochromocytoma is a rare and usually benign tumor arising from the adrenal gland that results in the increased production of catecholamines (epinephrine and norepinephrine). Total catecholamine levels are not recommended for diagnosis because catecholamines are highly labile and increase as a result of stress and pain. Therefore the recommendation is to assay plasma free metanephrines (metanephrines and normetanephrines), which are the metabolites of epinephrine and norepinephrine

75. a. Thyrotropin-releasing hormone (TRH) is a tripeptide produced from the hypothalamus that acts on the pituitary to produce thyroid-stimulating hormone (TSH). When exogenous TRH is administered to a person and there is no response, it is indicative of a nonfunctioning pituitary gland. Thyroid gland disorders arising from a problem with the pituitary gland are referred to as secondary conditions.

76. a. Thyroid hormone production occurs in five steps: (1) iodide trapping, (2) organification, (3) coupling, (4) storage, and (5) secretion.

77. d. Pheochromocytoma results in the excess production of catecholamines, which increase cardiac output and blood pressure to divert blood to muscle or brain, mobilize fuel from storage, and cause hypertension. If pheochromocytoma is untreated, death may occur from cardiovascular complications.

78. b. Estrogens are a group of steroids responsible for the development of female sex organs. The estrogens include estrone, estradiol, and estriol. Estradiol is the predominant form of estrogen.

79. b. The general relationship among an enzyme, its substrate, and its product is represented using the Michaelis-Menten theory, which is represented as $E + S \leftrightarrow ES \rightarrow E + P$, where E is the enzyme, S is the substrate, ES is the enzyme substrate complex, and P is the product.

80. d. Lipase and amylase are both markers of pancreatic function; however, lipase is considered more specific because it remains elevated longer in acute pancreatitis.

81. c. Alkaline phosphatase (ALP) belongs to a group of enzymes that catalyze the hydrolysis of phosphate esters in an alkaline medium. ALP catalyzes the conversion of p-nitrophenyl phosphate to a colored p-nitrophenol product.

82. b. One international unit of enzyme activity is the amount of enzyme that uses substrate at the rate of 1 μmole/min.

83. d. The recommended sample of choice for analysis of creatinine kinase (CK) is serum or heparin plasma. Anticoagulants other than heparin may inhibit CK activity.

84. c. Creatine kinase (CK) is an enzyme found in the heart, brain, skeletal muscle, and other tissues. Increased amounts of CK are released in the blood when muscle damage occurs, such as the muscle damage seen in acute myocardial infarction and Duchenne's muscular dystrophy.

85. c. Elevated alkaline phosphatase (ALP) levels may be seen with bone and liver disorders. In addition, ALP will also be increased physiologically during periods of bone growth, when bone fractures are healing, and in pregnancy.

86. a. Enzyme assays are recommended to be performed during the linear phase, so that a consistent change over time can be used to calculate the enzyme concentration.

87. a. The best tube to use for testing these enzymes is a red-top tube. The other anticoagulants may cause issues with some of the enzyme assays.

88. b. Amylase is an enzyme that can degrade complex carbohydrate molecules such as starch.

89. c. Parathyroid hormone (PTH) is responsible for maintaining calcium levels by acting on bone and the kidneys and by activating vitamin D. PTH acts on the bone to release calcium and phosphorus through osteoclastic activity. Once released from bone, PTH acts on the kidneys to allow absorption of calcium and excretion of phosphorous. High levels of PTH would most likely manifest with hypercalcemia and hypophosphatemia.

90. b. Calcium exists in three forms, 45% unbound (ionized), 45% bound to albumin, and 10% bound to other anions. Only the ionized (unbound form) is the physiologically active form.

91. d. Parathyroid hormone (PTH) is responsible for maintaining calcium levels by acting on bone and the kidneys and by activating vitamin D. PTH acts on the bone to release calcium and phosphorus through osteoclastic activity. Once released from bone, PTH acts on the kidneys to cause the kidneys to absorb calcium and excrete the phosphorous.

92. d. Hemolysis is the most common cause of hypercalcemia.

93. b. Calcitonin is a hormone produced by the C cells of the thyroid. Calcitonin is involved in calcium regulation and inhibits bone breakdown; thus it decreases calcium and phosphorus.

94. c. Sodium is the predominant plasma cation and maintains osmotic pressure.

95. a. Diabetes insipidus is a condition resulting from a deficiency in antidiuretic hormone that manifests with excessive thirst and excretion of large amounts of severely diluted urine. Because the body cannot conserve water, sodium levels rise and dehydration may occur.

96. c. In a state of acidosis there is an increased amount of hydrogen ions that combine with albumin. Because H ions are combining with albumin, less albumin is available to bind to calcium; therefore ionized calcium levels increase.

97. b. The anion gap is often reported with electrolyte measurements as a means of identifying shifts that may occur in these assays. Because the anion gap is a calculation parameter, it is an inexpensive and easy quality control check.

98. b. Hemolysis can often result from a tourniquet being on the arm too long.

99. d. A potassium value of 15 mEq/L is too high to be considered physiologic. The sample should be checked for a potential preanalytical interference, including hemolysis and incorrect collection tube (contamination via an anticoagulant).

100. a. The major intracellular cation is potassium. Sodium is the major extracellular cation.

CHAPTER 9

1. b. The sequence of a single strand of DNA gives rise to the sequence of its complementary strand. During replication the complementary strands are the "daughter" strand. Replication is semiconservative, meaning the new dsDNA is made up of a parent and daughter strand.

2. b. Nucleic acids include a sugar moiety (2-deoxyribose in the case of DNA), a phosphoric acid, and purine or pyrimidine base; deoxyribonucleic acid is DNA and ribonucleic acid is RNA. Nucleosides comprise a base and a sugar.

3. c. The "central dogma" proposes that DNA replicates from DNA, DNA is transcribed to RNA, and RNA is translated to produce proteins. Only genes (not all DNA sequences) are expressed as proteins, and specific sequences of nucleic acid make up a gene.

4. a. The coding sequence in a gene is divided into regions called exons. These coding regions specify the amino acid sequence in the resulting protein. Introns are the noncoding regions of a gene. The promoter region regulates initiation and rate of transcription.

5. c. DNA polymerase III synthesizes a daughter strand in the 5′ to 3′ direction only, because nucleotides are only able to be added to the 3′ carbon end of the sugar.

6. d. mRNA with its three-nucleotide codon will bind to the tRNA molecule's anticodone, which then carries the attached amino acid to a ribosome to be added to a growing peptide chain.

7. d. Mitochondrial DNA does not follow the Mendelian inheritance pattern.

8. b. The lagging strands are discontinuously assembled and require ligase to join the fragments.

9. a. RNA differs from DNA in that it has uracil that replaces thymine. RNA is also single stranded.

10. a. Response a is the only correct answer; b is incorrect because the gene-rich regions are euchromatin; answer c is incorrect because telomeres and centromeres are heterochromatin; d is incorrect because chromosomes are composed of DNA.

11. d. Restriction enzymes are sequence-specific endonucleases that cut dsDNA into fragments, resulting in either blunt-ended or sticky-ended pieces. These endonucleases are isolated from specific bacteria that use the enzymes as protection from invasion by foreign DNA.

12. c. Polymerases catalyze the synthesis of complementary nucleic acid polymers using a parent strand as a template. In vitro, these enzymes can extend an oligonucleotide primer that is annealed to a template strand.

13. b. Alleles linked when inherited are called haplotypes. The location of a gene on a chromosome is the locus, and the possible alternative forms of the gene at the locus are referred to as alleles. The variations in alleles are known as polymorphisms.

14. c. Messenger RNA (mRNA) is produced in the nucleus of the cell. After processing, the mature mRNA leaves the nucleus and enters the cytoplasm, where it is translated.

15. c. In the organic extraction method, cellular debris and protein are separated by organic solvent extraction from the hydrophilic soluble DNA fraction. The DNA will be in the aqueous phase of the biphasic solution.

16. a. Purity of extracted RNA and DNA can be evaluated by assessing the ratio of the absorbances at 260 nm and 280 nm (A260/A280). A ratio of 2.0 indicates a pure DNA extract.

17. c. Solid-phase extraction methods are amiable for high-throughput and adaptable for automated processing.

18. d. The sizes/molecular weight of the genomic DNA fragment can be estimated by gel electrophoresis using size standards.

19. a. Signal amplification techniques use nucleic acids to increase the signal for detection. The branched-chain DNA (bDNA) method is one of these techniques.

20. b. Denaturing the target duplexes into single strands is the first step in polymerase chain reaction (PCR). Next, the sample is allowed to cool and the primers anneal specifically to the complementary sequences on the target. The primers are extended by the polymerase.

21. c. RNA targets can be amplified into DNA sequences when they are initially transcribed into cDNA using reverse transcription. Some thermostable enzymes have both DNA polymerase and reverse transcription activities, so both steps can be performed in the same tube with the same enzyme.

22. d. Primers are provided in great excess and specifically anneal to a complementary sequence on the target DNA. Once the primers have annealed, the action of the polymerase synthesizes two additional DNA strands containing the primers as the 5′ ends.

23. a. The negative control or blank (all reactants minus target DNA) is one of the most important controls when providing quality control for a polymerase chain reaction (PCR) run. If the blank demonstrates DNA bands, the master mix has likely been contaminated with PCR reaction product from a previous run.

24. c. Southern blotting is the classic method for detecting large segments of DNA that are not easily amplified. The original sample DNA is digested by a restriction enzyme, separated by electrophoresis, and transferred to a solid support, followed by selective visualization of fragments by hybridization of labeled probes.

25. a. Hybridization probes are those that reversibly change fluorescence on duplex formation. Fluorescence resonance energy transfer techniques depend on the proximity between two distinct fluorescent labels. When the two labels are brought closer together through hybridization, fluorescence is released.

26. d. Real-time polymerase chain reaction (PCR) monitors the amount of product formed each cycle by systematically quantifying the fluorescence signal. The fluorescent signals depend on the amount of target DNA present in the sample.

27. d. Ultraviolet-induced cross-linking of DNA can minimize the effects of amplicon contamination during sample setup; laboratory surfaces should be regularly cleaned using amplicon-decontaminating agents, such as solutions of bleach, and closed analytical systems (i.e., reaction tubes that are analyzed without being opened) should be used to reduce contamination with amplicon.

28. c. The migration of a nucleic acid fragment through agarose gel depends on the size, shape, and charge of the fragment.

29. b. Polymerase chain reaction (PCR) requires several components: DNA polymerase, a buffer for the polymerase, primers, the four deoxynucleotide triphosphates, and a source of template DNA (the target). DNA endonuclease is not required for this method.

30. c. The purpose of primer extension is to produce amplicons, which are the resulting fragments from a polymerase chain reaction (PCR) cycle. The DNA polymerase takes the individual nucleotides and adds them to the 3′ end on each primer that has annealed to the target DNA strands. The target DNA strands act as the reference for the polymerase.

31. c. Ethidium bromide binds to nucleic acids by intercalating between bases. When ethidium bromide is irradiated with ultraviolet (UV) light it fluoresces. This fluorescence can be detected by holding a UV lamp next to the gel or using visualization software.

32. a. The term DNA microarray refers to a microscopic grouping of DNA molecules attached to a solid support mechanism. A DNA microarray is also referred to as a DNA chip or gene chip. A DNA microarray allows for the detection of gene expression or possible deletions using comparative genome hybridization (CGH).

33. a. Genomic sequencing has led to an increased understanding of protein interrelationships and expression in cells. Proteomics is the study of proteins on a cellular level. Like genomics, proteomics is a large-scale process, but it is probably more complicated than analysis at the gene and transcriptional levels.

34. c. The size of the target's genome does not affect hybridization, but the target nucleic acid sequence does, along with pH and temperature.

35. a. Primers should not be larger than 30 base pairs long. Primer design should take into account melting temperature (Tm) for both the forward and reverse primers.

36. a. After the generation of terminated fragments in the cycle sequencing steps, fragments are tagged with a fluorescent dye labeled terminator ddNTPs then separated by denaturing polyacrylamide gel or capillary electrophoresis.

37. d. In pyrosequencing, each incorporation event is accompanied by release of a pyrophosphate (PPi), so the quantity of PPi produced is equimolar to the amount of incorporated nucleotide. The conversion of PPi and adenosine 5′ phosphosulfate into adenosine triphosphate (ATP) by the ATP sulfurylase allows ATP to drive the conversion of luciferin into oxyluciferin, which generates visible light. The light produced is proportional to the number of nucleotides incorporated.

38. c. In autosomal recessive disease, two abnormal alleles at a given locus (by receiving one mutant allele from each carrier parent) are necessary to produce the disease phenotype. Affected individuals may be homozygous with two copies of the same mutation.

39. b. Imprinting refers to the differential marking of specific paternally and maternally inherited alleles during gametogenesis, resulting in differential expression of those genes.

40. c. DNA extracted from peripheral blood (or bone marrow) white cells is the preferred specimen for molecular techniques when they are used to diagnose inherited disorders. In inherited disorders, the DNA from any cell could theoretically be used because the DNA at the molecular level will be identical regardless of cell origin. However, DNA from peripheral blood white cells is the easiest tissue to obtain. Mature red blood cells cannot be used because they do not have a nucleus and therefore do not have any DNA.

41. d. A short tandem repeat (STR) consists of DNA sequences that have a core sequence of two to seven base pairs, which are repeated in tandem several times. An example of a trinucleotide repeat occurring four times is 5′ GTG-GTG-GTG-GTG 3′.

42. b. A locus is a location of a gene where polymorphic alleles are found. The alleles at a locus are the genotype for the locus.

43. a. Genes encoding the class I molecules, which includes *HLA A, B,* and *C* are considered class I genes. Class II consists of *DR, DQ,* and *DP.*

44. b. Hybrid capture is a signal-amplification assay that detects cytomegalovirus (CMV) and human papillomavirus (HPV) DNA in specimens. Hybrid capture methods use a bound antibody that is specific for RNA-DNA hybrid molecules that are formed during solution-phase hybridization of a DNA sample and an unlabeled RNA probe. The signal from the complex is amplified and detected.

45. b. Molecular techniques are designed to achieve high specificity for the organism that the test is designed to detect; however, the techniques are subject to false-negative results because of the presence of inhibitors. Additionally, detection of nucleic acid of a pathogen does not ensure that the organism is the cause of the disease. The organism might be forming part of the normal flora, colonizing a specific area, or causing infection but not disease.

46. d. The typical retroviral genome contains at least three genes: *gag, pol,* and *env.*

47. d. The translocation involving chromosomes 9 and 22 known as the Philadelphia chromosome is a hallmark in the diagnosis of chronic myelogenous leukemia (CML). The resulting protein has enhanced tyrosine kinase activity. t(9:22) may be seen in acute lymphoblastic leukemia (ALL) with a poor prognosis.

48. a. In a fluorescence in situ hybridization (FISH) assay, a fluorescent DNA probe is hybridized to a specific locus to produce a colored signal. A translocation would appear as the color produced from the combination of two different fluorescently labeled probes.

49. d. The proteins encoded by many tumor-suppressor genes are involved in the regulation of progression through the cell division cycle or in the regulation of DNA repair.

50. b. Oncogenes are derived from protooncogenes, which are normal cellular genes. The protooncogenes become oncogenic and are often associated with cancers when they have been altered by dominant mutations.

CHAPTER 10

1. d. Effective communication of change requires direct and active speaking and listening with all individuals involved in the change. Response a limits the employee number and limits the effective listening of those employees. Responses b and c are one-directional communication. Response d has the key component of "discussion" with all employees and is therefore the best answer.

2. b. Communication is the most appropriate answer for a manager, because this individual must coordinate multiple activities and people to accomplish the responsibilities of the profession. Informal discussions and decision making follow the foundation of communication.

3. a. Phase 1 deficiency requires a response to the CAP within 30 days of the citation, which indicates that responses b, c, and d are not appropriate.

4. d. The mission of the National Accrediting Agency for Clinical Laboratory Sciences (NAACLS) is to offer approval and accreditation of educational programs in the clinical laboratory sciences.

5. a. The COLA agency services include education, consultation, and accreditation. CAP also offers education, consultation, and accreditation. The Joint Commission offers accreditation, certification, and standards. AABB offers professional development, accreditation, and standards. ASCLS offers education, professional networking, and the body of knowledge for CLS.

6. b. COLA offers accreditation services for the whole laboratory. The Substance Abuse and Mental Health Services Administration offers guidelines and standards for monitoring of drug abuse and testing. AABB specializes in blood transfusion services. Clinical and Laboratory Standards Institute offers educational and training tools for laboratories. Because this question relates specifically to drug testing, SAMHSA is the best answer.

7. c.

8. b.

9. a. The Centers for Medicare & Medicaid Services (CMS) is the government agency responsible for the administration of CLIA certification. The U.S. Food and Drug Administration is the governing body for approval of new clinical laboratory testing procedures and methods. The Department of Transportation regulates shipments of human specimens, among other guidelines.

10. a. A job description lists the key activities defined through a job analysis and is the basis for evaluation of the individual performing that job.

11. b. Conventional wisdom states that a starting salary should not be listed in a job advertisement, because the organization should be able to "sell" the position through the professional benefits of the position. However, in this competitive environment, some advertisements now include starting salary. Yet b is still the correct answer, because the other listings are key components that are required for any job advertisement to be effective and informational to the reader.

12. d. Effective evaluations of individuals performing job tasks require an overview and knowledge of the job and work performed, the ability to interact with and observe the person on occasion (proximity), and a timeliness in scheduled review periods.

13. b. To evaluate a job, the evaluation instrument should contain components to assess the key activities of the job description.

14. a. Maslow's hierarchy of needs demonstrates that effective recognition can be perks such as reserved parking spots or conference attendance for continuing education.

15. d. Many accepted leadership tenets from historical observation show that individual and team recognition generate a sense of accomplishment, increased communication, and relief and well-being of employees.

16. d. Budget reviews require a return on investment for justification of capital expenditures. Replacement of old or nonfunctioning equipment, an operating cost-reduction if a new instrument is purchased, or new services and technology offered through new instrumentation are all appropriate justification categories for capital expenditures.

17. b. The *Family and Medical Leave Act* supplies guidelines for medical leave of absence. CAP, CLMA, and CLSI are agencies or organizations for professional laboratory networking, standards, or guidelines for accreditation.

18. a. The Code of Ethics as defined by ASCLS: "They contribute to the advancement of the profession by improving the body of knowledge, adopting scientific advances that benefit the patient, maintaining high standards of practice and education, and seeking fair socioeconomic working conditions for members of the profession."

19. b. The three Rs of customer service are relationships, response, and results.

20. b. Legal personnel issues is the key in this statement. Reimbursement does not fit into a personnel situation, whereas medical leaves, termination procedures, and interview questions are all applicable to personnel issues.

21. b. The *Fair Labor Standards Act* (FLSA) regulates overtime pay.

22. c. Diagnosis Related Groups (DRGs) is a system to classify hospital cases into one of approximately 500 groups for reimbursement based on the nature of the illness.

23. a. An effective manager will schedule the appropriate personnel to the workload requirements. Scheduling is an immediate and ongoing process versus workload management, which is a long-range planning process (b), and a free-for-all in a democratic schedule can create gaps in a schedule. A balance of experienced personnel on all shifts is an appropriate scheduling process.

24. b. An interview purpose is to assess the qualifications of an applicant and not to establish a friend network (a) or to determine the religious background (c). Generally an applicant with a prior arrest is not considered for an interview, but if interviewed, the goal is to determine the qualifications for the job.

25. d. Annual budget assumptions are based on direct and indirect costs to estimate expenses and projected reimbursement for tests and procedures to estimate revenue for the budget year.

26. c. Ambulatory Payment Categories are the U.S. government's method of paying for facility outpatient services through the Medicare program.

27. c. Managed health care plans reimburse by diagnosis codes assigned to each patient encounter or case.

28. b. Standard business practices and effective leaders and economists recommend a monthly review of budget variances.

29. b. To accurately assess a cost per billable for a test, a total test volume is required to perform this calculation.

30. c. The Health and Human Services Office of Inspector General (HHS OIG) developed the Medical Compliance Plan (MLP).

31. a. The Centers for Medicare & Medicaid Services (CMS) regulates all laboratory testing (except research) performed on humans in the United States through the Clinical Laboratory Improvement Amendments (CLIA). In total, CLIA covers approximately 239,000 laboratory entities.

32. a. The Office of Inspector General (OIG) set a template for laboratories to follow to ensure appropriate billing practices are followed and to curb fraud and abuse. "What is ordered, is tested, reported and billed."

33. b. The Clinical Laboratory Standards Institute publishes guidelines for technical procedures and is often referenced by the accreditation agencies (COLA, CAP) to laboratories.

34. b. A 24-hour, 7-days-per-week service contract can be expensive, but if an instrument goes down with no backup, the vendor must supply a repair technician immediately to remedy the problem and keep the instrument down time to a minimum. Response time will be slower for the other scenarios listed.

35. a. 10,000 billable tests in a 2-week pay period = 260,000 annually (26 × 10,000). The time it takes to produce the unit annually is 130,000 (260,000 × 0.5 unit). Each full-time equivalent (FTE) is equal to 2080 hr/yr. 130,000 divided by 2080 = 62.5 FTEs.

36. a. The definition of *productivity* is the measure of the efficiency of the person in converting inputs to useful outputs. This is measured by the actual hours worked by the paid or earned hours of the individual employee (which would include paid time off, holiday, sick, vacation, etc.).

37. b. Clinical laboratory has confidentiality guidelines (HIPAA), procedures (CLIA accreditation documentation), and chain of custody (drug screening documentation SAMSHA or similar). Posting of available jobs or open positions in the clinical laboratory does not fall under institutional legal issues.

38. a. PRN is a Latin term, *pro re nata,* that translates to "as needed" or "as the situation arises." In situations in which workload fluctuates, as-needed employees are very useful in scheduling for unexpected situations, to avoid overtime and allow for schedule flexibility.

39. a. The *Fair Labor and Standards Act* of 1938 set forth guidelines for hourly employees and regulations on payroll classifications. If a payroll is following the 8 and 80 guideline, the employer is required to pay an employee overtime for any work more than 8 hours in 1 day.

40. c. Management of employees in an effective and productive fashion requires much flexibility and creative scheduling. If all highly trained and experienced personnel are concentrated on one shift for a laboratory that is operating 24 hours per day, 7 days per week, it will place undue stress, confusion, and inexperience on the other two shifts, improperly allocating human resources and resulting in overtime costs, turnover of staff, and higher labor costs for those two shifts.

41. a. Through guidelines of the U.S. Bureau of Labor and Occupational Safety and Health Administration, all employers must offer the hepatitis B vaccine at employer cost to any employee who may have exposure to blood-borne pathogens.

42. b. A written technical procedure requires the methodology, quality control, and media and reagents needed to perform the test. Although a cost per billable could be added to any procedure, it is not required or necessary.

43. d. The College of American Pathologists, The Joint Commission, and the state health departments all have legal authority for laboratory inspection and accreditation.

44. b. Human resource guidelines on appropriate interview questions are based on U.S. laws, and it is illegal to ask a person's age, family status, or health care issues that could discriminate unfairly against any applicant technically and professionally proficient to perform the job listed.

45. a. The key to this answer is to apply the "most helpful during the interview" aspect to the answers. All answers listed could be perceived as a correct response, but the best answer is to observe how the applicant addresses problem solving by giving each applicant the same scenario and recording their verbal and nonverbal response rather than a yes/no answer.

46. d. Best educational practice includes the inclusion of learning objectives for each instructional unit. Learning objectives should explicitly describe what the student should be able to do after successful completion of the unit.

47. a. Bloom's taxonomy describes the various learning levels within the cognitive domain. Those levels are knowledge, comprehension, application, analysis, synthesis, and evaluation.

48. c. The three learning domains are cognitive, psychomotor, and affective. Affective traits are those associated with behavior and attitude.

49. b. Well-written learning objectives should be explicit and measurable. A student's ability to list the correct steps in a procedure in the correct order is an explicit, measurable learning objective.

50. c. The taxonomic levels that define examination questions are types I, II, and III. Type I questions are simple, recall questions. Type II questions involve the ability to apply learned knowledge to answer a question. Type III questions require applying and assimilating knowledge to solve a complex problem such as making an accurate diagnosis given a set of laboratory test results.

CHAPTER 11

1. c. Each liter contains 10 dL, so multiply 4 dL × 1 L/10 dL (or 0.1, which is equivalent) to cancel out the deciliter units.

$$4 \text{ dL} \times \frac{1 \text{L}}{10 \text{dL}} = 0.4 \text{ L}$$

2. b. Each liter contains 100,000 μL, so multiply 3 μL × 1 L/100,000 μL (or 0.000001, which is equivalent) to cancel out the microliter units.

$$3 \mu\text{L} \times \frac{1 \text{L}}{100,000 \text{ L}} = 0.000003 \text{ L}$$

3. c. Each gram contains 1000 mg, so multiply 10 mg × 1 g/1000 mg to get the number of grams. Then multiply the number of grams by the number of micrograms in each gram (10^6) to get the number of micrograms present.

$$10 \text{ mg} \times \frac{1 \text{ g}}{10^3 \text{ mg}} \times \frac{10^6 \text{ µg}}{1 \text{ g}} = 10 \times 10^3 \text{ g } or \text{ } 10,000 \text{ µg}$$

4. c. Each kilogram contains 1000 g, so multiply 0.85 kg by 1×10^3 g/1 kg to get the number of grams.

$$0.85 \text{ kg} \times \frac{1 \times 10^3 \text{ g}}{1 \text{ kg}} = 0.85 \times 10^3 \text{ g } or \text{ } 850 \text{ g}$$

5. c. Using the equation to convert degrees Celsius to degrees Fahrenheit:
F = 9/5 °C + 32
F = 9/5 25 + 32
F = 9/5 °C + 32
F = 45 + 32
F = 77

6. b. First convert degrees Fahrenheit to degrees Celsius:
C = 5/9 (°F − 32)
C = 5/9 (80 − 32)
C = 5/9 (48)
C = 26.7
Then convert the degrees Celsius to Kelvin:
K = °C + 273
K = 26.7 + 273
K = 299.7

7. b. A ⅕ dilution is equivalent to 1 part of urine in a total of 5 parts. The remaining 4 parts are the diluent, so to prepare a ⅕ dilution of a urine sample, use 1 part urine and 4 parts diluent.

8. b.

$$\frac{50 \text{g}}{L} \times \frac{1}{5} \times \frac{1}{10} = \frac{1 \text{g}}{L}$$

9. b. When making a dilution that changes concentrations, use the following formula (where *1* represents the stock solution and *2* represents the working solution):

V1 × C1 = V2 × C2
V1 × 0.8 = 300 × 0.2
V1 = 75 mL

This means that 75 mL of the stock solution was used. This 75 mL was diluted to a final volume of 300 mL, so to determine the amount of diluent needed, subtract the amount of stock solution from the final volume:

300 mL − 75 mL = 225 mL diluent needed

10. c. Molarity is the number of moles per liter of solution. In this problem, milliliters are given as units so convert this to L (1000 mL in 1 L):

$$\frac{2 \text{ mol}}{400 \text{ mL}} \times 1000 \text{ mL} = 5 \text{ M}$$

11. a. Multiply molarity (which is converted from M to mol/L) by volume to solve for moles.

$$300 \text{ ml} \times 2\text{M} = 300 \text{ mL} \times \frac{2 \text{ mol}}{1\text{L}} \times \frac{1\text{L}}{1000 \text{ mL}} = 0.6 \text{ moles}$$

12. c. Multiply the volume of the solution by the molarity (written as mol/L) by molecular weight (g/mol) to solve for grams:

$$\frac{1.5 \text{ mol}}{L} \times \frac{58.5 \text{ g}}{\text{mol}} \times 0.50 \text{ L} = 44 \text{ g}$$

13. a. Knowing that 4 M equals 4 mol/L, solve for volume by multiplying the weight of the sample by the inverse of the molarity by the inverse of molecular weight (to isolate liters in the numerator):

$$125.6 \text{ g} \times \frac{1 \text{ mol}}{74.5 \text{ g}} \times \frac{1\text{L}}{4\text{mol}} = 0.421 \text{ L}$$

14. b.

$$Gram \text{ } equivalent \text{ } weight = \frac{\text{MW} \times 1 \text{ mol}}{\text{valence}} = 49.0 \text{ g}$$

$$Eq = \frac{54.2}{49.0} = 1.11$$

$$N = \frac{1.11 \text{ Eq}}{2 \text{ L}} = 0.56 \text{ N}$$

15. b. First determine the amount of osmoles in the 3-kg solution by setting up a proportion:

$$\frac{0.67 \text{ osmol}}{1 \text{ kg}} = \frac{X \text{ osmol}}{3.0 \text{ kg}}$$

3.0 × 0.67 = X osmole
X = 2.01 osmole

The original solution contains 2.01 osmoles. NaCl dissociates into two osmotically active particles per molecule in solution. To determine the number of moles in the 2.01 osmoles, use the following formula:

$$osmoles = moles \times activeparticle$$
$$2.01 = moles\ of\ NaCl \times 2$$
$$Moles\ of\ NaCl = 1.005$$

Then convert the number of moles to grams:

$$1.005\ moles\ of\ NaCl = X grams\ of\ NaCl \times 1\ mol/58.5\ g$$
$$X = 59.1\ g$$

16. b. The formula used for the calculation of the mean is:

$$\bar{x} = \frac{\Sigma x}{n}$$

Where $\bar{x}$ equals the mean, Σx is the sum of all values and n equals the number of values in the set.

17. b. The mode of a data set is the number or value that is seen most frequently.

18. b. The standard deviation is the square root of the variance.

19. b. The formula used for the calculation of the mean is:

$$\bar{x} = \frac{\Sigma x}{n}$$

Where $\bar{x}$ equals the mean, Σx is the sum of all values, and n equals the number of values in the set.

$$\bar{x} = \frac{1683}{10} = 168$$

20. a. The mode is the most frequent result. In this data set, there are three results of 150.

21. c. Standard deviation $= \sqrt{\frac{\Sigma(x-\bar{x})^2}{n-1}}$

Where $\Sigma(x-\bar{x})^2$ is the sum of the difference between each value and the mean squared and $n - 1$ is the number of values (n) minus 1.
In this problem, the mean ($\bar{x}$) is 168 ([180+200+150 +170+150+165+205+150+168+145]/10).

x	$(x - \bar{x})$	$(x - \bar{x})^2$
180	12	144
200	32	1024
150	−18	324
170	2	4
150	−18	324
165	−3	9
205	37	1369
150	−18	324
168	0	0
145	−23	529
		$\Sigma(x - x)^2 = 4051$

$$\sqrt{\frac{\Sigma(x-\bar{x})^2}{n-1}}$$
$$\sqrt{\frac{4051}{9}} = 21.2$$

22. c. The midrange is the average of the lowest and highest values in the data set:

$$M = (4 + 14)/2$$
$$M = 9$$

23. a. When rounding, if the last digit is 5 and the preceding number is even, the final retained digit stays the same.

24. c. For addition and subtraction, the answer must have the same number of decimal places as the starting value with the fewest number of decimal places. In this data set, 3.45 has the fewest number of decimal places, with two decimal places. The sum of this data set would be 36.556, so the answer is rounded to 36.56 to reflect two decimal places.

25. c. The product of the significant figures is 24 (4 × 6). The sum of the exponents is 5 (3+2). The correct answer is 24×10^5.

26. a. Accuracy is the closeness of an individual result (or test value) to the true value.

27. c. The data from plots 5, 6, 7, and 8 all exceed the ×1 standard deviation mark, thus violating the 4_{1s} rule.

28. a. 1_{3s} is indicative of random error. The others are indicative of systematic error.

29. a. The sensitivity of a test is the ability of a test to minimize false-negative results. The specificity of the test describes the ability of the test to minimize false-positive results.

30. a. The clinical sensitivity of a test is calculated by dividing the true positives (TPs) by the total of the patients with the disease (the sum of the TPs and the false negatives [FN]). Response b represents the specificity of the test, c the positive predictive values, and d the negative predictive value.

Mock Examination

1. What is the preferred specimen for molecular techniques for diagnosis of inherited mutations?
   a. DNA extracted from peripheral blood mature red cells
   b. DNA extracted from peripheral blood white cells
   c. RNA extracted from peripheral mature red cells
   d. RNA extracted from fresh serum

2. The biochemical tests performed on a gram-positive bacillus were consistent with those of *Corynebacterium diphtheriae*. The MLS should now:
   a. Perform a spore stain of the colonies
   b. Determine if the isolate is toxigenic by performing an Elek test
   c. Perform an agglutination test to confirm the organism's identity
   d. Subculture the organism to Hektoen enteric medium and examine for black colonies

3. A decrease in serum haptoglobin accompanies which of the following?
   a. Extravascular hemolysis
   b. Intravascular hemolysis
   c. Extramedullary hematopoiesis
   d. Suppressed erythropoiesis

4. The presence of waxy casts in a microscopic examination of urine is consistent with a diagnosis of:
   a. Strenuous exercise
   b. Pyelonephritis
   c. Glomerulonephritis
   d. Chronic renal failure

5. The decreased release of thyroid-stimulating hormone (TSH) would result in which of the following actions from the hypothalamic-pituitary-thyroid axis?
   a. Decreased release of TSH from the pituitary gland
   b. Increased release of TSH from the thyroid gland
   c. Decreased release of thyroid hormones from the thyroid glands
   d. Increased release of thyroid hormones from the thyroid glands

6. Production of exotoxin A, which kills host cells by inhibiting protein synthesis and production of several proteolytic enzymes and hemolysins that destroy cells and tissue are factors that contribute to pathogenicity of which of the following organisms?
   a. *Pseudomonas aeruginosa*
   b. *Burkholderia cepacia*
   c. *Ralstonia pickettii*
   d. *Burkholderia mallei*

7. Which of the following factors binds to platelets via the glycoprotein Ib/IX receptor?
   a. von Willebrand factor
   b. Factor II
   c. Fibrinogen
   d. Thrombin

8. The respiratory culture of a patient with cystic fibrosis yielded gram-negative bacilli with the following reactions:

Oxidase: Positive	MacConkey agar: Positive
Glucose OF open: Positive	Gelatin hydrolysis: Positive
Pigment: Metallic green	Arginine dihydrolase: Positive
Growth at 42 °C: Positive	

   Which of the following is the most likely identification of this organism?
   a. *Burkholderia cepacia*
   b. *Pseudomonas aeruginosa*
   c. *Acinetobacter baumannii*
   d. *Stenotrophomonas xylosoxidans*

9. Which of the following cells can be described as neoplastic lymphocytes with noncleaved clumped nuclei and very basophilic cytoplasm with prominent vacuoles?
   a. Reed Sternberg cells
   b. Mantle cell lymphoma cells
   c. Small cell lymphocytic lymphoma cells
   d. Burkitt's lymphoma cells

10. When preparing fresh frozen plasma for transfusion, what compatibility testing is performed?
    a. Perform a reverse grouping on donor plasma
    b. Perform a reverse grouping on recipient plasma
    c. Plasma must be HLA-compatible
    d. No testing is required

11. The following OGTT results are indicative of what state?
    Fasting serum glucose: 124 mg/dL
    2-hour post load serum glucose: 227 mg/dL
    a. Normal
    b. Diabetes mellitus
    c. Addison's disease
    d. Hyperinsulinism

12. A Prussian blue stain of a bone marrow shows blue granules present inside of macrophages. Which of the following disorders can be ruled out by this result?
    a. Chronic disease
    b. Lead poisoning
    c. Iron deficiency
    d. Iron overload

13. A gram-negative diplococcus isolated from a patient's CSF specimen gives the following results:

Chocolate agar: Growth	Oxidase: Positive
SBA: Growth	CTA test: Glucose, yellow; maltose, yellow; lactose, red; sucrose, red

    This organism is most likely which of the following?
    a. *N. meningitides*
    b. *N. gonorrhoeae*
    c. *N. lactamica*
    d. *M. catarrhalis*

14. What characteristic red cell shape is associated with extravascular hemolysis?
    a. Burr cell
    b. Schistocyte
    c. Spherocyte
    d. Target cell

15. Two units of blood are ordered for a patient. Previous blood bank records indicate the patient had an anti-K 3 years ago. What is the next course of action for completing this order?
    a. Select three random units of ABO-compatible blood and crossmatch
    b. Perform an immediate spin crossmatch on two K-negative units
    c. Antigen type units for the K antigen and only crossmatch units positive for K
    d. Antigen type units for the K antigen and only crossmatch units negative for K

16. The antibody associated with type IV hypersensitivity is:
    a. IgA
    b. IgE
    c. IgG
    d. IgM
    e. None of the above

17. A child presents with an infected fingernail. The sample of the wound grows a pure culture. The gram-stained smear showed small gram-negative bacilli.
    Additional characteristics of this organism include:

Requires increased CO_2 for growth	Oxidase-positive
Catalase-, urease-, indole-negative	Pits the agar during growth

    The most likely identification of this organism is which of the following?
    a. *Weeksella virosa*
    b. *Legionella* spp.
    c. *Brucella melitensis*
    d. *Eikenella corrodens*

18. All of the following hormones *increase* serum glucose levels with the exception of:
    a. Glucagon
    b. Cortisol
    c. Epinephrine
    d. Insulin

19. Based on the following results, what is the most likely diagnosis?
    ALP and GGT moderately increase
    ALT, LD, and total bilirubin minimally increase
    a. Cirrhosis
    b. Biliary obstruction
    c. Infectious hepatitis
    d. Mumps

20. Which of the following conditions is usually associated with thrombosis?
    a. Factor XIII deficiency
    b. Factor V Leiden mutation
    c. Vitamin K deficiency
    d. PAI-1 deficiency

21. An antibody panel shows a pattern of anti-S, but anti-E cannot be ruled out on this initial panel. Which of the phenotyped cells below would be best to help in confirming only an anti-S is present?
    a. E−e+S−s+
    b. E+e+S+s+
    c. E+e+S+s−
    d. E+e−S−s+

22. The most critical step in obtaining accurate Gram stain results is the application of which of the following?
    a. Safranin
    b. Crystal violet
    c. Gram's iodine
    d. Acetone/ethanol

23. Which cell is capable of both phagocytosis and antigen processing?
    a. Basophil
    b. Lymphocyte
    c. Macrophage
    d. Segmented neutrophil

24. People who have anti-A and anti-B blood group antibodies detected in their serum are said to be of which blood group?
    a. AB
    b. O
    c. A
    d. B

25. Which of the following is true regarding indirect bilirubin?
    a. It requires an accelerator to react with the diazo reagent
    b. It is also called delta bilirubin
    c. It is calculated by adding the total bilirubin and direct bilirubin together
    d. It is elevated in liver obstruction

26. The examination question "What color is a positive spot indole test?" falls under which taxonomy level?
    a. Level I
    b. Level II
    c. Level III
    d. Level IV

27. A positive result was obtained when a Venereal Disease Research Laboratory test was performed on a patient's serum. The MLS should now:
    a. Report syphilis antibodies present
    b. Report positive for syphilis
    c. Perform a treponemal test
    d. Perform a nontreponemal test

28. An X and V factor requirement test was performed on a *Haemophilus* isolate using the following protocol:
    1. A TSB suspension of the organism was prepared
    2. The organism suspension was swabbed to a chocolate agar plate
    3. X and V factor disks were placed on the agar plate
    4. The plate was incubated for 24 hours at 35 ° C in CO_2

    On examination, the plate showed growth over the entire plate. In troubleshooting the protocol and results, the correct determination is:
    a. Organism should be identified as *H. aegyptius*
    b. TSB is *not* an appropriate medium for preparing the organism suspension
    c. Chocolate agar is *not* appropriate for use in the X and V factor requirement test
    d. The chocolate plate should *not* have been incubated in CO_2

29. Which of the following conditions is associated with abnormal von Willebrand factor (VWF) cleaving protease?
    a. Disseminated intravascular coagulation
    b. Hemolytic uremic syndrome
    c. March hemoglobinuria
    d. Thrombotic thrombocytopenic purpura

30. In salicylate overdose, what is the first acid-base disturbance present?
    a. Metabolic acidosis
    b. Metabolic alkalosis
    c. Respiratory acidosis
    d. Respiratory alkalosis

31. Which of the following red cell indices support microcytic hypochromic red cell morphology?

	MCV (fL)	MCH (pg)	MCHC (g/dL)
a.	118	35	34
b.	75	30	33
c.	92	30	34
d.	67	22	27

32. According to AABB Standards, what is the minimum information required to be on a sample label for transfusion testing purposes?
    a. First and last name of patient and date of collection
    b. First and last name of patient, date of collection, and identification of phlebotomist
    c. First and last name of patient, date of collection, identification of phlebotomist, and unique identifying number
    d. First and last name of patient, date of collection, identification of phlebotomist, unique identifying number, and date of patient's last transfusion

33. The L-pyrolidonyl-β-naphthylamide (PYR) hydrolysis test is a presumptive test for which of the following streptococci?
    a. Groups A and B
    b. *Streptococcus pneumoniae* and group C
    c. Group A and *Enterococcus*
    d. Group A and *Streptococcus bovis*

34. Which of the following ketones is(are) not detected using the reagent strip?
    a. Acetoacetic acid
    b. Acetone
    c. β-Hydroxybutyric acid
    d. All of the above are detected using the reagent strip

35. What is the transport temperature of packed red blood cells?
- a. Maintained at room temperature, not to exceed 25° C
- b. Transported at temperatures below 6° C
- c. Transported on ice not to exceed 10° C
- d. Transported on dry ice at temperature below 25° C

36. An anaerobic, box-shaped gram-positive bacillus is positive for the reverse CAMP test. This organism would also be:
- a. Lipase positive
- b. Indole positive
- c. Lecithinase positive
- d. Spore negative

37. If the cytoplasm of a cell is very basophilic or blue when stained with Wright stain, which of the following does it contain?
- a. Increased concentration of lysosomes
- b. Increased number of Golgi bodies
- c. Increased number of ribosomes
- d. Increased number of mitochondria

38. Which of the following is the best way to handle CAP Proficiency Testing samples?
- a. Be extra careful and run the test samples several times before reporting to make sure your results are correct
- b. Ensure that quality control and maintenance are acceptable before performing both patient testing and PT testing
- c. Double-check your answers before mailing by checking your results with those from another laboratory
- d. The most experienced MLS should do all proficiency testing to make sure it is right

39. A fastidious organism gave the following results:

SBA growth: Negative	Growth: After 7 days	Niacin: Yellow
Acid-fast stain: Positive	Colonies: Buff color	68° C catalase: No bubbles

The organism is most likely:
- a. *M. scrofulaceum*
- b. *M. xenopi*
- c. *M. bovis*
- d. *M. tuberculosis*

40. The most probable explanation for a patient who presents with an elevated osmolal gap, metabolic acidosis, and calcium oxalate crystals in the urine is:
- a. Methanol intoxication
- b. Ethanol overdose
- c. Ethylene glycol intoxication
- d. Cyanide poisoning

41. How do sickle cells or spherocytes interfere with the erythrocyte sedimentation rate (ESR)?
- a. Prevent rouleaux formation, so falsely decrease
- b. Encourage rouleaux formation, so falsely increase
- c. Agglutinate and increase red cell mass, so falsely increase
- d. Decrease plasma viscosity, so falsely decrease

42. What is the most likely cause of the ABO discrepancy below?

	Anti-A	Anti-B	A$_1$ cells	B cells	Autocontrol
Patient	3+	0	1+	4+	Negative

- a. Subgroup of A
- b. Cold-reacting antibody
- c. Neonatal patient
- d. Rouleaux

43. What is a point mutation?
- a. Mutation of the stop codon
- b. Replacement of one nucleotide in the normal gene with a different nucleotide
- c. Addition of one nucleotide in the normal gene
- d. Deletion of one nucleotide in the normal gene

44. Hemoglobin electrophoresis is performed on a patient with known homozygous Hb S who has received red cell transfusions in the past week. Which hemoglobins would be expected on the gel?
- a. Hb S and Hb F
- b. Hb A and Hb F
- c. Hb S, Hb A, and Hb F
- d. Hb S, Hb A, Hb F, and Hb A$_2$

45. Which of the following is the correct location of enteric "H" antigens?
- a. Flagella
- b. Capsule
- c. Cell wall
- d. Cytoplasm

46. You receive a blood gas sample on a patient who is in the emergency room for assessment of unexplained vomiting for the past 4 days and abnormal respirations. Which of the following interpretations best describes the patient's blood gas results?

pH: 7.50
Pco$_2$: 55 mm Hg

Po$_2$: 85 mm Hg
HCO$_3$$^-$: 35 mmol/L

- a. Partially compensated metabolic acidosis
- b. Partially compensated metabolic alkalosis
- c. Compensated metabolic alkalosis
- d. Compensated metabolic acidosis

47. The agency that is responsible for protecting workers' health and well-being is:
a. CAP
b. TJC
c. NAACLS
d. OSHA

48. A patient's sample shows a large spike on serum protein electrophoresis in the γ region. On further testing, the spike is shown to be mostly IgM. Which of the following is true regarding this patient's diagnosis?
a. Further testing is necessary to determine if the patient has multiple myeloma
b. The patient had a high-protein meal just before the test
c. Most likely has Waldenström's macroglobulinemia
d. May be in the early stages of combined variable immunodeficiency disease (CVID)

49. Which one of the following tests on donor units is not required?
a. Anti-EBV
b. Antibody screen
c. Anti-HCV
d. West Nile virus

50. The white count on an adult patient is 2.5×10^9/L. When the blood film is examined, the following results are obtained: 15% neutrophils and 75% lymphocytes. Reference ranges for these cell types, both relative and absolute, are as follows:

Cells	Relative %	Absolute no. ($\times 10^9$ /L)
Neutrophils	48-70	2.4-8.2
Lymphocytes	18-42	1.4-4.0

What conclusion can be made about the number of lymphocytes for this patient?
a. They are relatively increased but normal in absolute numbers
b. They are both relatively and absolutely increased
c. They are relatively decreased but absolutely increased
d. They are both relatively and absolutely decreased

51. Which of the following conditions is caused by an impairment of an enzyme needed to conjugate bilirubin?
a. Gilbert's disease
b. Physiologic jaundice of the newborn
c. Dubin-Johnson syndrome
d. Hemolytic jaundice

52. The most recent CBC results for a patient who has been treated for chronic myelogenous leukemia (CML) for several years show a blast count of 38% in the differential. The CML is now in which phase?

a. Accelerated phase
b. Dormant phase
c. Mobile phase
d. Terminal phase (blast crisis)

53. This type of resistance mechanism modifies the antibiotic targets and results in reduced affinity of antibiotics for their microbial target sites.
a. Cell-wall inhibition
b. Protein synthesis modification
c. Enzyme modification
d. Nucleic acid modification

54. Which of the following tests is used to monitor patients for early signs of renal disease?
a. Glucose measurement using the reagent strip
b. Protein measurement using the reagent strip
c. Specific gravity measurement using a refractometer
d. Microalbumin measurement using a sensitive reagent strip

55. A serum protein electrophoresis was performed on a patient. The MLS noted a sharp peak in the gamma-globulin fraction. This peak was similar to the albumin peak. This pattern is consistent with that of which of the following?
a. Cirrhosis
b. Acute inflammation
c. α_1-Antitrypsin deficiency, severe emphysema
d. Monoclonal gammopathy

56. A person of the genotype R_1R_1 could potentially produce antibodies to which of the following Rh antigens?
a. D
b. e
c. C
d. E

57. Which of the following groups of organisms is most correct for use in performing quality control on a TSI agar slant?
a. *Escherichia coli* and *Salmonella, Shigella,* and *Pseudomonas* spp.
b. *Escherichia coli* and *Klebsiella* and *Pseudomonas* spp.
c. *Proteus mirabilis, Enterobacter* spp., and *Escherichia coli*
d. *Shigella* and *Salmonella* spp.

58. Which of the following red blood cell precursors has a nucleus that can be described as pyknotic?
a. Basophilic normoblast
b. Orthochromic normoblast
c. Polychromatophilic normoblast
d. Pronormoblast

59. When testing the patient sample, it was reactive with all panel cells tested, including the autocontrol. Previous records indicate the patient underwent transfusion 1 month ago. What is the next course of action for pretransfusion testing?
    a. Perform an enzyme panel
    b. An autoadsorption test is necessary because of the patient's autoantibody
    c. An alloadsorption test should be performed to determine if an alloantibody is present
    d. It is necessary to perform both an adsorption and enzyme panel

60. Alkaline phosphatase values are expected to be increased in all of the following situations except:
    a. Child undergoing a growth spurt
    b. During a time of increased bone remodeling
    c. After a myocardial infarction
    d. Paget's disease

61. A patient comes to the emergency room with report of an upset stomach. He has a rash covering his body, and he is becoming increasingly hypotensive. The blood samples that you drew for culture were positive within 24 hours for gram-positive cocci in clusters. The most likely causative organism is which of the following?
    a. Group B streptococci
    b. *Staphylococcus aureus*
    c. *Enterococcus* sp.
    d. *Staphylococcus* sp. not *S. aureus*

62. A 13-year-old boy reports bone pain and headaches. His white count is 68.0×10^9/L, platelet count is 57×10^9/L, and hematocrit is 34%. His differential shows mostly nucleated cells that are identified as blasts. They are CD2, CD4, and CD8 positive. Which disorder does he most likely have?
    a. Acute myeloid leukemia without maturation
    b. Acute myeloid leukemia with maturation
    c. Immature B-cell acute lymphoblastic leukemia
    d. T-cell acute lymphoblastic leukemia

63. A patient sample tested positive for anti-dsDNA antibodies. The patient most likely has which of the following?
    a. Rheumatoid arthritis
    b. Syphilis
    c. Infectious mononucleosis
    d. Systemic lupus erythematosus

64. Which of the following analytes is helpful in distinguishing a condition affecting the liver from bone disease in the presence of an elevation of ALP?
    a. AST
    b. ALT
    c. ALP
    d. GGT

65. All of the following characteristics are consistent with the appearance of *normal* cerebrospinal fluid except:
    a. Crystal clear
    b. CSF protein of 20 mg/dL
    c. IgG index of 0.70 or less
    d. WBC count greater than 100/μL

66. Which of the following could result in a false-negative result for a DAT?
    a. Improper washing of cells
    b. AHG reagent not added
    c. Low pH of saline
    d. All of the above

67. An organism isolated from a stool culture gives the following reactions:

| Lactose: Colorless | VP: Colorless | Lysine: Purple |
| TSI: Red/black | Citrate: Blue | Indole: Colorless |

Which of the following is the next step in identifying the organism?
    a. Report *Salmonella* present
    b. Report no enteric pathogens isolated
    c. Perform serogrouping with *Salmonella* antisera
    d. Perform serogrouping with *Shigella* antisera

68. Which of the following is true about enzymes and their effect on red cell antigens and antibodies?
    a. The Rh, Duffy, MN, and Ss system antigen and antibody reactions are enhanced
    b. The Duffy, MN, and Ss system antigens are destroyed, so antigen and antibody reactions are not detectable
    c. Only the Duffy system antigens are affected by enzymes
    d. The Rh, Duffy, MN, and Ss system antigens are destroyed, so antigen and antibody reactions are not detectable

69. The underlying cause for anemia of chronic inflammation is that:
    a. Acute phase reactants impair iron mobilization
    b. Growth factors prevent iron incorporation into protoporphyrin
    c. Inflammation slows down cell division
    d. Iron stores in the bone marrow are depleted by acute phase reactants

70. In patients with developing subclinical hypothyroidism, TSH levels will likely be _____, and fT$_4$ will likely be _____.
    a. Decreased, increased
    b. Increased, decreased
    c. Decreased, normal
    d. Increased, normal

71. Which of the following would result in a permanent deferral for a whole blood donation?
a. Jaundice as a small child
b. Temperature above 37 ° C
c. Recipient of human growth hormone
d. Accidental needle stick 1 year previously; negative for infectious diseases

72. A 30-year-old pregnant female has an OGTT challenge test (screening test) performed at 26 weeks gestation. Her serum glucose result is 100 mg/dL at 1 hour. What should occur next?
a. Nothing, this confirms the diagnosis of GDM
b. This is suspicious for GDM, a diagnostic OGTT test should be performed
c. Nothing, this is the expected glucose level in a pregnant female
d. This is suspicious for hypoglycemia, a 5-hour OGTT should be performed

73. A PT and PTT on a patient fails to correct when mixed with normal pooled plasma. Which of the following is a possible explanation?
a. The patient has a factor deficiency of factor X
b. The patient has thrombocytopenia
c. A circulating inhibitor is present in the patient
d. This is a normal finding

74. Which of the following sets of results most closely indicates an exudate?
a. Clear, ratio of fluid to serum LD of 0.8, ratio of fluid to serum protein of 0.7, WBC count of 1000/μL
b. Cloudy, ratio of fluid to serum LD of 0.4, ratio of fluid to serum protein of 0.5, WBC count of 800/μL
c. Cloudy, ratio of fluid to serum LD of 0.8, ratio of fluid to serum protein of 0.7, WBC count of 2500/μL
d. Clear, ratio of fluid to serum LD of 0.45, ratio of fluid to serum protein of 0.40, WBC count of 800/μL

75. Immunoglobulins function by all of the following except:
a. Coat invading cells to act as opsonins
b. Reneutralize toxins produced by viruses
c. Activate complement cascade of cell lysis
d. Lyse viruses by activating T cells

76. Irradiated red blood cell transfusion would *not* be indicated for which of the following patient diagnoses?
a. Exchange transfusion
b. Bone marrow transplant
c. Severe combined immunodeficiency syndrome
d. Warm autoimmune hemolytic anemia

77. Which of the following lipid measurements is estimated using a formula, and not measured?
a. Total cholesterol
b. HDL
c. Triglycerides
d. LDL

78. Which of the following would be an acceptable alternative for a red cell transfusion if ABO group-specific blood was not available?
a. Group A recipient with group B donor
b. Group O recipient with group AB donor
c. Group O recipient with group A donor
d. Group AB recipient with group B donor

79. The laboratory manager's most appropriate approach to performing employee evaluations could best be described as?
a. Positive reinforcement
b. Destructive criticism
c. Retribution
d. Threatening

80. A latex agglutination test for cardiolipin is performed on a patient suspected of having which disease?
a. Rheumatoid arthritis
b. Syphilis
c. Infectious mononucleosis
d. The patient may be pregnant

81. Before release of a unit of red blood cells for transfusion, which records must be checked?
a. Donor's first and last name on the donor label
b. The intended recipient's first and last name, unique identifier number, and ABO/Rh
c. Name of person who performed the crossmatch
d. Date and time the blood was issued

82. Laboratory diagnosis of hookworm is usually made by:
a. Filariform and larvae in stool
b. Serology
c. Symptoms of nausea, malnutrition, diarrhea, and anemia
d. Ova in feces

83. Which red cell inclusion is often found in lead poisoning cases?
a. Basophilic stippling
b. Cabot rings
c. Heinz bodies
d. Howell Jolly bodies

84. The immunoglobulin typically found in secretions is:
a. IgA
b. IgD
c. IgE
d. IgG
e. IgM

85. Both blood and urine cultures are positive for an oxidase-negative, gram-negative bacilli that gave the following growth characteristics and biochemical reactions:

MacConkey agar: Colorless colonies	Citrate: Positive
TSI reactions: Alk/Acid, no gas, no H_2S	Lysine decarboxylase: Positive
Indole: Negative	Ornithine decarboxylase: Positive
Urea: Negative	Motility: Positive

These reactions are consistent with which of the following enteric pathogens?
   a. *Serratia marcescens*
   b. *Klebsiella pneumoniae*
   c. *Yersinia enterocolitica*
   d. *Proteus mirabilis*

86. The HIV virus belongs to which of the following groups of viruses?
   a. Rhinoviruses
   b. Herpesviruses
   c. Retroviruses
   d. Arboviruses

87. Which of the following is a CAP service that accounts for workload recording per billable test plus nonbillable expenses?
   a. CLIA
   b. COLA
   c. HFAP
   d. LMIP

88. Which of the following can occur days to weeks after transfusion?
   a. Transfusion-associated graft-versus-host disease
   b. Hemolytic transfusion reaction
   c. Posttransfusion purpura
   d. All of the above

89. Which of the following is associated with a decrease in cerebrospinal fluid glucose?
   a. Meningitis
   b. Increased serum glucose level
   c. Decreased use of glucose by brain cells
   d. Damaged blood-brain barrier glucose transport

90. Which of the following vitamins is less likely to accumulate at toxic levels?
   a. Vitamin A
   b. Vitamin C
   c. Vitamin D
   d. Vitamin E

91. A patient transfused with several units of red blood cells developed a febrile transfusion reaction. What component is most appropriate to prevent this reaction in the future?
   a. Red blood cells
   b. Irradiated red blood cells
   c. Leukocyte-reduced red blood cells
   d. CMV-seronegative red blood cells

92. An employee's demeanor falls under which of the following domains?
   a. Psychomotor
   b. Cognitive
   c. Affective
   d. Didactic

93. Features used in identifying *Cryptococcus neoformans* should include which of the following?
   a. Capsule formation, mucoid, creamy-white to yellow colonies, urea positive
   b. No capsule formation, produces mycelial forms, urea positive
   c. Capsule formation, mucoid, creamy-white to yellow colonies, urea negative
   d. No capsule formation, budding yeast cells, mucoid, creamy-white colonies, partially acid-fast

94. The growth factor erythropoietin is produced by which organ?
   a. Bone marrow
   b. Kidney
   c. Spleen
   d. Thymus

95. A neonate is to be transfused for the first time with group O red blood cells. Which of the following is performed for compatibility testing?
   a. Perform an antibody screen and crossmatch with mother's serum
   b. Perform an antibody screen and crossmatch with baby's serum
   c. Crossmatch is not necessary if initial antibody screen of mother's or baby's serum was negative
   d. An antibody screen or crossmatch is not necessary, issue group and Rh compatible blood

96. _____ protect from viral infection by recognizing and destroying infected cells and _____ protect us indirectly by producing cytokines to stimulate B cells.
   a. CD4+ cytotoxic T lymphocytes; CD8+ T helper lymphocytes
   b. CD8+ cytotoxic T lymphocytes; CD4+ T helper lymphocytes
   c. NK cells; CD8+ T helper lymphocytes
   d. NK cells; CD4+ cytotoxic T lymphocytes

97. Pernicious anemia can be distinguished from folate deficiency by which of the following findings?
    a. Presence of hypersegmented neutrophils
    b. Mean cell volume
    c. Bone marrow findings
    d. Presence of autoantibodies to intrinsic factor

98. Which of the following pairings of crystals and causes is not correct?
    a. Calcium oxalate crystals and antifreeze ingestion
    b. Uric acid crystals and patients receiving chemotherapy
    c. Cystine crystals and not clinically significant
    d. Amorphous phosphate crystals and not clinically significant

99. Which of the following hormones involved in calcium regulation acts by increasing the amount of calcium in the blood by enhancing absorption through the intestines, stimulation of osteoclasts, and suppressing loss in the urine?
    a. PTH
    b. Calcitonin
    c. Vitamin D
    d. Cortisol

100. Which of the following patients would be a candidate for RhIg?
    a. O-Positive mother who had a B-negative baby, first pregnancy, anti-K in mother
    b. B-Negative mother who had an O-positive baby, second pregnancy, no anti-D in mother
    c. A-Negative mother who had an O-negative baby, fourth pregnancy, anti-K in mother
    d. AB-Negative mother who had a B-positive baby, second pregnancy, anti-D in mother

ANSWERS TO MOCK EXAMINATION

1. b	35. c	69. a
2. b	36. c	70. d
3. b	37. c	71. c
4. d	38. b	72. c
5. c	39. d	73. c
6. a	40. c	74. c
7. a	41. a	75. d
8. b	42. a	76. d
9. d	43. c	77. d
10. d	44. d	78. d
11. b	45. a	79. a
12. c	46. b	80. b
13. a	47. d	81. b
14. c	48. c	82. d
15. d	49. a	83. a
16. e	50. a	84. a
17. d	51. a	85. a
18. d	52. d	86. c
19. b	53. c	87. d
20. b	54. d	88. d
21. d	55. d	89. d
22. d	56. d	90. c
23. c	57. a	91. c
24. b	58. b	92. c
25. a	59. c	93. a
26. a	60. c	94. b
27. c	61. b	95. c
28. c	62. d	96. b
29. d	63. d	97. d
30. d	64. d	98. c
31. d	65. d	99. a
32. c	66. d	100. b
33. c	67. c	
34. c	68. b	

Examination Preparation Worksheet

This worksheet is designed to help you formulate a study plan to prepare for the certification examination. To begin this process, it's important that you complete a mock examination to identify areas of strengths and weaknesses.

My score on the practice examination: _____

Content Areas: Hematology, Microbiology, Immunohematology, Clinical Chemistry, Hemostasis, Clinical Fluids, Immunology, Molecular, Laboratory Math	
Rank the areas that are your areas of strength based on your performance on questions:	**Rank the areas in terms of your comfort level:**
1.	1.
2.	2.
3.	3.
4.	4.
5.	5.
6.	6.
7.	7.
8.	8.
9.	9.

Part of the challenge in preparing for the certification examination in determining where to start! Most individuals tend to spend more time reviewing the subjects and topics that are most familiar and enjoyable; however, it's the other topics that need to be the focus in the early stages of preparation.

List the content areas that are the most challenging:

Making a Plan

Anticipated examination date: _____

Time (in weeks) to examination date: _____

The amount of time that you should spend reviewing in each area will vary depending on your schedule and how much review is needed. One to two weeks per content area is ideal if you have time each day to set aside as review time. An example of a 12-week plan is included below. It can be modified based on your schedule. Using a calendar to schedule specific study times will help you to stick with the plan. Some individuals may find it helpful to spend the review time at a library, bookstore, or coffee shop to help them focus on the review and minimize distractions.

For each content area, complete the following tasks:
- Complete practice questions during first 1-3 days of each period
- Prepare list of specific content items that were missed
- Spend the rest of this period reviewing those specific content areas
  - Prepare mini-study guides of each topic.
  - Critically review the questions that were missed. How can each answer choice be ruled out? Write a few sentences to explain the topic.
  - Prepare charts, diagrams, and flow charts.
  - Teach it to a friend.
- **Keep all of these notes in a notebook or in a binder to review again during the last week!**

Examination Date:	
Beginning to prepare	• Complete practice examination. • Identify areas of strengths and weaknesses. • Using a calendar, schedule study times leaving up to the examination date.
11-12 weeks out	Clinical Chemistry concentration
9-10 weeks out	Hematology concentration
7-8 weeks out	Immunohematology concentration
5-6 weeks out	Microbiology concentration
4 weeks out	Immunology and Lab Math concentration
3 weeks out	Hemostasis and Molecular concentration
2 weeks out	Clinical Fluids concentration Begin reading through the notes compiled during the review process.
Last week!	At the beginning of the week, complete a practice examination. Identify the questions that were missed and review those topics. Keep reading over the notes compiled during the review process.
Day before	Be sure to have all of your materials needed to take to the exam. Double-check the location, date, and time. Get some rest!

My Plan!	
Examination Date:	
Beginning to prepare	• Complete practice examination. • Identify areas of strengths and weaknesses. • Using a calendar, schedule study times leading up to the examination date.
11-12 weeks out	
9-10 weeks out	
7-8 weeks out	
5-6 weeks out	
4 weeks out	
3 weeks out	
2 weeks out	
Last week!	
Day before	Be sure to have all of your materials needed to take to the exam. Double-check the location, date, and time. Get some rest!

Color Insert Figure Credit Lines

Plates 1, 2, 3, 4, 5, 8, 9, 10, 12, 13, 14, 15, 16
Courtesy Joel Mortensen, PhD.

Plate 6
Photograph by Dr. W H Ewing, courtesy the Centers for Disease Control and Prevention, Public Health Image Library, http://phil.cdc.gov/.

Plate 7
Photograph by Dr. V R Dowell, Jr, courtesy the Centers for Disease Control and Prevention, Public Health Image Library, http://phil.cdc.gov/.

Plate 11
From Public Health Photo Library (PHL 960), http://phil.cdc.gov/phil/details.asp.

Plate 18
Photograph by Dr. Mae Melvin, courtesy the Centers for Disease Control and Prevention, Public Health Image Library, http://phil.cdc.gov/.

Plates 17, 19, 20, 21, 22, 23, 24, 25, 26
Courtesy the Centers for Disease Control and Prevention.

Plates 27, 28, 29, 30, 31, 32
From Rodak BF, et al: Hematology: clinical principles and applications, ed 4, St Louis, 2012, Saunders.

Note: Page numbers followed by "*f*" refer to illustrations; page numbers followed by "*t*" refer to tables; page numbers followed by "*b*" refer to boxes.